MIDWIFERY & WOMEN'S HEALTH NURSE PRACTITIONER CERTIFICATION REVIEW GUIDE

Third Edition

Beth M. Kelsey, EdD, APRN, WHNP-BC
Assistant Professor
DNP Program Director
School of Nursing
Ball State University
Muncie, Indiana

Jamille Nagtalon-Ramos, MSN, WHNP-BC, IBCLC
Associate Director
Women's Health Nurse Practitioner Program
School of Nursing
University of Pennsylvania
Philadelphia, Pennsylvania

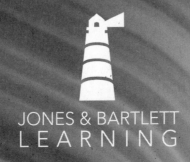

JONES & BARTLETT
LEARNING

World Headquarters
Jones & Bartlett Learning
5 Wall Street
Burlington, MA 01803
978-443-5000
info@jblearning.com
www.jblearning.com

Jones & Bartlett Learning books and products are available through most bookstores and online booksellers. To contact Jones & Bartlett Learning directly, call 800-832-0034, fax 978-443-8000, or visit our website, www.jblearning.com.

Substantial discounts on bulk quantities of Jones & Bartlett Learning publications are available to corporations, professional associations, and other qualified organizations. For details and specific discount information, contact the special sales department at Jones & Bartlett Learning via the above contact information or send an email to specialsales@jblearning.com.

Production Credits
Executive Publisher: William Brottmiller
Executive Editor: Amanda Martin
Acquisitions Editor: Teresa Reilly
Associate Acquisitions Editor: Rebecca Myrick
Production Editor: Amanda Clerkin
Marketing Communications Manager: Katie Hennessy
VP, Manufacturing and Inventory Control: Therese Connell
Composition: Cenveo Publisher Services
Cover Design: Kristin E. Parker
Manager of Photo Research, Rights & Permissions: Lauren Miller
Cover Image: © Eliks/ShutterStock, Inc.
Printing and Binding: Edwards Brothers Malloy
Cover Printing: Edwards Brothers Malloy

To order this product, use ISBN: 978-1-284-05302-9

Library of Congress Cataloging-in-Publication Data
Library of Congress Cataloging-in-Publication Data unavailable at time of printing.

6048

Printed in the United States of America
18 17 16 15 14   10 9 8 7 6 5 4 3 2 1

Contents

Preface

A comprehensive review essential for those preparing to take the midwifery (AMBC) or women's health nurse practitioner certification (NCC) examination. The *Midwifery & Women's Health Nurse Practitioner Certification Review Guide, Third Edition* was developed for both of these nursing specialties because of the many commonalities they share in providing health care for women throughout the life span. Experts in the field of women's health combined their expertise to provide a valuable resource that will assist women's health nurse practitioners and midwives in their pursuit of success on their respective certification examinations. Multiple resources have been utilized to ensure the integrity of this text so that it is representative of the content that may be encountered by both specialties during the examination process.

Many nurses preparing for certification examinations find that reviewing an extensive body of scientific knowledge requires a very difficult search of many sources that must be synthesized to provide a review base for the examination. The purpose of this review guide is to provide a succinct, yet comprehensive review of the core material.

The book has been organized to provide the reader with test-taking and study strategies first. This is a prerequisite for success in the certification examination arena.

The major content is then provided in chapters on General Health Assessment and Health Promotion, Principles of Pharmacology, Normal Gynecology and Well-Woman Care, Gynecological Disorders, Prenatal Care and Infant Assessment, Intrapartum and Postpartum, Midwifery Care of the Newborn, Common Health Problems in Primary Care, and Professional Issues.

Test questions are included at the end of each chapter as well as in the online TestPrep. These questions are intended to provide the reader with test taking practice and are representative of those found on the certification examinations. The correct answers with rationales are provided. A bibliography is included at the completion of each chapter for those who may need to review specific content in more detail.

The co-editors are certified women's health nurse practitioners. Kimberly K. Trout, a certified nurse midwife, authored/ co-authored three chapters. Both women's health nurse practitioners and nurse midwives reviewed all chapters.

It is assumed that the reader of this review guide has completed a course of study in either a women's health nurse practitioner and/or midwifery program. It is not intended to be a basic learning tool. The reader should be cognizant that practice guidelines, diagnostic criteria, and tests, treatment, and management recommendations/protocols are always evolving. The information is current at the time the guide went to print.

Jones & Bartlett Learning and the co-editors would like to thank the following individuals for their contributions to the first two editions of this review book:

Penelope Morrison Bosarge, MSN, RNC, WHNP
Patricia Burkhardt, DrPH, CNM
Mary C. Knutson, MN, RNC, ANP
Anthony A. Lathrop, MSN, CNM, RDMS
Anne A. Moore, DNP, APN, FAANP
Sandra K. Pfantz, DrPH, APRN
Susan P. Shannon, MS, CNM, RNC

1

Strategies for Studying and Test Taking

Beth M. Kelsey

If you are reading this chapter you are likely concerned about how best to prepare to take your certification examination. Understanding your current study and test-taking strategies is an important step in deciding where you may benefit from making some changes or additions to these strategies. Studying for a certification examination is somewhat different from studying for a single test in a course you are taking. Test-taking skills and strategies are very important to success. Preparing yourself to be a successful test taker is as important as studying for the test. The primary goal of this chapter is to assist potential test takers in knowing how to study for and take a certification test. Please use the described strategies in a way that meets your individualized study and test-taking needs.

Strategy 1: Know Yourself

Over years of test taking, each of us has developed certain study and testing behaviors, some of which are helpful and others of which present obstacles to success. Take control of your preparation for your certification exam by identifying study and test-taking behaviors you need to change, recognizing those behaviors you have in place that are beneficial, and developing skills to improve your study and test-taking abilities.

Strategy 2: Know the Content to Be Studied

The National Certification Corporation (NCC) is the certifying body for women's health nurse practitioners (WHNPs) and the American Midwifery Certification Board (AMCB) is the certifying body for nurse–midwives. Both the NCC and AMCB provide content outlines as well as information on examination content development on their websites. The website for NCC is http://www.nccwebsite.org and the website for AMCB is http://www.amcbmidwife.org.

The content of these certification examinations and the percentages for each area of content are based on periodic job analysis surveys of practicing advanced practice nurses representing the women's health nurse practitioner focus for NCC or the nurse–midwife focus for AMCB. Both NCC and AMCB use a rigorous process to ensure that test questions are reflective of current evidence-based practice and that the questions are constructed using psychometric test construction principles.

NCC offers lists of study resources that include textbooks and other widely used reference books. These lists are not meant to be inclusive but provide you with examples of resources you might consider along with the textbooks you have from your courses. Although you want a variety of resources, do not overload yourself with too many books to review because this will be very time consuming, overwhelming, anxiety provoking, and likely redundant in information that you need to know for the examination.

Strategy 3: Know Your Strengths and Weaknesses

Read through the exam content outline provided by the certification examination body.

Conduct a content self-assessment. Rate yourself on each content area. Use a simple rating scale such as the following:

1 = requires no review
2 = requires minimal review
3 = requires intensive review
4 = start from the beginning

Table 1-1 provides a sample exam content assessment (not all content included). Be honest with your self-assessment. It is far better to recognize your content weaknesses when you can study and remedy them rather than thinking during the exam how you wished you had studied more. Likewise with content strengths: if you know the material, do not waste time studying it.

■ **Table 1-1   Sample Content Self-Assessment**

Gynecology: Gynecologic Disorders	
Category: Provided by Test Giver (representative list—not all content included in table)	Rating: Provided by Test Taker
Abnormalities of puberty	3
Menstrual disorders	3
Vaginitis/vaginosis	1
Sexually transmitted infections	2
Pelvic pain	3
Infertility—etiologic factors, initial workup	4
Cervical cytology, HPV testing	2
Breast disorders	2

Strategy 4: Develop a Study Plan

Use the exam content outline and your content self-assessment to develop a study plan. This should require no more than 60 minutes and is well worth the time, with potential for reducing study stress and enhancing exam success.

The content outlines provided by NCC and AMBC include percentages for the major topic areas that approximate the number of questions that will be devoted to that content. This can change from year to year.

Develop your study plan to coordinate with the following:

- Examination content outline
- Percentages for content areas
- Content self-assessment of strengths and weaknesses
- Time available for study before you plan to take the exam

Prioritize your study needs, and start with weak areas first. Avoid the temptation to start with what you know best. Allow for a general review at the end of the study plan. There is no one correct answer to how much time you should spend studying. Spend as much time as you need, start the process early, know your strengths and weaknesses, plan, monitor your progress, and be flexible (Sefcik, Bice, & Prerost, 2013).

Table 1-2 illustrates a partial study plan developed on the basis of the exam content self-assessment in Table 1-1.

Strategy 5: Get Down to the Business of Studying

The quality of your studying is as important as the quantity of your studying. This is directly influenced by organization and concentration. If you expend effort on both of these aspects of exam preparation, you can increase your examination success.

Preparation for Studying: Getting Organized

Study habits are developed early in our educational experiences. Some of our habits enhance learning, whereas others do not. To increase study effectiveness, organization of study materials and time is essential. Organization decreases frustration, allows for easy resumption of study, and increases concentrated study time.

Create Your Own Study Space

Select a study area that is yours alone, free from distractions, comfortable, and well lighted. The ventilation and room temperature should be comfortable since a cold room makes it difficult to concentrate and a warm room may make you sleepy. All your study materials should be left in your study space. The basic premise of a study space is that it facilitates a mind-set that you are there to study. When you interrupt study, it is best to leave your materials just as they are. Do not close books or put away notes because you will just

■ **Table 1-2   Sample Study Plan: Gynecologic Disorders Content**

Study Day	Date	Content	Resources	Time
1		Infertility—etiologic factors, initial workup Rating 4 Abnormalities of puberty Rating 3	Chapter 7 Textbook A Chapter 14 Textbook B Class notes Chapter 3 Textbook A Class notes	6:00–7:30 p.m. 7:30–8:30 p.m.
2		Menstrual disorders Rating 3 Pelvic pain Rating 3	Chapter 4 Textbook A Class notes Chapter 5 Textbook A Class notes	6:00–7:00 p.m. 7:00–8:00 p.m.
3		Sexually transmitted infections Rating 2 Cervical cytology, HPV testing Rating 2	Chapter 6 Textbook A Class notes CDC STD Treatment Guidelines Class notes ASCCP Guideline Algorithms	6:00–7:00 p.m. 7:00–8:00 p.m.

have to relocate them, wasting your study time, when you do resume study.

Identify Your Peak Study Times and Maximize Them

Study in short bursts. Each of us has our own biologic clock that dictates when we are at our peak during the day. If you are a morning person, you are generally active and alert early in the day, slowing down and becoming drowsy by evening. If you are an evening person, you do not completely wake up until late morning and hit your peak in the afternoon and evening. Each person generally has several peaks during the day. It is best to study during those times when your alertness is at its peak.

Spread Out Study Time and Give Your Brain Breaks

Studying is more effective when spread out over a longer period of time. This is a concept called distributed effort or spaced studying (Medina, 2008) and is the opposite of cramming. In addition to spreading study time over several days or weeks, you also need to give your brain rests during any one study period. The best approach to breaks is to plan them and give yourself a conscious break. This approach eliminates the "day dreaming" or "wandering thought" approach to breaks that many of us use. It is better to get up, leave the study area, and do something non-study-related for longer breaks. For shorter breaks of 5 minutes or so, leave your desk, gaze out the window, or do some stretching exercises. When your brain says to give it a rest, accommodate it! You will learn more with less stress.

Focus on Major Concepts and Facts

Study the correct content. It is easy to become bogged down in the detail of the content you are studying. However, it is best to focus on the major concepts or the "state of the art" content. Leave the details, the suppositions, and the experience at the door of your study area. Concentrate on the major textbook facts and concepts that revolve around the subject matter being tested.

Use Your Study Plan Wisely

Your study plan is meant to be a guide, not a rigid schedule. You should take your time with studying. Do not rush through the content just to remain on schedule. Occasionally, study plans need revision. If you take more or less time than planned, readjust the plan for the time gained or lost. The plan can guide you, but you must go at your own pace.

Study Actively

Active study techniques have been shown to strengthen neural connections and improve ability to remember materials being studied. Three techniques for active study are recitation, visualization, and association (Hopper, 2013).

- *Recitation:* When you recite something in your own words you pay more attention. You also get immediate feedback. If you are able to explain something in your own words out loud, you understand it. Also when you hear something, you have used a different part of

your brain than when you read it. Having a study partner or group can facilitate the use of recitation if you ask each other questions and answer out loud.
- *Visualization:* Try to visualize the concepts you are studying in some way, such as by imagining a patient, either someone you have met or a made-up person, with a specific condition. Use illustration and pictures from textbooks as you study. Take notes or make flashcards to promote visualization. Convert connected information into a visual graph (pie, chart, concept map).
- *Association:* You can remember information more efficiently if you link new information to something you already know. Ask yourself: If I were to put this in a computer (brain) file, does a similar or related file already exist so that I don't have to create a new one? (Hopper, 2013).

Use your individual study quirks. Some people stand, others walk around, and some play background music. Whatever helps you to concentrate and study better, you should use.

Use Study Aids

Although there is no substitute for individual studying, several resources, if available, are useful in facilitating learning. One study aid already discussed is the detailed content outlines provided by NCC and AMCB. Review courses and review books such as this one can provide an effective means for organizing or summarizing your individual study. They generally provide the content parameters, the major concepts of the content that you need to know, and an opportunity to clarify not-well-understood content, as well as to review known material. Question and answer resources provide practice in test taking and are most helpful when answer rationales are also included to reinforce the correct information. Study groups are an excellent resource for summarizing and refining content. They provide an opportunity for thinking through your knowledge base, with the advantage of hearing another person's point of view. Each of these study aids increases understanding of content and, when used correctly, increases effectiveness of knowledge application.

Know When to Quit

It is best to stop studying when your concentration ebbs. It is unproductive and frustrating to force yourself to study. It is far better to rest or unwind, and then resume at a later point in the day. Avoid studying outside your morning or afternoon concentration peaks and focus your study energy on your right time of day or evening.

Strategy 6: Become Testwise

Purpose of a Test Question

Test questions are developed to examine different cognitive domains: knowledge, comprehension, application, analysis, synthesis, and evaluation. You will most likely see questions in the knowledge, comprehension, application, and analysis domains on the certification exam. A knowledge question requires the test taker to recall a fact; comprehension questions require the test taker to understand the meaning of the fact; application questions require the test taker to be able to apply knowledge in a concrete situation; and analysis questions require the test taker to be able to break down information, identifying parts, relationships, and organization (Wittman-Price & Godshall, 2009).

When taking a test, you want to be aware of whether you are being asked a fact or to use that fact. An example of a knowledge question is as follows:

Which of the following statements about herpes genitalis is true?
A. Suppressive therapy does not reduce viral shedding.
B. *Systemic symptoms are uncommon during recurrences.*
C. Topical acyclovir is as effective as oral acyclovir for recurrences.
D. Transmission of the virus is unlikely to occur during the prodromal phase.

To answer this question correctly, you must retrieve memorized facts. Understanding the fact, knowing why it is important, and analyzing what should be done with the fact are not needed.

An example of a question that tests comprehension is as follows:

A 24-year-old female presents with complaint of itching and pain in her genital area that started 2 days ago. She also complains of pain with urination. Physical examination reveals bilateral inguinal lymphadenopathy, vulvar edema with multiple vesicles and ulcerated lesions, and a large amount of watery vaginal discharge. The most likely diagnosis is:
A. *Genital herpes*
B. Genital warts
C. Syphilis
D. Trichomoniasis

To answer this question correctly, you must retrieve several facts about the signs and symptoms of herpes genitalis and understand that, put together, the findings are likely indicative of herpes rather than some other diagnosis.

An example of an application question is as follows:

A 24-year-old female presents with a history of herpes diagnosis 6 months ago and asks if there is anything she can do to deal with recurrent outbreaks. She has had two recurrences since her initial occurrence. Appropriate information for this patient would include:
A. Comfort measures and topical acyclovir are the best approach to managing her recurrences.
B. She can be assured that she is unlikely to have more than one or two recurrences a year.
C. *She can consider episodic therapy for recurrences or suppressive therapy with acyclovir.*
D. Suppressive medication is not recommended for someone who has less than four recurrences a year.

To answer this question correctly, you must know and comprehend facts about herpes recurrences and suppression and apply this information to an individual patient situation. You must think through each answer and decide its relevance and importance to the situation in question.

An example of an analysis question is as follows:

A 24-year-old female tells you her sex partner for the past year has a history of herpes genitalis. You order a herpes type-specific serologic test. The results show HSV-1 positive and HSV-2 negative. The accurate interpretation of these results is:
A. She has acquired a herpes infection from her sex partner.
B. She has not acquired a herpes infection from her sex partner.
C. She does not have the herpes virus type that causes genital herpes infection.
D. *She may or may not have acquired herpes infection from her partner.*

To answer this question correctly, you must be able to break down the information about the type-specific serologic test results and identify the parts and relationships with the information you have about the patient and her partner.

Question Format

Most standardized tests such as those used for nursing licensure and certification use multiple-choice questions (MCQs) composed of three or four answer options for which you are required to select the one best answer. Both NCC and AMCB certification exams use MCQs with either three or four answer options (American Midwifery Certification Board [AMCB], 2013; National Certification Corporation [NCC], 2014).

Successful test taking is dependent not only on content knowledge but on test-taking skill. If you are unable to impart your knowledge through the vehicle used for its conveyance, that is, the MCQ, your test-taking success is in jeopardy.

Components of MCQs

Multiple choice questions include the basic components of a stem and a set of answer options. The stem presents information needed by the test taker to select an answer. The stem may be short, consisting of just a phrase or a sentence or two, or it can be a paragraph in length. When the stem is more than a phrase or sentence in length, it usually includes a separate interrogatory question or statement that poses the question to be answered. The interrogatory question or statement helps to direct the test taker's thinking.

The answer options are three or four possible responses to the question. The correct option is called the *keyed response*, and all other options are called *distractors* (Sefcik et al., 2013). The keyed response may be the only correct answer or it may be the best answer. Higher-level questions usually have a best answer along with distractor options that may be partially correct or that may not address all of the data presented in the question stem.

Knowing the components of a test question helps you sift through the information presented and focus on the question's intent. Always focus on the information in the stem and, more specifically, what the interrogatory question/statement is asking. Avoid reading elements into the question that aren't specifically included in the stem and options (see **Table 1-3**).

Practice, Practice, Practice

Taking practice tests can improve performance. Although they can assist in evaluation of your knowledge, their primary benefit is to assist you with test-taking skills. You should use them to evaluate your thinking process; your ability to read, understand, and interpret questions; and your skills in completing the mechanics of the test.

Exam resources, including sample questions for the NCC and the AMCB, are available in the examination content information. The questions at the end of each chapter of this book and the separate test questions available online provide you with more than

■ **Table 1-3   Anatomy of a Test Question**

Stem	A woman using the contraceptive vaginal ring (NuvaRing) removes the ring during sex in the evening and realizes the next morning that she forgot to reinsert it.
Interrogatory statement	If this is week 1 or 2 for this ring, she should be advised to:
Options	a. Discard this ring and insert a new one immediately b. Discard this ring, wait for withdrawal bleed, and insert a new ring c. Reinsert this ring with no backup needed if it has been out for fewer than 8 hours d. *Reinsert this ring and use a backup method for 7 days*

900 multiple-choice questions. The answers to the questions at the end of each chapter are provided with reference to the information in the content of the chapter. The online questions come from well-known textbooks, websites that provide guidelines from national professional organizations, and some journal articles. The answers, rationales, and specific resource used are provided for each of these questions.

Strategy 7: Apply Basic Rules of Standardized Test Taking

Read All Directions Carefully

Be sure that you have completed all information needed to register for the exam and that you have all required documents and personal identification. Know what you are permitted to have in the testing area and what is not permitted. It is helpful to make a list of things you need for admission to the examination as well as permitted items you want to have with you during the exam.

The Night Before the Test

Follow your regular routine the night before a test. Eat familiar foods. Avoid the temptation to cram all night. Go to bed at your regular time.

The Day of the Test

Be prepared for exam day. It is important to familiarize yourself with the test site, the building, the parking, and travel route prior to the exam day. If you must travel, arrive early to allow time for this familiarization. On exam day, allow yourself plenty of time to arrive at the site, planning to get there 30 minutes before your scheduled exam time. Wear comfortable clothes and have a good breakfast that

morning. Know whether you are able to have food or drink in the exam area or will be able to have them available for a short break.

Know what to do if you experience any electronic or other difficulties during the examination. In addition to addressing the issue at the test site, you should also notify the certifying board.

Use Your Time Wisely and Effectively

Most standardized, computer-delivered exams have a digital clock on the computer indicating how much time you have remaining. This feature may be turned off and on during the exam if you find it to be anxiety producing. Know the number of questions on the exam and the total amount of time you have to complete the exam. For example, if there are 175 questions and you have 3 hours to complete the exam, you have approximately 1 minute per question, if there are 175 questions and you have 4 hours to complete the exam, you have approximately 1½ minutes per question. Remember that a good number of questions will likely take you less than 1 minute to answer. Skip or make an educated guess on difficult questions, and mark and return to them later.

Identify key words in the stem before looking at the options for each question. Confine your thinking to the information provided.

Read and consider all options. Be systematic and use problem-solving techniques. Relate options to the question and balance them against each other. Eliminate answers you know are wrong and focus on the remaining most likely correct responses.

Answer all of the questions on the exam. Currently, the NCC and AMCB certification examination scores are based on only the total number of correct answers selected. This means that you are not further penalized for an incorrect answer. So, go ahead and answer all of the test questions even if you are only guessing (AMCB, 2013; NCC, 2014).

Go back to questions you were not able to answer on the first pass through the test. You may have gained information from subsequent questions that is helpful in answering previous questions or you may be less anxious and more objective by the end of the test.

However, avoid second-guessing answers choices you have already made. Your first response is likely the best response. If you tend to second-guess your responses, only review questions that you could not answer on the first pass through the exam. Computer-based exams allow you to mark questions that you may want to address later in the exam.

Do not change an answer without a good reason. Good reasons might be realizing you misread the question the first time or running across information in later questions that either jogs your memory or gives you a better idea of what the correct answer might be (Lamonte, 2007; Sefcik et al., 2013).

Strategy 8: Psych Yourself Up

Adopt an "I Can" Attitude

Believing you can succeed is the key to success. Self-belief inspires and gives you the power to achieve your goals. Without a success attitude, the road to your goal is much harder. This "I can" attitude must permeate all your efforts in test taking, from studying to improving your test-taking skills, to actually completing the exam. Think positively. Performance is influenced not only by knowledge and skill, but by attitude as well. Those individuals who regard an exam as an opportunity or challenge will be more successful.

Take Control

By identifying your goal, deciding how to accomplish it, and developing a plan for achieving it, you take control. Do not leave your success to chance; control it through action and attitude.

Manage Anxiety

A little stress or anxiety can be productive, serving as a motivator to take a test seriously and to prepare for it adequately. Too much anxiety can have negative consequences that include not using study time productively, misreading questions, changing answers from right to wrong, and developing physical symptoms such as diarrhea, nausea, and palpitations.

Active anxiety-control strategies include relaxation techniques (i.e., guided imagery, meditation), stress management, attention to wellness behaviors (i.e., healthy eating, adequate sleep, regular exercise), combining individual review with small study groups for social support and increased confidence, completing practice questions, preparing well in advance, and taking the time to review all of the examination day processes (Lamonte, 2007; McDowell, 2008).

For persons with severe test anxiety, interventions such as cognitive therapy, systematic desensitization, study skills counseling, and biofeedback have all been used with some success. Techniques derived from these approaches can influence the results achieved by changing attitudes and approaches to test taking and thereby reducing anxiety.

Persevere, Persevere, Persevere!

Endurance must underlie all your efforts. Call forth those reserve energies when you have had all you think you can take. Rely on

yourself and your support systems to help you maintain a sense of direction and keep your goal in the forefront.

Reward Yourself

Reward yourself during your exam preparation and once the exam has been completed. You alone hold the key to success; use what you have wisely.

Know How You Will Manage Failure

An initial failure on the certification exam is a possibility. Keep in mind that passing or not passing the test is not a measure of an individual's self-worth or a reflection of an individual's true value. An initial failure does not mean that the individual will not be an excellent nurse practitioner or midwife. If you do not pass the test on the first try, do not dwell on the failure. Recognize what you need to change in your preparation and move forward. Failure is a time to begin again; use it as a motivator to do better.

SUMMARY

This chapter provided concepts, strategies, and techniques for improving study and test-taking skills. Your first task in improvement is to know yourself: how you study and how you take a test. You should use your strengths and remedy the weaknesses. Next, you need to organize your study and concentrate on using your strengths and new and improved skills to be successful. Create a study space, develop a plan of action, and then implement that plan during your periods of peak concentration. Before taking the exam, be sure you understand the components of a test question, can identify key words and phrases, and have practiced. Apply the test-taking rules during the exam process.

Finally, believe in yourself, your knowledge, and your talent. Believing you can accomplish your goal facilitates the fact that you will.

Bibliography

American Midwifery Certification Board. (2013). *Information for candidates of the National Certification Examination in Nurse-Midwifery and Midwifery*. Linthicum, MD: Author.

Hopper, C. (2013). *Practicing college learning strategies* (6th ed.). Orlando, FL: Houghton Mifflin.

Lamonte, M. (2007). Test-taking strategies for CNOR certification. *AORN Journal, 85*(2), 315–331.

McDowell, B. (2008). KATTS: A framework for maximizing NCLEX-RN performance. *Journal of Nursing Education, 47*(4), 183–186.

Medina, J. (2008). *Brain rules*. Seattle, WA: Pear Press.

National Certification Corporation. (2014). *2014 candidate guide women's health nurse practitioner*. Chicago, IL: Author.

Sefcik, D., Bice, G., & Prerost. (2013). *How to study for standardized tests*. Burlington, MA: Jones & Bartlett Learning.

Wittman-Price, R., & Godshall, M. (2009). *Certified nurse educator (CNE) review manual*. New York, NY: Springer.

2

General Health Assessment and Health Promotion

Beth M. Kelsey

Health History

- Purpose and correlation to physical examination
  1. Begins the client–clinician relationship
  2. Identifies the client's main concerns
  3. Provides information for risk assessment and health promotion
  4. Provides focus for physical examination and diagnostic/screening tests
  5. Provides information about cultural variations in health beliefs and practices
- Components of the health history
  1. Reason for visit/chief complaint—brief statement in client's own words of reason for seeking health care
  2. Presenting problem/illness—chronological account of problem(s) for which client is seeking care
     a. Description of principal symptoms should include *OLD-CARTS* mnemonic:
        (1) *Onset*
        (2) *Location*
        (3) *Duration*
        (4) *Characteristics*
        (5) *Aggravating/Associated factors*
        (6) *Relieving factors*
        (7) *Temporal factors*
        (8) *Severity*
     b. Include pertinent negatives in symptom descriptions; when a symptom suggests that an abnormality may exist or develop in that area, include documentation of absence of symptoms that may help eliminate some of the possibilities
     c. Describe impact of illness/problem on client's usual lifestyle
     d. Summarize current health status and health promotion/disease prevention needs if client has no presenting problem
  3. Past health history
     a. General state of health as client perceives it
     b. Childhood illnesses
     c. Major adult illnesses
     d. Psychiatric illnesses
     e. Accidents/injuries
     f. Surgeries/other hospitalizations
     g. Blood transfusions—dates and number of units
  4. Current health status
     a. Current medications—prescription, over-the-counter, herbal
     b. Allergies—name of allergen, type of reaction
     c. Tobacco, alcohol, illicit drugs—type, amount, frequency
     d. Nutrition—24-hour diet recall, recent weight changes, eating disorders, special diet
     e. Screening tests—dates and results
     f. Immunizations—dates
     g. Sleep patterns
     h. Exercise/leisure activities
     i. Environmental hazards
     j. Use of safety measures—safety belts, smoke detectors
     k. Disabilities—functional assessment if indicated
  5. Family health history—provides information about possible genetic, familial, and environmental associations with client's health
     a. Age and health or age and cause of death of immediate family members—parents, siblings, children, spouse/significant other
     b. Specific conditions to ask about—heart disease, hypertension, stroke, diabetes, cancer, epilepsy, kidney disease, thyroid disease, asthma, arthritis, blood diseases, tuberculosis, alcoholism, allergies, congenital anomalies, mental illness, genetic disorders
     c. Indicate if client is adopted and/or does not know family health history
  6. Psychosocial/cultural health history
     a. Living situation
     b. Support system
     c. Stressors (including violence)
     d. Typical day
     e. Religious/spiritual beliefs and practices
     f. Outlook on present and future
     g. Special issues to address with adolescent clients include *HEADSS:* Home, Education, Activities, Drugs, Sex, Suicide

h. Cultural assessment considerations
   (1) Cultural/ethnic identification—place of birth, length of time in country
   (2) Communication—language spoken, use of nonverbal communication, use of silence
   (3) Space—degree of comfort with distance between self and other, degree of comfort with touching by another
   (4) Social organization—family structure and roles, influence of religion/spirituality
   (5) Time—past, present, or future oriented; view of time—clock-oriented or social-oriented
   (6) Environmental control—internal or external locus of control, belief in supernatural forces
   (7) Use of culturally based healing practices or remedies

7. Obstetric history—may include in separate section, past health history, or review of systems—includes all pregnancies regardless of outcome
   a. Gravidity—total number of pregnancies including a current pregnancy
   b. Parity—total number of pregnancies reaching 20 weeks or greater gestation
      (1) Include term, preterm, and stillbirth deliveries
      (2) Include length of each pregnancy; type of delivery; weight and sex of infant; length of labor; complications during prenatal, intrapartum, or postpartum periods; infant complications; cause of stillbirth if known
   c. Abortions—spontaneous and induced
   d. GTPAL—*Gravida, Term, Preterm, Abortion, Living* children is a commonly used method of obstetric history notation
   e. Any infertility evaluation and treatment

8. Menstrual history—may include in separate section or in review of systems
   a. Age at menarche, regularity, frequency, duration, and amount of bleeding
   b. Date of last normal menstrual period
   c. Use of pads, tampons, douching
   d. Abnormal uterine bleeding
   e. Premenstrual symptoms
   f. Dysmenorrhea
   g. Perimenopausal symptoms
   h. Age at menopause, use of hormone therapy, postmenopausal bleeding

9. Sexual history/contraceptive use—may include in separate section, under current health status, or in review of systems
   a. Age at first sexual intercourse—consensual/nonconsensual
   b. History of sexual abuse or sexual assault
   c. Sexual orientation/gender identity
   d. Current sexual relationship(s)
      (1) Frequency of sexual intercourse
      (2) Satisfaction or concerns with sexual relationship(s)
      (3) Dyspareunia, orgasmic or libido problems
   e. Sexually transmitted infection (STI)/human immunodeficiency virus (HIV) infection risk assessment
      (1) Total number of sexual partners and number in past 3 months
      (2) Types of sexual contact—vaginal, oral, and/or anal
      (3) Use of condoms or other barrier methods
      (4) Previous history of sexually transmitted infections
      (5) Use of injection drugs or sex with partner who has used injection drugs
      (6) Sex while drunk, stoned, or high
      (7) Previous testing for HIV
   f. Current and future desire for pregnancy
   g. Contraceptive use
      (1) Establish if pregnancy is not a concern—hysterectomy, sterilization, not sexually active, only sexually active with females, menopausal
      (2) Current method, length of time used, satisfaction, problems or concerns
      (3) Previous methods used, when, length of time used, satisfaction, problems or concerns, reason for discontinuation

10. Review of systems—used to assess common symptoms for each major body system to avoid missing any potential or existing problems—special focus for women's reproductive health includes:
    a. Endocrine—menses, breasts, pregnancy, thyroid, menopause
    b. Genitourinary
       (1) In utero exposure to diethylstilbestrol (DES) if born before 1971
       (2) History or symptoms of uterine or ovarian problems
       (3) History or symptoms of STI or pelvic infection
       (4) History or symptoms of vaginal infections
       (5) History of abnormal Pap tests—date, abnormality, treatment
       (6) History or symptoms of urinary tract infection
       (7) Symptoms of urinary incontinence

11. Concluding question—Is there anything else I need to know about your health in order to provide you with the best health care?

- Risk factor identification
  1. Consider prevalence (existing level of disease) and incidence (rate of new disease) in general population and in your client population
  2. Determine risks specific to client related to the following:
     a. Gender
     b. Age
     c. Ethnic or racial background
     d. Family history
     e. Environmental exposures
     f. Lifestyle
     g. Geographic area
     h. Inadequate preventive health care

- Problem-oriented medical record—organized sequence of recording information using SOAP format
  1. SOAP format
     a. *S*—subjective information obtained during history
     b. *O*—objective information obtained through physical examination and laboratory/diagnostic test results
     c. *A*—assessment of objective and subjective data to determine a diagnosis with rationale or a prioritized differential diagnosis

d. *P*—plan to include diagnostic tests, therapeutic treatment regimen, client education, referrals, and date for reevaluation

2. Problem list—list each identified existing or potential problem and indicate both onset and a resolution date

3. Progress notes—use SOAP format for information documented at follow-up visits

Physical Examination (General Screening Examination)

- Purpose and correlation to health history
  1. Begins laying on of hands—diagnostic and therapeutic
  2. Findings may indicate need for further health history information
  3. Takes into account normal physical variations of different age and racial/ethnic groups
- Techniques of examination
  1. Inspection—observation using sight and smell
     a. Takes place throughout the history and physical examination
     b. Includes general survey and body-system-specific observations
  2. Auscultation—use of hearing usually with stethoscope to listen to sounds produced by the body
     a. Diaphragm best for high-pitched sounds (e.g., S_1, S_2 heart sounds)
     b. Bell best for low-pitched sounds (e.g., large blood vessels)
  3. Percussion—use of light, brisk tapping on body surfaces to produce vibrations in relation to density of underlying tissue and/or to elicit tenderness
     a. Provides information about size, shape, location, and density of underlying organs or tissue
     b. Percussion sounds are distinguished by intensity (soft–loud), pitch (high–low), and quality
     c. Tympany—loud, high-pitched, drum-like sound (e.g., gastric bubble, gas-filled bowel)
     d. Hyperresonance—very loud, low-pitched, boom-like sound (e.g., lungs with emphysema)
     e. Resonance—loud, low-pitched, hollow sound (e.g., healthy lungs)
     f. Dull—soft-to-moderate, moderate-pitched, thud-like sound (e.g., liver, heart)
     g. Flat—soft, high-pitched sound, very dull (e.g., muscle, bone)
  4. Palpation—use of hands and fingers to gather information about body tissues and organs through touch
     a. Finger pads, palmar surface of fingers, ulnar surface of fingers/hands, and dorsal surface of hands are used
     b. Light palpation—about 1 cm in depth, used to identify muscular resistance, areas of tenderness, and large masses or areas of distention
     c. Deep palpation—about 4 cm in depth, used to delineate organs and to identify less obvious masses
- Standard precautions—minimum infection prevention practices that apply to all patient care, regardless of suspected or confirmed infection status (Centers for Disease Control and Prevention [CDC], 2011a)
  1. Precautions based on principle that all blood, body fluids, secretions, excretions except sweat, nonintact skin, and mucous membranes may contain transmissible infectious agents
  2. Hand hygiene
  3. Use of personal protective equipment (e.g., gloves, gowns, masks)
  4. Safe needle injection practices
  5. Safe handling of potentially contaminated equipment or surfaces
  6. Respiratory hygiene/cough etiquette
- Screening examination
  1. General appearance—posture, dress, grooming, personal hygiene, body or breath odors, facial expression
  2. Anthropometric measurements
     a. Height and weight
     b. Body mass index (BMI) provides measurement of total body fat; weight (kg)/height (m²); tables available to calculate BMI based on the individual's height and weight
        (1) Underweight—BMI less than 18.5
        (2) Normal weight—BMI 18.5 to 24.9
        (3) Overweight—BMI 25 to 29.9
        (4) Obesity—BMI 30 to 39.9
        (5) Extreme obesity—BMI 40 or greater
     c. Waist circumference
        (1) Provides measurement of abdominal fat as an independent prediction of risk for type 2 diabetes, dyslipidemia, hypertension, and cardiovascular disease in individuals with BMI between 25 and 39.9 (overweight and obesity)
        (2) Has little added value in disease risk prediction in individuals with BMI 40 or greater (extreme obesity)
        (3) Measure with horizontal mark at uppermost lateral border of right iliac crest and cross with vertical mark at midaxillary line; place tape measure at the cross and measure in horizontal plane around abdomen while patient is standing
        (4) In adult female increased relative risk is indicated at greater than 35 in. (88 cm)
  3. Skin, hair, and nails
     a. Skin—color, texture, temperature, turgor, moisture, lesions
     b. Hair—color, distribution, quantity, texture
     c. Nails—color, shape, thickness
     d. Skin lesion characteristics—size, shape, color, texture, elevation, exudate, location, and distribution
        (1) Primary lesions—occur as an initial, spontaneous reaction to an internal or external stimulus (macule, papule, pustule, vesicle, wheal)
        (2) Secondary lesions—result from later evolution or trauma to a primary lesion (ulcer, fissure, crust, scar)
     e. ABCDEs of malignant melanoma—*a*symmetry, *b*orders irregular, *c*olor blue/black or variegated, *d*iameter greater than 6 mm, *e*levation
  4. Head, eyes, ears, nose, and throat
     a. Head and neck
        (1) Skull and scalp—no masses or tenderness
        (2) Facial features—symmetrical and in proportion

(3) Trachea—midline

(4) Thyroid—palpable with no masses or tenderness, rises symmetrically with swallowing

(5) Neck—full range of motion (ROM) without pain

(6) Lymph nodes

    (a) Preauricular, postauricular, occipital, tonsillar, submandibular, submental, superficial cervical, posterior and deep cervical chains, supraclavicular

    (b) Normal findings—less than 1 cm in size, nontender, mobile, soft, and discrete

b. Eyes

(1) Visual acuity

    (a) Snellen chart for central vision; normal 20/20

    (b) Rosenbaum card or newspaper for near vision

    (c) Impaired near vision—presbyopia

    (d) Impaired far vision—myopia

(2) Peripheral vision—estimated with visual fields by confrontation test

(3) External eye structures—eyebrows equal; lids without lag or ptosis; lacrimal apparatus without exudate, swelling, or excess tearing; conjunctiva clear with small blood vessels and no exudate; sclera white or buff colored

(4) Eyeball structures

    (a) Cornea and lenses—no opacities or lesions

    (b) Pupils—*P*upils *E*qual, *R*ound, *R*eact to *L*ight, and *A*ccommodate (PERRLA)

(5) Extraocular muscle (EOM) function—symmetrical movement through the six cardinal fields of gaze without lid lag or nystagmus

(6) Ophthalmoscopic examination—red reflex present with no clouding or opacities; optic disc yellow to pink color with distinct margins; arterioles light red and two-thirds of the diameter of veins with bright light reflex; veins dark red and larger than arterioles with no light reflex; no venous tapering at the arteriole-venous crossings

c. Ears

(1) Hearing evaluation

    (a) Whispered voice—able to hear softly whispered words in each ear at 1 to 2 feet

    (b) Weber test—tests for lateralization of sound through bone conduction; normally hear sound equally in both ears

    (c) Rinne test—compares bone and air conduction of sound; normally air-conducted (AC) sound is heard for twice as long as bone-conducted (BC) sound (AC: BC = 2:1)

    (d) Weber and Rinne tests may help in differentiating conductive and sensorineural hearing loss

    (e) Precision, test-retest reproducibility, and accuracy of Weber and Rinne tests have been questioned

(2) External ears—symmetrical, no inflammation, lesions, nodules, or drainage

(3) Tragus tenderness may indicate otitis externa; mastoid process tenderness may indicate otitis media

(4) Otoscopic examination

    (a) External canal—no discharge, inflammation, lesions, or foreign bodies; varied amount, color, and consistency of cerumen

    (b) Tympanic membrane—intact, pearly gray, translucent, with cone of light at 5:00 to 7:00; umbo and handle of malleus visible; no bulging or retraction

d. Nose and sinuses

(1) Nasal mucosa pinkish red; septum midline

(2) Frontal and maxillary sinuses nontender

e. Mouth and oropharynx

(1) Mouth—lips, gums, tongue, mucous membranes all pink, moist, without lesions or inflammation; teeth—none missing, free from caries or breakage

(2) Oropharynx—tonsils, posterior wall of pharynx without lesions or inflammation

5. Respiratory system

a. Chest symmetrical, anterior/posterior diameter less than transverse diameter; respiratory rate 16 to 20 breaths per minute, rhythm regular; no rib retraction or use of accessory muscles; no cyanosis or clubbing of fingers

b. Anterior and posterior respiratory expansion—symmetrical movement when client inhales deeply

c. Tactile fremitus—decreased with emphysema, asthma, pleural effusion; increased with lobar pneumonia, pulmonary edema

d. Percussion—resonant throughout lung fields

e. Auscultation—vesicular over most of lung fields; bronchovesicular near main bronchus and bronchial over trachea

(1) Adventitious sounds—crackles (intermittent, nonmusical, brief sound), caused by air flowing by fluid; rhonchi (low-pitched, snoring quality), caused by air passing over solid or thick secretion; wheezes (high-pitched, shrill quality), caused by air flowing through constricted passageways; pleural friction rub (grating or creaking sound), caused by inflammation of pleural tissue

(2) Transmitted voice sounds/vocal resonance—normally voice sounds are muffled or indistinct; bronchophony, egophony, whispered pectoriloquy indicate fluid or a solid mass in lungs

6. Cardiovascular system

a. Blood pressure (BP)—less than 120/80 mm Hg and pulse 60 to 90 beats per minute (bpm), regular, not bounding or thready

b. Heart

(1) Apical impulse—4th to 5th left intercostal space (ICS) medial to the midclavicular line (MCL), no lifts or thrills

(2) Auscultation at 2nd right ICS; 2nd, 3rd, 4th, 5th left ICS at the sternal border; and 5th left ICS at the MCL

    (a) Assess rate and rhythm

    (b) Identify S_1 and S_2 at each site—S_1 heard best at apex, S_2 heard best at base

    (c) Identify extra heart sounds at each site

        i. Physiologic split S_2—may normally be heard during inspiration

        ii. Fixed split S_2—heard in inspiration and expiration; may be heard with atrial septal defect or right ventricular failure

iii. Increased S_3—early diastole, low-pitched; may be normal in children, young adults, and in late pregnancy; not normal in older adults

iv. Increased S_4—late diastole, low-pitched; may be normal in well-trained athletes and older adults; heard with aortic stenosis and hypertensive heart disease

v. Murmurs—systolic murmur may be physiologic (pregnancy) or pathologic (diseased valves); diastolic murmur usually indicates valvular disease

    a) Note timing, duration, pitch, intensity, pattern, quality, location, radiation, respiratory phase variations

    b) Murmur of mitral stenosis—early/late diastole, low-pitched, grade I to IV; heard loudest at apex without radiation; no respiratory phase variation

vi. Clicks and snaps—heard with heart valve abnormalities

vii. Pericardial friction rub—grating sound heard throughout cardiac cycle; heard with pericarditis

c. Neck vessels

  (1) No jugular venous distention

  (2) Carotid arteries—strong, symmetrical, no bruits

d. Extremities (peripheral arteries)

  (1) No erythema, pallor, or cyanosis; no edema or varicosities; skin warm; capillary refill time less than 2 seconds; normal hair distribution; no muscle atrophy

  (2) Pulses strong and symmetrical—brachial, radial, femoral, dorsalis pedis, posterior tibial

  (3) Lymph nodes less than 1 cm, nontender, mobile, soft, and discrete—axillary, epitrochlear, inguinal

7. Abdomen

a. Symmetrical, no lesions or masses; no visible pulsations or peristalsis

b. Active bowel sounds; no vascular bruits or friction rubs

c. No guarding, tenderness, or masses on palpation

d. Liver border—edge smooth, sharp, nontender; no more than 2 cm below right costal margin

e. Spleen and kidneys—usually not palpable

f. Aorta—slightly left of midline in upper abdomen, less than 3 cm width

g. Percussion—tympany is predominant tone, dullness over organs or any masses

h. Liver span—normally 6 to 12 cm at the right MCL

i. Splenic dullness—6th to 10th ICS just posterior to midaxillary line on left side

j. No tenderness on fist percussion over the costovertebral angle; costovertebral angle tenderness (CVAT) may indicate kidney problem

8. Musculoskeletal system

a. No gross deformities; body aligned, extremities symmetrical, normal spinal curvature, no involuntary movements

b. Muscle mass and strength equal bilaterally, full range of motion without pain

c. No inflammation, nodules, swelling, crepitus, or tenderness of joints

9. Neurologic system

a. Cranial nerves (CN)—CN II through XII routinely tested, CN I tested if abnormality is suspected

  (1) CN I (olfactory)—test ability to identify familiar odors

  (2) CN II (optic)—test visual acuity, peripheral vision, and inspect optic discs

  (3) CN III, IV, VI (oculomotor, trochlear, abducens)—observe for PERRLA, EOM function, and ptosis

  (4) CN V (trigeminal)—palpate strength of temporal and masseter muscles, test for sharp/dull and light touch sensation on forehead, cheeks, and chin

  (5) CN VII (facial)—observe for any weakness, asymmetry, or abnormal movements of face

  (6) CN VIII (acoustic)—assess auditory acuity, perform Weber and Rinne tests

  (7) CN IX and X (glossopharyngeal and vagus)—observe ability to swallow, symmetry of movement of soft palate and uvula when client says "ah," gag reflex, any abnormal voice quality

  (8) CN XI (spinal accessory)—observe and palpate strength and symmetry of trapezius and sternocleidomastoid muscles

  (9) CN XII (hypoglossal)—observe tongue for any deviation, asymmetry, or abnormal movement

b. Cerebellar function—smooth coordinated gait, able to walk heel to toe, balance maintained with eyes closed (Romberg test), rapid rhythmic alternating movements smooth and coordinated

c. Sensory function—able to identify superficial pain and touch, able to identify vibration on bony prominences and passive position change of fingers and toes, normal response to discriminatory sensation tests, all findings symmetrical

d. Deep tendon reflexes—brisk and symmetrical (biceps, brachioradialis, triceps, patellar, Achilles)

10. Mental status

a. Physical appearance and behavior—well groomed, emotional status appropriate to situation, makes eye contact, posture erect

b. Cognitive abilities—alert and oriented, able to reason, recent and remote memory intact, able to follow directions

c. Emotional stability—no signs of depression or anxiety, logical thought processes, no perceptual disturbances

d. Speech and language skills—normal voice quality and articulation, coherent, able to follow simple instructions

e. Mini Mental Status Examination (MMSE)—standardized screening tool used for mental status assessment

f. Depression screening tools—Beck Depression Inventory, Zung Self-Rating Depression Scale, Geriatric Depression Scale

- Detailed female reproductive examination

1. Breasts

a. The female breast extends from the second to the sixth ribs and from the sternal border to the midaxillary line

b. Inspect breasts with client in sitting position and hands pushing against hips; view breasts from all sides to assess for symmetry and skin changes
   (1) Tanner sexual maturity rating in adolescent
   (2) Skin—smooth, color uniform, no erythema, masses, retraction, dimpling, or thickening
   (3) Symmetry—breast shape or contour is symmetrical; some difference in size of breasts and areola is common and usually normal
   (4) Nipples—pointing in same direction, no retraction or discharge, no scaling; long-standing nipple inversion is usually normal variation
c. Palpate axillary, supraclavicular, infraclavicular lymph nodes with patient in sitting position and arms relaxed at sides
d. Palpate breasts with client lying down, arm above head, small pillow under shoulder/lower back on side being examined if needed to provide even breast tissue distribution
   (1) Include entire area from midaxillary line, across inframammary ridge and fifth/sixth rib, up lateral edge of sternum, across clavicle, back to midaxillary line
   (2) Palpate using finger pads of middle three fingers with overlapping dime-shaped circular motions in a vertical strip pattern over entire area including nipples; do not squeeze nipples unless client indicates she has spontaneous nipple discharge
   (3) Palpate each area of breast tissue using three levels of pressure—light, medium, and deep
   (4) Follow same procedures for client with implants because correctly placed implants are located behind breast tissue
   (5) Include palpation of chest wall, skin, and incision area in client with mastectomy
   (6) Breast tissue—consistency varies from soft fat to firmer glandular tissue, physiologic nodularity may be present, there may be a firm ridge of compressed tissue under lower edge of breasts
   (7) Describe any palpable mass or lymph nodes in terms of location according to clock face as examiner faces client—size, shape, mobility, consistency, delimitation, and tenderness
   (8) Describe any nipple discharge in terms of whether spontaneous/not spontaneous, bilateral/unilateral, single or multiple ducts, color, and consistency
2. Pelvic examination
   a. Prepare equipment/supplies prior to examination
   b. Conduct pelvic examination with attention to preventing contamination of equipment such as examination lights and lubricant containers
   c. Positioning—client lying supine with head and shoulders elevated, lithotomy position, buttocks extending slightly beyond edge of table, draped from midabdomen to knees, drape depressed between knees to allow eye contact
   d. Inspection and palpation of external structures—mons pubis, labia majora and minora, clitoris, urethral meatus, vaginal introitus, paraurethral (Skene's) glands, Bartholin's glands, perineum
      (1) Tanner sexual maturity rating in adolescent
      (2) Mons pubis—pubic hair inverted triangular pattern, skin smooth with uniform color
      (3) Labia majora—may be gaping or closed and dry or moist, tissue soft and homogenous, covered with hair in postpubertal female
      (4) Labia minora—moist and dark pink, tissue soft and homogenous
      (5) Clitoris—approximately 2 cm or less in length and 0.5 cm in diameter
      (6) Urethral meatus—irregular opening or slit
      (7) Vaginal introitus—thin vertical slit or large orifice, irregular edges from hymenal remnants, moist
      (8) Skene's and Bartholin's glands—opening of Skene's glands just posterior to and on each side of urethral meatus, opening of Bartholin's glands located posteriorly on each side of vaginal orifice and not usually visible
      (9) Perineum—consists of tissue between introitus and anus, smooth, may have episiotomy scar
      (10) Note presence of any abnormal hair distribution, discoloration, erythema, swelling, atrophy, lesions, masses, discharge, malodor, fistulas, tenderness
   e. Pelvic floor muscles—form supportive sling for pelvic contents and functional sphincters for vagina, urethra, and rectum; able to constrict introitus around examining finger; no anterior or posterior bulging of vaginal walls, incontinence, or protrusion of cervix or uterus when client bears down
   f. Inspection of internal structures
      (1) Vaginal walls—pink, rugated, homogenous, may have thin, clear/cloudy, odorless discharge
      (2) Cervix—midline, smooth, round, pink, about 2.5-cm diameter, protrudes 1–3 cm into vagina; points posteriorly with anteverted uterus, anteriorly with retroverted uterus, horizontally with midposition uterus; nabothian cysts may be present; os small and round (nulliparous); may be oval, slit-like, or stellate if parous; may have area of darker red epithelial tissue around os if squamocolumnar junction is on ectocervix
      (3) Note presence of discoloration, erythema, swelling, atrophy, friable tissue, lesions, masses, discharge that is profuse, malodorous, thick, curdy, frothy, gray, green, yellow, or adherent to vaginal walls
   g. Palpation of internal structures
      (1) Vaginal walls—smooth, nontender
      (2) Cervix—smooth, firm, mobile, nontender, about 2.5-cm diameter, protrudes 1–3 cm into vagina
      (3) Uterus—smooth, rounded contour, firm, mobile, nontender; 5.5 to 8 cm long and pear shaped in nulliparous female, may be 2 to 3 cm larger in parous female; position anteverted, anteflexed, midplane, retroverted, or retroflexed
      (4) Adnexa—fallopian tubes nonpalpable; ovaries ovoid, smooth, firm, mobile, slightly tender; size during reproductive years 3 cm × 2 cm × 1 cm

(5) Note presence of enlargements, masses, irregular surfaces, consistency other than firm, deviation of positions, immobility, tenderness

h. Rectovaginal examination

(1) Purpose—palpate retroverted uterus; screen for colorectal cancer in females 50 years of age and older; assess pelvic pathology

(2) Repeat the maneuvers of the bimanual examination with index finger in vagina and middle finger in rectum

(3) Rectum—smooth, nontender without masses; firm anal sphincter tone

(4) Rectovaginal septum—smooth, intact, nontender, without masses

- Male-focused reproductive health assessment

1. Health history

a. Reason for visit and any presenting problems/illness

b. Review of past health history, current health status, family health history, psychosocial/cultural health history as appropriate for reason for visit

c. Review of systems—endocrine, genitourinary

d. Sexual health history

(1) Age at first intercourse—consensual/nonconsensual

(2) History of sexual abuse or sexual assault

(3) Sexual orientation/gender identity

(4) Current sexual relationship(s)—frequency of sexual intercourse; satisfaction or concerns with sexual relationship(s); libido; ability to achieve and sustain erection; ability to achieve orgasm; dyspareunia

(5) STI/HIV risk assessment—total number of sexual partners and number in past 3 months; types of sexual contact (vaginal, oral, anal); use of condoms; previous history of STIs; use of injection drugs or sex with partner who uses injection drugs; sex while drunk, stoned, or high; previous testing for HIV

(6) Contraceptive use by female partner(s) if not desiring pregnancy

(7) Fertility/infertility concerns

(8) Any current penile discharge, lesions, scrotal swelling, or pain

2. Physical examination

a. Tanner sexual maturity rating in adolescent

b. Pubic hair—skin smooth with uniform color, hair course in triangular pattern pointing toward umbilicus

c. Penis—skin smooth without hair, no lesions, no tenderness; prepuce (foreskin) if present retracts easily, may have some smegma under prepuce; glans penis without lesions or erythema; urethral meatus on ventral surface at tip of glans penis, without lesions or erythema

d. Scrotum—loose, wrinkled skin darker pigment than rest of body; no lesions; may appear asymmetrical with left testis lower than right testis

e. Testes—oval, smooth, rubbery, move freely when palpated, sensitive to pressure but not tender

f. Epididymis—posterolateral surface of testes, comma shaped, smooth, softer than testes, nontender

g. Spermatic cords—starts at lower end of epididymis and extends to external inguinal ring; smooth; nontender

Nongynecological Diagnostic Studies/ Laboratory Tests

- Complete blood count (CBC) with differential

1. Red blood cell (RBC) count—measurement of red blood cells per cubic millimeter of blood

a. Normal findings (adult female)—4.2 to 5.4 million/mm^3

b. Low values—hemorrhage, hemolysis, dietary deficiencies, hemoglobinopathies, bone marrow failure, chronic illness, medications

c. High values—dehydration, diseases causing chronic hypoxia such as congenital heart disease, polycythemia vera, medications

2. Hematocrit (Hct)/Hemoglobin (Hgb)—rapid indirect measurement of RBC count

a. Hct—percentage of total blood volume that is made up of RBCs

(1) Normal findings (nonpregnant adult female)—37% to 47%

(2) Normal findings (pregnant adult female)—33% or greater in first and third trimesters, 32% or greater in second trimester

b. Hgb—measurement of total hemoglobin (which carries oxygen) in the blood

(1) Normal findings (nonpregnant adult female)—12 to 16 g/dL

(2) Normal findings (pregnant adult female)—11 g/dL or greater in first and third trimesters, 10.5 g/dL or greater in second trimester

c. Low values—anemia, hemoglobinopathies, cirrhosis, hemorrhage, dietary deficiency, bone marrow failure, renal disease, chronic illness, some cancers

d. High values—erythrocytosis, polycythemia vera, severe dehydration, severe chronic obstructive pulmonary disease

e. Heavy smokers and individuals living at higher elevations may also have higher Hgb levels

3. Red blood cell indices—provide information about size, weight, and Hgb concentration of RBCs; useful in classifying anemias

a. Mean corpuscular volume (MCV)—average volume or size of a single RBC

(1) Normal finding—80 to 95 mm^3, normocytic

(2) Microcytic/abnormally small—seen with iron-deficiency anemia and thalassemia

(3) Macrocytic/abnormally large—seen with megaloblastic anemias such as vitamin B$_{12}$ deficiency and folic acid deficiency

b. Mean corpuscular hemoglobin (MCH)—average amount or weight of Hgb within an RBC

(1) Normal finding—27 to 31 pg/cell

(2) Causes for abnormalities same as with MCV

c. Mean corpuscular hemoglobin concentration (MCHC)—average concentration or percentage of Hgb within a single RBC

(1) Normal finding—32 to 36 g/dL, normochromic

(2) Decreased concentration or hypochromic—seen with iron-deficiency anemia and thalassemia

4. White blood cell (WBC) count with differential—provides information useful in evaluating individual with infection, neoplasm, allergy, or immunosuppression
   a. Normal finding for total WBC (adult)—5000 to 10,000/mm³
   b. Increased WBC count—seen with infection, trauma, inflammation, some malignancies, dehydration
   c. Decreased WBC count—seen with some drug toxicities, bone marrow failure, overwhelming infections, immunosuppression
   d. May be elevated in late pregnancy and during labor
   e. Neutrophils—increased with acute bacterial infections and trauma; increased immature forms (band or stab cells) referred to as a "shift to left," seen with ongoing acute bacterial infection
   f. Basophils and eosinophils—increased with allergic reactions and parasitic infections; not increased with bacterial or viral infection
   g. Lymphocytes and monocytes—increased with chronic bacterial and acute viral infections
5. Peripheral blood smear—microscopic examination of smear of peripheral blood to examine RBCs, platelets, and leukocytes
6. Platelet count—used to evaluate abnormal bleeding or blood clotting
   a. Normal finding (adult)—150,000 to 400,000/mm³
   b. Low count (thrombocytopenia)—hypersplenism, hemorrhage, leukemia, cancer chemotherapy, infection
   c. High count (thrombocytosis)—some malignant disorders, polycythemia vera, rheumatoid arthritis
- Urinalysis—dipstick and/or microscopic evaluation of urine
  1. Includes evaluation of appearance, color, odor, pH, protein, specific gravity, leukocyte esterase, nitrites, ketones, crystals, casts, glucose, WBCs, and RBCs
  2. Obtain midstream clean catch specimen so culture can be performed if urinalysis indicates infection
  3. Normal findings
     a. No nitrites, ketones, crystals, casts, or glucose
     b. Clear, amber yellow, aromatic
     c. pH 4.6 to 8.0
     d. Protein 0 to 8 mg/dL
     e. Specific gravity (adult)—1.005 to 1.030
     f. Leukocyte esterase negative
     g. WBCs 0 to 4 per high-power field (HPF)
     h. RBCs at 2 or less
- Blood glucose—used for diagnosis and evaluation of diabetes mellitus
  1. Fasting glucose
     a. No caloric intake for at least 8 hours
     b. Normal finding (adult)—less than 100 mg/dL
     c. Impaired fasting glucose—100 to 125 mg/dL
     d. Diagnostic for diabetes—126 mg/dL or greater
  2. Two-hour postload glucose during oral glucose tolerance test (OGTT)
     a. Sample obtained 2 hours after a glucose load containing the equivalent of 75 g of glucose dissolved in water
     b. Normal finding—less than 140 mg/dL
     c. Impaired glucose tolerance—140 mg/dL to 199 mg/dL
     d. Diagnostic for diabetes—200 mg/dL or greater

3. American Diabetes Association (ADA) criteria for the diagnosis of diabetes mellitus with blood glucose tests
   a. Classic symptoms of hyperglycemia plus random nonfasting glucose concentration of 200 mg/dL or greater
   b. Fasting glucose of 126 mg/dL or greater
   c. Two-hour post glucose 200 mg/dL or greater
   d. Repeat testing on a subsequent day to confirm diagnosis
4. HbA_{1c} or A_{1c}
   a. May be used for the diagnosis of diabetes
   b. Threshold for diagnosis of diabetes is 6.5% or greater, prediabetes is 5.7% to 6.4%
   c. Gold standard for measurement of long-term (previous 60–90 days) glycemic control in individuals with diabetes
   d. Reliable tool for evaluating need for drug therapy and monitoring effectiveness of therapy
   e. Good diabetic control—less than 7%
- Blood urea nitrogen (BUN) and creatinine—used in evaluation of renal function
  1. BUN—indirect measure of renal and liver function
     a. Normal finding (adult)—10 to 20 mg/dL
     b. Increased levels—hypovolemia, dehydration, reduced cardiac function, gastrointestinal bleeding, starvation, sepsis, renal disease
     c. Decreased levels—liver failure, malnutrition, nephrotic syndrome
  2. Serum creatinine—indirect measure of renal function
     a. Normal finding (adult female)—0.5 to 1.1 mg/dL
     b. Increased levels—renal disorders, dehydration
     c. Decreased levels—debilitation and decreased muscle mass
- Lipid profile—determines risk for coronary heart disease and evaluation of hyperlipidemia
  1. Includes total cholesterol, triglycerides, high-density lipoproteins (HDL), and low-density lipoproteins (LDL)
  2. Fast for 12 to 14 hours prior to obtaining sample
  3. Total cholesterol normal level (adult)—less than 200 mg/dL; may be elevated in pregnancy
  4. Triglycerides normal finding (adult female)—35 to 135 mg/dL; may be elevated in pregnancy
  5. HDL—removes cholesterol from peripheral tissues and transports to liver for excretion
     a. Normal level (adult)—40 mg/dL or greater
     b. Low levels associated with increased risk for heart and peripheral vascular disease
  6. LDL—cholesterol carried by LDL can be deposited into peripheral tissues
     a. Normal finding (adult)—less than 130 mg/dL
     b. High levels associated with increased risk for heart and peripheral vascular disease
- Thyroid function studies
  1. Thyroid-stimulating hormone (TSH)—used to diagnose hyperthyroidism and primary hypothyroidism, differentiate primary from secondary hypothyroidism, and monitor thyroid replacement or suppression therapy
     a. Normal finding (adult)—0.4 to 4.7 mU/mL
     b. Increased levels—seen with primary hypothyroidism and thyroiditis

    c. Decreased levels—seen with secondary hypothyroidism, hyperthyroidism, suppressive doses of thyroid medication

    d. Debate on lowering upper limit of normal to 3.0 mU/mL to detect mild thyroid disease

  2. Free thyroxine (FT_4)—used in diagnosis of thyroid disease

    a. Normal finding (adult female)—0.58 to 1.64 ng/dL

    b. Increased levels—hyperthyroidism and acute thyroiditis

    c. Decreased levels—hypothyroidism

  3. Total thyroxine (T_4)

    a. Normal finding (adult female)—4.5 to 12.0 μg/dL

    b. Measurement affected by increases in thyroxine-binding globulin (TBG)

    c. Causes for increased TBG include pregnancy, oral contraceptive use, and estrogen therapy

- Blood type and Rh factor—used to determine blood type prior to donating or receiving blood and to determine blood type in pregnant women

  1. Blood types are grouped according to presence or absence of antigens A, B, and Rh on RBCs

  2. Individual without a particular antigen may develop antibodies to that antigen if exposed through blood transfusion or fetal-maternal blood mixing

  3. Blood type O negative (universal donor because no antigens on RBCs), AB positive (universal recipient because no antibodies to react to transfused blood)

- Infectious disease tests

  1. Rubella (German measles)

    a. Hemagglutination inhibition (HAI) test—used to detect immunity to rubella and diagnose rubella infection

      (1) Titer of 1:10 or greater indicates immunity to rubella

      (2) High titers (1:64 or greater) may indicate current rubella infection

    b. Rubella IgM antibody titer—used if pregnant woman has a rash suspected to be from rubella; if titer is positive, recent infection has occurred; IgM antibodies appear 1 to 2 days after onset of rash and disappear 5 to 6 weeks after infection

  2. HIV tests—used for diagnosis of human immunodeficiency virus infection

    a. Sensitive screening tests—enzyme immunoassay (EIA) or rapid test

    b. Reactive screening tests must be confirmed by supplemental test—Western blot or immunofluorescence assay (IFA)

    c. HIV antibody detectable in 95% of individuals within 6 months of infection

    d. Polymerase chain reaction (PCR)—used to confirm indeterminate Western blot results or negative results in persons with suspected HIV infection

    e. HIV plasma ribonucleic acid (RNA) testing may be used if suspect recent HIV infection before development of immune response; positive HIV RNA testing should be confirmed with subsequent antibody testing to document seroconversion

  3. Hepatitis B (HBV) tests

    a. Hepatitis B surface antigen (HBsAg)—rises before onset of clinical symptoms, peaks during first week of symptoms, and returns to normal by time jaundice subsides

      (1) Indicates active HBV infection—individual is infectious

      (2) Individual is considered a carrier if HBsAg persists

    b. Hepatitis B surface antibody (HBsAb)—appears 4 weeks after disappearance of surface antigen

      (1) Indicates end of acute infectious phase and signifies immunity to subsequent infection

      (2) Also used to denote immunity after administration of hepatitis B vaccine

  4. Hepatitis C (HCV) tests

    a. HCV antibody assay (rapid fingerstick/venipuncture blood test or laboratory test)

    b. Follow reactive antibody test with HCV RNA test; positive HCV RNA test indicates current HCV infection; negative HCV RNA test indicates either past resolved HCV infection or false HCV antibody positivity

  5. Tuberculosis (TB) tests

    a. Usually positive within 6–8 weeks after infection

    b. Does not indicate whether infection is active or dormant

    c. Centers for Disease Control and Prevention (CDC) definition of positive purified protein derivative (PPD) skin test

      (1) High-risk population 5 mm induration or greater

      (2) Moderate-risk population 10 mm induration or greater

      (3) General population 15 mm induration or greater

    d. Once positive reaction, usually persists for life

    e. False negative PPD test may result from incorrect administration (must be intradermal) or immunosuppression

    f. False positive PPD test may result if individual had prior immunization with bacillus Calmette–Guérin (BCG) vaccine

    g. PPD test is contraindicated if history of BCG vaccination or active TB since severe local reaction can occur

    h. TB blood test (interferon-gamma release assay—IRGA) measures how immune system reacts to bacteria causing TB; result reported as positive or negative; preferred method for person who has had BCG vaccination or will have trouble returning in 48–72 hours to read PPD skin test

- Sickle cell screening (Sickle Cell Prep, Sickledex)—used to screen for sickle cell disease and trait

  1. Positive test—presence of Hgb S indicates sickle cell disease or trait

  2. Hgb electrophoresis is definitive test to be performed if screening test is positive; identifies Hgb type and quantity

- Liver function studies

  1. Bilirubin

    a. Normal findings (adult)—total bilirubin 0.3 to 1.0 mg/dL; direct (conjugated) bilirubin 0.1 to 0.3 mg/dL; indirect (unconjugated) bilirubin 0.2 to 0.8 mg/dL

    b. Elevated direct bilirubin level—occurs with gallstones and obstruction of extrahepatic duct

    c. Elevated indirect bilirubin level—seen with hepatocellular dysfunction (hepatitis, cirrhosis) and hemolytic anemias

  2. Albumin

    a. Normal finding (adult)—3.5 to 5.0 g/dL

    b. Increased levels—dehydration

    c. Decreased levels—seen with liver disease, malabsorption syndromes, nephropathies, severe burns, malnutrition, and inflammatory disease

3. Liver enzymes
   a. Alkaline phosphatase (ALP)
      (1) Normal finding—30 to 120 U/L
      (2) Elevated levels—liver disease, bone disease, and myocardial infarction
   b. Aspartate aminotransferase (AST), alanine aminotransferase (ALT), lactic dehydrogenase (LDH), and 59 nucleotidase
      (1) Normal findings—AST 0–35 U/L, ALT 4–36 U/L, LDH 100–190 U/L
      (2) Useful in differentiating cause for ALP elevation
   c. Gamma-glutamyl transpeptidase (GGT)
      (1) Normal finding—8–38 U/L
      (2) Elevated levels with liver disease, myocardial infarction, pancreatic disease, and heavy or chronic alcohol use
- Stool for occult blood
  1. Annual screen for individuals 50 years of age or older and for evaluation of gastrointestinal conditions that may cause gastrointestinal (GI) bleeding
  2. Positive test—may indicate GI cancer or polyps; peptic ulcer disease; inflammatory or ischemic bowel disease; GI trauma; bleeding caused by medications
  3. Several interfering factors can cause false positives or negatives
     a. Red meat and some raw fruits/vegetables if consumed within 3 days prior to or during the test period can result in false positive
     b. Large amounts of vitamin C consumed within 3 days prior to or during the test period can result in false negative
  4. Positive test requires further evaluation with sigmoidoscopy, colonoscopy, or barium enema

General Health Promotion

- Nutrition
  1. Evaluation of nutritional status
     a. Anthropometric measurements—height, weight, BMI, waist circumference
     b. General appearance—skin, hair, muscle mass
     c. Biochemical measurements—Hgb/Hct, lipid analysis, serum albumin, serum glucose, serum folate
     d. 24-hour diet recall or 3- to 4-day food diary
     e. Use of vitamin, mineral, and herbal supplements
  2. *Dietary Guidelines for Americans* (U.S. Department of Health and Human Services [USDHHS], 2010)
     a. Principles for promoting calorie balance and weight management
        (1) Focus on total number of calories consumed
        (2) Monitor food intake
        (3) Choose smaller portions or lower-calorie options when eating out
        (4) Prepare, serve, and consume smaller portions of foods and beverages, especially those high in calories
        (5) Eat a nutrient-dense breakfast
        (6) Limit screen time (e.g., video games, television)
     b. Foods and food components to reduce
        (1) Limit sodium intake to 2300 mg/day (approximately 1 teaspoon of salt); 1500 mg for individuals 51 years and older, African Americans, and those with hypertension, diabetes, chronic kidney disease
        (2) Choose a diet low in fat (20% to 35% of calories), saturated fats (< 10% of calories), trans fats as low as possible, and cholesterol (300 mg or less/day)
        (3) Choose and prepare foods and beverages with little added sugar
        (4) Drink alcoholic beverages only in moderation (no more than one drink daily for women); one drink = 12 ounces of beer, 5 ounces of wine, 1.5 ounces of hard liquor
        (5) Limit consumption of foods that contain refined grains
     c. Foods and nutrients to increase
        (1) Eat a variety of nutrient-dense foods from the basic food groups
        (2) Eat a variety of $2\frac{1}{2}$ cups of vegetables and 2 cups of fruit each day (reference 2000 calories intake)
        (3) Eat 6 ounces of grains with at least one-half whole grain products each day
     d. Eat 3 cups of fat-free or low-fat milk or equivalent milk products each day
     e. Eat $5\frac{1}{2}$ ounces of meat and beans, choosing low-fat lean meats, more fish, beans, peas, nuts, and seeds
  3. Calcium and vitamin D requirements for women
     a. Institute of Medicine (2010)
        (1) 14 to 18 years of age—1300 mg/day of calcium; same amount if pregnant or lactating
        (2) 19 to 50 years of age—1000 mg/day of calcium; same amount if pregnant or lactating
        (3) 51 years of age and older—1200 mg/day of calcium
        (4) 14 to 70 years of age—600 IU/day of vitamin D
        (5) 71 years of age and older—800 IU/day of vitamin D
     b. National Osteoporosis Foundation (2013)
        (1) Adults age 50 and younger—1000 mg/day of calcium; 400 to 800 IU/day of vitamin D
        (2) Adults age 51 and older—1200 mg/day of calcium; 800 to 1000 IU of vitamin D
     c. Sources of calcium—milk, yogurt, soybeans, tofu, canned sardines and salmon with edible bones, cheese, fortified cereals and orange juice, supplements
     d. Sources of vitamin D—fortified milk, egg yolks, saltwater fish, liver, supplements, regular exposure to direct sunlight
  4. Folate requirements for women of childbearing age
     a. 0.4 mg folic acid/day
     b. Women of childbearing age who have had an infant with neural tube defect or who have seizure disorders or insulin-dependent diabetes may benefit from a higher dose of 4 mg folic acid/day starting 1 to 3 months before trying to become pregnant
     c. Sources—dried beans, leafy green vegetables, citrus fruits and juices, fortified cereals; most multivitamins contain 0.4 mg folic acid
  5. Iron requirements for nonpregnant women
     a. 14 to 18 years of age—15 mg/dL each day
     b. 19 to 50 years of age—18 mg/dL each day
     c. 51 years of age or older—8 mg/dL each day
     d. Sources—meat, fish, poultry, fortified cereals, dried fruits, dark green vegetables, supplements

6. Special concerns
   a. Eating disorders—reviewed elsewhere in this text
   b. Vegetarians—plan diet to avoid deficiencies in protein, calcium, iron, vitamin B_{12}, and vitamin D
   c. Older adults—consider effects of chronic illness, medications, isolation, decrease in ability to taste and smell, limited income

- Physical activity
  1. There is strong evidence that regular physical activity lowers risk for heart disease, stroke, high blood pressure, adverse lipid profile, type 2 diabetes, metabolic syndrome, colon and breast cancers; prevents weight gain and promotes weight loss; improves cardiovascular and muscular fitness; reduces depression; improves cognitive function in older adults
  2. Sixty percent of Americans are not regularly physically active and 25% report no physical activity at all
  3. Physical Activity Guidelines for Americans (USDHHS, 2008)
     a. Engage in at least 150 minutes of moderate intensity or 75 minutes of vigorous intensity aerobic physical activity each week; performed for at least 10 minutes per episode; spread throughout the week
     b. Moderate intensity exercise achieves 50% to 69% of maximum heart rate—maximum average heart rate equals 220 minus age
     c. Examples of aerobic physical activity—brisk walking, running, bicycling, jumping rope, swimming
     d. Engage in muscle-strengthening activities of moderate or high intensity involving all major muscle groups 2 or more days each week
     e. Examples of muscle-strengthening activities—weight lifting, exercises with elastic bands or use of body weight (push-ups, tree climbing) for resistance
     f. Include bone-strengthening activity in exercise regimen—running, brisk walking, weight training, tennis, dancing

- Routine screening recommendations
  1. Breast self-examination (BSE)/breast self-awareness
     a. BSE—self-examination performed in a systematic way on a regular basis
     b. Breast self-awareness—knowing normal appearance and feel of one's breasts, no systematic or regular technique of self-examination
     c. American Cancer Society (ACS)—beginning in their 20s, inform of benefits and limitations of BSE and provide instruction for women who choose to do BSE; it is acceptable for women to choose not to do BSE or to do BSE irregularly
     d. American College of Obstetricians and Gynecologists (ACOG)—educate women age 20 and older about breast self-awareness; woman may or may not choose to do BSE
  2. Clinical breast examination
     a. ACS—every 3 years from age 20 to 39 years
     b. American College of Obstetricians and Gynecologists (ACOG)—every 1 to 3 years from age 20 to 39 years
     c. ACS and ACOG—yearly clinical breast examination for women age 40 and older
  3. Mammogram
     a. ACS and ACOG—yearly beginning at age 40 years
     b. ACS and ACOG—no definitive age to discontinue mammogram screening; base on woman's health and if would be candidate for treatment of breast cancer
  4. Magnetic resonance imaging (MRI)
     a. ACS and ACOG—not recommended for routine breast cancer screening in women with average risk (< 15% lifetime risk)
     b. ACS—combination of yearly mammogram and MRI for women at high risk (> 20% lifetime risk) starting at 30 years of age
     c. ACS—discuss risks and benefits of combined yearly mammogram and MRI for women at moderately increased risk (15% to 20%)
     d. ACOG—combination of yearly mammogram and MRI in women with *BRCA* gene mutation beginning at age 25 or younger based on earliest age of onset in family
     e. Risk assessment tools—BRCAPRO, Claus model, Tyrer-Cuzick model
  5. Pap test (ACS and ACOG)
     a. Begin at age 21 years
     b. Age 21 to 29 years—screen every 3 years with cytology alone, do not use HPV testing for screening in this age group
     c. Age 30 to 65 years—screen with HPV test and cytology every 5 years (preferred); screen with cytology alone every 3 years (acceptable)
     d. Age > 65 years—no screening following adequate negative prior screening; do not resume screening even if woman reports new sexual partner; women with history of CIN2 or a more serious diagnosis should continue routine screening for at least 20 years after spontaneous regression or treatment
     e. No screening after hysterectomy with cervix removed unless history of CIN2 or more severe diagnosis in past 20 years or cervical cancer ever
  6. Chlamydia screening—CDC—yearly screening for all sexually active females 24 years of age or younger
  7. Blood pressure—National High Blood Pressure Education Program (NHBPEP) of the National Heart, Lung, and Blood Institute (NHLBI)—at least every 2 years for adults
  8. Lipids
     a. *Third Report of the Expert Panel on Detection, Evaluation, and Treatment of High Blood Cholesterol in Adults (Adult Treatment Panel III or ATP III)* (National Cholesterol Education Program, 2001) recommendations for cholesterol screening—fasting lipid profile (total cholesterol, LDL, HDL, triglycerides) once every 5 years beginning at age 20 years
     b. United States Preventive Services Taskforce (USPSTF, 2008)
        (1) Screen women aged 45 years and older for lipid disorders if they are at increased risk for coronary heart disease (Grade A Strong Recommendation)
        (2) Screen women aged 20 to 45 years for lipid disorders if they are at increased risk for coronary heart disease (Grade B Recommendation)
        (3) Screen with total cholesterol and HDL on nonfasting or fasting samples

(4) No recommendation on interval of screening, states every 5 years is reasonable

c. Lipid level recommendations

(1) Total cholesterol

(a) Desirable level—less than 200 mg/dL

(b) Borderline high—200 to 239 mg/dL

(c) High—240 mg/dL or greater

(2) LDL

(a) Optimal level—less than 100mg/dL; less than 70 mg/dL if very high risk for coronary heart disease (CHD)

(b) Near optimal/above optimal—100 to 129 mg/dL

(c) Borderline high—130 to 159 mg/dL

(d) High—160 to 189 mg/dL

(e) Very high—190 mg/dL or greater

(3) HDL

(a) Low—less than 40 mg/dL (considered a risk for CHD)

(b) High—60 mg/dL or greater (protective against CHD)

(4) Triglycerides

(a) Normal—less than 150 mg/dL

(b) Borderline high—150 to 199 mg/dL

(c) High—200 mg/dL or greater

d. CHD risk factors for women include being 55 years of age or older, family history of premature CHD (male relative < 55 years, female relative < 65), cigarette smoking, hypertension, HDL at less than 40 mg/dL, diabetes mellitus

e. Desirable cholesterol is less than 200 mg/dL, HDL 60 mg/dL or greater, LDL at less than 130 mg/dL

9. Fecal occult blood test (ACS and ACOG)

a. Yearly beginning at age 50

b. Use multiple stool sample take-home test

10. Tests that find colorectal polyps and cancer (ACS and ACOG)

a. ACS and ACOG—beginning at age 50 years colonoscopy every 10 years; flexible sigmoidoscopy every 5 years; double-contrast barium enema every 5 years; or computed tomography (CT) colonography (virtual colonoscopy) every 5 years

b. More frequent testing and starting at younger age for those with risk factors including inflammatory bowel disease and personal or family history of colonic polyps or colon cancer

11. Diabetes—American Diabetes Association (2010)

a. Every 3 years starting at age 45

b. More frequent testing and starting at a younger age if BMI > 25 and one or more other risk factors

c. Risk factors—obesity; hypertension; dyslipidemia; cardiovascular disease; polycystic ovarian syndrome; diabetes in first-degree relative; African American, Asian, Hispanic, Native American, Pacific Islander; history of gestational diabetes or baby weighing more than 9 lbs at birth

d. Use HbA_{1c}, fasting glucose, or 2-hour 75-g glucose tolerance test

12. Thyroid function

a. USPSTF—routine screening for thyroid function is not warranted in asymptomatic individuals

b. ACOG—TSH periodically for women with an autoimmune condition or strong family history of thyroid disease

13. Tuberculosis

a. CDC and ACOG—perform on all individuals at high risk

b. See discussion elsewhere in this text for more information on tuberculosis and risk factors

14. Vision—American Academy of Ophthalmology recommendations for screening for visual acuity and glaucoma by an ophthalmologist

a. Every 3 to 5 years for African Americans age 20 to 39 years

b. Every 2 to 4 years for individuals age 40 to 64 years and every 1 to 2 years beginning at age 65 regardless of race

c. Yearly for diabetic individuals regardless of age

15. Dental—American Dental Association recommends that adults should have routine dental care and preventive services including oral cancer screening at least once every year

16. Bone mineral density (BMD)—National Osteoporosis Foundation (2013)

a. Screen all women 65 years of age or older for osteoporosis/osteopenia with BMD test

b. Screen postmenopausal women younger than 65 years of age with risk factors associated with increased fracture risk

c. Risk factors—low BMI, history of low-trauma fracture, smoking, alcohol intake ≥ 3 drinks/day, family history of hip fracture or osteoporosis

17. HIV—CDC (Branson et al., 2006)

a. Screen all adolescents and adults seen in any healthcare setting unless decline (opt-out screening)

b. Screen individuals at high risk for HIV infection at least annually

c. Include in routine panel of prenatal screening tests for all pregnant women unless decline (opt-out screening)

d. Repeat screening in third trimester in areas with elevated rates of HIV infection among pregnant women

18. Hepatitis C virus (HCV)—CDC (2012, 2013)

a. Screen all individuals born between 1945 and 1965 once if no other risk factors

b. Screen all individuals who have received blood products with clotting factor before 1987 or who have had blood transfusion or organ transplant before July 1992

c. Screen all individuals who currently inject or have ever injected drugs

d. Screen all individuals who have HIV infection

e. Screen all individuals who have been on hemodialysis for several years

f. Screen health or public safety workers who have needle, sharp object, or mucosal exposure to HCV-positive blood

g. Screen infants born to mother with hepatitis C

• Immunizations

1. Hepatitis B

a. Effective in 95% of cases in preventing hepatitis B virus (HBV) infection

b. High-risk groups for whom HBV vaccination is recommended include, but are not limited to, individuals who have multiple sex partners; men who have sex with men; household contacts or sex partners of those with HBV infection; injection drug users; healthcare workers or workers otherwise at occupational risk; inmates of long-term correctional institutions

   c. Three-dose series with the second and third doses at 1 and 6 months after the first dose

   d. If 3-dose series is interrupted, the series does not need to be restarted; give second dose as soon as possible and third dose at least 8 weeks later

2. Influenza

   a. Recommended yearly for all individuals age 6 months and older

   b. Recommended for all women who will be in the second or third trimester of pregnancy during the influenza season; administration of inactivated influenza vaccine is considered safe at any stage of pregnancy and during lactation

   c. Inactivated influenza vaccine (IIV) given intramuscularly or intradermally in one dose

   d. Live attenuated influenza vaccine (LAIV) given intranasally—only use for healthy, nonpregnant individuals younger than 50 years of age

3. Pneumococcus (pneumococcal polysaccharide vaccine—PPSV23)

   a. Recommended one time for all immunocompetent individuals age 65 and older

   b. Recommended for adults 64 years of age or younger who have chronic illness, functional or anatomic asplenia, immunocompromising conditions, organ or bone marrow transplant recipients; who are residents of nursing homes or long-term care facilities; or who smoke cigarettes

   c. A single revaccination 5 or more years after the initial vaccination is recommended for individuals who received the initial vaccine when they were younger than 65 years old; individuals with functional or anatomic asplenia; organ or bone marrow transplant recipients; and immunocompromised individuals

   d. Pneumococcal conjugate 13-valent vaccination (PCV13) is indicated in addition to PPSV23 for individuals with immunocompromising conditions, functional or anatomic asplenia, cerebrospinal fluid leaks, and cochlear implants

4. Rubella

   a. Recommended for all nonpregnant women of childbearing age who lack documented laboratory evidence of immunity or prior immunization after 12 months of age; documentation of provider-diagnosed rubella is not considered acceptable evidence of immunity

   b. Contraindications—pregnancy (advise not to become pregnant for 4 weeks after vaccination); known severe immunodeficiency; individuals with HIV infection who are severely immunocompromised

   c. May be given to breastfeeding women

5. Tetanus, diphtheria, and acellular pertussis (Td/Tdap)

   a. Recommended 3-dose vaccination series including a Tdap dose for adults with unknown or incomplete history of primary Td vaccination

   b. Recommended one dose of Tdap for all adults who have not previously received Tdap

   c. Recommended one dose of Tdap vaccine for pregnant women during each pregnancy regardless of number of years since prior Td or Tdap vaccination; preferred timing between 27 and 36 weeks' gestation to offer optimal protection to infant in first few months of life when high risk for severe illness or death from pertussis

   d. Booster Td vaccination every 10 years for adults

6. Varicella

   a. Recommended for all nonpregnant adolescents and adults without evidence of immunity, given in two doses 4 to 8 weeks apart

   b. Evidence of immunity—documentation of 2-dose vaccination, history of varicella based on diagnosis by healthcare provider, history of herpes zoster based on diagnosis of healthcare provider, laboratory evidence of immunity or confirmation of disease, U.S. born before 1980 except for pregnant women and healthcare personnel

   c. Pregnant women should be assessed for evidence of immunity and, if not immune, give first dose of vaccine upon completion or termination of pregnancy and second dose 4 to 8 weeks later

   d. May be given to breastfeeding women

   e. Contraindications—pregnancy (advise not to become pregnant for 4 weeks after vaccination), known severe immunodeficiency; individuals with HIV infection who are severely immunocompromised

7. Zoster (shingles)

   a. Recommended one-time dose for all individuals 60 years of age or older regardless of previous history of herpes zoster (shingles)

   b. Contraindications—pregnancy; known severe immunodeficiency; individuals with HIV infection who are severely immunocompromised

8. Hepatitis A

   a. Recommended for individuals who live in or are traveling to countries with high levels of hepatitis A infection; men who have sex with men; illicit drug users (injection or noninjection); those with occupational exposure risks; food handlers; and individuals with chronic liver disease or clotting factor disorders

   b. Two doses at least 6 months apart

   c. Combination hepatitis A and hepatitis B vaccine given in three doses with second dose 1 month after first dose and third dose 6 months after first dose

9. Human papillomavirus (HPV)

   a. Bivalent HPV vaccine (HPV2) targeting HPV types 16 and 18 and quadrivalent HPV vaccine (HPV4) targeting HPV types 6, 11, 16, 18 available

   b. Recommended as routine vaccination for females 11 to 12 years of age; may be given as young as 9 years of age

   c. Three doses with second dose 2 months after first dose and third dose 6 months after first dose

   d. Recommended as a catch-up vaccination for females 13 to 26 years of age who did not receive it when younger

   e. Individuals already infected with one or more HPV types will still get protection from types not yet acquired

f. Routine pregnancy testing prior to initiation of HPV vaccination series is not recommended; if found to be pregnant after initiation, delay the remainder of the 3-dose series until completion of pregnancy

g. HPV4 recommended for males in 3-dose series at 11 to 12 years of age as routine vaccination, catch-up ages 13 to 21 years of age, and through age 26 for men who have sex with men

10. Meningococcal

a. Recommended initial vaccination age 11 to 12 as one-time dose

b. Recommended booster vaccination at age 16; booster not needed if initial vaccination done at age 16 or older

c. Recommended for all college freshmen living in dormitories; military recruits; individuals with anatomic or functional asplenia; individuals traveling to regions where meningococcal disease is common

11. Immunizations during pregnancy and lactation

a. Live attenuated-virus vaccines should *not* be given during pregnancy—LAIV; varicella; zoster; measles, mumps, rubella (MMR)

b. Varicella, zoster, and MMR may be given during lactation, IIV preferred over LAIV

c. Inactivated virus vaccines, bacterial vaccines, toxoids, and tetanus immunoglobulin may be given if indicated

- Smoking cessation

1. Overall, 17.3% of adult women currently smoke cigarettes (CDC, 2011b)

2. In women of reproductive age, 18.6% currently smoke cigarettes (CDC, 2011b)

3. Of female high school students, 14.8% currently smoke cigarettes (CDC, 2010a)

4. Smoking-cessation interventions should be individualized in relation to the smoker's physical and psychological dependence and the stage of readiness for change

5. Behavior-modification strategies—provide self-help materials and/or refer to a smoking-cessation class

6. Five As of smoking cessation—*Ask* about tobacco use, *Advise* to quit, *Assess* willingness to attempt to quit, *Assist* in quit attempt, *Arrange* follow-up

7. Pharmacologic aids

a. Nicotine replacement therapy (gum, patches, inhalers, nasal spray, lozenges)—helps to reduce the physical withdrawal symptoms that occur with smoking cessation

(1) Major side effects—local skin reactions with patch; mouth and throat irritation with gum, lozenge, and inhaler; nasal irritation with spray; headache; dizziness; nausea

(2) Contraindications—serious cardiac arrhythmias, severe angina, recent myocardial infarction, concurrent smoking, pregnancy Category D

(3) Avoid using for at least 1 hour before breastfeeding

(4) Client education

(a) Individual must stop smoking before initiating nicotine replacement therapy

(b) Provide specific instructions for the chosen route of delivery

b. Bupropion hydrochloride sustained release tablets—reduces cravings smokers experience; exact manner of action unknown; probably acts on brain pathways involved in nicotine addiction and withdrawal

(1) Major side effects—insomnia, dry mouth, nausea, skin rash

(2) Contraindications—seizure disorder, eating disorder, use of a monoamine oxidase (MAO) inhibitor, concomitant use of other forms of bupropion

(3) Pregnancy Category C; not recommended during breastfeeding

(4) Client education

(a) Individual should initiate medication 1 to 2 weeks before smoking cessation

(b) Recommended duration of therapy is up to 6 months

c. Varenicline tablets—reduces withdrawal symptoms; blocks effect of nicotine if individual resumes smoking; nicotinic acetylcholine receptor partial agonist

(1) Major side effects—nausea, changes in dreaming, constipation, gas, vomiting, neuropsychiatric symptoms

(2) Contraindications—precautions with psychiatric disorders and renal impairment

(3) Pregnancy Category C; not recommended during breastfeeding

(4) Client education

(a) Individual should initiate medication 1 week before smoking cessation

(b) Concomitant use of nicotine replacement may increase side effects

(c) Discontinue medication and report any agitation, depression, and suicidal ideation

- Safety—address use of seat belts, safety helmets, smoke alarms, occupational safety, and other injury prevention

- Sexuality

1. Sexual history—see section "Health History" earlier in this chapter

2. PLISSIT model used by clinicians who are not sex therapists or psychiatrists/psychologists to address sexual concerns and to make appropriate referrals—*Permission* giving, *Limited Information* giving, *Specific Suggestions*, *Intensive Therapy*

3. Sexual practices

a. Sexuality includes a wide range of behaviors—sexual intercourse, fantasy, self-stimulation, noncoital pleasuring, erotic stimuli other than touch, communication about needs and desires

b. Sexual lifestyle—bisexuality, heterosexuality, homosexuality, long-term monogamy, serial monogamy, multiple partners, celibacy

4. Sexual response cycle

a. Masters and Johnson (four phases)—excitement (arousal), plateau, orgasm, resolution

b. Kaplan (three phases)—desire, excitement, orgasm

c. Basson (nonlinear model)—demonstrates that emotional intimacy, sexual stimuli, and relationship satisfaction affect female sexual response

5. Female sexual dysfunction
   a. Etiology may include relationship factors, medical conditions, medication side effects, psychological factors, sexual abuse history
   b. Must cause personal distress to be considered a sexual dysfunction
   c. May be persistent or recurrent, lifelong or acquired, generalized or situational
   d. Assessment—thorough health history, focused sexual and gynecological history, complete physical examination, focused gynecological examination
   e. Management—PLISSIT model for education, counseling, referral; treatment of related medical problems; change in medications
   f. Classification of female sexual dysfunction
      (1) Sexual desire disorders—hypoactive sexual desire (HSSD), most common female sexual dysfunction disorder; sexual aversion disorder
      (2) Sexual arousal disorder—inability to attain or maintain sufficient sexual excitement; may have lack of lubrication or feeling of erotic genital sensations
      (3) Sexual orgasmic disorder—difficulty, delay in, or absence of orgasm following sufficient stimulation and arousal
      (4) Sexual pain disorders
         (a) Dyspareunia—genital pain associated with sexual intercourse
         (b) Vaginismus—involuntary contraction of musculature of the outer third of the vagina that interferes with vaginal penetration
         (c) Noncoital sexual pain disorder—genital pain induced by noncoital sexual stimulation (e.g., endometriosis, vestibulitis, genital mutilation, or trauma)
6. Male sexual dysfunction
   a. Erectile disorder—inability to obtain or maintain an adequate erection suitable for sexual activity; factors may include performance anxiety, neurologic and vascular disorders, diabetes, hormonal deficiency, alcoholism, medications
   b. Premature ejaculation—inability to delay ejaculation to a point that is mutually desirable for both partners; factors may include sexual inexperience and anxiety

Preconception Care

- Historical factors linking birth defects and certain drugs
  1. Thalidomide
  2. Radiation exposure
  3. DES
- Goals of preconception care
  1. Assistance in preventing unintended pregnancies
  2. Identification of risk factors that could affect reproductive outcomes
  3. Identification and management of medical conditions that could be affected by pregnancy or could affect reproductive outcomes (e.g., diabetes)
  4. Initiation of education and desired preventive interventions prior to conception
- Timing of preconception care—integrate into well-woman visits for all reproductive-age women
- Components of preconception care
  1. Assessment—family history, medical/surgical history, infectious disease history, obstetric history, environmental history, cultural health beliefs/practices, psychosocial history including violence, nutrition assessment, paternal health history
  2. Education/counseling and interventions
     a. Health promotion/disease prevention/risk reduction
        (1) Rubella, varicella, hepatitis B, HPV, Td/Tdap, influenza vaccinations if needed
        (2) Nutrition counseling for weight loss or gain as needed
        (3) Smoking cessation
        (4) Discontinuation of alcohol use
        (5) Treatment for substance abuse/addiction
        (6) Limit environmental/occupational exposures that may be teratogenic
        (7) Folic acid supplementation
        (8) Optimal glucose control for diabetics
        (9) Dietary management for phenylketonuria
        (10) STI testing and treatment as indicated
        (11) HIV counseling and testing as indicated
        (12) Medication changes as needed to avoid teratogens such as some antiseizure medications
     b. Resources/referrals
        (1) Genetic testing and counseling as indicated—repeated spontaneous abortions, ethnic background that is high risk for autosomal recessive disorder, previous infant with congenital anomaly, age 35 years or older
        (2) Dietary counseling
        (3) Substance abuse treatment
        (4) Domestic violence resources
- Transmission of genetic diseases
  1. Autosomal dominant inheritance
     a. Only one mutated copy of gene in each cell needed for person to be affected
     b. Affected person usually has one affected parent
     c. Disorder tends to occur in every generation of affected family
     d. Huntington disease, neurofibromatosis type 1
  2. Autosomal recessive inheritance
     a. Two mutated copies of gene present in each cell of affected person
     b. Affected person usually has unaffected parents (carriers) who each carry a single copy of the mutated gene
     c. Disorder not typically seen in every generation of affected family
     d. Cystic fibrosis, sickle cell anemia
  3. X-linked dominant inheritance
     a. Caused by mutations in genes on the X chromosome
     b. Females more frequently affected than males, males can be affected
     c. Often have affected males and females in each generation
     d. Fathers cannot pass X-linked dominant traits to sons
     e. Fragile X syndrome

4. X-linked recessive inheritance
    a. Caused by mutations in genes on the X chromosome
    b. Males more frequently affected than females, females may be affected
    c. Often have affected males but not females in each generation
    d. Fathers cannot pass X-linked recessive traits to sons
    e. Hemophilia
5. Other disorders may be caused by combination of effects of multiple genes or by interactions between genes and the environment—heart disease, diabetes, schizophrenia, certain types of cancer

Parenting

- Definitions
    1. Parent(s)—the person or persons responsible for a child's care and long-term welfare
    2. Infant–parent attachment—process by which parent and infant develop an affectionate, reciprocal relationship that endures over time
- Conditions promoting attachment
    1. Parental emotional well-being and ability to trust
    2. Social support system
    3. Competent level of communication and caregiving skills
    4. Proximity with the infant
- Risk factors for abuse or neglect
    1. Immaturity of parent(s)—adolescent parents at high risk
    2. Isolation/lack of support system
    3. Parent rejected or abused as child
    4. Emotional instability
    5. Lack of knowledge about development and care of children
    6. Low self-esteem
    7. Stressful situations—intimate partner abuse, poverty, unemployment
- Anticipatory guidance (birth to 1 year)
    1. Growth and development
        a. Physical growth—height and weight
        b. Motor development—early reflexive responses, gross and fine motor skills
        c. Cognitive development—sensorimotor and language
        d. Psychosocial development—temperament, emotional development, attachment
    2. Immunization schedule and health maintenance visits
    3. Nutritional needs—nutritional requirements, introduction of solid foods, weaning
    4. Safety promotion/injury prevention—Shaken Baby Syndrome, use of infant car seats, accident prevention, prevention of abduction, prevention of second-hand smoke exposure

Aging

- Definition
    1. Aging—process of growing older, regardless of chronologic age
    2. Senescence—mental and physical decline associated with the aging process
- Etiology/incidence
    1. Theories of aging—biologic, sociologic, and developmental
    2. By the year 2030, 25% of Americans will be older than 65 years
    3. Poverty—elderly women living alone or ethnic minorities tend to be poorer than elderly men are; they are more likely to have only public healthcare coverage or no insurance
    4. Elder abuse and neglect—approximately 4% of elderly individuals are victims of abuse each year
- Signs and symptoms
    1. Dry skin, pruritus, delayed wound healing
    2. Decreased visual and hearing acuity
    3. Decreased taste and smell sensations
    4. Decreased exercise tolerance
    5. Decreased muscle strength
    6. Changes in sleep–wake cycle
    7. Cognitive and memory changes
- Differential diagnosis—other medical conditions that may account for signs and symptoms
    1. Hypothyroidism
    2. Glaucoma, cataracts
    3. Chronic cardiac and pulmonary disorders
    4. Depression
    5. Alzheimer's disease
- Physical findings
    1. Anthropometric—percentage of total body fat increases, waist-to-hip ratio increases, height may decrease because of thinning of cartilage between vertebrae and changes in posture (kyphosis)
    2. Skin—skin thinner and less elastic; thinning and graying of hair; increase in benign skin lesions; thick, ridged nails
    3. Head, eyes, ears, nose, throat (HEENT)
        a. Arcus senilis—opaque ring at margins of cornea with decreased tear production
        b. Increased cerumen, increased hair in ear canals
        c. Dry buccal mucosa with atrophy of salivary glands; decreased taste sensation
    4. Respiratory—rib cage less mobile, increased anterior-posterior (AP) diameter
    5. Cardiovascular/peripheral vascular—slower heart rate, increase in systolic BP, may have carotid bruits, peripheral vessels distended and tortuous
    6. Breasts—size and elasticity decrease
    7. Abdomen—decreased muscle tone, may have less pain with abdominal pathology
    8. Musculoskeletal—decrease in muscle mass, kyphosis
    9. Neurologic—slower reaction time, may have decreased response to pain stimuli
    10. Reproductive organs—sparse pubic hair; smaller labia; shorter, narrow vaginal canal with thin, smooth vaginal walls; shorter cervix; smaller uterus; and atrophy of the ovaries
- Diagnostic tests and findings
    1. Most laboratory values not significantly changed by aging in the absence of disease process
    2. Decreased glucose tolerance common in older people—fasting glucose levels increase after age 50 years
    3. Mammography—American Cancer Society (ACS) and American College of Obstetricians and Gynecologists (ACOG) do not

currently recommend a cut-off point for screening related to age

- Management—ACOG periodic (yearly or as appropriate) health examination recommendations for women 65 years of age and older include:
  1. Health history to include health status update; dietary assessment; physical activity; tobacco, alcohol, drug use/abuse; medications; abuse/neglect; sexual practices; pelvic prolapse; urinary or fecal incontinence; menopausal symptoms
  2. Physical examination—height and weight; BMI; blood pressure; hearing and visual acuity; examination of oral cavity, thyroid, heart, lungs, breasts, abdomen, and skin; pelvic and rectovaginal examination; other as indicated
  3. When age or health issues are such that woman would choose not to intervene on conditions detected during routine examination it is reasonable to discontinue pelvic examinations
  4. Laboratory/diagnostic procedures—dipstick urinalysis, mammography, and fecal occult blood test every year; lipid profile and TSH every 5 years; diabetes testing every 3 years; colonoscopy every 10 years; BMD screening no more frequently than

every 2 years in absence of new risk factors; hepatitis C screening one time for individuals born between 1945 and 1965 and unaware of infection status
5. Other screening tests as indicated by risk factors
6. Counseling—sexuality, diet, exercise, psychosocial concerns, cardiovascular risk factors, hormone replacement therapy, injury prevention, dental care, glaucoma testing, advance directives
7. Immunizations—Td booster every 10 years with one Tdap dose if none previously, influenza vaccination annually, pneumococcal vaccination once, zoster (shingles) vaccination once
8. Pharmacologic considerations
   a. Age-related decreases in hepatic metabolism and renal elimination, changes in body fat distribution, and central nervous system changes may have an impact on drug absorption, distribution, metabolism, and excretion
   b. Polypharmacy—increased risk for adverse reactions, drug interactions, noncompliance, and increased cost with use of multiple medications

Questions

Select the best answer.

1. A 17-year-old client presents at the clinic with the following reason for seeking care. "I have been sick for 3 days. I feel sick to my stomach and have diarrhea." Which of the following would be most appropriate to document as her reason for visit/chief complaint?
   a. Flu-like symptoms
   b. Gastrointestinal distress
   c. "I feel sick to my stomach and have diarrhea"
   d. Possible pregnancy, needs further evaluation

2. Which of the following would be considered a subjective assessment finding to be placed in the S section of SOAP format charting?
   a. Motile trichomonads
   b. Mucopurulent discharge
   c. *Trichomoniasis vaginitis*
   d. Vaginal itching

3. Which of the following includes a pertinent negative that needs to be documented?
   a. 16-year-old female who has never been sexually active; no history of STIs
   b. 25-year-old female with abdominal pain; no nausea, vomiting, or diarrhea
   c. 40-year-old female with depression; past history of suicidal attempt
   d. 60-year-old female with stress incontinence; no breast mass or nipple discharge

4. Appropriate information in the review of systems section of the health history would include:
   a. Alert, cooperative, well groomed
   b. Had measles and chicken pox as a child
   c. Occasional loss of urine with coughing
   d. Walks 2 miles a day for exercise

5. Which of the following would most appropriately be documented in the A section of SOAP charting format?
   a. Breast self-examination instructions provided
   b. CBC ordered
   c. Client states she would like to quit smoking
   d. Mucopurulent cervicitis

6. The bell of the stethoscope should be used when listening for:
   a. Bowel sounds
   b. Carotid bruits
   c. Lung sounds
   d. S_1 and S_2 heart sounds

7. Evaluation of extraocular muscle (EOM) movement includes:
   a. Ophthalmoscopic examination
   b. PERRLA evaluation
   c. Six cardinal fields of gaze
   d. Visual fields by confrontation

8. The adventitious lung sound most commonly associated with chronic bronchitis is:
   a. Crackles
   b. Pleural rub
   c. Rhonchi
   d. Wheezes

9. When auscultating lung sounds, the normal finding over most of the lung fields is:
   a. Bronchial
   b. Resonant
   c. Tympanic
   d. Vesicular

10. Increased tactile fremitus would be an expected finding with:
    a. Asthma
    b. Emphysema
    c. Lobar pneumonia
    d. Pleural effusion

11. The sound heard over the cardiac area if there is pericarditis is mostly likely to be a/an:
    a. Diastolic murmur
    b. Fixed split S_2
    c. Friction rub
    d. Increased S_4

12. Which of the following is an abnormal abdominal examination finding in an adult?
    a. Abdominal aorta 2.5 cm in width
    b. Liver border nonpalpable
    c. Liver span 8 cm at the right MCL
    d. Splenic dullness at the left anterior axillary line

13. One of the cranial nerves for which you would test both motor and sensory function is:
    a. CN II—optic nerve
    b. CN V—trigeminal nerve
    c. CN VI—abducens nerve
    d. CN XI—spinal accessory nerve

14. A client with an Hgb of 10.2 g/dL and RBC indices indicating both microcytosis and hypochromia most likely has:
    a. Folic acid deficiency
    b. Iron deficiency
    c. Severe dehydration
    d. Vitamin B_{12} deficiency

15. A client with an increased WBC count related to infectious hepatitis would most likely have an elevated level of:
    a. Basophils
    b. Eosinophils
    c. Lymphocytes
    d. Neutrophils

16. Expected thyroid function test findings with primary hypothyroidism include:
    a. Decreased TSH and decreased FT_4
    b. Decreased TSH and increased FT_4
    c. Increased TSH and decreased FT_4
    d. Increased TSH and increased FT_4

17. A pregnant woman presents with a recent-onset rash. Which of the following laboratory results would be reassuring that this is not likely rubella?
    a. HAI titer of 1:10 at her initial visit 1 month earlier
    b. HAI titer of 1:128 at the current visit
    c. Increased IgG antibody levels at the current visit
    d. Increased IgM antibody levels at the current visit

18. A client who had hepatitis B 6 months ago currently has no symptoms but has a positive test for HbsAg. This most likely indicates that she:
    a. Has immunity to future infection
    b. Has persistent active infection
    c. Is a chronic carrier of hepatitis B
    d. Is in the early stage of reinfection

19. A false-negative TB PPD test may be the result of:
    a. Dormant infection
    b. Immunosuppression
    c. Intradermal injection
    d. Prior BCG vaccination

20. An individual with cholecystitis would most likely have a/an:
    a. Decreased alkaline phosphatase
    b. Decreased indirect bilirubin
    c. Increased albumin level
    d. Increased direct bilirubin

21. Measuring waist circumference is most appropriate when the client's BMI places her in which of the following categories:
    a. Underweight
    b. Normal weight
    c. Overweight
    d. Extreme obesity

22. Which of the following lab values is not normally affected by pregnancy?
    a. Cholesterol
    b. Mean corpuscular volume (MCV)
    c. Total thyroxine (T_4)
    d. Triglycerides

23. HPV testing is indicated for:
    a. 18-year-old female whose sex partner has a history of genital warts
    b. 24-year-old female with current genital warts as adjunct to routine Pap test
    c. 30-year-old female with no history of genital warts as adjunct to routine Pap test
    d. 67-year-old female with new sex partner in past year who has history of genital warts

24. Appropriate management for a 45-year-old white woman who has no diabetes risk factors and no symptoms of diabetes with a fasting glucose of 130 mg/dL would include:
    a. Inform client she has impaired glucose tolerance
    b. Order HbA_{1c} level
    c. Repeat glucose testing on another day
    d. Repeat glucose screening in 3 years

25. A pregnant female who received a Tdap vaccination postpartum with her last pregnancy 3 years ago should have:
    a. Td booster in first or second trimester
    b. Td booster in 7 years
    c. Tdap vaccination between 27and 36 weeks' gestation
    d. Tdap vaccination at 6–8 weeks postpartum

26. Tests for cerebellar function include:
    a. Deep tendon reflex evaluation
    b. Short-term memory evaluation
    c. Discriminatory sensation tests
    d. Romberg test for balance

27. Which of the following statements is correct regarding autosomal recessive inheritance of a genetic disorder?
    a. Both parents are unaffected but are carriers of the mutated gene
    b. Disorder tends to occur in every generation of the affected family
    c. Male offspring are more likely to be affected than females
    d. One parent has the genetic disorder with the mutated gene

28. Client education concerning the use of bupropion hydrochloride for smoking cessation should include:
    a. Discontinue smoking prior to initiation of this medication
    b. The medication should not be used for more than 8 weeks
    c. Initiate the medication at least 1 week prior to smoking cessation
    d. Side effects may include drowsiness and weight gain

29. Which of the following statements regarding influenza vaccination during pregnancy is true?
    a. Influenza vaccination should be given only if the woman has health problems that place her at high risk for complications with influenza
    b. Influenza vaccination may be safely given in any trimester of pregnancy
    c. Intranasal influenza vaccine is recommended for pregnant women to reduce chances of side effects
    d. Influenza vaccination is contraindicated during pregnancy

30. Which of the following heart sounds may be a normal finding for a woman in the third trimester of pregnancy?
    a. Diastolic murmur
    b. Fixed split S_2
    c. S_3
    d. S_4

31. Pelvic findings on examination of a 22-year-old nulliparous woman are uterus 7 cm in length and ovaries 3 cm × 2 cm × 1 cm. These findings are consistent with:
    a. Enlarged uterus and enlarged ovaries
    b. Normal size uterus and enlarged ovaries
    c. Enlarged uterus and normal size ovaries
    d. Normal size uterus and normal size ovaries

32. A laboratory test finding of increased immature neutrophils (shift to the left) is consistent with a/an:
    a. Acute bacterial infection
    b. Acute viral infection
    c. Allergic reaction
    d. Chronic bacterial infection

33. An elderly woman has had gastroenteritis with vomiting and diarrhea for the past 3 days. Her mucous membranes appear dry, and she says she has not urinated yet today. Expected laboratory test findings related directly to her current condition might include:
    a. Decreased urine specific gravity
    b. Decreased hematocrit
    c. Increased blood glucose
    d. Increased blood urea nitrogen

34. The blood type in which an individual has no antigens on their RBCs is:
    a. AB+
    b. AB–
    c. O+
    d. O–

35. A woman who describes finding her partner sexually attractive but is not able to maintain sufficient sexual excitement and lubrication during sexual activity has:
    a. Hypoactive sexual desire disorder
    b. Sexual arousal disorder
    c. Sexual orgasmic disorder
    d. Vaginismus

36. The second and third doses of the human papillomavirus (HPV) vaccination should be given:
    a. 1 month and 3 months after the initial dose
    b. 1 month and 6 months after the initial dose
    c. 2 months and 6 months after the initial dose
    d. 3 months and 12 months after the initial dose

37. An abnormal finding on ophthalmoscopic examination would be:
    a. Arterioles smaller than veins
    b. Optic disc that is yellow
    c. Presence of a red reflex
    d. Tapering of the veins

38. When examining the cervix of a 20-year-old female, you note that most of the cervix is pink but there is a small ring of dark-red tissue surrounding the os. This is most likely:
    a. An endocervical polyp
    b. Due to cervical dysplasia
    c. Due to cervical infection
    d. The squamocolumnar junction

39. The laboratory test that is done for definitive diagnosis of sickle cell disease is:
    a. Hgb electrophoresis
    b. Peripheral blood smear
    c. RBC indices
    d. Sickle cell preparation

40. A woman who is currently pregnant, has had two full-term deliveries, and has had one first-trimester abortion would be considered:
    a. Gravida 2 Para 2
    b. Gravida 3 Para 2
    c. Gravida 3 Para 3
    d. Gravida 4 Para 2

41. The best position for palpating the axilla is with the woman:
    a. Lying down with her arm above the head on the side you are examining
    b. Lying down with her arm at her side on the side you are examining
    c. Sitting up with her arm raised above her head on the side you are examining
    d. Sitting up with her arm down on the side you are examining

42. Which of the following would be considered a positive PPD result?
    a. General population—5 mm induration
    b. General population—10 mm induration
    c. Moderate-risk population—5 mm induration
    d. High-risk population—5 mm induration

43. Abnormal findings on a urinalysis would include:
    a. pH 5.0
    b. Specific gravity 1.5
    c. WBCs 3 per HPF
    d. Protein 4 mg/dL

44. Which of the following types of vaccines should *not* be given during pregnancy?
    a. Bacterial vaccines
    b. Inactivated virus vaccines
    c. Live attenuated virus vaccines
    d. Immunoglobulins

45. Which of the components of the PLISSIT model would best describe instructing a couple on the use of water-soluble lubrication for dyspareunia caused by vaginal dryness?
    a. Permission giving
    b. Limited information

c. Specific suggestions

d. Intensive therapy

46. Good dietary sources for folic acid include:

a. Chicken

b. Dried beans

c. Egg yolks

d. Milk

47. Expected physical findings with aging include:

a. Decrease in total body fat

b. Increase in benign skin lesions

c. Increase in heart rate

d. Increased response to pain stimuli

48. Which of the following would *not* be an expected pelvic examination finding in a 70-year-old woman?

a. Narrow vaginal canal

b. Palpable ovaries

c. Small uterus

d. Thin vaginal walls

Answers with Rationales

1. c. "I feel sick to my stomach and have diarrhea"
    In the health history, the reason for visit/chief complaint should be documented as a brief statement in the client's own words.

2. d. Vaginal itching
    Subjective information is obtained as part of the health history and is what the client or caregiver tells you.

3. b. 25-year-old female with abdominal pain; no nausea, vomiting, or diarrhea
    The description of presenting symptoms should include pertinent negatives. When a symptom suggests that an abnormality may exist or may develop in that area, include documentation of absence of symptoms that may help eliminate some of the possibilities.

4. c. Occasional loss of urine with coughing
    The review of systems is used to assess common symptoms for each major body system to avoid missing any potential or existing problems.

5. d. Mucopurulent cervicitis
    The A section of SOAP charting format is your diagnosis or prioritized list of problems determined from your assessment of subjective and objective data.

6. b. Carotid bruits
    The bell of the stethoscope is best for listening to low-pitched sounds such as those heard over large blood vessels.

7. c. Six cardinal fields of gaze
    Extraocular muscle (EOM) function is evaluated by assessing symmetry, lid lag, and nystagmus as the client holds her head still and follows your finger through the six cardinal fields of gaze.

8. c. Rhonchi
    Rhonchi are low-pitched, snoring-quality adventitious lung sounds that may be heard when air passes over thick secretions in the large airways found in such conditions as chronic bronchitis.

9. d. Vesicular
    The lung sound over most of the lung fields is vesicular with inspiratory sounds lasting longer than expiratory sounds.

10. c. Lobar pneumonia
    Tactile fremitus refers to the palpable transmission of vibrations through the bronchus to the chest wall when the client is speaking. There is increased transmission through consolidated tissue, as is found with lobar pneumonia.

11. c. Friction rub

A pericardial friction rub may be heard over the cardiac area as a grating sound throughout the cardiac cycle when there is inflammation of the pericardium.

12. d. Splenic dullness at the left anterior axillary line
    Splenic dullness may be percussed at the 6th to 10th intercostal space just posterior to the midaxillary line on the left side with the client in supine position. Splenic dullness at the anterior axillary line is indicative of an enlarged spleen.

13. b. CN V—trigeminal nerve
    The cranial nerves with both motor and sensory functions are CN V trigeminal nerve, CN VII facial nerve, CN IX glossopharyngeal, and CN X vagus. Routinely, the only cranial nerve in which you test both motor and sensory function is CN V.

14. b. Iron deficiency
    Red blood cell indices provide information about size, weight, and Hgb concentration of RBCs and are useful in classifying anemia when the individual has a low Hgb level. Iron-deficiency anemia is characterized by abnormally small (microcytic) and pale (hypochromic) RBCs.

15. c. Lymphocytes
    The WBC count with differential provides information useful in evaluating the individual with infection, neoplasm, allergy, or immunosuppression. Lymphocytes and monocytes are increased with acute viral infections and chronic bacterial infections.

16. c. Increased TSH and decreased FT_4
    An increased thyroid-stimulating hormone (TSH) level is seen with primary hypothyroidism and thyroiditis. A decreased free thyroxine (FT_4) is seen with hypothyroidism.

17. a. HAI titer of 1:10 at her initial visit 1 month earlier
    The hemagglutination inhibition (HAI) test is used to detect immunity to rubella and to diagnose rubella infection. Titers of 1:10 or greater indicate immunity to rubella. High titers (1:64 or greater) may indicate current rubella infection.

18. c. Is a chronic carrier of hepatitis B
    Hepatitis B surface antigen (HBsAg) rises before onset of clinical symptoms, peaks during the first week of symptoms, and returns to normal by the time jaundice subsides. An individual is considered to be a carrier (remains infectious) if HBsAg persists.

19. b. Immunosuppression
    False-negative TB PPD tests may result from incorrect administration (must be intradermal) or immunosuppression.

20. d. Increased direct bilirubin
    An elevated direct (conjugated) bilirubin level occurs with gallstones and obstruction of the extrahepatic duct.

21. c. Overweight

Waist circumference provides measurement of abdominal fat as an independent prediction of risk for type 2 diabetes, dyslipidemia, hypertension, and cardiovascular disease in individuals with body mass index (BMI) between 25 and 39.9 (overweight and obesity). Waist circumference has little added value in disease risk prediction in individuals with BMI of 40 or greater (extreme obesity).

22. b. Mean corpuscular volume (MCV)

Cholesterol and triglyceride levels may be elevated during pregnancy. Total thyroxine (T_4) levels are affected by the amount of thyroxine-binding globulin (TBG), which is increased during pregnancy. The MCV is the average volume or size of a single RBC. Although Hgb/Hct may be lower during pregnancy, the size of the RBCs should not change unless the woman has iron-deficiency anemia, thalassemia, vitamin B_{12} deficiency, or folic acid deficiency.

23. c. 30-year-old female with no history of genital warts as adjunct to routine Pap test

ACOG and ACS recommend screening women age 30 to 65 years with combination Pap test and HPV test every 5 years. Screening in this age group with Pap test alone every 3 years is also acceptable.

24. c. Repeat glucose testing on another day

A fasting glucose of 126 mg/dL or greater is diagnostic of diabetes in individual. Repeat testing should be done on a subsequent day to confirm the diagnosis.

25. c. Tdap vaccination between 27 and 36 weeks' gestation

One dose of Tdap vaccine is recommended during each pregnancy. The preferred timing is between 27 and 36 weeks to offer optimal protection to the infant in the first few months of life when at high risk for severe illness or death from pertussis.

26. d. Romberg test for balance

The cerebellum coordinates motor activity, maintains equilibrium, and helps to control posture.

27. a. Both parents are unaffected but are carriers of the mutated gene

In autosomal recessive inheritance of a genetic disorder, the affected individual has two mutated copies of the responsible gene in each cell. The affected individual usually has unaffected parents (carriers) who each carry a single copy of the mutated gene.

28. c. Initiate the medication at least 1 week prior to smoking cessation

Individuals should initiate buproprion hydrochloride sustained release tablets 1 to 2 weeks before they stop smoking. This medication reduces cravings that smokers experience.

29. b. Influenza vaccination may be safely given in any trimester of pregnancy

Administration of inactivated influenza vaccine (IIV) is recommended for all women who will be in the second or third trimester of pregnancy during the influenza season. IIV is considered safe at any stage in pregnancy and during lactation. Live attenuated influenza vaccine (LAIV) given intranasally is contraindicated in pregnancy.

30. c. S_3

An increased S_3 may be audible in late pregnancy. This heart sound is heard early in diastole during rapid ventricular filling.

31. d. Normal size uterus and normal size ovaries

The uterus is 5.5 to 8 cm long and pear shaped in the nulliparous woman. During the reproductive years, the ovaries are approximately 3 cm × 2 cm × 1 cm.

32. a. Acute bacterial infection

Neutrophils are increased with acute bacterial infections and trauma. Increased immature neutrophil forms (band or stab cells), referred to as a "shift to the left," are seen with ongoing acute bacterial infection.

33. d. Increased blood urea nitrogen

Blood urea nitrogen (BUN) is an indirect measure of renal and liver function. Increased levels may be seen with hypovolemia, dehydration, reduced cardiac function, gastrointestinal bleeding, starvation, sepsis, and renal disease.

34. d. O−

Blood types are grouped according to presence or absence of antigens A, B, and Rh on RBCs. Blood type O negative has no antigens on RBCs.

35. b. Sexual arousal disorder

Sexual arousal disorder is the inability to attain or maintain sufficient sexual excitement. The individual with sexual arousal disorder may have normal sexual desire but may have lack of lubrication or feeling of erotic genital sensations.

36. c. 2 months and 6 months after the initial dose

The recommended schedule for the 3-series HPV vaccination is initial dose, second dose 2 months after the initial dose, and third dose 6 months after the initial dose.

37. d. Tapering of the veins

The normal retinal artery wall is transparent except for the column of blood going down the middle, so a vein crossing beneath the artery can be seen up to the column of blood on either side (arteriovenous crossing). When there is narrowing of the retinal artery (as with hypertension) the arterial wall thickens and becomes less transparent. The vein crossing under the narrowed artery appears to taper down on either side of the artery.

38. d. The squamocolumnar junction

The squamocolumnar junction is the area where squamous epithelium (pink) and columnar epithelium (dark red) of the cervix meet. The junction may be inside the cervical os so that only squamous epithelium is visible, or a ring of columnar tissue may be visible to a varying extent around the os.

39. a. Hgb electrophoresis

The sickle cell preparation is used to screen for sickle cell disease and trait. A positive test indicates the presence of Hgb S, indicating either sickle cell disease or trait. The Hgb electrophoresis is the definitive test performed if the screening test is positive. It identifies Hgb type and quantity.

40. d. Gravida 4 Para 2

Gravida denotes the total number of pregnancies including a current pregnancy. *Para* denotes total number of pregnancies reaching 20 weeks or longer gestation.

41. d. Sitting up with her arm down on the side you are examining

Palpate the axillary lymph nodes and breast tissue that extends into the axillary area (tail of Spence) with the woman sitting with arms relaxed at her side. The examiner supports the lower arm and uses the palmar surface of fingers to palpate the entire area.

42. d. High-risk population—5 mm induration

In the individual considered to be high risk for tuberculosis, a PPD skin test resulting in a 5-mm or greater area of induration is a positive reaction.

43. b. Specific gravity 1.5

Normal values are as follows: specific gravity 1.005 to 1.030, pH 4.6 to 8.0, WBCs 0–4 per high-power field (HPF), and protein 0 to 8 mg/dL.

44. c. Live attenuated virus vaccines

Live attenuated viruses virus vaccines are contraindicated during pregnancy. Rubella, measles, mumps, varicella, zoster, and the intranasal form of influenza vaccine (LAIV) are all live attenuated viruses.

45. c. Specific suggestions

Instructing a couple on the use of water-soluble lubrication for dyspareunia caused by vaginal dryness is a specific suggestion to treat an identified problem.

46. b. Dried beans

Dried beans, leafy green vegetables, citrus fruits and juices, and fortified cereals are good dietary sources of folic acid.

47. b. Increase in benign skin lesions

Skin changes seen with aging include skin being thinner and less elastic, thinning and graying of hair, increase in benign skin lesions, and thicker, ridged nails.

48. b. Palpable ovaries

Three to 5 years after menopause ovaries are atrophic and are usually not palpable.

Bibliography

American Cancer Society. (2013). Can breast cancer be found early? Retrieved from http://www.cancer.org/cancer/breastcancer/detailedguide/breast-cancer-detection

American College of Obstetricians and Gynecologists. (2009, March 20). Routine screening for hereditary breast and ovarian cancer recommended. *ACOG News Release*.

American College of Obstetricians and Gynecologists. (2010). Smoking cessation during pregnancy. *ACOG Committee Opinion, 471*, 1–4.

American College of Obstetricians and Gynecologists. (2013). *Well-woman care: Assessments and recommendations*. Washington, DC: Author.

American Diabetes Association. (2010). Position statement: Diagnosis and classification of diabetes mellitus. *Diabetes Care*, 33 (Suppl. 1), S62–S69.

Bickley, L. (2013). *Bates' guide to physical examination and history taking* (11th ed.). Philadelphia, PA: Lippincott Williams & Wilkins.

Branson, B., Handsfield, H., Lampe, M., Janssen, R., Taylor, A. W., Lyss, S. B., & Clark, J. E. (2006). Revised recommendations for HIV testing of adults, adolescents, and pregnant women in healthcare settings. *Morbidity and Mortality Weekly Report*, 55(RR14), 1–17.

Bridges, B., Woods, L., & Coyne-Beasley, T. (2013). Advisory Committee on Immunization Practices (ACIP): Recommended immunization schedule for adults aged 19 years and older—United States, 2013. *Morbidity and Mortality Weekly Report*, 62, 9–18.

Centers for Disease Control and Prevention. (2010a). Tobacco use among high school students, United States— 2000–2009. *Morbidity and Mortality Weekly Report*, 59(33), 1063–1068.

Centers for Disease Control and Prevention. (2010b). Updated guidelines for using interferon gamma release assays to detect *Mycobacterium tuberculosis infection—*United States, 2010. *Morbidity and Mortality Weekly Report*, 59(RR05), 1–25.

Centers for Disease Control and Prevention. (2011a). *Guide to infection prevention in outpatient settings: Minimum expectations for safe care.* Retrieved from http://www.cdc.gov/hai/pdfs/guidelines/ambulatory-care-04-2011.pdf

Centers for Disease Control and Prevention. (2011b). Vital signs: Current cigarette smoking among adults aged > 18 years, United States. *Morbidity and Mortality Weekly Report*, 60(35), 1207–1212.

Centers for Disease Control and Prevention. (2012). Recommendations for the identification of chronic hepatitis C virus infection among persons born during 1945–1965. *Morbidity and Mortality Weekly Report*, 61(RR04), 1–18.

Centers for Disease Control and Prevention. (2013). Testing for HCV infection: An update of guidance for clinicians and laboratorians. *Morbidity and Mortality Weekly Report*, Early Release 62, 1–4.

Chernecky, C., & Berger, B. (2013). *Laboratory tests and diagnostic procedures* (6th ed.). St. Louis, MO: Saunders Elsevier.

Ferri, F. (2014). *Ferri's clinical advisor 2014*. Philadelphia, PA: Mosby Elsevier.

Giger, J. (2013). *Transcultural nursing assessment and intervention* (6th ed.). St. Louis, MO: Mosby.

Institute of Medicine. (2010). *Dietary reference intakes for calcium and vitamin D*. Washington, DC: Author.

Kingsberg, S., Iglesia, C., Kellogg, S., & Krychman, M. (2011). *Handbook on female sexual health and wellness*. Washington, DC: Association of Reproductive Health Professionals.

Lister Hill National Center for Biomedical Communications. (2013). *Handbook: Help me understand genetics*. Washington, DC: National Institutes of Health.

National Cholesterol Education Program. (2001). *Third report of the Expert Panel on Detection, Evaluation, and Treatment of High Blood Cholesterol in Adults (Adult Treatment Panel III)*. Bethesda, MD: National Heart, Lung, and Blood Institute.

National Heart, Lung, and Blood Institute. (2003). *The seventh report of the Joint National Committee on Prevention, Detection, Evaluation, and Treatment of High Blood Pressure*. Washington, DC: National Institutes of Health.

National Heart, Lung, and Blood Institute. (2012). How are overweight and obesity diagnosed. Retrieved from http://www.nhlbi.nih.gov/health/health-topics/topics/obe/diagnosis.html

National Osteoporosis Foundation. (2013). *Clinician's guide to prevention and treatment of osteoporosis*. Washington, DC: Author.

Rhoads, J., & Petersen, S. (2014). *Advanced health assessment and diagnostic reasoning* (2nd ed.). Burlington, MA: Jones & Bartlett Learning.

Saslow, D., Boetes, C., Burke, W., Harms, M., Leach, M. O., Lehman, C. D., . . . American Cancer Society Breast Cancer Advisory Group. (2007). American Cancer Society guidelines for breast cancer screening with MRI as an adjunct to mammography. *CA Cancer Journal for Clinicians, 57,* 75–89.

Saslow, D., Solomon, D., Lawson, H., Killackey, M., Kulasingam, S. L., Cain, J., . . . ACS-ASCCP-ASCP Cervical Cancer Guideline Committee. (2012). American Cancer Society, American Society for Colposcopy and Cervical Pathology, and American Society for Clinical Pathology screening guidelines for the prevention and early detection of cervical cancer. *CA Cancer Journal for Clinicians, 62*(3), 147–172.

Seidel, H., Ball, J., Dains, J., Benedict, G., Flynn, J. A., Solomon, B. S., & Stewart, R. B. (2011). *Mosby's guide to physical examination* (7th ed.). St. Louis, MO: Mosby.

Smith, R., Cokkinides, V., & Brawley, O. (2012). Cancer screening in the United States: A review of current American Cancer Society guidelines and cancer screening issues. *CA Cancer Journal for Clinicians, 62,* 129–142.

Tharpe, N., Farley, C., & Jordan, R. (2013). *Clinical practice guidelines for midwifery and women's health* (4th ed.). Burlington, MA: Jones & Bartlett Learning.

U.S. Department of Health and Human Services. (2008). *Physical activity guidelines for Americans.* Washington, DC: Author.

U.S. Department of Health and Human Services. (2010). *Dietary guidelines for Americans* (7th ed.). Washington, DC: Author.

U.S. Preventive Services Task Force. (2008). Screening for lipid disorders in adults: U.S. Preventive Services Task Force recommendation statement. Retrieved from http://www.uspreventive servicestaskforce.org/uspstf08/lipid/lipidrs.htm

3

Principles of Pharmacology

Beth M. Kelsey

© Kheng Guan Toh/ShutterStock, Inc.

Pharmacokinetics (Study of How the Body Processes Drugs)

- Absorption
  1. Movement of drug from site of entry into the systemic circulation
  2. Bioavailability—percentage of active drug that is absorbed and available at the target tissue
  3. Affected by cell membranes, blood flow, drug solubility, pH of drug, variables with the gastrointestinal tract, drug concentration, dosage form, route of administration
- Distribution
  1. Movement of drug into body fluids and body tissues
  2. Affected by permeability of capillaries and tissues, systemic circulation, size of drug molecule, affinity for lipid and aqueous tissues, protein binding, and pH
  3. Plasma protein binding—drugs may attach to proteins (mainly albumin) in the blood; only unbound drug is active; as free drug is excreted more of drug is released from binding to replace what is lost; competition for binding sites by different drugs and hypoalbuminemia can affect amount of free drug that is available
  4. Blood–brain barrier affects drug distribution—endothelial cells of capillaries surrounding brain are packed tightly together, limits passive transport from blood into cerebral tissue, drug must be highly lipophilic to pass into brain
  5. Placental barrier affects drug distribution
     a. Several layers of placental tissue separate maternal and fetal circulation, not an absolute barrier to drugs; almost all drugs taken by mother pass through placenta to fetus to some degree and reach steady state levels in fetus between 50% to 100% of maternal concentration
     b. General determinants of drug transfer across placenta include lipid solubility, extent of plasma protein binding, and degree of ionization of weak acids and bases

c. Placenta has enzyme systems that metabolize some drugs and P-glycoprotein that actively transports some drug substrates away from fetal circulation
  6. Steady state—when rate of drug elimination equals rate of drug availability (absorption)
  7. Half-life—time it takes for plasma concentration of a drug to be reduced by 50%; used to determine time required to reach steady state and dosage interval
  8. Volume of distribution—apparent volume in which drug is dissolved; relates to concentration of drug in plasma and the amount in the body; may be used to calculate loading dose need to immediately achieve a desired steady state drug level
- Metabolism
  1. Chemical inactivation of drug by conversion to a more water-soluble compound (metabolite) that can be excreted from the body
  2. Chemical alterations are produced by microsomal enzymes mainly in the liver
  3. Hepatic first pass effect—orally administered drug goes from GI tract through portal system to liver before going to the general circulation; some metabolism of drug may occur as it is taken up by hepatic microsomal enzymes
  4. Drug interactions can impact metabolism by enzyme induction or inhibition
  5. Variation in drug metabolism may be impacted by genetics, age, pregnancy, liver disease, diet, alcohol, circadian rhythm
  6. Prodrugs—drugs that must be metabolized to become effective (active metabolites); developed to improve stability, increase absorption, or prolong duration of drug activity; e.g., valacyclovir is not effective, but its active metabolite, acyclovir is
- Excretion
  1. Removal of drug from body via the kidneys, intestines, sweat and salivary glands, lungs, or mammary glands
  2. Urinary excretion—net effect of glomerular filtration, active tubular secretion, and partial reabsorption
  3. Enterohepatic recirculation—some fat-soluble drugs may be reabsorbed into the bloodstream from the intestines and returned to the liver

- Pharmacokinetic changes during pregnancy
  1. Absorption—not significantly affected
  2. Distribution
     a. Increase in plasma volume may result in lower serum levels of drug
     b. Reduction in plasma proteins (albumin) may result in higher levels of free (unbound) drug
  3. Metabolism
     a. Hepatic enzyme systems (e.g., CYP3A4, CYP1A2) are affected by rising levels of estrogen and progesterone and may result in either faster or slower metabolism of some drugs
     b. Blood flow through the liver is not changed significantly so there is no change in first-pass effects
  4. Excretion—increase in glomerular filtration rate (GFR) may result in faster elimination of drugs excreted primarily through the kidneys

Pharmacodynamics (Study of Mechanism of Drug Action on Living Tissue)

- Drug effects produced by
  1. Drug-receptor interaction
  2. Drug-enzyme interaction
  3. Nonspecific drug interaction
- Drug receptors—cellular protein, enzyme, or membrane that when bound to a drug initiates a physiologic response or blocks a response that receptor normally stimulates
  1. Agonist—drug combines with receptor to stimulate a response
  2. Antagonist—drug interferes with receptor action or with other drug agonists present
- Drug–response relationship—study of relationship between concentration of drug in circulation and response obtained
  1. Affinity—propensity of a drug to bind itself to a given receptor site
  2. Efficacy—ability to initiate biologic activity as a result of such binding
- Therapeutic effect
  1. All pharmacologic responses have a maximum effect at which no further response is achieved regardless of drug concentration
  2. Therapeutic range (window)—plasma concentration of drug that produces desired action without toxic effects
  3. Therapeutic index (TI)—ratio of lethal doses in 50% of population over the median minimum effective dose in 50% of the population; higher TI = safer drug

Adverse Reactions—Unintended, Undesired Effects of Drug

- Predictable—may occur related to
  1. Age
  2. Body mass
  3. Gender
  4. Pathologic state
  5. Circadian rhythm
  6. Genetic factors
  7. Psychologic factors
- Unpredictable types include:
  1. Drug allergy
  2. Idiosyncrasy
  3. Tolerance
  4. Drug dependence
- Iatrogenic responses include:
  1. Blood dyscrasias
  2. Hepatic toxicity
  3. Renal damage
  4. Teratogenic effects
  5. Dermatologic effects

Drug Interactions

- Modification of an expected drug response due to exposure to another drug or substance at approximately the same time—may be pharmacokinetic or pharmacodynamic
- Pharmacokinetic—inhibition of absorption, enzyme inhibition, or induction increasing risk for drug toxicity or resulting in reduced drug effect, altered renal elimination
- Pharmacodynamic—additive if two drugs have similar pharmacodynamic effects, antagonistic if have opposing pharmacodynamics effects
- Drug–food interactions may decrease bioavailability by interfering with absorption or increase bioavailability via inhibition of enzymatic activity in intestinal wall
- Drug-herb interactions may decrease or increase bioavailability of drug

Drug Contraindications

- Allergies, medical conditions, concurrent use of another drug, age, pregnancy, lactation may be drug contraindications
- Food and Drug Administration (FDA) Pregnancy Safety Classifications
  1. Category A—studies indicate no risk to fetus
  2. Category B—studies indicate no risk in animal fetus; information in pregnant women unavailable
  3. Category C—adverse effects reported in animal fetus; information in pregnant women is unavailable
  4. Category D—possible fetal risk in humans reported; in selected cases potential benefits may outweigh risks for use of drug
  5. Category X—fetal abnormalities reported and positive evidence of fetal risk in humans is available; these drugs should not be used in pregnancy
- FDA pregnancy and lactation prescription drug labeling is in process of revision to include risk summary, clinical considerations to support patient care decisions and counseling, and a data section with detailed information; revision will eliminate pregnancy categories A, B, C, D, and X

- Lactation and drugs
  1. Properties of drug that determine how much of drug will be in breast milk include pH, protein binding, liposolubility, and molecular weight
  2. Infant pharmacokinetics have influence—drug metabolism variables such as gastric acid production, liver function, amount of body fat, renal excretion

Pharmacotherapy (Applying Knowledge of Benefits and Risks of Drug Therapy to Individual Care)

- Effects of age
- Gender differences in drug metabolism
- Health status
- Family history—genetic factors
- Lifestyle behaviors
- Polypharmacy
- Drug regimen adherence

Client Education

- Purpose of drug, mechanism of action, effectiveness
- Benefits and risks
- Dosage and administration
- Major side-effects/adverse reactions
- Plan for follow-up

Selected Drug Review

- Metronidazole
  1. Class: nitroimidazole
  2. Indications for use include but are not limited to treatment of:
     a. Trichomonas vaginalis
     b. Bacterial vaginosis
     c. Pelvic inflammatory disease (PID) in combination with other antibiotics
     d. Pseudomembranous colitis caused by clostridium difficile
     e. Gastric or peptic ulcer associated with Helicobacter pylori
  3. Pharmacokinetics
     a. Absorption
        (1) Oral route—excellent, bioavailability at least 90%
        (2) Intravaginal route—absorbed systemically, peak serum concentrations are < 2% of levels achieved with oral doses
     b. Distribution
        (1) Widely distributed throughout body tissues and fluids
        (2) Crosses placenta and enters breast milk
     c. Metabolism—majority in liver
     d. Excretion
        (1) Majority through urine, some fecal excretion
        (2) Mean elimination half-life—8 hours

4. Pharmacodynamics
   a. Disrupts DNA and protein synthesis of susceptible organisms
   b. Amebicidal, bactericidal, anti-protozoal
   c. Selectivity for anaerobic bacteria
5. Adverse reactions
   a. More common with oral than vaginal route
   b. GI—nausea, vomiting, dry mouth, metallic taste, anorexia, abdominal cramping
   c. Headache
   d. Hypersensitivity
   e. Mild leukopenia or neutropenia—not persistent after treatment
   f. Peripheral neuropathy—high doses, prolonged use
   g. Seizures—high doses, prolonged use
6. Drug interactions
   a. Disulfiram—acute psychosis and confusion if metronidazole taken within 2 weeks of taking disulfiram
   b. Alcohol (including medications with significant alcohol content)—may cause nausea/vomiting, headache, flushing, abdominal cramps
   c. Warfarin—metronidazole can potentiate action
   d. Cimetidine—can decrease hepatic metabolism of metronidazole and increase serum levels
   e. Phenobarbital/phenytoin—can increase hepatic metabolism of metronidazole, clinical significance uncertain
7. Contraindications/precautions
   a. Hypersensitivity
   b. History of drug-induced hematological dyscrasias
   c. Hematological disease
   d. Severe hepatic disease/impairment
   e. Renal impairment/renal failure
   f. Pre-existing seizure disorder
8. Use in pregnancy and lactation—Category B in pregnancy, interrupt nursing for 12-24 hours after drug dose to allow excretion of drug
9. Client education
   a. Take with food to decrease GI irritation
   b. Avoid alcohol/alcohol-containing substances during and for 48 hours after last dose
   c. Chew gum or suck on ice/hard candy to help reduce dry mouth and metallic taste
   d. May cause darkening of urine
   e. Report any central nervous system symptoms
   f. If taking for trichomoniasis, refrain from sex until self and partner treatment is complete
- Fluconazole
  1. Class: triazole
  2. Indications for use include but are not limited to treatment of:
     a. Candidiasis—oropharyngeal, esophageal, vulvovaginal
     b. Fungal meningitis—cryptococcosis, candida species, histoplasmosis
  3. Pharmacokinetics
     a. Absorption—rapidly absorbed in GI tract, bioavailability over 90%
     b. Distribution
        (1) Widely distributed into body tissues and fluids

    (2) Vaginal secretion, saliva, and sputum concentrations about 10 times that of plasma concentrations

    (3) Distribution in breast milk and across placenta unknown

  c. Metabolism—liver via interaction with CYP 450 enzyme system, no first pass metabolism

  d. Excretion

    (1) Majority through urine (60–80%) as unchanged drug

    (2) Mean elimination half-life—30 hours

4. Pharmacodynamics

  a. Highly selective inhibitor of fungal CY450 enzyme

  b. Alters fungal cell membrane function and cell wall synthesis

  c. Broad spectrum of antifungal activity

  d. Emerging resistance of non-candida albican species

5. Adverse reactions

  a. Headache

  b. GI effects—nausea, abdominal pain

6. Drug interactions

  a. Cisapride (Propulsid)—prolonged QT interval

  b. Cyclosporin—nephrotoxicity

  c. Carbamazepine (Tegretol)—increased carbamazepine levels, decreased fluconazole levels

  d. Phenytoin (Dilantin)—nystagmus, ataxia

  e. Sulfanylureas—hypoglycemic reactions

  f. Theophylline—increased theophylline levels

  g. Warfarin—increased warfarin levels

7. Contraindications/precautions

  a. History of heart arrhythmia

  b. Hepatic disease

  c. Renal impairment/renal failure

  d. Hypersensitivity

  e. Multiple drug interactions

8. Use in pregnancy and lactation

  a. Category C in pregnancy

  b. Available human data do not suggest increased risk of congenital anomalies following a single maternal dose of 150 mg

  c. Recommended treatment for vulvovaginal candidiasis in pregnancy is topical azole for 7 days

  d. Distributed in breast milk at concentrations similar to those in plasma

  e. Considered compatible with breast feeding

9. Client education

  a. Symptoms should start to go away about 24 hours after taking medication

  b. It may take several days for symptoms to go away completely

  c. Notify provider of all medications as several drug interactions are possible

  d. Avoid overuse/unnecessary use of antibiotics

- Acyclovir

1. Class: nucleoside analogue

2. Indications for use include treatment of:

  a. Herpes simplex

  b. Herpes genitalia

  c. Herpes zoster

  d. Varicella

3. Pharmacokinetics (oral)

  a. Absorption—poorly absorbed, 15–20% bioavailability, however therapeutic levels are achieved

  b. Distribution—widely distributed, crosses placenta and enters breast milk

  c. Metabolism—mostly in liver

  d. Excretion

    (1) 90% in urine as unchanged drug

    (2) Mean elimination half-life—3-4 hours

4. Pharmacodynamics

  a. Selectively activated in infected cells

  b. Inhibits viral DNA synthesis

  c. Only effective against rapidly replicating herpes virus

  d. Does not eliminate latent herpes virus

5. Adverse reactions

  a. GI effects—nausea/vomiting, diarrhea

  b. Headache

  c. Skin rash

  d. Acute renal failure—rare with oral route

6. Drug interactions—increased risk for renal toxicity with nephrotoxic drugs

7. Contraindications/precautions—renal or hepatic function impairment

8. Use in pregnancy and lactation

  a. Category B in pregnancy

  b. May use to treat first episode of genital herpes or severe recurrent herpes

  c. May consider treatment in late pregnancy to reduce frequency of recurrences at term

  d. Lactation—use if indicated, some excretion in breast milk

9. Client education

  a. Take with full glass of water

  b. Space doses evenly

  c. Start at first sign of recurrent episode

  d. Additional education for suppressive regimens

10. Other nucleoside analogues—same indications, mechanism of action, adverse reactions, contraindications/precautions

  a. Famcyclovir—converted to active form via first-pass metabolism, better bioavailability

  b. Valacycolvir—prodrug converted to acyclovir, better bioavailability, less frequent dosing

---

Questions

Select the best answer.

1. Which of the following pharmacokinetic changes could decrease the effect of a medication?

  a. Decrease in plasma protein binding

  b. Increase in hepatic first pass effect

  c. Increase in enterohepatic recirculation

  d. Increase in bioavailability

2. The drug category in which adverse effects have been reported in an animal fetus and information in pregnant women is unavailable is:
   a. Category B
   b. Category C
   c. Category D
   d. Category X
3. Plasma protein binding most significantly affects drug:
   a. Absorption
   b. Distribution
   c. Metabolism
   d. Excretion
4. The half-life of a drug is used to:
   a. Calculate the loading dose needed to immediately achieve the desired steady state
   b. Determine the time required to reach steady state and dosage interval
   c. Estimate the therapeutic index
   d. Predict the likelihood of an adverse reaction
5. Acyclovir is not effective in eliminating latent herpes virus because it:
   a. Has a short elimination half-life of 3–4 hours
   b. Has only a 15–20% bioavailability
   c. Is a prodrug that is converted to active form by first-pass metabolism
   d. Is only effective against rapidly replicating herpes virus
6. A patient taking metronidazole and cimetidine at the same time is at increased risk for:
   a. Bothersome side effects from the metronidazole
   b. Decreased effectiveness of cimetidine

   c. Renal impairment
   d. Severe disulfiram type reaction
7. The term used to describe a drug that initiates a physiologic response when it is bound to a drug receptor is:
   a. Agonist
   b. Antagonist
   c. Metabolite
   d. Prodrug
8. The term used to describe the propensity of a drug to bind with a specific receptor is:
   a. Affinity
   b. Bioavailability
   c. Efficacy
   d. Potency
9. Fluconazole is effective in a one-time dose because it:
   a. Is rapidly absorbed in the GI tract
   b. Has a bioavailability over 90%
   c. Is widely distributed into body tissues and fluids
   d. Has a mean elimination half-life of 30 hours
10. Which of the following statements in regard to pharmacokinetic changes during pregnancy is correct?
    a. First-pass metabolism of drugs is increased during pregnancy because of increased blood flow through the liver
    b. Drug elimination may be faster because of an increase in glomerular filtration rate
    c. Higher levels of drug protein binding may occur with decreased albumin levels
    d. Drug absorption may be decreased because of increased plasma volume

Answers with Rationales

1. b. Increase in hepatic first-pass effect
   Orally administered drugs go from the gastrointestinal tract through the portal system to the liver before going to the general circulation. Some metabolism (chemical inactivation) of drug may occur as it taken up by hepatic microsomal enzymes
2. b. Category C
   The FDA pregnancy safety classification of Category C for a drug indicates that adverse effects have been reported in animal fetus and information in pregnant women is unavailable.
3. b. Distribution
   Drugs may attach to proteins (mainly albumin) in the blood (plasma protein binding). Only unbound drug is active and able to move out of the blood into body fluids and body tissues (distribution).
4. b. Determine the time required to reach steady state and dosage interval
   Half-life of a drug is the time it takes for plasma concentration of a drug to be reduced by 50%. It can be used to determine the time required to reach steady state and dosage interval.
5. d. Is only effective against rapidly replicating herpes virus
   Acyclovir is selectively activated in infected cells and works by inhibiting viral DNA synthesis. Because it is only effective

against rapidly replicating herpes virus it is not effective in eliminating latent herpes virus.
6. a. Bothersome side effects from the metronidazole
   Cimetidine can decrease hepatic metabolism of metronidazole and increase serum levels.
7. a. Agonist
   One mechanism of drug effect is through drug-receptor interaction. A receptor can be a cellular protein, enzyme, or membrane that when bound to a drug initiates a physiologic response or blocks a response that the receptor normally stimulates. The term agonist refers to a drug that when combined with the receptor stimulates a physiologic response. The term antagonist refers to a drug that when combined with the receptor blocks the response.
8. a. Affinity
   Affinity is the propensity of a drug to bind itself to a given receptor site. Efficacy is the ability of the drug to initiate biologic activity as a result of such binding.
9. d. Has a mean elimination half-life of 30 hours
   Half-life is the time it takes for plasma concentration to be reduced by 50% and is used to determine both time required to reach a steady state and dosage interval. Based on a half-life of

30 hours the recommended dose of fluconozole for uncomplicated vulvovaginal candidiasis is 150 mg oral tablet in a single dose.

10. b. Drug elimination may be faster because of an increase in glomerular filtration rate

Glomerular filtration rate (GFR) begins increasing early in pregnancy, peaks at 9 to 16 weeks, and plateaus at a rate about 50% above that of pre-pregnancy at 34 to 36 weeks. Increased GFR can result in faster elimination of some drugs resulting in a lower serum concentration during pregnancy.

Bibliography

Corbett, R., & Owens, L. (2011). Introductory pharmacology for clinical practice. *Journal of Midwifery and Women's Health*, 56 (3), 190–197.

King, T., & Brucker, M. (2011). *Pharmacology for women's health.* Sudbury, MA: Jones & Bartlett Learning.

U.S. Food and Drug Administration. (2009). Summary of proposed rule on pregnancy and lactation labeling. Retrieved from http://www.fda.gov/drugs/developmentapprovalprocess/developmentresources/labeling/ucm093310.htm

Wynne, A., & Woo, T. (2011). *Pharmacotherapeutics for nurse practitioner prescribers* (3rd ed.). Philadelphia, PA: F. A. Davis.

4

Normal Gynecology and Well-Woman Care

Beth M. Kelsey

© Kheng Guan Toh/ShutterStock, Inc.

Reproductive Anatomy and Physiology

- Reproductive organs
  1. Breast—a modified sweat/mammary gland responsible for lactation; located within the superficial fascia of the anterior chest wall over the pectoral muscles; extends from clavicle and second rib down to sixth rib and from sternum across the midaxillary line; supported by fibrous tissue (Cooper's ligaments); a triangle of breast tissue (tail of Spence) extends laterally across the anterior axillary fold
     a. Body—composed of lobes, lobules, and alveoli
        (1) Lobes—sections of breast composed of glandular tissue and surrounded by fatty and connective tissue radiating around the nipple; 15 to 20 each breast
        (2) Lobules—small glands within each lobe containing tiny, hollow sacs called alveoli responsible for milk production
        (3) Each lobe empties into a single lactiferous duct that opens out through the nipple; lactiferous ducts enlarge behind the nipple to form small reservoirs called lactiferous sinuses
        (4) Unique proliferation occurs under influence of estrogen during puberty
     b. Nipple—composed of pigmented erectile tissue, areola, and Montgomery's glands; terminus into which lactiferous sinuses secrete milk
        (1) Areola—circular pigmented area that surrounds the nipple
        (2) Montgomery's glands—sebaceous glands that circle the nipple located within the areola
     c. Lymphatics—most drain toward the axilla
        (1) Central nodes along chest wall, high in axilla between anterior and posterior axillary folds; most likely to be palpable; pectoral, subscapular, lateral nodes drain into central nodes
        (2) Central nodes drain into infraclavicular and supraclavicular nodes; internal mammary chain also drains into infraclavicular nodes
  2. External genitalia—composed of the vulva and its associated structures
     a. Vulva—visible external structures bordered by symphysis pubis anteriorly, buttocks posteriorly, and thighs laterally; develops as a secondary sex characteristic under the influence of estrogen during puberty
        (1) Mons pubis—fatty tissue prominence overlying symphysis pubis, covered by coarse hair in an inverted triangular pattern
        (2) Labia majora—two longitudinal folds of adipose tissue extending from the mons pubis downward enclosing four structures:
           (a) Labia minora—thin folds inside/parallel to the labia majora; forms prepuce anteriorly, encloses the vestibule, and terminates in the fourchette above the perineum
           (b) Clitoris—small erectile body of tissue; abundant supply of sensory nerve endings; rich vascular supply; important for female sexual response
           (c) Vestibule—contains urethral/vaginal openings, hymen, Skene's glands on each side of the urethral meatus, Bartholin's glands with openings located posteriorly on each side of vaginal orifice
           (d) Perineum—located between the fourchette anteriorly and the anus posteriorly
     b. Pelvic musculature—consists of perineal muscles and pelvic floor muscles
        (1) Perineal muscles
           (a) Bulbocavernosus—surrounds vagina acting as weak sphincter
           (b) Ischiovernosus—surrounds clitoris; responsible for clitoral erection
           (c) Superficial/deep transverse perineal muscles—converge with urethral sphincter
           (d) External anal sphincter

(2) Pelvic floor muscles

    (a) Levator ani—pubococcygeus, iliococcygeus, and ischiococcygeus muscles

    (b) Pubococcygeus—pubovaginalis, puborectalis, and pubococcygeus proper

3. Internal pelvic structures—develop primarily as a result of stimulation by estrogen initiated during puberty; structures reach their adult size/appearance by approximately age 16

  a. Vagina—muscular/membranous canal that connects the external genitalia to the uterus

    (1) Length—approximately 7 cm anterior, 10 cm posterior

    (2) Stratified squamous epithelium

    (3) Rugae—transverse folds in sidewalls; allows for distention during coitus and childbirth

    (4) pH—acidic because of prevalence of lactobacilli; due to influence of estrogen initiated during puberty

  b. Uterus—pear-shaped organ that is composed of the following:

    (1) Cervix—round, firm terminus to the uterus that protrudes into the vagina; approximately 2.5 cm in length

      (a) Os—opening in cervix that provides access to the uterine cavity; external os is proximal to the vagina, internal os is proximal to the uterine cavity

      (b) Squamocolumnar junction—juncture of the squamous epithelium covering the cervical body (portio) and the columnar epithelium lining the endocervix

      (c) Transformation zone—area around the squamocolumnar junction where squamous metaplasia occurs

      (d) Squamous metaplasia—process whereby columnar cells of the endocervix are replaced by mature squamous epithelium

    (2) Uterine body—extends upward from cervix and lies in the pelvic cavity; contains cavity or potential space that can accommodate pregnancy

      (a) Located between bladder and rectum

      (b) Approximately 8 cm in length, 5 cm in width, 2.5 cm in thickness

      (c) Composed externally of thick myometrial muscles (myometrium)

      (d) Composed internally of columnar epithelium (endometrium); shed during menstruation

      (e) Fundus—top portion where fallopian tubes insert

      (f) Isthmus (lower uterine segment)—immediately superior to cervix

      (g) Corpus—main body

  c. Fallopian tubes—ciliated oviducts that transport ova from the ovaries to the uterus

    (1) Length—approximately 10 cm

    (2) Interstitial portion—within uterus

    (3) Isthmus—main body

    (4) Ampulla—adjacent to the ovary; receives ova at ovulation

    (5) Fimbriated ends/infundibulum

  d. Ovaries—pair of endocrine organs located at the end of fallopian tubes

    (1) Responsible for secretion of steroid hormones—estrogen/progesterone

    (2) Approximately 3 cm × 2 cm × 1 cm

    (3) Cyclic release of ovum

  e. Lymphatics—lymph from vulva and lower vagina drains into inguinal nodes; lymph from internal genitalia and upper vagina drains into pelvic and abdominal nodes

• Puberty/adolescence—*adolescence* defined means "to grow up"; *puberty* denotes the biology of adolescence, beginning around age 9 years and culminating in development of regular menstrual cycles; some variations with ethnicity, race, and nutritional status

1. Hormonal changes—begin as hypothalamic-pituitary-ovarian axis matures

  a. Gonadotropin-releasing hormone (GnRH)—released from hypothalamus

  b. Gonadotropins—follicle-stimulating hormone (FSH) and luteinizing hormone (LH) released from anterior pituitary gland in response to GnRH

  c. Estrogen—primarily released by ovary in response to FSH; results in development of secondary sex characteristics and ultimately in menstruation

2. Physical changes—physical characteristics of breast/pubic hair development/distribution delineate progressive advancement of physiologic maturity

  a. Growth spurt—girls may grow from 6 to 11 cm taller; greatest height velocity (peak of growth spurt) occurs around age 12 or just prior to onset of menses

  b. Thelarche—breast development; begins with breast budding around age 9, progresses to conical shape followed by fully developed breast with round contour around age 17

  c. Adrenarche—growth of pubic and axillary hair; results from secretion of adrenal androgens; usually starts after breast development begins

  d. Menstruation—results from shedding of estrogen-primed endometrium; average age is 12.5 years following peak height velocity

  e. Tanner stages—used to assess progressive sexual maturity changes that occur in breast development and pubic hair growth

• Reproductive years

1. Effect of hormones

  a. Estrogen—steroid hormone responsible for development of secondary sex characteristics; produced by ovarian follicles, adrenal cortex, corpus luteum; predominant in follicular phase of menstrual cycle

    (1) Estradiol—most potent; derived from ovarian follicles, particularly dominant follicle; primary estrogen of reproductive age

    (2) Estrone—estrogen of menopause; converted from androstenedione produced by adrenal gland and ovarian stroma

    (3) Estriol—least potent; estrogen of pregnancy; derived from conversion of estrone and estradiol in liver, uterus, placenta, and fetal adrenal gland

    (4) Breasts develop fully to round adult contour—development/growth of ductal system, lobular, alveolar growth

(5) External genitalia—some further increase in size of labia majora, clitoris, completed in middle to late 20s

(6) Internal pelvic structures

(a) Vagina lengthens to approximately 10 cm; pH less than 4.5; rugae appear

(b) Uterus—proliferative endometrium; thin, clear cervical mucus

(c) Ovaries—follicular development; approximately 3 cm long, 2 cm wide, and 1 cm thick

b. Progesterone—steroid hormone produced by ovarian corpus luteum and conversion of adrenal pregnenolone/pregnenolone sulfate; predominant in luteal phase of menstrual cycle

(1) Uterus—secretory endometrium; thickens cervical mucus

(2) Ovary—supplied by corpus luteum; level of 3 ng/mL or greater indicates ovulation

(3) Breast—subcutaneous fluid retention

c. Prostaglandins—group of lipid compounds derived from fatty acids at a number of different sites in body via enzymatic action (prostaglandin synthesase enzymes) acting at target sites near area of secretion; regulate contraction and relaxation of smooth muscle

(1) Produced by endometrium; peak levels in late secretory phase

(2) Stimulates uterine myometrial contractions

d. Gonadotropin-releasing hormone—released from hypothalamus

(1) Stimulates anterior pituitary gland to release FSH/LH

(2) Pulsatile release

e. Follicle-stimulating hormone—gonadotropin; released by anterior pituitary gland in response to GnRH from hypothalamus

(1) Ovary—stimulates follicular growth

(2) Positive/negative feedback from ovarian hormones determines level

f. Luteinizing hormone—gonadotropin, released by anterior pituitary gland in response to GnRH from hypothalamus

(1) "Surge" responsible for physical act of ovulation

(2) Induces steroidogenesis and increases synthesis of androgens by the internal cells of ovary

(3) Promotes follicular atresia in nondominant follicles

(4) Promotes final growth of Graafian follicle

(5) Promotes luteinization of granulosa cells

g. Peptide hormones—produced by ovaries and pituitary gland

(1) Activin, inhibin, follistatin

(2) Contribute to regulation of FSH and menstrual cycle

h. Prolactin—anterior pituitary gland hormone

(1) Progressive release during pregnancy

(2) Stimulates synthesis of milk proteins in mammary tissue

(3) Stimulates epithelial growth in breast during pregnancy

i. Androgens

(1) Androgens are common precursors of estrogens

(2) Dehydroepiandrosterone (DHA) is produced in the adrenal gland, ovarian stroma, and peripheral tissues

(3) DHA is converted to testosterone in peripheral tissues

(4) Androstenedione is produced in the adrenal gland and ovarian stroma

(5) Androstenedione is converted to testosterone and estrone in peripheral tissues

(6) Testosterone is produced in the adrenal gland, ovarian stroma, and through conversion of androstenedione and DHA in peripheral tissues

(7) Testosterone is aromatized to estradiol in peripheral tissues

2. Menstrual cycle—timed from day 1 of one menstrual bleed to day 1 of next menstrual bleed; average 28 days plus or minus 2 days; duration 4 to 6 days plus or minus 2 days; volume average 40 cc

a. Ovarian cycle—defined by ovarian changes

(1) Follicular phase

(a) Begins day 1 menses

(b) Variable length (time frame)

(c) Increased FSH/LH

(d) Increased E_2 from dominant follicle

(e) Decreased FSH

(f) LH surge (peak 10 to 12 hours before ovulation)

(g) Thin cervical mucus

(2) Ovulation

(a) Prostaglandins and proteolytic enzymes break down the follicular wall

(b) Follicle ruptures releasing oocyte

(c) Occurs 32–44 hours after LH surge begins

(d) Maximal production of thin, stretchy, cervical mucus (spinnbarkeit)—refers to ability of cervical mucus to be "stretched" between two fingers; increased stretch equals increased influence of estrogen

(e) Peak sexual desire

(f) Increase in basal body temperature (BBT) of 0.2°F to 0.5°F

(3) Luteal phase

(a) Begins after ovulation occurs

(b) Approximately 14 days plus or minus 2 days in length

(c) Corpus luteum (CL) formed from ruptured follicle; secretes progesterone—peak 7 to 8 days postovulation

(d) Thickened cervical mucus

(e) Maintained increase in BBT

(f) If no pregnancy, CL regresses and progesterone decreases

(g) Ends with onset menses

b. Uterine cycle—defined by endometrial changes

(1) Proliferative phase—estrogen influence

(a) Endometrium grows/thickens

(b) Lasts approximately 10 days from end of menses to ovulation

(2) Secretory phase—progesterone influence

(a) Average 12 to 16 days

(b) From ovulation to menses

(c) Endometrial hypertrophy

(d) Increased vascularity

(e) Favorable for implantation of fertilized ovum

(3) Menstruation—declining progesterone from CL
  (a) Endometrium undergoes involution, necrosis, sloughing
  (b) Average 3 to 6 days

- Menopause
  1. Definitions
     a. Menopause—permanent cessation of ovulation and menses; average age in United States is 51 years; genetically predetermined; confirmed after 12 consecutive months without a period
     b. Menopause transition—span of time when menstrual cycle and endocrine changes begin to occur and ending with the final menstrual period
     c. Perimenopause—extends from beginning of menopause transition until 12 months after final menstrual period
     d. Postmenopause—refers to the years following menopause
     e. Premature menopause (primary ovarian insufficiency)—cessation of ovulation and menses before age 40; spontaneous or induced
  2. Physiology
     a. As menopause transition begins, the rhythmic ovarian and endometrial responses of the menstrual cycle decline and eventually stop
     b. Number of responsive follicles decreases with resultant decreased production of estradiol throughout menopause transition
     c. With decreasing estradiol, FSH levels increase
     d. At the end of the menopause transition, ovary contains no follicles and endometrium atrophies so that reproductive capability is terminated
     e. After menopause, estrone becomes principal estrogen
     f. Estrone produced through aromatization of androstenedione; androstenedione is an androgen produced by adrenal cortex and ovarian stroma; converted to estrone in peripheral fat cells
     g. After menopause, both FSH and LH levels are elevated
     h. Generally rely on cessation of menses, hypoestrogenic symptoms, and age for diagnosis of menopause
  3. Laboratory findings
     a. FSH—greater than 40 mIU/mL
     b. LH—threefold elevation after menopause (20–100 mIU/mL)
     c. Estradiol—less than 20 pg/mL
  4. Possible menstrual changes during menopause transition
     a. No change
     b. Cycles shorter or longer than usual
     c. Bleeding lighter/shorter or heavier/longer than usual
  5. Physical changes
     a. Reproductive organs
        (1) Labia—decrease in subcutaneous fat and tissue elasticity
        (2) Vagina
           (a) Thinning of epithelium; decreased rugae, decreased vascularization and elasticity, increase in pH of greater than or equal to 5.0

(b) May have pruritus, leukorrhea, friability, increased susceptibility to infection
(c) May have dyspareunia
(d) May have changes in orgasm experience (increased time to reach, shorter duration, decreased strength of contractions) with diminished genital sensation, less vaginal expansion, and decreased vasocongestion
        (3) Cervix—decrease in size, os may become flush with vaginal walls, may become stenotic
        (4) Uterus and ovaries—decrease in size and weight; ovaries usually not palpable
     b. Urinary tract
        (1) Decreased muscle tone—urethra and trigone area of bladder
        (2) Atrophic changes in urethra and periurethral tissue—urinary urgency, frequency, and dysuria may occur
        (3) Cross-sectional epidemiological studies report increase in prevalence of urinary incontinence in women ages 45–55
        (4) Longitudinal studies show that the development or worsening of urinary incontinence is not associated with menopause
     c. Breasts—reduction in size and flattened appearance; decrease in glandular tissue
     d. Skin
        (1) Thinning/decreased activity of sebaceous and sweat glands
        (2) Hyperpigmentation/hypopigmentation
        (3) Scalp, pubic, and axillary hair becomes thinner and drier
     e. Bone integrity—increased bone loss associated with decrease in estrogen
  6. Vasomotor symptoms—hot flashes
     a. Observed in 75% of women during perimenopause and postmenopause
     b. Mechanism responsible not known; gonadotropin-related effect on the central thermoregulatory function of the hypothalamus (measurable increase in core body temperature, increase in body surface temperature, peripheral vasodilation, then decrease in core temperature)
     c. Sudden feeling of warmth to intense heat followed by visible redness of upper body and face
     d. May be associated with profuse sweating and palpitations
     e. May awaken during the night, leading to insomnia, sleep disturbance, cognitive (memory) and affective (anxiety) disorders with loss of REM sleep
     f. Range of duration 6 months to 10 years; average duration 3 to 5 years; highest occurrence first 2 years postmenopause
  7. Cardiovascular system effects
     a. Lipid levels—increase in low-density lipoproteins (LDL-C), very low density lipoproteins (VLDL-C), and triglycerides, possible decrease in high-density lipoproteins (HDL-C)
     b. Regulation of clotting processes—increase in certain fibrinolytic and procoagulation factors
     c. Vasoactive substances—increase in endothelin and decrease in angiotensin-converting enzyme (vasoconstrictors),

increase in nitric oxide and decrease in prostacyclin (vasodilators)

    d. Extent of impact of decreased estrogen levels on cardiovascular disease not definitively established

8. Alterations in mood

    a. Majority of women do not have psychological problems attributable to menopause

    b. Depression in menopause often related to history of previous depression or premenstrual syndrome

    c. Depression/irritability may be related to sleep disturbances caused by hot flashes

    d. Perceived health shown to be a major factor related to depression in perimenopausal women; individual characteristics and self-perception appear to be important determinants of each woman's experience of the perimenopause

    e. More research is needed to establish hormonal influences on mood changes that occur during the perimenopause

9. Cognitive function

    a. Memory impairment may be indirectly related to decreased estrogen secondary to hot flashes and sleep disturbance

    b. No evidence that memory or cognitive skills decline directly as a result of normal menopause transition

    c. Women's Health Initiative Memory Study (WHIMS)—risk of dementia increased in healthy women aged 65 to 79 years using estrogen or estrogen with progesterone therapy

    d. Unclear how estrogen or estrogen with progesterone therapy affects cognitive function in younger menopausal women

Well-Woman Visit

- Includes health history, physical examination, screening tests, counseling, and immunizations based on age, risk factors, and individual's concerns
- General health history and physical examination
- General nutrition and physical activity counseling, screening tests, and immunization recommendations
- Adolescent (13–20 years of age)—focus on reproductive/sexual health

  1. Health history

    a. Menstrual, gynecologic, and obstetric history

    b. Psychosocial assessment—family and peer relationships; emotional, physical, or sexual abuse by family or partner; drug/alcohol use

    c. Sexuality/sexual history—sexual orientation, gender identity, sexual practices, sexual satisfaction, dyspareunia, use of contraception, use of condoms; exchange of sex for drugs or money

  2. Physical examination

    a. Pelvic and breast examination not routinely recommended

    b. Perform if indicated by health history/risk factors

    c. May consider external-only genital examination

  3. Screening tests

    a. Chlamydia test if sexually active (urine or self-collected vaginal specimen)

    b. Human immunodeficiency virus (HIV) screening test if sexually active

    c. Other as indicated by history/risk factors

  4. Counseling/education

    a. Expected body changes during puberty

    b. Reproductive life planning—plan for having children, timing, use of contraception, preconception care

    c. Safer sex practices—abstinence, condom use, limiting partners, sexually transmitted infection (STI) screening; acquaintance rape prevention; Internet/phone safety

    d. Other as indicated by health history/physical examination/risk factors

  5. Immunizations—human papillomavirus (HPV) vaccination series for cervical cancer prevention

- Ages 21–39 years—focus on reproductive/sexual health

  1. Health history

    a. Menstrual, gynecologic, and obstetric history

    b. Psychosocial assessment—emotional, physical, or sexual abuse by family or partner current or past; drug/alcohol use

    c. Sexuality/sexual history—sexual orientation, gender identity, sexual practices, sexual satisfaction, dyspareunia, use of contraception, use of condoms; exchange of sex for drugs or money

  2. Physical examination

    a. Clinical breast examination—every 1 to 3 years

    b. Pelvic examination—periodic, if need Pap test or otherwise indicated

    c. Other as indicated by health history/risk factors

  3. Screening tests

    a. Chlamydia test if sexually active (age 25 or younger) or if older and has risk factors

    b. HIV screening if sexually active

    c. Pap test

      (1) Age 21–29 years—cytology alone every 3 years

      (2) Age 30–65 years—cytology with HPV test every 5 years or cytology alone every 3 years

    d. Other as indicated by health history/risk factors

  4. Counseling/education

    a. Reproductive life planning—plan for having children, timing, use of contraception, preconception care

    b. Safer sex practices—abstinence, condom use, limiting partners, STI screening

    c. Breast health—breast self-awareness (may include breast self-examination if woman chooses)

    d. Purpose of Pap tests and how often to schedule

    e. Other as indicated by health history/physical examination/risk factors

  5. Immunizations—HPV vaccination series for cervical cancer prevention if not done earlier and 26 years of age or younger

- Age 40 years of age or older—focus on reproductive/sexual health

  1. Health history

    a. Menstrual, gynecologic, and obstetric history; menopausal symptoms; pelvic prolapse; urinary or fecal incontinence

    b. Psychosocial assessment—emotional, physical, or sexual abuse by family or partner current or past; drug/alcohol use

    c. Sexuality/sexual history—sexual orientation, gender identity, sexual practices, sexual satisfaction, dyspareunia, use of contraception, use of condoms; exchange of sex for drugs or money

2. Physical examination
   a. Clinical breast examination—yearly
   b. Pelvic examination—if need Pap test or otherwise indicated
   c. Other as indicated by health history/risk factors
3. Screening tests
   a. Pap test—cytology with HPV test every 5 years or cytology alone every 3 years; discontinue after age 65 unless risk factors indicated by previous Pap test results
   b. Mammogram—yearly, no definitive age to discontinue, based on woman's health and if would be candidate for treatment of breast cancer
   c. HIV screening if sexually active
   d. Other as indicated by health history/risk factors
4. Counseling/education
   a. Safer sex practices—abstinence, condom use, limiting partners, sexually transmitted infections (STI) screening
   b. Breast health—breast self-awareness (may include breast self-examination if woman chooses); purpose of screening mammograms
   c. Purpose of Pap tests, how often to schedule, when can discontinue
   d. Expected physical and hormonal changes during perimenopause
   e. Management of menopausal symptoms—see section titled "Menopause" earlier in this chapter; "Perimenopause and Menopause Symptom Management" later in this chapter
   f. Other as indicated by health history/physical examination/ risk factors

Breast Health

- Clinical breast examination
- Breast self-examination (BSE)
  1. Studies indicate breast self-examination alone does not reduce number of cancer deaths; it should not be used in place of clinical breast examination and mammography (National Cancer Institute, 2014)
  2. American Cancer Society (ACS, 2013)—beginning in their 20s, inform of benefits and limitations of BSE and provide instruction for women who choose to do BSE; it is acceptable for women to choose not to do BSE or to do BSE irregularly
  3. American College of Obstetricians and Gynecologists (ACOG, 2011)—educate women age 20 and older about breast self-awareness; woman may or may not choose to do BSE
  4. BSE technique
     a. Inspection—in front of mirror
        (1) Hands pressed on hips
        (2) Observe for symmetry, dimpling, contour, skin changes
     b. Palpation
        (1) In upright position with arm slightly raised, palpate the underarm area on each side
        (2) Reclining with pillow under shoulder; arm raised
        (3) Pads of three middle fingers used, overlapping dime-sized circular motions at three levels of pressure over entire area of both breasts

(4) Use vertical up and down pattern across entire chest wall; clavicle to inframammary fold, sternum to posterior axillary line

- Screening mammography
  1. ACS and ACOG—yearly beginning at age 40 years
  2. ACS and ACOG—no definitive age to discontinue mammogram screening; base on woman's health and if would be candidate for treatment of breast cancer
  3. Ten percent to 15% false-negative rate for detection of malignancies
- *BRCA1/BRCA2* breast cancer gene testing
  1. 5% to 10% of breast cancer is hereditary—result from gene mutation inherited from a parent
  2. *BRCA1* and *BRCA2* mutations are the most common
  3. Lifetime risk of breast cancer if have *BRCA1* mutation on average is 55% to 65% but may be as high as 80%; risk with *BRCA2* mutation is around 45%; lifetime risk without mutation is 12%
  4. Discuss pros and cons of *BRCA1/BRCA2* mutation testing with women who have strong family history of breast cancer/ovarian cancer, family history of breast cancer at younger age, male relative with breast cancer
  5. ACOG—combination of yearly mammogram and MRI in women with *BRCA* gene mutation beginning at age 25 or younger based on earliest age of diagnosis of breast cancer in family
  6. Prophylactic bilateral mastectomy and/or chemoprevention may be considered to reduce cancer risks

Sexuality

- Sexual orientation
  1. General term used to describe individuals' physical and/or romantic attractions to other people
  2. Most common labels are heterosexual (straight), homosexual (gay or lesbian), bisexual
  3. *Sexual identity* refers to one's self-label as heterosexual, homosexual, bisexual, or something else
- Gender identity
  1. Internal sense that one is female, male, or some variation of both
  2. *Transgender* refers to individuals whose internal feelings of being male or female differ from the sexual anatomy with which they were born
  3. Transgender individuals may be heterosexual, homosexual, or bisexual
- Sexual drive—biological component of desire, based on neuroendocrine mechanisms
- Sexual motivation—intrapsychic and interpersonal component, influenced by quality of relationship, emotional/psychological health, past sexual history, cultural and religious values
- Female sexual response
  1. Linear model (Masters & Johnson, 1966)—applied to both men and women; excitement (sensory stimulation leads to vasocongestion), plateau (increased vasocongestion and pelvic floor muscle tension), orgasm (widespread genitopelvic muscle contraction), resolution (return to nonstimulated state)

2. Nonlinear model (Bassoon, 2001)—focuses on women; emotional intimacy and physical satisfaction, not necessarily orgasm, may be goal; recognizes female sexual motivation is complex and not an innate physiologic phenomenon

Diagnostic Studies and Laboratory Tests

- Pap test
  1. Purpose—a screening technique
     a. Increases detection and treatment of precancerous and early cancerous lesions of the uterine cervix
     b. Early detection decreases morbidity and mortality from invasive cervical cancer
  2. Procedure
     a. Instruct patient to avoid douching, intercourse, and use of vaginal creams for 48 hours prior to Pap test screening
     b. Avoid scheduling when on menses
     c. Speculum may be lubricated with water or small amount of water-soluble lubricant prior to insertion
     d. Entire squamocolumnar junction (transformation zone) must be sampled with spatula/broom to avoid false negative related to sampling technique
     e. Endocervical sampling must be obtained with broom/cytobrush
     f. Rapid fixation with cytologic fixative is essential to avoid air-drying artifact unless specimen is transferred to aqueous solution
- Wet mounts (preparations)
  1. Purpose—to detect organisms responsible for symptoms of vulvovaginal infections through microscopic evaluation of vaginal discharge
  2. Procedure
     a. Obtain specimen from posterior and lateral vaginal walls
     b. Prepare initial slide with saline to detect clue cells, epithelial cells, red blood cells (RBCs), white blood cells (WBCs), trichomonads, yeast hyphae, and spores
     c. Second specimen can be prepared with potassium hydroxide (KOH) to facilitate visualization of yeast buds and pseudohyphae
     d. Addition of KOH may also be used to detect presence of amines (whiff test)
- Human papillomavirus (HPV) tests
  1. Purpose
     a. Triage of atypical squamous cells of undetermined significance (ASC-US) Pap test results to determine follow-up; co-screening with Pap test for women 30–65 years of age
     b. Not recommended for screening of women younger than 21 years of age or for co-screening in women 21–29 years of age
  2. Procedure
     a. DNA-based tests are most commonly used
     b. Some RNA-based tests are now available
     c. Specimen collected with Pap test

- Colposcopy
  1. Purpose—to allow inspection of vagina and cervix using a binocular microscope; detects lesions/abnormalities that may be biopsied for histologic examination
  2. Procedure
     a. Position speculum and colposcope for complete visualization of cervix and vagina
     b. Swab cervix/vagina to remove secretions; wash cervix/vagina with 2% acetic acid to allow for easier identification of abnormalities
     c. Look for areas of abnormality
        (1) Aceto white areas
        (2) Abnormal vascular patterns—punctation, mosaic pattern, "corkscrew vessels"
        (3) Leukoplakia—visible before application of acetic acid
     d. Biopsy any abnormal areas
     e. Apply pressure to biopsy site(s) with large swab to stop bleeding
     f. Apply silver nitrate or Monsel's solution if bleeding continues
     g. Endocervical sampling
        (1) Indicated if not able to see the entire transformation zone or if glandular abnormalities reported on Pap test
        (2) 360-degree sample of endocervical canal with cytology brush or curette
- Endometrial sampling
  1. Purpose—evaluate abnormal bleeding (perimenopause, postmenopause); rule out/confirm endometritis
  2. Procedure
     a. If pregnancy is a possibility, time to avoid potential disruption of implantation
     b. Inform woman she may experience cramping during time biopsy instrument is in uterus
     c. Perform bimanual examination—determine uterine position and size
     d. Cleanse ectocervix and vagina
     e. Apply tenaculum to stabilize cervix/provide traction
     f. Consider paracervical block if encounter cervical stenosis or spasm
     g. Gently pass flexible, endometrial suction cannula through cervix up to fundus
     h. Withdraw stilette/aspirate with syringe while rotating the cannula, moving from fundus down and repeating several times
     i. Transfer contents of cannula/syringe into fixative
     j. Remove tenaculum and control bleeding—pressure, silver nitrate, Monsel's solution
- Vulvar biopsy
  1. Purpose—sample areas of vulva that appear abnormal for diagnostic purposes
  2. Procedure
     a. Identify vulvar lesion(s) to biopsy and inject local anesthetic
     b. Rotate punch biopsy instrument with downward pressure to obtain specimen
     c. Elevate incised specimen and remove with scissors
     d. Place specimen in histologic solution
     e. Control bleeding—pressure, silver nitrate, Monsel's solution

- Pregnancy test
  1. Purpose—to detect human chorionic gonadotropin (hCG) in blood/urine
  2. Urine hCG tests
     a. Highly sensitive urine tests provide accurate qualitative (positive/negative) results with hCG levels as low as 5 to 50 mIU/mL
     b. May detect pregnancy as early as 28 days from last menstrual period
     c. First morning urine is best as will be most concentrated
     d. Cross-reactions with other hormones not a problem with highly sensitive urine tests
  3. Serum hCG radioimmunoassay (RIA) or immunometric assay
     a. Provides level of hCG (quantitative); not any advantage for use as qualitative (positive/negative) test over highly sensitive urine tests in most situations
     b. Single level useful if concern about ectopic pregnancy—should be able to visualize intrauterine pregnancy when level is 1500–2000 mIU/mL
     c. Serial testing of serum hCG allows following rise or fall of levels—assists in diagnosis of ectopic pregnancy, evolving spontaneous abortion, possible retained products of conception, surveillance for persistent trophoblastic proliferation after uterine evacuation of hydatidiform mole
- Serum hormonal levels
  1. Purpose—to evaluate and monitor treatment of infertility; to assist in differential diagnosis of gonadal dysfunction; to assist in diagnosis of certain neoplasms
  2. Estradiol—pg/mL
     a. Follicular phase—20 to 150
     b. Midcycle—150 to 750
     c. Luteal phase—30 to 450
     d. Postmenopause—20 or less
  3. Follicle-stimulating hormone—mIU/mL
     a. Follicular phase—5 to 25
     b. Midcycle—20 to 30
     c. Luteal phase—5 to 25
     d. Postmenopause—40 to 250
  4. Luteinizing hormone—mIU/mL
     a. Follicular phase—5 to 25
     b. Midcycle—75 to 150
     c. Luteal phase—5 to 40
     d. Postmenopause—30 to 200
  5. Progesterone—ng/mL
     a. Follicular phase—less than 2
     b. Luteal phase—2 to 20
     c. Postmenopause—less than 0.2
- Pelvic ultrasound
  1. Purpose—use of high-frequency sound waves to evaluate internal organs/structure for diagnostic purposes
     a. Distinguish between solid and cystic pelvic masses
     b. Confirm viability and location of gestation/products of conception
     c. Determine endometrial thickness
     d. Evaluate size/location of uterine myomas
     e. Evaluate adnexal masses/fullness

      (1) Ectopic pregnancy
      (2) Ovarian cysts—serial evaluation
     f. Predict ovulation—infertility evaluation
     g. Evaluate fetal growth
     h. Detect fetal anomalies/abnormalities
  2. Procedure
     a. Transabdominal pelvic ultrasound—use if pelvic structures to be examined extend into abdomen; instruct patient to have full bladder, pass transducer over tissue/organs to be examined
     b. Transvaginal ultrasound—better resolution than transabdominal; instruct patient to empty bladder, use vaginal probe placed in sterile sheath (glove, condom)
- Laparoscopy
  1. Purpose—to provide direct visualization of internal reproductive organs for diagnosis and treatment of certain conditions and for female sterilization procedures
     a. Provides for inspection of internal reproductive organs
     b. Diagnostic for endometriosis
     c. Assists in diagnosis of
        (1) Pelvic pain
        (2) Infertility
        (3) Ectopic pregnancy
        (4) Ovarian cysts/neoplasia
        (5) Uterine fibroids
        (6) Pelvic adhesions
     d. Therapeutic uses
        (1) Tubal ligation
        (2) Appendectomy
        (3) Infertility procedures—harvesting ova for in vitro fertilization (IVF) or gamete intrafallopian transfer (GIFT) procedure
        (4) Lysis of adhesions
        (5) Laser/fulguration of endometrial implants
        (6) Removal of ectopic pregnancy
  2. Procedure
     a. Local, regional, or general anesthesia administered
     b. Incision into peritoneal cavity
     c. CO_2 or nitrous oxide instilled—distends abdominal cavity, allows visibility of organs
     d. Laparoscope inserted—facilitates inspection
     e. Additional incision(s) made to facilitate instrumentation if procedure performed
     f. Patient may experience abdominal/referred shoulder pain following procedure related to CO_2 instillation
     g. Major complications are not common (0.2–2%)—laceration of vessels, intestinal and urinary tract injuries, cardiorespiratory problems resulting from pneumoperitoneum
- Mammogram
  1. Purpose—radiographic examination of the breast to determine presence of small cancerous, precancerous, and benign lesions; screening and diagnostic use
     a. Digital mammography—detectors convert X-rays into electric signals, produce images that can be seen on computer screen; most centers now use digital mammography
     b. Digital mammography and conventional film mammography similar overall in ability to detect breast cancer

c. Digital mammography may offer better detection in women who are premenopausal, perimenopausal, and/or have dense breast tissue

d. Mammmographic findings standardized terminology—Breast Imaging Reporting and Data System (BI-RADS)—six assessment categories (0–5) provide overall assessment of likelihood findings represent a malignancy

2. Procedure

a. Instruct patient to avoid use of any underarm deodorant spray or powder prior to procedure

b. Typically two views taken of each breast for screening mammogram

c. Target specific area with multiple views and magnifications if suspicious lesion found on clinical breast examination or screening mammogram—diagnostic mammogram

d. Referral and/or biopsy recommended on any clinically suspicious lesion regardless of mammography results

- Breast ultrasound

1. Purpose—use of high-frequency sound waves as adjunct to mammography to assist in diagnosis of breast disease; not a screening tool

a. Helpful in differentiating cystic from solid masses

b. May be used as a guide for needle aspiration, needle core biopsy, and in localization procedures

2. Procedure—handheld, real-time, high-frequency probe passed over tissue to be examined

- Breast biopsy

1. Purpose—determine whether breast mass found on examination or through imaging contains benign or malignant cells

2. Procedure—fine-needle aspiration: obtains fluid/cells from breast mass

a. Local anesthesia not usually necessary; cleanse area

b. Secure breast mass with one hand; introduce 20- or 22-gauge needle attached to 10- to 20-mL syringe

c. Withdraw all fluid from cyst and prepare slide of specimen if fluid is not clear

d. If no fluid obtained, mass is likely solid; pass needle through mass several times with suction to obtain cellular specimen, prepare slide

e. Apply firm pressure over site for 5–10 minutes to prevent hematoma

3. Procedure—tissue biopsy: provides definitive diagnosis with histologic findings providing foundation for treatment plan

a. Wire-guided excisional biopsy—wire placed percutaneously in vicinity of abnormality by radiologist, needle may be placed over wire for better localization, surgeon uses wire to guide removal of abnormal tissue

b. Stereotactic core needle biopsy—woman placed prone on table with breast in dependent position, breast imaged to localize lesion, core biopsy needle advanced into lesion, cores of tissue obtained for evaluation

- Screening/diagnostic tests for sexually transmitted infections (STIs)

1. *Chlamydia trachomatis*

a. Nucleic acid amplification test (NAAT)—test recommended by Centers for Disease Control and Prevention (CDC)

b. NAAT provides option of testing with urine, vaginal (provider or patient obtained), or endocervical sample; some approved for liquid-based cytology specimens; few approved for rectal or oropharyngeal specimens

c. Other tests—direct fluorescent antibody (DFA), enzyme immunoassay (EIA), DNA probe, tissue culture

2. *Neisseria gonorrhoeae* (GC)

a. NAAT provides same testing ability as with *Chlamydia*

b. Culture with antimicrobial sensitivity testing should be used with suspected or documented treatment failure

3. *Treponema pallidum* (syphilis)

a. Dark field microscopy examination and direct fluorescent antibody tests of lesion exudate or tissue are definitive methods of diagnosing early syphilis

b. Serology—provides for presumptive diagnosis

(1) Nontreponemal tests

(a) Venereal Disease Research Laboratories (VDRL)

(b) Rapid plasma reagin (RPR)

(c) Become positive 1 to 2 weeks past chancre

(d) Reported as nonreactive or reactive

(e) Reactive test also reported quantitatively as titer

(f) Nonspecific

(g) False positives associated with mononucleosis, collagen vascular disease, and some other medical conditions; usually see low titer 1:8

(h) Reactive nontreponemal tests must be confirmed with a treponemal test

(i) Titers are also used for follow-up after treatment

(j) Nontreponemal tests usually become nonreactive with time after treatment

(2) Treponemal tests

(a) Fluorescent treponemal antibody absorption test (FTA-ABS)

(b) *Treponema pallidum* immobilization test (TPI)

(c) Reported as positive or negative; not quantitative

(d) Specific

(e) Treponemal tests usually remain positive indefinitely after treatment

4. Genital herpes simplex (herpes simplex virus [HSV])

a. Tissue culture or polymerase chain reaction (PCR) are the CDC-recommended tests for patients presenting with genital lesions

(1) PCR assays are more sensitive than culture

(2) Sensitivity varies with stage of infection—highest if sample vesicular lesion

b. Cytologic tests—Pap test and Tzanck preparation are insensitive and nonspecific; should not be relied on for diagnosis

c. Type-specific serologic tests—serum; detect presence of HSV-1 and HSV-2 antibodies; may take 4 to 12 weeks for seroconversion; useful if history suggestive of HSV but no current lesions, negative culture of lesions but suspect HSV infection, partner with known HSV infection, or patient with HIV infection

5. Condyloma acuminata (genital warts)

a. Generally diagnosed by inspection

b. Biopsy rarely indicated—consider if diagnosis uncertain, atypical lesion appearance, no response to therapy, worsening during therapy, compromised immunity

c. HPV testing is not recommended because test results would not change management

d. Acetic acid application is not recommended because skin color change is not specific for HPV infection

6. Chancroid—culture/DNA probe

7. Trichomoniasis

  a. Microscopic evaluation of vaginal secretions with saline wet mount

    (1) Motile, flagellated protozoa

    (2) Greater than 10 WBC/high-power field

  b. Vaginal pH greater than 4.5

  c. NAAT testing—higher sensitivity than wet mount for trichomoniasis

8. Hepatitis B (HBV)

  a. Serologic testing

  b. Hepatitis B surface antigen (HBsAg)—seen with acute active infection; chronic active infection/carrier state

  c. Hepatitis B surface antibody (HBsAb)—seen with convalescence; indicates immunity to HBV

  d. Hepatitis B core antibody (HBcAb)—indicates past infection; chronic hepatitis

  e. Hepatitis B e-antigen (HBeAg)—seen with acute infection; indicates infectivity

  f. Hepatitis B e-antibody (HBeAb)—seen with convalescence; indicates decreased infectivity

9. Human immunodeficiency virus (HIV)

  a. Sensitive screening tests—conventional enzyme immunoassay (EIA) or rapid test; detect antibodies against HIV 1 and HIV 2; detectable in at least 95% of individuals within 3 months after infection

  b. Reactive screening tests must be confirmed by supplemental immunofluorescence assay (IFA) or virologic test—HIV-1 RNA assay

  c. HIV-1 RNA assay may be used to identify acute infection when antibody tests are negative

- Bone density testing/bone densitometry

1. Purpose—diagnosis and monitoring treatment of osteopenia and osteoporosis; assessment (T-score)—bone density compared to a young normal adult

  a. Normal—bone mineral density (BMD) within 1 standard deviation (SD) of young normal adult; T-score above –1

  b. Osteopenia—BMD between 1 and 2.5 SD below that of young normal adult; T-score between –1 and –2.5

  c. Osteoporosis—BMD 2.5 SD or more below that of young normal adult; T-score at or below –2.5

2. Procedure for dual-energy X-ray absorptiometry (DEXA) scan—most-used technique, low radiation exposure

  a. Patient lies supine while imager passes over body

  b. Process takes about 10 to 15 minutes

  c. Computer calculates density of patient's bones

  d. Image/regions scanned for osteoporosis diagnosis—hip, spine, radius; use of other sites such as heel or finger may predict fracture risk but cannot be used for diagnosis

Fertility Control

- Contraceptive efficacy

1. Risk of pregnancy—unintended pregnancy in first year of use

2. Perfect use—pregnancy rate when used consistently and correctly at all times

3. Typical use—pregnancy rate during actual use, includes inconsistent and incorrect use

4. User characteristics that influence efficacy—frequency of intercourse, age, regularity of menstrual cycles

5. Typical use effectiveness comparisons

  a. Less than one pregnancy per 100 women in one year—progestin-only contraceptive implant, intrauterine contraception, male and female sterilization

  b. Between 6 and 12 pregnancies per 100 women in one year—depo medroxyprogesterone acetate (DMPA), combination hormonal contraceptives (pills, patch, vaginal ring), progestin-only contraceptive pills, diaphragm

  c. 18 or more pregnancies per 100 women in one year—male and female condom, sponge, withdrawal, spermicides, fertility awareness methods

6. Drug interactions that may decrease contraceptive efficacy

  a. Drugs that increase production of liver enzyme cytochrome P-450 may cause more rapid clearance of other drugs metabolized by this enzyme

  b. Drugs that increase cytochrome P-450—rifampin, rifapentine, some anticonvulsants, some antiretrovirals, griseofulvin, St. John's wort

  c. Contraceptives that may have decreased efficacy—all combination hormonal contraceptive methods, progestin-only contraceptive pills, progestin-only contraceptive implants

  d. Depo medroxyprogesterone acetate (DMPA) efficacy is not affected

7. Maintaining efficacy when switching methods

  a. Use quick-start method—if switching among different combination hormonal contraceptives (CHC), progestin-only methods, or intrauterine contraceptives (IUC), start the new method the same day as discontinuing the other method

    (1) Start new method the same day an IUC or progestin-only implant is removed

    (2) Continue current method until day that IUC or progestin-only implant is placed

    (3) Start new method at time progestin-only injection is due

    (4) Backup contraception is not needed if follow quick-start method when switching among these methods

  b. If not using quick start to switch methods, follow backup contraception instructions for the new method

  c. If gap of time between stopping one method, starting another method, and unprotected intercourse occurs

    (1) Offer emergency contraception

    (2) Start new method no later than next day

    (3) Use backup method for 7 days

    (4) Perform urine pregnancy test in 2 to 3 weeks to detect emergency contraception failure

- Safety of contraceptive methods
  1. Major health risks associated with contraceptive use are uncommon, risk of death extremely low
  2. Most major health risks occur in women with underlying medical conditions
  3. Thorough health assessment for potential increase in risk with selected method is key
  4. Educate women about risks and danger signs
  5. CDC Medical Eligibility Criteria for Contraceptive Use (CDC, 2010)—individual characteristics or known preexisting medical/pathologic condition affecting eligibility for use of a contraceptive method classified under one of four categories
     a. Category 1—condition for which there is no restriction on use of the method
     b. Category 2—condition where advantages of using method generally outweigh theoretical or proven risks
     c. Category 3—condition where theoretical or proven risks usually outweigh advantages of using method
     d. Category 4—condition that represents an unacceptable health risk if method is used
- Combination oral contraceptives (COC)
  1. Description—pill taken daily for contraception; combination of estrogen and progestin; also has noncontraceptive applications
     a. Monophasic pills—deliver constant amount of estrogen/progestin throughout cycle
     b. Multiphasic pills—vary amount of estrogen and/or progestin delivered throughout cycle
     c. Patterns of use—monthly cycling (21/7), shortened pill-free interval, extended cycle
  2. Mechanism of action
     a. Estrogen—inhibits ovulation through suppression of FSH, potentiates action of progestin, stabilizes endometrium for less unscheduled bleeding and spotting
        (1) Ethinyl estradiol (E_2)—most prevalent synthetic estrogen in COC
        (2) Estradiol valerate (E_2V)—newer synthetic estrogen available in one brand of COC
        (3) Mestranol—weaker estrogen; utilized in only a few older 50-mcg COC formulations
     b. Progestin—inhibits ovulation through suppression of LH surge; inhibits sperm penetration by thickening cervical mucus; progestins available vary in bioavailability, dose needed for ovulation inhibition, and half-life
        (1) One method of categorizing progestins is by historical generation of introduction in COCs available in the United States
        (2) First three generations include progestins that are derivitives of testosterone designated as 19-nortestosterones with class names of estranes and gonanes
        (3) First-generation progestins—lowest potency, short half-life, lower doses more likely to have unscheduled bleeding and spotting: norethindrone, northindrone acetate, ethynodiol diacetate
        (4) Second-generation progestins—more potent and longer half-life designed to decrease unscheduled bleeding and spotting, associated with more androgen-related side effects—norgestrel, levonorgestrel
        (5) Third-generation progestins—designed to maintain potency of second-generation but with less androgenic side effects—desogestrel, norgestimate, gestodene (not available in United States)
        (6) Fourth-generation progestins—one is analog of spironolactone, a potassium-sparing diuretic; progestogenic effect, antiandrogenic properties—drospirenone; another is a 19-nortestosterone with slightly different structure to maintain strong progestin effect and exert an antiandrogenic effect—dienogest
  3. Effectiveness/first-year failure rate
     a. Perfect use—0.3%
     b. Typical use—9%
  4. Advantages
     a. Ease of use
     b. Reversible
     c. Effective
     d. May reduce incidence of/afford protection against
        (1) Acne
        (2) Dysmenorrhea
        (3) Pelvic inflammatory disease
        (4) Endometriosis
        (5) Iron-deficiency anemia
        (6) Osteoporosis
        (7) Benign breast conditions
        (8) Functional ovarian cysts
        (9) Ovarian cancer, endometrial cancer, colorectal cancer
        (10) Menstrual migraine headaches—extended-cycle regimens
        (11) Premenstrual syndrome/premenstrual dysphoric disorder
        (12) May be used as emergency contraception
  5. Disadvantages/side effects
     a. Does not prevent transmission of STI/HIV
     b. Requires user compliance/daily dosing schedule
     c. Side effects /adverse effects may include:
        (1) Estrogenic effects
           (a) Nausea
           (b) Increased breast size/breast tenderness
           (c) Chloasma
           (d) Telangiectasia
           (e) Cervical eversion/ectopy
           (f) Increased blood pressure
           (g) Increased cholesterol concentration in gallbladder bile
           (h) Migraine headaches
           (i) Increased triglycerides
           (j) Hepatocellular adenoma
           (k) Arterial thrombosis
           (l) Venous thromboembolism
        (2) Progestogenic side effects/adverse effects
           (a) Breast tenderness
           (b) Fatigue
           (c) Depressive symptoms
           (d) Increased insulin resistance
           (e) Constipation/bloating
           (f) Precipitation of gallbladder sludge or stones

(g) Cyclic weight gain

(h) Nausea

(3) Androgenic side effects /adverse effects

    (a) Increased appetite/weight gain

    (b) Hirsutism

    (c) Acne, oily skin

    (d) Increased LDL-C

6. Contraindications (CDC categories 3 and 4)

  a. Category 4 for COC use—do not use method if following conditions exist:

    (1) Smoker 35 years of age or older, 15 or more cigarettes/day

    (2) Multiple risk factors for arterial cardiovascular disease

    (3) Hypertension (160/100 mm Hg) or hypertension with vascular disease

    (4) Acute deep vein thrombosis (DVT) or pulmonary embolism (PE)

    (5) History of DVT or PE and one or more risk factors for recurrence

    (6) Major surgery with prolonged immobilization

    (7) Known thrombogenic mutations

    (8) History of or current ischemic heart disease, stroke, complicated valvular heart disease

    (9) Migraine headaches with aura at any age; migraine headaches at 35 years of age or older with/without aura

    (10) Breast cancer within past 5 years

    (11) Diabetes with nephropathy, retinopathy, neuropathy, other vascular disease; or longer than 20 years duration

    (12) Active viral hepatitis, severe cirrhosis, hepatocellular adenoma, malignant hepatoma

    (13) Systemic lupus erythematosus (SLE) with positive or unknown antiphospholipid antibodies

    (14) Peripartum cardiomyopathy—normal or mildly impaired cardiac function and less than 6 months postpartum; moderately or severely impaired cardiac function

    (15) Solid organ transplantation with complications

    (16) Less than 21 days postpartum (breastfeeding and nonbreastfeeding)

  b. Category 3 for COC use—use of the method not generally recommended for the following conditions unless other more appropriate methods are not available or acceptable:

    (1) 21 to 42 days postpartum, nonbreastfeeding, other risk factors for venous thromboembolism (VTE)

    (2) 21 to < 30 days postpartum, breastfeeding, with or without other risk factors for VTE

    (3) 30 to 42 days postpartum, breastfeeding, with other risk factors for VTE

    (4) Smoker 35 years of age or older, fewer than 15 cigarettes/day

    (5) Hypertension—adequately controlled or 140–159/90–99 mm Hg

    (6) Known hyperlipidemia—consider type, severity, and other cardiovascular risk factors

    (7) Migraine headache without aura and younger than 35 years of age that starts or worsens with COC use

    (8) History of breast cancer with no evidence of disease for 5 years

    (9) Symptomatic gallbladder disease; history of cholestasis related to past COC use

    (10) Mild cirrhosis

    (11) History of bariatric surgery with malabsorptive procedure

    (12) History of DVT or PE with no risk factors for recurrence

    (13) Peripartum cardiomyopathy with normal or mildly impaired cardiac function and 6 or more months postpartum

    (14) Moderate or severe inflammatory bowel disease with associated risks for DVT or PE

7. Management

  a. Health assessment prior to initiation of method

    (1) Elicit information from thorough history concerning any contraindications/risks/specific noncontraceptive benefits for use of COCs

    (2) Blood pressure

    (3) Breast examination, pelvic examination, Pap test, STI tests are not needed prior to starting COC but may be indicated for other reasons

  b. Follow-up

    (1) May consider visit within 3 months because this is when most side effects leading to discontinuation occur

    (2) Do not tie dispensing policies to follow-up visits

    (3) Encourage to return if problems develop or wish to change method

  c. Special considerations

    (1) Drug interactions—drugs that may decrease the effectiveness of COC include:

      (a) Most broad-spectrum antibiotics (e.g., ampicillin, metronidazole, doxycycline, fluconazole) do *not* lower hormone levels or reduce COC effectiveness

      (b) A few broad-spectrum antibiotics do induce cytochrome P-450 enzyme activity and may reduce COC effectiveness—rifampin, rifapentine, griseofulvin

      (c) Some anticonvulsants induce cytochrome P-450 enzyme activity—carbamazepine, flebamate, oxcarbazine, primidone, phenobarbital, phenytoin, topiramate

      (d) Other anticonvulsants do not induce cytochrome P-450 enzyme and do not affect COC efficacy—clonazepam, gabapentin, pregabalin, valporic acid

      (e) Anticonvulsants may be used for treatment of other conditions—neuropathic pain, bipolar disease, schizophrenia, migraine headaches

      (f) Some antiretroviral drugs induce cytochrome P-450 enzyme and may affect COC efficacy—protease inhibitors

      (g) St. John's wort is a cytochrome P-450 enzyme inducer that may increase hepatic metabolism of COC

      (h) Orlistat—blocks fat absorption and may reduce intestinal absorption of COC as well as induce diarrhea

    (2) Drug interactions—COC may potentiate effect of some drugs

      (a) Benzodiazepines—diazepam and chlordiazepoxide

      (b) Tricyclic antidepressants

(c) Theophylline

(d) Potassium-sparing drugs may interact with drospirenone-containing COCs and cause hyperkalemia—angiotensin-converting-enzyme (ACE) inhibitors, angiotensin-II antagonists, potassium-sparing diuretics, heparin, aldosterone antagonists, chronic daily use of nonsteroidal anti-inflammatory drugs (NSAIDs); check potassium level during first cycle of COC and if normal no future testing is necessary

(3) Management of unscheduled bleeding/spotting

(a) Common side effect first 3 months of use; usually decreases over time

(b) Reinforce to take pills daily at the same time

(c) May consider timing of unscheduled bleeding in cycle to decide on pill formulation change if persists

(d) Spotting/bleeding before complete active pills—increase progestin content for more endometrial support

(e) Continued spotting/bleeding following scheduled bleeding—increase estrogen content of first pills in pack or decrease progestin content of first pills for more estrogen to proliferate endometrium

(f) Unscheduled spotting/bleeding with extended-cycle use—take at least 21 active pills, take 2–3 days off for withdrawal bleed to start, restart active pills, and take for at least 21 days before stops again

(g) If problem persists, consider another cause for bleeding (e.g., infection, polyps)

(4) Management of absence of withdrawal bleeding

(a) Occurs in about 5% of women after several years of COC use

(b) Rule out pregnancy or other potential causes of amenorrhea

(c) No intervention required if woman is okay with no menses

(d) Change to 30–35 mcg estrogen if on 20-mcg COC or triphasic formulation with lower levels of progestin in early pills

8. Instructions for use

a. General instructions

(1) Quick start—reasonably certain not pregnant, take first pill on day of office visit; backup method for 7 days

(2) First day start—take first pill on first day of menses; no backup method needed

(3) Sunday start—take first pill on first Sunday after menses starts; use backup method for 7 days

(4) Take pill at approximately same time each day

(5) If nausea occurs, take pill with meals or at bedtime

(6) Use backup method (condoms) if efficacy/absorbency compromised by severe vomiting/diarrhea

(7) Emergency contraception instructions

(8) Use condoms for prevention of STI/HIV

b. Missed pills—simplified instructions

(1) If less than 12 hours late, take pill immediately and continue with other pills at usual time

(2) If more than 12 hours late, take the last missed pill right away and the pill that should be taken at that time

(a) Use emergency contraception if had unprotected intercourse in previous 5 days

(b) Use condoms or abstain until have taken 7 pills in a row

c. Warning signs (ACHES)

(1) *A*bdominal pain (severe)

(2) *C*hest pain (sharp, severe, shortness of breath)

(3) *H*eadache (severe, dizziness, unilateral)

(4) *E*ye problems (scotoma, blurred vision, blind spots)

(5) *S*evere leg pain (calf or thigh)

- Transdermal contraceptive system

1. Description—patch applied to skin; delivers continuous daily systemic dose of progestin (norelgestromin) and estrogen (ethinyl estradiol), new patch applied each week for 3 weeks followed by 1 week without patch to induce withdrawal bleeding

2. Mechanism of action—same as COC

3. Effectiveness/first-year failure rate

a. Perfect use—0.3%

b. Typical use—9%

4. Advantages

a. Ease of use—no daily dosing regimen

b. Reversible

c. Effective

d. Good menstrual cycle control

5. Disadvantages and side effects

a. Does not prevent transmission of STI/HIV

b. Skin irritation at application site

c. Other side effects similar to those of COC

6. Contraindications (CDC categories 3 and 4)—same as with COC except history of bariatric surgery not relevant

7. Management

a. Health assessment prior to initiation—same as with COC

b. Follow-up—same as with COC

c. Special considerations

(1) May be less effective in women who weigh 90 kg (198 lbs) or more

(2) Probably same drug interactions as with COC

8. Instructions for using the method

a. Quick start—reasonably certain not pregnant, apply patch on day of office visit or when convenient; backup method for 7 days

b. First day start—apply patch on first day of menses; no backup method needed

c. Sunday start—apply patch on first Sunday after menses starts; use backup method for 7 days

d. Apply patch to buttocks, abdomen, upper torso front or back (excluding breasts), upper outer arm—rotate application site

e. Apply new patch on same day each week for total of 3 weeks

f. Do not wear patch on week 4; withdrawal bleeding will occur

g. Use condoms for STI/HIV prevention

h. Apply new patch if current patch partially or completely pulls away from skin

i. Contact healthcare provider if warning signs occur—same as COC warning signs

- Contraceptive vaginal ring (NuvaRing)
  1. Description—soft, malleable, clear plastic ring; delivers continuous, systemic dose of estrogen (ethinyl estradiol) and progestin (etonogestrel); worn in vagina for 3 weeks followed by 1 week without ring to induce withdrawal bleeding
  2. Mechanism of action—same as COC
  3. Effectiveness/first-year failure rate
     a. Perfect use—0.3%
     b. Typical use—9%
  4. Advantages
     a. Ease of use—no daily dosing regimen
     b. Reversible
     c. Effective
     d. Good menstrual cycle control
  5. Disadvantages and side effects
     a. Does not prevent transmission of STI/HIV
     b. Side effects similar to those of COC
     c. Vaginal discharge/vaginal irritation
  6. Contraindications (CDC categories 3 and 4)—same as with COC except history of bariatric surgery not relevant
  7. Management
     a. Health assessment prior to initiation—same as with COC
     b. Follow-up—same as with COC
     c. Special considerations—probably same drug interactions as with COC
  8. Instructions for using the method
     a. Quick start—reasonably certain not pregnant, insert ring on day of office visit or when convenient; backup method for 7 days
     b. First day start—insert ring on first day of menses; no backup method needed
     c. Days 2 to 5 of menstrual cycle—insert ring and use backup method for 7 days
     d. Wash hands before inserting
     e. Fold ring and gently insert into vagina
     f. Exact position of ring in vagina is not important
     g. Leave ring in vagina for 3 weeks then remove
     h. Insert new ring in 7 days
     i. If ring is expelled or removed for 3 hours or more, use backup method for next 7 days after ring is reinserted in vagina
     j. If ring is left in vagina for more than 3 weeks but less than 4 weeks, it should be removed; insert new ring after 1 week ring-free period
     k. If ring is left in vagina more than 4 weeks, it may not protect from pregnancy; use backup method until new ring in vagina for 7 days
     l. Use condoms for STI/HIV prevention
     m. Contact healthcare provider if warning signs occur—same as COC warning signs
- Progestin-only pills (POP)
  1. Description—pill taken daily for purposes of contraception; composed of synthetic progestins in lower doses than those used in combination oral contraceptive pills
  2. Mechanism of action
     a. Inhibits ovulation—inconsistent, variable in different women

b. Produces atrophic endometrium
c. Thickens cervical mucus
  3. Effectiveness/first-year failure rate
     a. Perfect use—0.3%
     b. Typical use—9%
  4. Advantages
     a. Ease of use
     b. Reversible
     c. Effective
     d. Contains no estrogen for women in whom it is contraindicated or who cannot tolerate estrogenic side effects
     e. Can be used during lactation and immediately postpartum
  5. Disadvantages and side effects
     a. Effectiveness may be compromised by same drug interactions as COCs because of low-dose formulation
     b. Decreased availability/increased expense compared to COC
     c. Strict daily dosing schedule
     d. Possible side effects include:
        (1) Increased incidence of functional follicular cysts
        (2) Menstrual cycle irregularities
        (3) Mastalgia
        (4) Depression
     e. No protection against STI/HIV
  6. Contraindications (CDC categories 3 and 4)
     a. Category 4 for POP use—do not use method if breast cancer within past 5 years
     b. Category 3 for POP use—use of the method not generally recommended for the following conditions unless other more appropriate methods are not available or acceptable:
        (1) History of breast cancer with no evidence of disease for 5 years
        (2) Severe cirrhosis, benign hepatocellular adenoma, malignant hepatoma
        (3) History of bariatric surgery with malabsorptive procedure
        (4) Ischemic heart disease or stroke occurring while on POP
        (5) Migraine with aura at any age that starts or worsens with POP use
        (6) SLE and positive or unknown antiphospholipid antibodies
        (7) Taking ritonivar-boosted protease inhibitors as part of HIV/AIDS treatment; some anticonvulsants; rifampin or rifabutin
  7. Management
     a. Health assessment prior to initiation of method—refer to the section titled "Combination oral contraceptives (COC)" earlier in this chapter
     b. Follow-up—refer to the section titled "Combination oral contraceptives (COC)" earlier in this chapter
     c. Special considerations—ectopic pregnancy more likely if pregnancy occurs
  8. Instructions for using the method
     a. General instruction
        (1) Start pills on cycle day 1 (first day of menses)
        (2) Take pill at same time each day every day; no placebo/off week

(3) If more than 3 hours late taking pill, use backup method for 48 hours

(4) Advise may have irregular periods or may have amenorrhea

b. Warning signs

(1) Severe low abdominal pain

(2) No bleeding after series of regular cycles

(3) Severe headache

- Progestin-only injectable contraception (depo medroxyprogesterone acetate, or DMPA)

1. Description—intramuscular (IM) or subcutaneous (SC), injectable progestin administered in 3-month intervals for contraception

2. Mechanism of action

a. Inhibits ovulation through suppression of FSH and LH

b. Produces atrophic endometrium

c. Thickens cervical mucus

3. Effectiveness/first-year failure rate

a. Perfect use—0.2%

b. Typical use—6%

4. Advantages

a. Ease of use

b. Effective

c. Long-term contraceptive option

d. Does not require compliance with daily/event regimen

e. Minimal drug interaction profile—only drug that may decrease effectiveness is aminoglutethimide used in Cushing's disease treatment

f. Results in absence of menstrual bleeding in up to 50% of women by end of first year of use (four injections); by end of second year, 70% are amenorrheic

g. Contains no estrogen for women in whom it is contraindicated or who cannot tolerate estrogenic side effects

h. Can be used during lactation and immediately postpartum

i. May decrease the following

(1) Intravascular sickling in patients with sickle cell disease

(2) Incidence of seizures in affected individuals

(3) Pain from endometriosis. SC formulation approved for treatment of pain associated with edometriosis.

(4) Risk for pelvic inflammatory disease

(5) Risk for endometrial cancer

5. Disadvantages/side effects

a. Menstrual cycle irregularities

b. Mastalgia

c. Depression

d. No protection against STI/HIV

e. Not immediately reversible—requires 3 months to be eliminated

f. Requires routine 3-month injection schedule

g. Weight gain

(1) Average 5.4 lbs first year

(2) 13.8 lbs after 4 years

h. 6- to 12-month delayed return to fertility in some women

i. Decreased bone density in long-term (greater than 5 years) user—returned to normal following discontinuance

j. May decrease HDL-C, increase LDL-C and total cholesterol

6. Contraindications (CDC categories 3 and 4)

a. Category 4 for DMPA use—do not use method if breast cancer within past 5 years

b. Category 3 for DMPA use—use of the method not generally recommended for the following conditions unless other more appropriate methods are not available or acceptable:

(1) Multiple risk factors for arterial cardiovascular disease

(2) Hypertension (160/100 mm Hg) or with vascular disease

(3) Current/history of ischemic heart disease or stroke

(4) Migraine with aura at any age that starts or worsens with DMPA use

(5) History of breast cancer with no evidence of disease for 5 years

(6) Unexplained vaginal bleeding before evaluation

(7) Diabetes with nephropathy, retinopathy, neuropathy, other vascular disease; or longer than 20 years duration

(8) Severe cirrhosis, benign hepatocellular adenoma, malignant hepatoma

(9) SLE with positive or unknown antiphospholipid antibodies

(10) SLE with severe thrombocytopenia—initiation category 3, continuation category 2

(11) Rheumatoid arthritis or long-term corticosteroid therapy with history of or risk factors for nontraumatic fractures

7. Management

a. Health assessment prior to initiation of method

(1) Refer to the section titled "Combination oral contraceptives (COC)" earlier in this chapter

(2) Include relevant health history

(3) Baseline weight assessment

b. Follow-up

(1) Return every 3 months for injection

(2) Determine last menstrual period, ask about any concerns with bleeding pattern

(3) Assess for side effects/problems

(4) Weight and blood pressure

8. Instructions for using the method

a. Explain importance of adherence to 3-month injection schedule—contraceptive efficacy maintained for at least 14 weeks after injection

b. Administer first injection within first 5 days of menstrual period; no backup method needed

c. If irregular menses, rule out pregnancy—menstrual/coital history and pregnancy test; use backup method for 7 days after injection

d. Counsel patients regarding possibility of irregular bleeding; use of backup contraception if more than 3 months between injections; use of condoms for STI/HIV prevention

e. If late for injection—if more than 17 weeks since previous injection, rule out pregnancy, offer emergency contraception if unprotected intercourse in previous 5 days, give injection, and advise to use backup method for 7 days

f. Procedure for injection

(1) IM formulation—deep intramuscular injection in deltoid or gluteal muscle

(2) SC formulation—anterior thigh or abdominal wall

(3) Do not massage injection site (alters absorption/efficacy)

(4) Observe patient for 20 minutes following first injection to rule out allergic reaction

g. Warning signs
(1) Frequent intense headache
(2) Heavy bleeding
(3) Depression
(4) Abdominal pain (severe)
(5) Signs of infection at injection site (prolonged redness, bleeding, pain, discharge)

- Progestin-only implants—etonogestrel (Implanon and Nexplanon)
1. Description—long-term (3 years) contraceptive; single rod-shaped implant placed subdermally inner side of upper arm; provides low-dose sustained release of the progestin etonogestrel; Nexplanon rod is radiopaque
2. Mechanism of action
a. Suppresses LH—ovulation inhibited in almost all users
b. Produces atrophic endometrium
c. Thickens cervical mucus
3. Effectiveness/first-year failure rate
a. Perfect use—0.05%
b. Typical use—0.05%
c. Unknown if overweight/obesity may reduce efficacy
4. Advantages
a. Ease of use
b. Effective
c. Reversible—most users ovulate within 6 weeks after removal
d. Contains no estrogen for women with contraindications to estrogen or who cannot tolerate estrogenic side effects
e. Can be used during lactation and immediately postpartum
f. Affords long-term contraception (3 years)
g. Reduced dysmenorrhea and pain from endometriosis
5. Disadvantages and side effects
a. Requires clinician insertion and removal, removal requires minor surgical procedure
b. Specific information on drug interactions is not available, very low dose progestin, potential for reduced efficacy with same drugs as listed for COC
c. Pain, bruising, infection (potential) at insertion site
d. Irregular, prolonged, more frequent uterine bleeding especially in first few months; may have amenorrhea
e. No protection against STI/HIV
f. Implant may be visible or palpable
g. Possible side effects include:
(1) Increased incidence of functional ovarian cysts
(2) Headache
(3) Emotional lability
(4) Breast tenderness
(5) Loss of libido
(6) Vaginal secretion changes—dryness, leukorrhea
(7) Acne
6. Contraindications (CDC categories 3 and 4)
a. Category 4 for etonogestrel implant use—do not use method if breast cancer within past 5 years
b. Category 3 for use etonogestrel implant—use of the method not generally recommended for the following conditions unless other more appropriate methods are not available or acceptable:

(1) Ischemic heart disease or stroke occurring while using method
(2) Migraine headaches with aura at any age if starts or worsens after implant insertion
(3) Unexplained vaginal bleeding before evaluation
(4) History of breast cancer with no evidence of disease for 5 years
(5) Severe cirrhosis, benign hepatocellular adenoma, malignant hepatoma
(6) SLE with positive or unknown antiphospholipid antibodies
7. Management
a. Health assessment prior to initiation of method—same as COC
b. Follow-up—no routine follow-up visit required
8. Instructions for using the method
a. Discuss possible bleeding changes prior to insertion
b. Inform patient must be replaced every 3 years for effective contraception
c. Insert within days 1 to 5 of menses; no backup method needed
d. If irregular menses, rule out pregnancy with menstrual and coital history and pregnancy test
e. If inserted other than days 1 to 5 of menses, use backup method for 7 days
f. Discuss use of condoms for STI prevention
g. Warning signs to report
(1) Abdominal pain (severe)
(2) Arm pain or signs of infection
(3) Heavy vaginal bleeding
(4) Missed menses after period of regularity
(5) Onset of severe headaches

- Emergency contraception
1. Definition—method used to prevent conception after unprotected coitus; levonorgestrel pill (Plan B or generic), ulipristal pill (Ella), combination of ethinyl estradiol and norgestrel or levonorgestrel pills (COC), or copper-releasing intrauterine contraception (IUC)
2. Mechanism of action
a. Emergency contraception pill (ECP)
(1) Inhibits or delays ovulation
(2) May alter sperm/ova transport
(3) May inhibit implantation of a fertilized egg
(4) Will not disrupt an established pregnancy—minimal endometrial effect
b. Copper-releasing IUC
(1) Prevents fertilization (regular use)
(2) Interferes with implantation
3. Effectiveness
a. ECP
(1) Depends on preexisting fertility
(2) Reduces risk of pregnancy by at least 75%
(3) Levonorgestrel ECP may have reduced effectiveness in obese women
b. Copper-releasing IUC—reduces risk of pregnancy by more than 99%

4. Advantages
   a. Provides means of emergency contraception in event of any of the following:
      (1) Unplanned intercourse
      (2) Method failure—condom breaks/leaks; IUC expelled; cap/diaphragm dislodged/improperly placed
      (3) Missed COC pills
      (4) Late using contraceptive method—injection, patch, vaginal ring, pills
      (5) ECP may be provided with instructions for use for women using any contraceptive method
      (6) Levonorgestrel ECP available without prescription if age 17 years or older
   b. Can provide continuous contraception (IUC)
5. Disadvantages and side effects
   a. ECP
      (1) Nausea/vomiting—less common with levonorgestrel or ulipristal pills than with COC
      (2) Change in next menses—timing, length, intermenstrual bleeding
   b. Copper-releasing IUC
      (1) Irregular, heavy bleeding
      (2) Uterine cramping/abdominal pain
      (3) Refer to the section titled "Intrauterine contraception (IUC)" later in this chapter
6. Precautions and risks
   a. Contraindications for ECP—no CDC category 3 or 4 contraindications
   b. Contraindications for copper-releasing IUC—see the section titled "Intrauterine contraception (IUC)" later in this chapter
7. Management
   a. Health assessment prior to initiation of method
      (1) Health history—menstrual, first episode of unprotected sex in cycle to determine if need pregnancy test, last episode of unprotected sex to ensure within time frame for emergency contraception
      (2) Urine pregnancy test if episode of unprotected sex more than 1 week ago
      (3) If using IUC—see the section titled "Intrauterine contraception (IUC)" later in this chapter for required history and examination
      (4) Discuss/provide ongoing contraception
   b. Follow-up—no routine follow-up visit required
8. Instructions for using the method
   a. ECP
      (1) Take as soon as possible after unprotected sex and within 120 hours for maximum effectiveness
      (2) If using COC for emergency contraception, take in 2 doses 12 hours apart
      (3) If using COC for emergency contraception, consider taking antinausea medicine 1 hour before the first dose
      (4) If you vomit within 2 hours of taking pills, contact clinician, may need a repeat dose
      (5) ECP will not provide any ongoing protection from pregnancy

      (6) Provide with contraception of choice—resume current method or begin new method immediately; wait until next day to start or restart oral contraceptives to prevent nausea/vomiting
      (7) If starting a hormonal contraceptive method immediately have a pregnancy test in 3 weeks to rule out pregnancy that may have occurred with ECP failure
      (8) Have a pregnancy test if no period within 3 weeks of ECP
   b. Copper-releasing IUC (Copper T 380A)
      (1) Can be inserted up to 5 days after unprotected sex
      (2) No evidence that progestin-releasing IUC offers effective emergency contraception
- Intrauterine contraception (IUC)
  1. Description—device placed in uterus for purpose of long-acting contraception
     a. Copper-releasing IUC (Copper T 380A)
        (1) T-shaped plastic device with copper wrapped around both vertical stem and horizontal arms
        (2) Effective for at least 10 years
     b. Levonorgestrel Intrauterine Systems (LNG IUS)—two types available
        (1) T-shaped plastic frame with steroid reservoir in vertical stem that contains levonorgestrel
        (2) 13.5 mcg or 20 mcg of levonorgestrel released daily into uterine cavity
        (3) Effective for 3 years (13.5 mcg daily LNG release), 5 years (20 mcg daily LNG release)
  2. Mechanism of action
     a. Copper T 380A
        (1) Copper may inhibit sperm capacitation
        (2) Alters tubal/uterine transport of ovum
        (3) Enzymatic influence on endometrium
     b. LNG IUS—progestin influence
        (1) Thickens cervical mucus
        (2) Produces atrophic endometrium
        (3) Slows ovum transport through tube
        (4) Inhibits sperm motility and function
  3. Effectiveness/first-year failure rate
     a. Perfect use
        (1) Copper T—0.6%
        (2) LNG IUS—0.2%
     b. Typical use
        (1) Copper T—0.8%
        (2) LNG IUS—0.2%
  4. Advantages
     a. Ease of use
     b. Not coitally dependent
     c. Effective
     d. Reversible
     e. Cost-effective (if used longer than 1 year)
     f. LNG IUS can decrease blood loss and dysmenorrhea during menses
     g. Effective choice for women who cannot use estrogen-containing methods
     h. Can be used during lactation and immediately postpartum

5. Disadvantages and side effects
   a. Altered menstrual bleeding patterns
      (1) Increased amount and length of menstrual bleeding—Copper T; first few months of LNG IUS
      (2) Increased dysmenorrhea—Copper T
      (3) Absence of bleeding—LNG IUS
   b. Risk of pelvic inflammatory disease (PID)—increased risk first 20 days following insertion
   c. Risk of spontaneous expulsion
      (1) May go undetected by the woman
      (2) More likely at time of menses
6. Contraindications (CDC categories 3 and 4)
   a. Category 4 for IUC use—do not use method if following conditions exist:
      (1) Known/suspected pregnancy
      (2) Postpartum or postabortion sepsis
      (3) Unexplained vaginal bleeding prior to insertion and before evaluation
      (4) Gestational trophoblastic disease with persistently elevated hCG levels or malignant disease
      (5) Cervical cancer prior to insertion and awaiting treatment
      (6) Current breast cancer within past 5 years—LNG IUS only
      (7) Any uterine anatomical abnormalities distorting uterine cavity incompatible with IUC insertion
      (8) Current PID, purulent cervicitis, chlamydia, or gonorrhea—initiation but not continuation
      (9) Endometrial cancer—initiation but not continuation
      (10) Known pelvic tuberculosis—initiation but not continuation
   b. Category 3 for IUC use—use of the method not generally recommended for the following conditions unless other more appropriate methods are not available or acceptable:
      (1) Ischemic heart disease occurring after insertion—LNG IUS only
      (2) Migraine headache with aura starting after insertion—LNG IUS only
      (3) Gestational trophoblastic disease with decreasing or undetectable hCG levels
      (4) History of breast cancer with no evidence of disease for 5 years—LNG IUS only
      (5) High likelihood of exposure to chlamydia or gonorrhea—initiation but not continuation
      (6) AIDS—unless clinically well on antiretroviral therapy—initiation but not continuation
      (7) Severe cirrhosis, benign hepatocellular adenoma, or malignant hepatoma—LNG IUS only
      (8) SLE with positive or unknown antiphospholipid antibodies—LNG IUS only
      (9) SLE with severe thrombocytopenia—initiation of Copper T IUC only
      (10) Solid organ transplantation with complications—initiation but not continuation
      (11) Pelvic tuberculosis—continuation
7. Management
   a. Health assessment prior to initiation of method
      (1) History to include
         (a) STI/PID, vaginitis symptoms
         (b) STI risk factors
         (c) HIV status/exposure
         (d) Pap test history of abnormal results
         (e) Heavy menses/anemia
         (f) Menstrual history
      (2) Physical examination to include
         (a) Speculum examination to assess for possible vaginal/cervical infection
         (b) Chlamydia and GC tests/wet prep (if history/physical examination indicates)
         (c) Pregnancy test if indicated
         (d) Bimanual examination—contour, size, consistency, mobility, position of uterus
      (3) Placement technique
         (a) Wash cervix and vagina with antiseptic
         (b) Apply tenaculum to anterior or posterior lip of cervix and apply gentle traction to straighten axis of uterus
         (c) Sound uterus prior to placing IUC—should sound to length of 6 to 9 cm for best placement
         (d) Place IUC per manufacturer's instructions
         (e) Trim IUC threads to 3 to 4 cm
         (f) Have patient remain supine until feels well—then monitor as sits up as may have vasovagal reaction from instrumentation of cervical os
   b. Follow-up
      (1) Speculum examination after first menses following placement check for IUC threads
      (2) Assessment for any signs/symptoms of pelvic infection
   c. Special considerations
      (1) Timing of insertion
         (a) Not necessary to wait for menses if evidence that patient is not pregnant
         (b) May be inserted within 48 hours after delivery (vaginal and cesarean)
         (c) May be inserted 4 or more weeks postpartum
         (d) Insertion after 48 hours and before 4 weeks postpartum is associated with increased risk of uterine perforation
         (e) May be inserted immediately following first- or second-trimester abortion
      (2) Menstrual abnormalities (spotting, bleeding)
         (a) Nonsteroidal anti-inflammatory drugs (NSAIDs) may reduce bleeding if initiated at start of menses
         (b) Hemoglobin/hematocrit (Hgb/Hct) if excessive or prolonged bleeding—if low, consider iron supplementation
         (c) Assess for other causes if persistent abnormal bleeding or bleeding associated with pain—cervicitis, pregnancy including ectopic, pelvic infection
         (d) Remove IUC if patient desires and provide alternative contraception; may consider switch to LNG IUS if having excessive bleeding with Copper T 380A and wants to continue IUC as method
      (3) Cramping and pain
         (a) If severe—rule out perforation
         (b) If mild—NSAID/other analgesic or remove IUC
         (c) May indicate infection, pregnancy
      (4) Expulsion—2% to 10% within first year
         (a) Symptoms—cramping, spotting, dyspareunia, lengthening of threads

(b) Partial expulsion
    i. Remove IUC
    ii. Rule out pregnancy/infection
    iii. Replace IUC if patient desires
    iv. Doxycycline for 5 to 7 days
(c) Complete expulsion
    i. Pregnancy test
    ii. Replace IUC if patient desires

(5) Pregnancy
(a) Ultrasound evaluation to rule out ectopic pregnancy
(b) Remove IUC promptly regardless of plans for pregnancy—reduces risk for spontaneous abortion and preterm delivery
(c) Spontaneous abortion—treat with doxycycline/ampicillin for 7 days
(d) Patient wants to continue pregnancy
    i. Advise concerning risk for spontaneous septic abortion if IUC not removed
    ii. If threads not visible—ultrasound to see if IUC still present
    iii. If unable to remove IUC—monitor closely for infection during pregnancy

(6) Perforation, embedding
(a) Perforation occurs 1 in 1000 insertions
    i. May/may not be associated with severe pain at time of insertion
    ii. Ultrasound to determine location—may require laproscopic removal
    iii. If protrusion through cervix, can be removed in office with local anesthetic
(b) Embedding
    i. Can remove IUC from uterus with forceps if visualized
    ii. May need to be removed with dilatation and curettage (D&C)

(7) PID
(a) Most IUC-related PID occurs within the first 20 days after insertion
(b) No evidence supporting the use of prophylactic antibiotics to reduce postinsertion infection
(c) Treat PID with appropriate antibiotics
(d) Not necessary to remove IUC unless has current high risk for STI

(8) *Actinomyces*-like organisms on Pap test
(a) Pap test does not diagnose actinomycosis infection
(b) *Actinomyces* are normal female genital tract organisms
(c) Colonization of *Actinomyces* more likely in IUC user
(d) Pelvic actinomycosis is very rare but serious infection
(e) Asymptomatic—inform IUC user of Pap test report, no treatment necessary, advise to contact healthcare provider if has infection symptoms
(f) Symptomatic—endometritis
    i. Treat with antibiotics—sensitive to penicillin and several other antibiotics
    ii. Remove IUC—*Actinomyces* preferentially grow on foreign bodies

8. Instructions for using the method
a. Check IUD threads
    (1) After each menses
    (2) If increased cramping
    (3) If absent—use backup birth control and notify healthcare provider
    (4) If longer
        (a) May be in process of expulsion
        (b) Use backup birth control and notify healthcare provider
b. Signs of infection—notify healthcare provider if
    (1) Pelvic pain
    (2) Vaginal discharge
    (3) Unexplained vaginal bleeding
c. Monitor menses—notify healthcare provider if any of the following:
    (1) Heavy, irregular bleeding
    (2) Missed menses—may have amenorrhea with LNG IUS
    (3) Increased cramping
d. Warning signs (PAINS)
    (1) *Period late/missed; abnormal spotting or bleeding*
    (2) *Abdominal pain*
    (3) *Infection—vaginal discharge*
    (4) *Not feeling well—fever, aches, chills*
    (5) *String missing, shorter or longer*

- Vaginal spermicides
1. Description—cream, foam, suppository, tablet, film, gel, or other preparation that destroys sperm when placed in vagina
2. Mechanism of action
a. Nonoxynol-9 is active ingredient
b. Destroys sperm cell membrane
3. Effectiveness/first-year failure rate
a. Perfect use—18%
b. Typical use—28%
4. Advantages
a. Accessible
b. Inexpensive
c. Readily available backup method
d. No systemic effects
5. Disadvantages and side effects
a. Coitally dependent
b. Does not protect against STI/HIV
c. Potential for allergy/sensitivity/irritation
d. Must follow instructions carefully for effective use
6. Contraindications (CDC categories 3 and 4)
a. Category 4—do not use method if following condition exists—high risk for HIV (relates to frequent spermicide use two or more time a day, vulvovaginal epithelium disruption, and theoretical increased susceptibility to HIV infection)
b. Category 3—use of method not generally recommended for following condition unless other more appropriate methods are not available or acceptable—HIV/AIDS (relates to frequent spermicide use, disruption of cervical mucosa, potential increased viral shedding, and HIV transmission)
7. Management
a. No health assessment needed prior to initiation of method
b. Individuals with skin sensitivities may want to test/avoid use

    c. Vaginal abnormalities (septa, prolapse) may preclude use

  8. Instructions for using method

    a. Use spermicide with each act of intercourse

    b. Read all instructions carefully

    c. Leave spermicide in place (no douching) for at least 6 hours following last intercourse

    d. Follow instructions regarding how long prior to intercourse the spermicide may be inserted—if too much time has lapsed, pregnancy may occur

    e. Place spermicide deep within vagina

    f. Allow adequate time for spermicide to dissolve (if film, tablets, or suppositories)

    g. With foam use—shake canister well, as directed, prior to filling applicator

    h. Use with condom for increased effectiveness

- Male condom
  1. Description—latex/polyurethane/natural membranous sleeve placed over erect penis prior to intercourse to prevent transmission of semen/sperm into vaginal vault
  2. Mechanism of action—barrier; prevents transmission of semen/sperm into vagina
  3. Effectiveness/first-year failure rate
     a. Perfect use—2%
     b. Typical use—18%
  4. Advantages
     a. Accessible
     b. Cost-effective
     c. Prevents/reduces transmission of STI (except membrane condoms)
     d. Active involvement of male partner
     e. Prevents allergic reaction to semen
     f. Arrests development of antisperm antibodies in infertility patients
     g. May help prevent premature ejaculation
     h. Does not require visit to healthcare provider
  5. Disadvantages
     a. Decreased penile sensitivity
     b. Interrupts act of love making
     c. Some men cannot maintain erection during condom use
     d. Requires active involvement of male partner
     e. Possibility of condom rupture
  6. Contraindications—latex allergy, can use polyurethane
  7. Management—no health assessment needed prior to initiation of method
  8. Instructions for using method
     a. Natural membrane condoms may not protect against STI/HIV
     b. Use water-soluble lubricants (e.g., K-Y Jelly, Astroglide, egg whites); avoid oil-based lubricants with latex condoms (e.g., baby oil, vegetable or mineral oils, petroleum jelly)
     c. Use new condom with each act of intercourse
     d. Unroll condom over penis completely (to the base) prior to any genital contact
     e. Immediately after ejaculation, hold rim of condom and withdraw penis from vagina while it is still erect
     f. If condom slips/breaks
        (1) Before ejaculation—apply new condom

      (2) After ejaculation—consider emergency contraception

- Female condom
  1. Description—nitrile sheath placed in the vagina that acts as a barrier to prevent direct contact with seminal fluid during intercourse; smaller ring at closed end lies inside vagina and wider ring at open end of sheath remains outside the vagina; has silicone-based lubricant on inside
  2. Mechanism of action—barrier, protects vagina/vulva from direct contact with penis/seminal fluid
  3. Effectiveness/first-year failure rate
     a. Perfect use—5%
     b. Typical use—21%
  4. Advantages
     a. Prevents/reduces transmission of STI
     b. Does not require use of spermicide
     c. Accessible
     d. Controlled by the woman
     e. Stronger than latex and less likely to tear or break
     f. Does not require visit to healthcare provider
  5. Disadvantages and side effects
     a. Coitally dependent
     b. Noisy—less of problem with switch from polyurethane to nitrile
     c. May be aesthetically unappealing
     d. Expensive
  6. Contraindications—nitrile allergy
  7. Management
     a. No health assessment needed prior to initiation of method
     b. Women with vaginal anatomy abnormalities may not be able to use this method
  8. Instructions for using the method
     a. Hold pouch with open end down—inner ring should be at bottom of pouch
     b. Squeeze inner ring together and insert inner ring and pouch into vagina
     c. Push inner ring deep into vagina
     d. Outer ring should rest outside vulva
     e. Remove condom immediately after intercourse
     f. Squeeze outer ring together and twist to prevent spillage
     g. Discard the whole condom
     h. Use new condom with each act of intercourse
     i. Do not use male condom when using female condom—may adhere together causing dislodgement

- Diaphragm
  1. Description—reusable latex dome that covers anterior vaginal wall, including cervix; spermicide placed in dome covers cervix affording increased contraceptive protection; sizes 50-mm to 95-mm diameter; different types of inner construction of circular rim include:
     a. Flat spring
        (1) Good for women with firm vaginal tone
        (2) Gentle spring strength
     b. Coil spring
        (1) Good for women with average vaginal tone
        (2) Firm spring strength
     c. Arcing spring
        (1) Good for women with lax vaginal tone

(2) Firm spring strength

d. Wide seal

    (1) Good for women with average/lax vaginal tone

    (2) Available as arcing or coil spring

2. Mechanism of action

    a. Barrier—prevents direct cervical contact with seminal fluid

    b. Spermicide—destroys sperm cell membrane

3. Effectiveness/first-year failure rate

    a. Perfect use—6%

    b. Typical use—12%

4. Advantages

    a. Cost effective—may be used for 1 to 2 years

    b. Affords some protection against STIs—possible decreased incidence of PID

    c. No systemic effects

    d. May use with male condom for increased effectiveness

5. Disadvantages

    a. Requires sizing by trained clinician and instructions in use

    b. May have sensitivity to latex/spermicide

    c. Increased risk of bacterial vaginosis and urinary tract infection (UTI)

        (1) Due to increased colonization with Escherichia *coli*

        (2) Related to use of spermicide

        (3) Mechanical irritation/compression against urethra

    d. Does not afford absolute protection from STI/HIV

    e. Risk of toxic shock—2 to 3/100,000 per year

6. Contraindications (CDC categories 3 and 4)

    a. Category 4 for diaphragm use—do not use method if following conditions exist:

        (1) Allergy to latex; does not apply to nonlatex diaphragms

        (2) High risk for HIV—related to concerns about frequent spermicide use disrupting vaginal epithelium rather than diaphragm

    b. Category 3 for diaphragm use—use of method not generally recommended for the following conditions unless other more appropriate methods are not available or acceptable:

        (1) History of toxic shock syndrome

        (2) HIV/AIDS—related to concerns about frequent spermicide use disrupting vaginal epithelium rather than diaphragm

7. Management

    a. Health assessment prior to initiation of method

        (1) Health history to determine whether special circumstances or contraindications

        (2) Vaginal examination to determine any abnormal anatomy that may preclude proper fit and retention—prolapse, cystocele, rectocele, vaginal septum

        (3) Proper fit by trained clinician—determine appropriate size and type for woman's anatomy; choose largest size comfortable for individual woman, too small will not remain in place during intercourse, too large may cause discomfort, vaginal ulceration, and increased risk for UTI

        (4) Wait 6 weeks postpartum or until uterine involution complete and 6 weeks post second trimester abortion to fit and use

    b. Follow-up—no routine follow-up required, recheck fit following childbirth or if patient gains/loses 10 lbs or more

8. Instructions for using the method

    a. Insert just prior to intercourse or up to 6 hours before

    b. Coat inner dome with 1 tablespoon of spermicide

    c. Pinch sides of diaphragm and insert fully into vagina

        (1) Tuck anterior rim behind symphysis

        (2) Be certain that dome covers cervix

    d. If repeated intercourse, insert another application of spermicide in vagina; do not remove diaphragm

    e. Leave diaphragm in place for at least 6 hours following last intercourse

    f. Do not leave in place for more than 24 hours

    g. After each use wash diaphragm with plain soap and water and store in clean, cool, dark environment; do not use talcum powder on diaphragm

    h. Do not use with oil-based lubricants or vaginal medications

    i. Replace diaphragm every 1 to 2 years

    j. Assess for holes/tears periodically by filling with water and inspecting for leaks

    k. Consider emergency contraception if diaphragm is dislodged during or less than 6 hours after sex

    l. Warning signs (toxic shock)

        (1) High fever

        (2) Nausea, vomiting, diarrhea

        (3) Syncope, weakness

        (4) Joint/muscle aches

        (5) Rash resembling sunburn

- Cervical cap (FemCap)

1. Description—reusable silicone cap, fits over cervix providing barrier contraception; spermicide placed in dome affords additional contraceptive efficacy; three sizes—22 mm, 26 mm, 30 mm; strap on convex side of cap aids in removal

2. Mechanism of action

    a. Barrier—prevents direct cervical contact with seminal fluid

    b. Spermicide—destroys sperm cell membrane

3. Effectiveness/first-year failure rate

    a. Perfect use

        (1) Parous women—21%

        (2) Nulliparous women—10%

    b. Typical use

        (1) Parous women—40%

        (2) Nulliparous women—20%

4. Advantages

    a. Cost-effective—may be used for 1 to 2 years

    b. Affords some protection against STIs

    c. Possible decreased incidence of PID

    d. Possible decreased incidence of cervical dysplasia/neoplasia

    e. No systemic effects

    f. May be left in place for 48 hours

    g. Does not require insertion of more spermicide with repeat intercourse

    h. Does not increase incidence of bladder infection

    i. May use with male condom to increase effectiveness

5. Disadvantages

    a. Requires trained clinician for sizing

    b. Sensitivity to silicone/spermicide

    c. Not every woman can be fitted appropriately—short cervix, asymmetry

    d. May become dislodged during intercourse

  6. Contraindications (CDC categories 3 and 4)

    a. Category 4 for cervical cap use—do not use method if following condition exists—high risk for HIV—related to concerns about frequent spermicide use disrupting vaginal epithelium rather than the cervical cap

    b. Category 3 for cervical cap use—use of method not generally recommended for the following conditions unless other more appropriate methods are not available or acceptable:

      (1) HIV/AIDS—related to concerns about frequent spermicide use disrupting vaginal epithelium rather than the cervical cap

      (2) History of toxic shock syndrome

  7. Management

    a. Health assessment prior to initiation of method

      (1) Visualization of cervix to rule out abnormalities/anatomy that may prevent proper fit—extensive lacerations, asymmetry, short cervix

      (2) Palpation of cervix—length, position, symmetry

      (3) Size generally determined by obstetric history—smallest size if never pregnant, middle size if miscarried or had cesarean section, largest size if has had vaginally delivered full-term baby

      (4) Wait 6 weeks postpartum or until uterine involution complete and 6 weeks post second trimester abortion to fit and use

    b. Follow-up—no routine follow-up required, reevaluate cap fit if patient complains of dislodgement during intercourse

    c. Special considerations—do not use less than 6 weeks postpartum, immediate postabortion, or during menses

  8. Instructions for using method

    a. Insert cap at least 30 minutes prior to intercourse to create suction

    b. Fill one-third of cap with spermicide

    c. Compress rim prior to insertion

    d. Advance into vagina so rim can slide over cervix

    e. Check that cap covers cervix

    f. Not necessary to reinsert spermicide with repeated intercourse

    g. Leave in place for at least 6 hours and no more than 48 hours after sex

    h. Warning signs (toxic shock)—refer to the section titled "Diaphragm" earlier in this chapter

    i. Do not use after recent spontaneous or induced abortion

    j. Do not use during menses or any other vaginal bleeding

- Lea's shield—not currently available in United States

  1. Description—reusable oval-shaped silicone device fits over cervix and part of upper vagina providing barrier contraception; airflow valve lets air between cervix and shield escape, creating a seal between shield and vagina; flexible ring used to help with removal; spermicide placed inside device affords additional contraceptive efficacy; one size

  2. Mechanism of action

    a. Barrier—prevents direct cervical contact with seminal fluid

    b. Spermicide—destroys sperm cell membrane

  3. Effectiveness/first-year failure rate

    a. Perfect use—8%

    b. Typical use—no information

  4. Advantages

    a. No fitting required—one size fits all

    b. Reusable—good for about 6 months

    c. No systemic effects

    d. May afford some protection against some STIs

  5. Disadvantages and side effects

    a. Prescription required

    b. Increased risk of bacterial vaginosis and UTI

    c. Does not afford absolute protection from STI/HIV

    d. Potential risk of toxic shock—same as with diaphragm

    e. May have sensitivity to silicone or spermicide

  6. Contraindications (CDC recommendations not specifically provided)—considered same as for diaphragm and cervical cap

  7. Management

    a. No health assessment needed prior to initiation of method

    b. Special considerations

      (1) Abnormal vaginal anatomy—prolapse, cystocele, rectocele may prevent proper placement

      (2) Do not use if delivery within past 6 weeks, recent abortion, or vaginal bleeding

  8. Instructions for using the method

    a. Apply spermicide around rim of shield

    b. Fold shield and insert as high in vagina as possible

    c. Check that cervix is covered by shield

    d. Leave in place for at least 6 hours following intercourse

    e. Use additional spermicide in vagina if repeat intercourse

    f. Do not leave in place more than 40 hours

    g. Consider emergency contraception if shield becomes dislodged during intercourse

    h. After use wash with soap and water and air dry

    i. Replace every 6 months

    j. Warning signs (toxic shock)—see the section titled "Diaphragm" earlier in this chapter

- Contraceptive sponge

  1. Description—small pillow-shaped polyurethane sponge containing 1 g of nonoxynol-9 spermicide, concave side fits over cervix, polyester loop facilitates removal, one size

  2. Mechanism of action

    a. Barrier—prevents direct cervical contact with seminal fluid

    b. Spermicide—destroys sperm cell membrane

  3. Effectiveness/first-year failure rate

    a. Perfect use

      (1) Nulliparous—9%

      (2) Parous—20%

    b. Typical use

      (1) Nulliparous—12%

      (2) Parous—24%

  4. Advantages

    a. No prescription required

    b. No systemic effects

    c. May be used with male condom for additional contraceptive and STI protection

    d. Protects up to 24 hours regardless of how many times intercourse occurs

5. Disadvantages
   a. Significant decrease in efficacy for parous women versus nulliparous woman
   b. Potential risk of toxic shock—same as with diaphragm
   c. May have sensitivity to polyurethane or spermicide
   d. Abnormal vaginal anatomy—prolapse, cystocele, rectocele may prevent proper placement
6. Contraindications (CDC recommendations not specifically provided)—consider same as for diaphragm and cervical cap
7. Management
   a. No health assessment needed prior to initiation of method
   b. Wait 6 weeks postpartum to use
8. Instructions for using the method
   a. Moisten sponge with tap water prior to use
   b. Insert deep into vagina
   c. Check to be sure cervix is covered by sponge
   d. Leave in place for at least 6 hours after last intercourse
   e. If repeated intercourse, no additional spermicide needed
   f. Do not wear the sponge for more than 24 to 30 hours
   g. Discard sponge after use
   h. Do not use after recent spontaneous or induced abortion
   i. Do not use during menses or any other vaginal bleeding
   j. Warning signs (toxic shock)—refer to the section titled "Diaphragm" earlier in this chapter
- Fertility awareness methods
   1. Description—method of contraception using abstinence during estimated fertile period based on all or some of the following methods
      a. Menstrual cycle pattern (calendar method)
      b. Basal body temperature (BBT)—determines ovulation
      c. Evaluation of cervical mucus (ovulation/Billings method)—determines ovulation
      d. Sympto-thermal method—combines BBT with evaluation of cervical mucus and cervical position/consistency
      e. Standard days method—consider fertile days 8 through 19 of each menstrual cycle
   2. Mechanism of action—intercourse is avoided during fertile period
      a. Ovum remains fertile for 24 hours
      b. Sperm viability approximately 72 hours
      c. Most pregnancies occur when intercourse occurs before ovulation
   3. Effectiveness/first-year failure rate
      a. Perfect use
         (1) Calendar method—9%
         (2) BBT—2%
         (3) Ovulation method—3%
         (4) Sympto-thermal—0.4%
         (5) Standard days method—5%
      b. Typical use for all methods—24%
   4. Advantages
      a. Minimal cost
      b. Natural
      c. No systemic effects
      d. No localized side effects, e.g., latex allergy
      e. Can be utilized for contraception and conception planning

5. Disadvantages
   a. Requires motivation from both partners
   b. Requires periodic abstinence
   c. No protection against STI/HIV
6. Precautions and risks
   a. Not reliable for women with the following conditions:
      (1) Irregular menses (consider sympto-thermal and ovulation methods)
      (2) Perimenopausal
      (3) Recently postpartum
      (4) Have had recent menarche
   b. Not a suitable method for
      (1) Women who cannot accurately evaluate their fertile period
         (a) Inability to use/read thermometer
         (b) Inability to understand cervical mucus/changes
         (c) Inability to time intercourse based on calendar evaluation
      (2) Couples unwilling to abstain during fertile time period
      (3) If nonconsensual coitus is likely to occur
7. Management
   a. Health assessment prior to initiation of method
      (1) History to reflect pattern of menses
      (2) Evaluation of client's willingness/ability to check cervical mucus/consistency/position
   b. Follow-up—BBT/sympto-thermal chart evaluation
8. Instructions for using the method
   a. Calendar method
      (1) Keep record of menstrual cycle intervals for several months
      (2) From the shortest cycle length, subtract 18 days—this determines first fertile day
      (3) From the longest cycle length, subtract 11 days—this determines last fertile day
      (4) Use these numbers to determine days of abstinence for every cycle
   b. Basal body temperature (BBT) method
      (1) Take temperature each morning before rising
         (a) BBT thermometer
         (b) Temperature can be oral, vaginal, or rectal (maintain same route)
      (2) Record on BBT chart
      (3) Temperature increase of 0.4°F or higher at ovulation—remains elevated for at least 3 days
      (4) Abstain from intercourse until 3-day temperature increase occurs
   c. Ovulation method
      (1) Inspect cervical mucus/secretions on underwear, toilet tissue, with fingers, beginning day after menses
      (2) Determine consistency—elastic, slippery, wet by touch indicates preovulatory
         (a) Amount increases; becomes thinner and more elastic around time of ovulation
         (b) After ovulation, mucus becomes thick, tacky, and cloudy

(3) Abstain from intercourse during "wet days" at onset of increased, slippery, thin mucus discharge until 4 days past the peak day (last day of clear, stretchy, slippery secretions)

(4) Abstain from intercourse during menses because of inability to assess mucus

d. Sympto-thermal method—combines cervical mucus evaluation, BBT, and assessment of consistency/position of cervix in vagina

(1) May also use calendar method and other symptoms such as ovulatory pain "mittelschmertz" as additional indicators

(2) Abstain until last combined methods indicates "safe" time

e. Standard days method

(1) Abstain from intercourse days 8 through 19 of each menstrual cycle

(2) CycleBeads are color-coded string of beads to help woman keep track of cycle days

- Lactational amenorrhea method
1. Description—method of contraception for women who are breastfeeding without supplementation or with minimal supplementation and have not had a postpartum menstrual cycle
2. Mechanism of action—high prolactin
   a. FSH normal; LH decreased—no ovarian follicular development
   b. Inhibits pulsatile GnRH
   c. Results in anovulation
3. Effectiveness/first-year failure rate
   a. Perfect use—0.5% to 1.5% (if amenorrheic)
   b. Typical use—data not available
4. Advantages
   a. Requires no pills or other devices
   b. No cost
   c. Highly effective until infant nutritional requirements mandate supplementation (approximately 6 months)
   d. Not coitally dependent
   e. Advantageous for infant
      (1) Nutritional
      (2) Bonding
5. Disadvantages
   a. Woman must breastfeed completely or with minimal supplementation—may lead to exhaustion
   b. Decreased estrogen due to absence of follicular development
      (1) Atrophic vaginitis
      (2) Decreased vaginal lubrication
      (3) Dyspareunia
   c. Affords no protection against STI/HIV
   d. Efficacy decreases with resumption of menses
6. Management
   a. No health assessment needed prior to initiation of method
   b. Special considerations—should not use vaginal estrogen cream to treat atrophic vaginitis
      (1) Absorption can inhibit milk production
      (2) Recommend use of vaginal lubricants
7. Instructions for using the method
   a. Use no or only minimal supplementation

b. Choose an alternative contraceptive method when any of the following occur
   (1) Menses
   (2) Regular supplementation is being used
   (3) Long periods without breastfeeding (e.g., baby sleeping through night)
   (4) Baby is 6 months old
c. Ovulation may occur before onset of menses
d. Milk expression by hand or pump does not have same fertility-inhibiting effect as breastfeeding
e. Do not use vaginal estrogen cream for atrophic vaginitis—absorption may inhibit milk production
f. Use vaginal lubricants as needed

- Coitus interruptus (withdrawal)
1. Description—contraceptive method whereby male withdraws penis from vagina prior to ejaculation
2. Mechanism of action—sperm not introduced into vagina
3. Effectiveness/first-year failure rate
   a. Perfect use—4%
   b. Typical use—22%
4. Advantages
   a. Requires no devices
   b. No systemic effects
   c. No expense
   d. May result in decreased transmission of HIV (man to woman)
5. Disadvantages and side effects
   a. Requires self-control on part of male partner
   b. Requires ability to predict time of ejaculation
   c. Does not afford protection from STI
6. Precautions and risks—should not be used by men with premature ejaculatory disorder
7. Management—no health assessment needed prior to initiation of method
8. Instructions for using the method
   a. Male partner should void prior to intercourse
   b. Withdraw penis prior to ejaculation, do not ejaculate near female's external genital area
   c. If intercourse is going to be repeated in short period of time, male should urinate again and wipe off tip of penis to remove any sperm remaining from previous intercourse
   d. Although pre-ejaculate itself contains little or no sperm, repeated intercourse may result in increased amounts of sperm in the pre-ejaculatory fluid

- Abstinence
1. Description—contraception based on abstaining from penile-vaginal intercourse
2. Mechanism of action—sperm not introduced into vagina
3. Effectiveness/first-year failure rate
   a. Perfect use—0%
   b. Typical use—data not available
4. Advantages
   a. No cost
   b. Prevention of STIs
5. Disadvantages—requires motivation and acceptance by both partners

6. Management—no health assessment needed prior to initiation of method
7. Instructions for using the method
    a. Avoid any penile-vaginal contact
    b. Consider alternative means of intimacy/sexual expression (e.g., mutual masturbation, massage, kissing)
    c. Penile-anal intercourse may result in some sperm entering vagina during withdrawal
    d. Penile-anal, oral-genital, and digital-genital contact may result in STI/HIV transmission
    e. Avoid alcohol or drug use; may affect commitment to method

- Female sterilization
1. Description—permanent contraception for woman achieved through surgical means; commonly performed on outpatient basis or postpartum prior to discharge
2. Mechanism of action
    a. Fallopian tubes are obstructed to prevent union of sperm and ovum
    b. Transabdominal occlusion methods—laparoscopy or suprapubic mini-laparoscopy approach; general or local anesthesia
        (1) Surgical ligation—Pomeroy procedure
        (2) Surgical ligation and attachment to uterine body—Irving procedure
        (3) Electrocauterization
        (4) Section of tube excised
            (a) Pritchard procedure
            (b) Fimbriectomy
        (5) Occluded—compressed with silastic band (Falope Ring) or clip (Filshie)
    c. Transcervical occlusion methods (Essure)
        (1) Micro-insert device inserted in tubes transcervically through hysteroscope
        (2) Office procedure with local anesthesia
3. Effectiveness/first-year failure rate
    a. Perfect use—0.5%
    b. Typical use—0.5%
4. Advantages
    a. Affords permanent contraception
    b. Highly effective
    c. Cost-effective over long term
    d. Not coitally dependent
5. Disadvantages
    a. Invasive surgical procedure requiring anesthesia
    b. Reversal is difficult, expensive, and often unsuccessful
    c. No protection against STI/HIV
    d. Initially expensive
    e. Probability of pregnancy being ectopic is higher if method fails
6. Precautions and risks
    a. Surgical procedure
        (1) Operative complications—bladder/uterine/intestinal injury may occur
        (2) Anesthetic complications—death (rare)
    b. Wound infection

c. If pregnancy occurs following procedure, increased risk of ectopic
7. Management
    a. Health assessment prior to initiation of method
        (1) Assess if patient candidate for surgery
        (2) Assess psychological readiness for permanent contraceptive method
        (3) Follow federal and state regulations regarding informed consent process
    b. Follow-up—assess for appropriate healing and signs/symptoms of infection 1–2 weeks after procedure
8. Instructions for using the method
    a. Nothing by mouth at least 8 hours prior to procedure
    b. Need transportation assistance from hospital/clinic to home
    c. Rest for at least 24 hours recommended following procedure
    d. Light lifting only for 1 week
    e. No coitus for 1 to 2 weeks
    f. Notify healthcare provider of any signs/symptoms of infection
    g. Continue another method of contraception for 3 months after transcervical occlusion method
    h. Confirm correct placement and tubal occlusion with hysterosalpingogram 3 months after transcervical occlusion method
    i. If suspect pregnancy, see healthcare provider as soon as possible to evaluate for possible ectopic pregnancy

- Male sterilization
1. Description—permanent contraception involving occlusion of vas deferens, preventing transmission of sperm through semen
    a. Approaches to vas deferens
        (1) Conventional vasectomy—local anesthesia, skin and muscle overlying vas deferens is incised with scalpel, vas deferens occluded, incisions closed with absorbable suture
        (2) No-scalpel vasectomy—local anesthesia; ringed clamp secures vas deferens, midline puncture of scrotum with dissecting forceps rather than incision; vas deferens occluded; sutures not needed; less risk of infection, hematoma, pain than conventional method
    b. Methods of occlusion
        (1) Ligation with sutures and excision of section of vas deferens most common
        (2) Other methods include electrosurgical or thermal cautery, application of clips, or a combination of methods
2. Mechanism of action—sperm not present in ejaculate
3. Effectiveness/first-year failure rate
    a. Perfect use—0.10%
    b. Typical use—0.15%
4. Advantages
    a. Cost-effective
    b. Highly effective
    c. Affords permanent contraception
    d. Not coitally dependent
    e. No systemic effects/artificial devices
5. Disadvantages
    a. Initial expense
    b. Should be considered irreversible

c. Invasive surgical procedure

d. No protection against STI/HIV

6. Precautions and risks

   a. Surgical procedure

   b. Wound infection

   c. Prostate cancer—conflicting studies, those that were positive show only weak association of vasectomy and prostate cancer, prostate cancer screening recommendations in men who have had vasectomy is same as for men in general population

7. Management

   a. Health assessment prior to initiation of procedure

     (1) Assess psychological readiness for permanent contraceptive method

     (2) Assess general health and inguinal area, scrotum, and testicles

     (3) Follow federal and state regulations regarding informed consent process

   b. Follow-up—confirm vasectomy success with semen analysis 3 months post procedure if possible

8. Instructions for using the method

   a. Rest for approximately 48 hours following procedure

   b. Apply ice pack to scrotum for minimum of 4 hours after procedure

   c. Notify healthcare provider if have signs/symptoms of infection

     (1) Fever greater than 100.4°F

     (2) Increasing pain not relieved by analgesics

     (3) Redness, inflammation, swelling, drainage, or discharge at incision site

     (4) Stitches causing extreme pulling sensation

   d. Wear scrotal support for 2 days

   e. Avoid intercourse for 2 to 3 days

   f. Avoid strenuous exercise or heavy lifting for 1 week

   g. Continue using other contraception for at least 3 months; obtain semen analysis to confirm azospermia

- Special considerations in contraceptive management

1. Postpartum contraception

   a. On average the first ovulation occurs 45 days postpartum in nonlactating women; however, it may occur as early as 25 days postpartum

   b. Lactational amenorrhea method (LAM) is a highly effective temporary method of contraception up to 6 months postpartum if following recommended parameters

   c. Venous thromboembolism (VTE) risk is increased for first few weeks postpartum, generally declining to baseline levels by 42 days postpartum

   d. Initiation of combination hormonal contraceptive methods in lactating women

     (1) Less than 21 days postpartum (CDC category 4)

     (2) 21 to < 30 days postpartum (CDC category 3)—whether or not has other VTE risk factors

     (3) 30 to 42 days postpartum—with other VTE risk factors (CDC category 3), without other VTE risk factors (CDC category 2)

     (4) Greater than 42 days postpartum (CDC category 2)

   e. Initiation of combination hormonal contraceptive methods for nonlactating women

     (1) Less than 21 days postpartum (CDC category 4)

     (2) 21 to 42 days postpartum with other VTE risk factors (CDC category 3), without other VTE risk factors (category 2)

     (3) Greater than 42 days postpartum (CDC category 1)

   f. Initiation of progestin-only contraceptive methods for lactating women

     (1) Less than 21 days postpartum (CDC category 2)

     (2) 21 to < 30 days postpartum (CDC category 2) whether or not has other VTE risk factors

     (3) 30 or greater days postpartum (CDC category 1)

   g. Initiation of progestin-only contraceptive methods for nonlactating women (CDC category 1)—may initiate immediately postpartum

   h. Initiation of intrauterine contraception—lactating, nonlactating, including postcesarean delivery

     (1) Less than 10 minutes after delivery of placenta—LNG-IUS (CDC category 2), copper-releasing IUC (CDC category 1)

     (2) 10 minutes after delivery of placenta to less than 4 weeks (both CDC category 2)

     (3) 4 weeks or greater postpartum (both CDC category 1)

2. Contraception for women older than 40 years

   a. Most contraceptive options safe for women older than 40 without category 3 or 4 contraindications

   b. Combination hormonal contraception (CHC)—pills, patch, vaginal ring

     (1) Safe option for nonsmoking, nonobese, healthy perimenopausal women

     (2) Noncontraceptive benefits may be especially attractive to the perimenopausal woman—relief of vasomotor symptoms, menstrual regulation

     (3) May reduce risk of endometrial hyperplasia/cancer associated with anovulatory cycles during perimenopausal years

   c. Progestin-only methods (DMPA, POP, implants)

     (1) No specific age-related contraindications

     (2) May provide some relief from vasomotor symptoms

     (3) May reduce risk of endometrial hyperplasia/cancer

     (4) DMPA may diminish bone mineral density in perimenopausal women; however, these women do not undergo the typical rapid loss of bone mineral density following menopause

   d. Intrauterine contraceptives

     (1) Long-acting reversible method option as effective as sterilization

     (2) Levonorgestrel IUS (LNG IUS) may also be therapeutic for perimenopausal women with heavy bleeding

   e. Barrier methods—safe option

   f. Sterilization—most prevalent contraceptive method among married women in United States

   g. Fertility awareness methods—may be less effective during menopause because of irregular ovulation and menstrual cycles

h. Approaches used in deciding when to discontinue contraception

(1) There are no definitive answers to when to discontinue contraception

(2) CHC

  (a) Continue to age 50–55 years

  (b) Must be off of method for 14 days to eliminate effect on FSH and estradiol levels

  (c) FSH and estradiol levels are unreliable predictors because of normal fluctuations seen during perimenopause

(3) Progestin only method including LNG IUS—two options

  (a) Continue until age 55

  (b) At age 50–54 check FSH on two occasions at least 1–2 months apart; if both levels are ≥ 30 mIU/mL, continue method one more year and then stop

(4) Nonhormonal methods—copper-releasing IUC and barrier methods—two options

  (a) Continue until amenorrhea for 1 year

  (b) If younger than age 50, continue until amenorrhea for 2 years or 1 year of amenorrhea and 2 FSH levels ≥ 30 mIU/mL at least 1–2 months apart

- Abortion

1. Medication abortion

a. Mifepristone plus misoprostol

(1) Mifepristone—19-norsteroid, progesterone antagonist

  (a) Blocks action of progesterone needed to establish and maintain placental attachment

  (b) Softens cervix

  (c) Stimulates prostaglandin synthesis by cells of early decidua

(2) Misoprostol—prostaglandin analog

  (a) Softens cervix

  (b) Stimulates uterine contractions

  (c) Common short-term side effects—nausea, vomiting, diarrhea, temporary elevation of body temperature

  (d) Prenatal exposure to misoprostol associated with major congenital anomalies, absolute risk low (about 1%)

(3) 96% to 98% effective through 9 weeks of gestation (oral mifepristone 200 mg followed by buccal misoprostol 800 mcg regimen)

(4) Contraindications—known or suspected ectopic pregnancy, IUC in place, chronic adrenal failure, current long-term systemic corticosteroid therapy, history of allergy to medication, hemorrhagic disorders, anticoagulant therapy, inherited porphyrias

(5) Method requires two clinic visits

  (a) Mifepristone orally at initial visit

  (b) Misoprostol buccally at home 24 to 48 hours after mifepristone

  (c) 1- to 2-week follow-up appointment to assess for complete abortion

  (d) May repeat misoprostol or provide aspiration if abortion is not complete at 1 week

  (e) Aspiration abortion if pregnancy persists 2–3 weeks after initiation of medication abortion

b. Methotrexate plus misoprostol

(1) Methotrexate—folic acid analog

  (a) Inhibits enzyme necessary for DNA synthesis

  (b) Acts on rapidly dividing cells of placenta

(2) 92% to 96% effective through 49 days of gestation

(3) May take up to 1 month for expulsion of gestational sac

(4) Precautions

  (a) Known teratogen when taken in large doses

  (b) Discontinue breastfeeding for 72 hours after methotrexate administration

  (c) Avoid use of folic acid supplements for 1 week after procedure—may inhibit action of methotrexate

(5) Contraindications

  (a) Chronic renal or hepatic disease

  (b) Coagulopathy or current severe anemia

  (c) Acute inflammatory bowel disease

  (d) Uncontrolled seizure disorder

(6) Two clinic visits

  (a) Methotrexate IM or orally at initial visit

  (b) Misoprostol buccally at home 3 to 7 days later

  (c) Follow-up appointment same as with mifepristone–misoprostol regimen

2. Surgical methods

a. Vacuum aspiration (first trimester)

(1) Suction curettage

(2) Local anesthetic

b. Dilation and evacuation (D&E)—can be performed up to 20 weeks' gestation

3. Preabortion health assessment and counseling

a. History

(1) LMP and menstrual history

(2) Surgical history including gynecological surgeries

(3) Contraceptive history

(4) Medical history

(5) Current medications/history of allergic responses

b. Physical examination

(1) Size of uterus

(2) Note uterine/cervical position

(3) Presence of uterine/cervical/adnexal abnormalities

  (a) Fibroids

  (b) Adnexal masses (rule out ectopic)

(4) Laboratory tests

  (a) Pregnancy test—urine/serum

  (b) Hgb/Hct

  (c) Blood type and Rh

  (d) STI evaluation if warranted (e.g., sexual assault/patient concern)

c. Counseling

(1) Discuss all pregnancy options

(2) Discuss options for termination—medication, surgical

4. Postabortion health assessment and counseling

a. Contraceptive counseling

b. Rh immunization if patient Rh negative—give at first visit with medication abortion

c. Prophylactic antibiotics may be given to surgical patients

d. Tissue examined to rule out molar pregnancy

5. Potential postabortion complications
   a. Infection
   b. Retained products of conception
   c. Trauma to uterus/cervix
   d. Excessive bleeding
   e. Warning signs
      (1) Fever
      (2) Persistent/increasing lower abdominal pain
      (3) Prolonged/excessive vaginal bleeding
      (4) Purulent vaginal discharge
      (5) No return of menses within 6 weeks

Perimenopause and Menopause Symptom Management

- HT encompasses both estrogen therapy (ET) and estrogen-progestogen therapy (EPT)
- Indications
  1. Relief of menopausal symptoms related to estrogen deficiency—vasomotor instability, vulvar/vaginal atrophy
  2. Prevention of osteoporosis
  3. Other potential benefits—reduction in risk for colon cancer
- Contraindications
  1. Active or history of deep vein thrombosis or pulmonary embolism
  2. Active or recent (past year) arterial thromboembolic disease (e.g., stroke, myocardial infarction)
  3. Known or suspected breast cancer
  4. Known or suspected estrogen-dependent cancer
  5. Liver dysfunction or disease
  6. Undiagnosed abnormal uterine bleeding
  7. Known or suspected pregnancy
  8. HT with only local (no systemic) effects may be considered with above contraindications
- Potential risks
  1. Endometrial hyperplasia/cancer—estrogen only
  2. Breast cancer
     a. Relationship with HT inconclusive
     b. Possible small, but significant increase of breast cancer with long-term HT
  3. Thromboembolic disorders—coronary heart disease, stroke, VTE
     a. Relationship with HT inconclusive
     b. Women who start HT at or close to time of menopause do not incur the same risks as those who start several years after menopause
     c. Oral ET affects cardiovascular markers—positive effects are increase in HDL-C and decrease in LDL-C levels; negative effects are increase in triglycerides and C-reactive protein levels
     d. Transdermal ET has no effect on cardiovascular markers
     e. VTE risk is lower with transdermal ET than with oral ET
- Assessment prior to initiation of HT
  1. Health history with attention to specific contraindications and precautions

2. General physical examination, gynecological examination with Pap test if indicated, breast examination, mammogram
3. Base decisions concerning HT use on woman's symptoms, treatment goals, benefit-risk analysis

- Routine follow-up after HT initiation
  1. Reevaluate in 3 months—assess therapeutic effectiveness and any problems
  2. Annual follow-up thereafter if no problems
     a. Evaluate continuing need for HT and discontinue as appropriate
     b. Consider nonhormonal drugs for osteoporosis prevention if long-term therapy needed
- Regimen options
  1. Recommendations for progestogen use for endometrial protection with standard estrogen dosing
     a. 12–14 days each month of 5 mg of medroxyprogesterone acetate (MPA) or equivalent
     b. Daily doses of 2.5 mg MPA or equivalent
     c. Levonorgestrel intrauterine system
     d. Vaginal progesterone gel 45 mg daily or 12–14 days each month
  2. Continuous-combined regimen EPT
     a. Estrogen and progestin every day
     b. Lower cumulative dose of progestin than with cyclic regimens
     c. May initially have unpredictable bleeding
     d. After several months endometrium atrophies and amenorrhea usually results
     e. No estrogen-free period during which vasomotor symptoms can occur
  3. Continuous-cyclic regimen
     a. Estrogen every day
     b. Progestin added 10 to 14 days each month
     c. No estrogen-free period during which vasomotor symptoms can occur
     d. Withdrawal bleeding when progestin withdrawn each month, may start 1–2 days earlier depending on dose and type of progestin used
  4. Cyclic regimen
     a. Estrogen days 1 to 25
     b. Progestin added last 10 to 14 days
     c. Followed by 3 to 6 days of no therapy
     d. Withdrawal bleeding when progestin withdrawn each month
     e. Less popular option because of vasomotor symptoms on hormone-free days
  5. Continuous unopposed estrogen—for woman without uterus
  6. Types of estrogen—17β-estradiol, estradiol acetate, conjugated estrogen, estropipate (estrone), estradiol hemihydrate, estriol (plant based)
  7. Types of progestogens—medroxyprogesterone acetate, norethindrone, norethindrone acetate, norgestrel, progesterone, micronized progesterone (plant based), levonorgestrel intrauterine system

8. Routes of administration
   a. Oral
      (1) Estrogen, progestogen, or combination
      (2) First-pass metabolism determines bioavailability
      (3) Increased HDL-C and decreased LDL-C
      (4) Increased triglycerides
      (5) Increased C-reactive protein
   b. Transdermal patches
      (1) Estrogen and progestogen combined or estrogen only
      (2) May use lower doses as not dependent on GI absorption and no first-pass hepatic metabolism
      (3) No significant impact on HDL-C, LDL-C, triglycerides, or C-reactive protein
      (4) May have less adverse effects on gallbladder and coagulation factors than oral estrogen
   c. Vaginal estrogen creams and tablets
      (1) Treatment of vulvar and vaginal atrophy
      (2) Will not provide relief from vasomotor symptoms
      (3) Little or no systemic absorption
      (4) Do not need cyclic progestogen with low-dose vaginal estrogen
   d. Estrogen vaginal ring (Estring)
      (1) Little or no systemic absorption
      (2) Approved for treatment of vulvar/vaginal atrophy
      (3) Will not relieve vasomotor symptoms
      (4) 90 days duration
      (5) Do not need cyclic progestogen
   e. Estrogen vaginal ring (Femring)
      (1) Systemic absorption
      (2) Approved for treatment of vasomotor symptoms and vulvar/vaginal atrophy
      (3) 90 days duration
      (4) Requires added progestogen if have intact uterus
   f. Topical sprays, gels, and emulsions—17β-estradiol
      (1) Systemic absorption
      (2) No significant impact on HDL or triglycerides
      (3) May have less adverse effects on gallbladder and coagulation factors than oral estrogen
      (4) Need cyclic progestogen with intact uterus
      (5) Topical progesterone preparations may not provide sufficient endometrial protection
9. Progestogen-only may be used if estrogen is contraindicated
   a. Effective in relieving vasomotor symptoms; may have a positive impact on calcium balance
   b. Not effective in relief of vulvovaginal symptoms; may have adverse effect on lipid metabolism
10. Androgens—no FDA-approved androgen products for treatment of menopausal vasomotor symptoms or for sexual dysfunction
11. Combination of conjugated estrogen and an estrogen agonist/antagonist (bazedoxifene)—FDA approved for treatment of moderate to severe vasomotor symptoms and prevention of osteoporosis
12. Bioidentical hormones
   a. Hormones chemically identical to hormones produced by women during their reproductive years—17β-estradiol, estrone, estradiol, progesterone, testosterone
   b. Bioidentical hormone therapy (BHT) provides one or more of these hormones as active ingredients
   c. 17β-estradiol is available in several FDA-approved ET products in oral, transdermal, transcutaneous, and vaginal preparations
   d. Progesterone is available in an FDA-approved oral capsule and vaginal gels
   e. Custom compounded BHT uses commercially available hormones with the type and amount prescribed by the clinician
   f. Custom compounded BHT products are *not* FDA approved; there is no evidence that they are safer than conventional HT; the same contraindications apply to their use
   g. No evidence that saliva testing is effective for customizing hormone dosing regimens

- Side effects of HT
   1. Breast tenderness—estrogen or progestogen (usually subsides after first few weeks)
   2. Nausea—estrogen (relieved if taken at mealtime or bedtime)
   3. Skin irritation with transdermal patches
   4. Fluid retention and bloating—estrogen or progestogen
   5. Alterations in mood—progestogen
- Management of side effects may include:
   1. Lowering dose
   2. Altering route of administration
   3. Changing to different formulation
- Management of bleeding during HT
   1. Continuous-cyclic regimen—usually experience some uterine bleeding; starts last few days of progestin administration or during progestin-free days; earlier bleeding, heavy or persistent bleeding may indicate endometrial hyperplasia and warrants endometrial evaluation
   2. Continuous-combined regimen—erratic spotting and light bleeding of 1 to 5 days duration in first year; need endometrial evaluation if bleeding heavier or longer than usual or if resumes after several months of amenorrhea
   3. Use of levonorgestrel IUD for progestogen may result in less bleeding
- Nonhormonal management of vasomotor symptoms
   1. Serotonin norepinephrine reuptake inhibitors (SNRIs) and selective serotonin reuptake inhibitors (SSRIs) may diminish hot flash severity and frequency; a 7.5-mg formulation of paroxetine has been approved by FDA for this purpose
   2. Gabapentin, an anticonvulsant medication, has been shown to be effective in reduction of severity and frequency of hot flashes—not FDA approved for this purpose
   3. Avoid caffeine, alcohol, cigarettes, spicy foods, and big meals
   4. Engage in regular, moderate exercise—may also help alleviate insomnia
   5. Wear layers and natural fibers
   6. Sleep in a cool room
   7. Keep an insulated bottle of ice water available
   8. Use stress management and relaxation techniques
   9. Black cohosh—some data support beneficial effect on vasomotor symptoms similar to estrogen; multiple products and formulations available; rare side effects of intestinal upset, headache, dizziness with larger doses; safety for use beyond 6 months not established

10. Current data do not support the use of isoflavones (soy and red clover), evening primrose oil, licorice root, or St. John's wort for relief of vasomotor symptoms
- Nonhormonal management of vulvovaginal symptoms
  1. Ospemifene—oral estrogen agonist/antagonist FDA approved for treatment of dyspareunia related to vulvovaginal atrophy; makes vaginal tissue thicker and less fragile

2. Use water-soluble lubricants and vaginal moisturizers
3. Engage in regular sexual activity
4. Use noncoital methods of sexual expression—massage, mutual masturbation if penetration is painful

---

Questions

Select the best answer.

1. Which of the following lab values would be expected with menopause?
   a. Decreased FSH, increased LH, decreased estradiol
   b. Decreased LH, increased FSH, increased estradiol
   c. Increased FSH, increased LH, decreased estradiol
   d. Increased LH, decreased FSH, increased estradiol
2. Which of the following physical examination and screening tests should be part of the routine well-woman visit every year for females ages 40 to 60 years?
   a. Chlamydia test
   b. Clinical breast examination
   c. Pelvic examination
   d. Pap test
3. The most prevalent contraceptive method among married women in the United States is:
   a. Combination oral contraceptives
   b. Condoms
   c. Sterilization
   d. Withdrawal
4. A 54-year-old female with vaginal dryness causing irritation and dyspareunia has no problem with hot flashes and has a bone densitometry T-score of 1.0. The best treatment for her would be:
   a. Continuous-combined regimen HT
   b. Cyclic HT with added testosterone
   c. Estrogen vaginal ring
   d. Progestin-only therapy
5. An advantage of continuous-combined HT over continuous-cyclic HT regimens is:
   a. No estrogen-free period during which vasomotor symptoms can occur
   b. Predictable withdrawal bleeding each month
   c. Lower cumulative dose of progestin
   d. Less negative impact on triglyceride levels
6. Which of the following women should have an endometrial biopsy/evaluation?
   a. Woman on continuous-cyclic HT regimen with amenorrhea
   b. Woman on continuous-cyclic HT regimen with bleeding starting last few days of progestogen administration each month
   c. Woman on continuous-combined HT regimen with irregular bleeding in the first year of use
   d. Woman on continuous-combined HT regimen with spotting that occurs after several months of amenorrhea
7. The sebaceous glands located within the areola are called:
   a. Bartholin's glands
   b. Cowper's glands
   c. Montgomery's glands
   d. Skene's glands
8. The lymph nodes that drain directly into the infraclavicular nodes are the:
   a. Central nodes
   b. Lateral nodes
   c. Subscapular nodes
   d. Supraclavicular nodes
9. A vaginal pH less than 4.5 is an expected finding:
   a. In a healthy reproductive-age woman
   b. In a menopausal woman with atrophic vaginitis
   c. In a reproductive-age woman with trichomoniasis
   d. In a healthy prepubertal-age girl
10. The predominant vaginal organism responsible for an acidic pH is:
    a. *Doderlein bacilli*
    b. *Gardnerella*
    c. *Haemophilus*
    d. *Lactobacilli*
11. Squamous metaplasia of the cervix occurs within the:
    a. Columnar epithelium
    b. Internal cervical os
    c. Squamous epithelium
    d. Transformation zone
12. Which of the following is true concerning the luteal phase of the menstrual cycle?
    a. It begins at the time of the LH surge
    b. It corresponds with the uterine proliferative phase
    c. There is thickened cervical mucus
    d. It lasts an average of 10 days from time of ovulation to menses
13. Estrogen is released by the ovary in response to:
    a. FSH
    b. GnRH
    c. hCG
    d. LH
14. The predominant estrogen after menopause is:
    a. Estradiol
    b. Estriol
    c. Estrone
    d. Estropipate
15. Which of the following androgens can be converted to estradiol?
    a. Androstenedione
    b. Cortisol
    c. DHA
    d. Testosterone

16. Which phase of the menstrual cycle is the most variable?
    a. Follicular
    b. Luteal
    c. Ovarian
    d. Secretory

17. Which hormone is dominant during the proliferative phase of the menstrual cycle?
    a. Estrogen
    b. LH
    c. Progesterone
    d. Prolactin

18. A 28-year-old woman who has a positive test for *BRCA1* mutation and is negative for *BRCA2* mutation should be advised:
    a. Her lifetime risk for breast cancer is twice that of a woman without the gene mutation
    b. Because she does not have the *BRCA2* mutation she is not at increased risk for breast cancer
    c. She should start having a yearly combination mammogram and MRI
    d. Her only prophylactic option is a bilateral mastectomy after menopause

19. A 52-year-old female asks you if she should take estrogen to help her memory because she is sometimes forgetful and has difficulty concentrating. Her mother had dementia at age 65. The best initial response would be:
    a. Advise her that she may benefit from taking estrogen for about 5 years
    b. Ask about other menopausal symptoms such as hot flashes and night sweats
    c. Tell her the WHIMS study showed an increase in dementia for women her age who took estrogen
    d. Tell her that her memory changes are likely caused by depression

20. A 50-year-old female who had a hysterectomy 5 years ago for dysfunctional uterine bleeding presents with complaints of severe hot flashes and night sweats for the past few months. Her lipid profile is significant for cholesterol of 220 mg/dL and triglycerides of 350 mg/dL. The most appropriate therapy for her vasomotor symptoms at this time would be:
    a. Continuous-combined oral HT
    b. Estrogen agonist/antagonist (ospemifene)
    c. Transdermal estrogen patch
    d. Vaginal estrogen cream

21. Which of the following estrogen replacement options does *not* require opposition by a progestogen in a woman with an intact uterus?
    a. Bioidentical oral estrogen formulation
    b. Estring vaginal ring
    c. Plant-based (estriol) oral estrogen
    d. Transdermal estrogen patch

22. Adding potassium hydroxide (KOH) to a wet mount slide before viewing it under the microscope is useful in the detection of:
    a. Clue cells
    b. Pseudohyphae
    c. Trichomonads
    d. White blood cells

23. A 45-year-old-female is concerned that she may be pregnant because she is 12 days late for her period. The best initial pregnancy test to obtain is:
    a. Qualitative sensitive urine hCG test
    b. Qualitative serum hCG test
    c. Quantitative sensitive urine hCG test
    d. Quantitative serum hCG test

24. The American Cancer Society recommends yearly mammogram screening beginning at age:
    a. 35
    b. 40
    c. 45
    d. 50

25. A woman who was treated for primary syphilis 1 year ago now has the following test results: VDRL nonreactive and FTA-ABS positive. These findings indicate:
    a. She most likely was not adequately treated for her primary syphilis 1 year ago
    b. She has most likely become reinfected since her treatment 1 year ago
    c. She most likely has some other condition that is causing a false-positive FTA-ABS
    d. She most likely was treated adequately for her syphilis and has not become reinfected

26. When evaluating cervical mucus, the term *spinnbarkeit* refers to:
    a. Amount
    b. Cellularity
    c. Clarity
    d. Elasticity

27. A 24-year-old female presents to your office with a request for combination oral contraceptives. Her current medications include a bronchodilator for asthma. Management for this client should include advising her that:
    a. Combination oral contraceptives are not recommended for women with asthma
    b. Combination oral contraceptives may potentiate the action of her bronchodilator
    c. She should use a backup method if using the bronchodilator several days in a row
    d. Use of progestin-only contraceptive injections may reduce her asthma attacks

28. Which of the following contraceptive methods would be best for a woman with a seizure disorder who is taking phenytoin?
    a. Combination oral contraceptives
    b. Transdermal contraceptive patch
    c. Progestin-only oral contraceptives
    d. Progestin-only contraceptive injections

29. A client calls the clinic on Tuesday morning. She had unprotected sex Friday night and is interested in emergency contraception. Appropriate information for this client would include:
    a. Emergency contraception pills are very effective for a medication abortion in early pregnancy
    b. If she is not midcycle when she had sex, she does not need emergency contraception
    c. It is too late for emergency contraceptive pills, but insertion of an IUC is an option

d. She can use emergency contraception pills even if she has had other unprotected sex since her last period

30. The levonorgestrel-releasing IUC may be a better choice than the copper-releasing IUC for a woman who:
    a. Has never been pregnant
    b. Has dysmenorrhea
    c. Is currently breastfeeding
    d. Is sure she does not want more children

31. A 28-year-old female who has had an IUC for 2 years has a Pap test showing actinomycosis. She has no symptoms of infection. Appropriate management would include:
    a. Removing the IUC and repeating the Pap test in 6 months
    b. Removing the IUC, treating with doxycycline, and repeating the Pap test in 1 year
    c. Keeping the IUC and repeating the Pap test in 3 years
    d. Keeping the IUC, treating with doxycycline, and repeating the Pap test in 3 months

32. Which of the following diaphragms would be best for a woman with very firm vaginal tone?
    a. Arcing spring
    b. Coil spring
    c. Flat spring
    d. Wide seal

33. The type of skin lesion seen initially with toxic shock syndrome is:
    a. Diffuse sunburn-like rash
    b. Multiple vesicles on chest and extremities
    c. Petechiae on mucomembranous tissues
    d. Ulcerative lesions in genital area

34. Advantages of the cervical cap over the diaphragm include:
    a. It is has a lower failure rate
    b. It is easier to insert
    c. It can remain in place for 48 hours
    d. Spermicide is not needed

35. Which of the following statements concerning a transcervical (Essure) sterilization procedure is correct?
    a. The fallopian tubes are occluded with a silastic band
    b. The success of reversals is higher than with other sterilization methods
    c. It is effective within 1 to 2 weeks after the procedure
    d. The patient needs to return for a hystosalpingogram 3 months after the procedure

36. The main mechanism of action of misopristol in medically induced abortion is:
    a. Blocking the action of progesterone
    b. Inhibiting enzymes necessary for DNA synthesis
    c. Stimulating synthesis of prostaglandin by cells of the early decidua
    d. Stimulating uterine contractions

37. Potential disadvantages of progestin-only implants include:
    a. May have increased side effects in women who are underweight
    b. May cause a significant decrease in bone mineral density
    c. May cause irregular bleeding and spotting
    d. Return to fertility after discontinuation may take several months

38. The CDC-recommended test for *Chlamydia* is:
    a. Nucleic acid amplification test (NAAT)
    b. Polymerase chain reaction (PCR) test
    c. Tissue culture
    d. Tzanck preparation test

39. Which endogenous estrogen is known as the "estrogen of pregnancy"?
    a. Estradiol
    b. Estriol
    c. Estrone
    d. Estropipate

40. Increased production of _____ is associated with primary dysmenorrhea.
    a. Androstenedione
    b. Arachidonic acid
    c. Cortisol
    d. Prostaglandin

41. An 18-year-old female presents with genital warts. Appropriate tests to consider at this visit include:
    a. *Chlamydia* test
    b. HPV test
    c. Pap test
    d. Type-specific herpes serologic test

42. Which of the following is *not* an FDA-approved indication for the use of hormone therapy (HT)?
    a. Prevention of cardiovascular disease
    b. Prevention of osteoporosis
    c. Relief of moderate to severe symptoms of vaginal atrophy
    d. Relief of moderate to severe vasomotor symptoms

43. An advantage of the transdermal patch over oral delivery of estrogen for the woman experiencing menopausal symptoms is that the transdermal delivery method:
    a. Does not require addition of a progestogen
    b. Has less adverse effects on coagulation factors
    c. Improves vulvovaginal symptoms more quickly
    d. Increases HDL-C and decreases LDL-C levels

44. A woman who is requesting contraception and who also wants to get pregnant in 1 year should avoid using:
    a. Combination oral contraceptives
    b. Fertility awareness methods
    c. Progestin-only oral contraceptives
    d. Progestin-only contraceptive injections

45. A woman plans to use the calendar method for contraception. She has charted her menstrual cycles for several months and has noted her longest cycle to be 30 days and her shortest cycle to be 27 days. She should abstain from sexual intercourse each cycle from day ___ through day ___.
    a. 9; 19
    b. 10; 15
    c. 11; 18
    d. 12; 16

46. Which of the following statements by a client indicates she needs additional information about use of the contraceptive vaginal ring?
    a. I should insert a new ring every 7 days
    b. I should expect to have regular periods while using the ring

c. My partner can use a male condom while I am wearing the ring

d. The exact position of the ring in the vagina is not important

47. According to CDC, initiating progestin-only contraceptive injections (DMPA) is a category 3 when which of the following conditions exists?

   a. Age 35 years or older and smoking more than 15 cigarettes daily

   b. History of deep vein thrombosis or pulmonary emboli

   c. Unexplained vaginal bleeding prior to evaluation

   d. Use of drugs that alter liver enzymes

48. A 4-week-postpartum woman who is breastfeeding on demand without supplements presents in your office to discuss her contraceptive options. She plans to continue breastfeeding for at least 6 months. Information for this woman concerning the lactational amenorrhea method of contraception should include:

   a. The expected failure rate for this method of contraception is about 20%

   b. This method is considered effective for only 3 months postpartum

   c. The woman can rely on this method as long as she is not having periods

   d. Another method of contraception should be considered when the infant begins sleeping through the night

49. A 4-week-postpartum woman who is breastfeeding now and plans to start weaning the baby in the next month is in your office to discuss her contraceptive options. She has a BMI of 35 (obese). Of the following, the best contraceptive choice for her at this time would be:

   a. Combination oral contraceptives

   b. Fertility awareness method

   c. Lactational amenorrhea method

   d. Progestin-only pills

50. A woman using a diaphragm for contraception has sexual intercourse at 8:00 p.m. on Friday, at 2:00 a.m. on Saturday, and again at 8:00 a.m. on Saturday. When can she safely remove her diaphragm for effective contraception while minimizing problems related to leaving the diaphragm in for extended periods of time?

   a. 10:00 a.m. on Saturday

   b. 2:00 p.m. on Saturday

   c. 10:00 p.m. on Saturday

   d. 8:00 a.m. on Sunday

51. An individual who either has acute active hepatitis B infection or who is a carrier (chronic active state) would have a positive test for:

   a. Hepatitis B surface antigen

   b. Hepatitis B surface antibody

   c. Hepatitis B e-antigen

   d. Hepatitis B e-antibody

52. Which of the following statements is true concerning rapid HIV tests when compared with EIA blood tests sent to a lab?

   a. It may take longer after exposure for a rapid HIV test to be positive

   b. Positive results of rapid HIV test are definitive, so a confirmatory test is not necessary

   c. EIA blood test sent to lab can detect presence of virus as well as antibodies

   d. Sensitivity of both types of tests is the same

53. A 58-year-old female has a bone densitometry test with the results of T-score –2.0. This indicates the following:

   a. She has bone density that is greater than that of most women her age

   b. She has bone density that is equal to that of a young normal adult

   c. She has bone loss that is at the level for a diagnosis of osteopenia

   d. She has bone loss that is at the level for a diagnosis of osteoporosis

54. A female patient presents with no symptoms but concern because she had sexual intercourse 3 weeks ago with a new partner who has recently told her he had a history of genital herpes. She wants to know if there is a test she can have at this visit to see if she has been infected. The best response would be:

   a. A Pap test can be done at this visit that will show if she has been infected

   b. A blood test can be done at this visit to see if she has been recently infected

   c. If she does not develop lesions in the next 4 to 8 weeks, she is not infected

   d. She can have a blood test in 1 to 2 months to determine whether she has herpes antibodies

55. The anatomic area that contains the urethral/vaginal openings, hymen, Skene's glands, and Bartholin's glands is called the:

   a. Labia majora

   b. Perineum

   c. Vestibule

   d. Vulva

56. Findings on a pelvic examination of a 25-year-old nulliparous female include uterus 8 cm in length, right ovary 3 cm × 2 cm, and left ovary not palpable. These findings indicate a/an:

   a. Normal uterus, normal ovaries

   b. Normal uterus, enlarged right ovary

   c. Enlarged uterus, normal ovaries

   d. Enlarged uterus, enlarged right ovary

57. Which of the following occurs first during female puberty?

   a. Beginning breast development

   b. Beginning pubic hair development

   c. Growth spurt peak

   d. Menstruation

58. Which of the following structures produces gonadotropin-releasing hormone (GnRH)?

   a. Anterior pituitary gland

   b. Hypothalamus

   c. Posterior pituitary gland

   d. Ovaries

59. Which of the following list of events is in the correct chronological order?

   a. LH surge, ovulation, rise in BBT, thickened cervical mucus

   b. Ovulation, LH surge, thickened cervical mucus, rise in BBT

   c. Rise in BBT, thickened cervical mucus, ovulation, LH surge

   d. Thickened cervical mucus, rise in BBT, LH surge, ovulation

60. According to CDC recommendations, which of the following would be considered a category 4 situation for the indicated contraceptive method?
    a. Levonorgestrel IUC for woman with endometriosis
    b. Copper IUC for woman with history of breast cancer
    c. Progestin-only pills for woman with past history of deep vein thrombosis
    d. Vaginal contraceptive ring for woman older than 35 years of age who smokes 1 pack of cigarettes per day (ppd)

61. An advantage of the female condom is:
    a. It can be used with a male condom for added protection
    b. It can be used for repeated acts of intercourse
    c. It may be used by individuals with latex allergy
    d. It has a lower failure rate than the male condom does

62. Noncontraceptive benefits of combination oral contraceptives include all of the following *except*:
    a. Decrease in risk for benign breast disease
    b. Decrease in risk for cervical cancer
    c. Decrease in risk for endometrial cancer
    d. Decrease in risk for ovarian cancer

63. For which of the contraceptive methods is there the *least* difference between the perfect use and typical use failure rates?
    a. Combination oral contraceptives
    b. Diaphragm
    c. Intrauterine contraceptive
    d. Male condom

64. A woman who weighs 200 lbs or more may have decreased effectiveness with which of the following contraceptive methods?
    a. Progestin-only injectable contraception
    b. Contraceptive vaginal ring
    c. Levonorgestrel intrauterine system
    d. Transdermal contraceptive system

65. The mechanism by which drugs that increase production of cytochrome P-450 may decrease the effectiveness of combination oral contraceptives (COC) is:
    a. Decrease in absorption in the gastrointestinal tract
    b. Decrease in enterohepatic recirculation
    c. Increase in first-pass metabolism in the liver
    d. Increase in protein binding at receptor sites

66. A 20-year-old female who has a BMI of 38 (obese) presents for her first DMPA injection. Concerns in administering DMPA to this woman include:
    a. She may need a larger dose than the usual 150 mg
    b. She should return for repeat injections every 2 months
    c. You should massage the injection site well to ensure absorption
    d. You should choose a site that ensures deep IM injection

67. Instructions for progestin-only oral contraceptive users should include:
    a. If you are more than 3 hours late taking a pill, use a backup method for 48 hours
    b. If two pills are missed in the third week of the pack, throw away the pack and start a new one
    c. If you miss pills in the fourth week of the pack, you do not have to use a backup method
    d. If you miss two pills in the first week of the pack, make them up and use a backup method for 7 days

68. A 60-year-old female currently on a cyclic HT regimen is at your office for a routine well-woman examination. She states she has been healthy in the last year and is having no problems with HT. On bimanual examination, a 4-cm nontender right ovary is palpated. Appropriate management would include:
    a. Discontinue HT and repeat the bimanual examination in 2 months
    b. Have her return in 1 year because this is a normal finding for a 63-year-old woman
    c. Refer her to a gynecologist for further evaluation
    d. Switch to a continuous HT regimen and reexamine her in 2 months

69. The structure in the breast that is responsible for milk production is the:
    a. Areola
    b. Alveoli
    c. Lobule
    d. Lactiferous sinus

70. The hormone that stimulates synthesis of milk is:
    a. Aldosterone
    b. Estrogen
    c. Progesterone
    d. Prolactin

71. The menopausal woman may experience some changes in sensation or the orgasmic experience during sexual activity related to:
    a. Decreased vasocongestion and decreased vaginal expansion
    b. Decreased vasocongestion and increased vaginal expansion
    c. Increased vasocongestion and decreased vaginal expansion
    d. Increased vasocongestion and increased vaginal expansion

72. Which of the following contraceptive choices should *not* be recommended for the perimenopausal woman who is having irregular menses?
    a. Combination oral contraceptives
    b. Diaphragm
    c. Fertility awareness methods
    d. LNG intrauterine system

73. The term that best describes an individual's physical and/or romantic attractions to other people is:
    a. Gender identity
    b. Sexual drive
    c. Sexual motivation
    d. Sexual orientation

74. A 26-year-old female is planning to use basal body temperatures for contraception. Which of the following statements would indicate that she needs further instruction on this method?
    a. I will take my temperature the same time each day before getting out of bed
    b. I know that I am about to ovulate when my temperature rises at least 0.4 degrees Fahrenheit
    c. I will need to use a special thermometer to take my basal body temperature
    d. A rise of 0.4 degrees Fahrenheit above my baseline for 3 days indicates it is safe to have sex

75. A woman who has been using a copper-releasing intrauterine contraceptive (IUC) presents with a positive pregnancy test. After determining that the pregnancy is intrauterine and the IUC

is in place, information that should be provided to the woman includes:

   a. Removing the IUC may increase the chance of a spontaneous abortion

   b. The baby is at risk for congenital defects related to copper exposure

   c. The IUC should be removed promptly regardless of her plans for the pregnancy

   d. There is no risk to the baby if she leaves the IUC in place until delivery

76. Instructions/information for a new user of combination oral contraceptives should include:

   a. Combination oral contraceptives may decrease the effectiveness of some antibiotics

   b. Discontinue your pills immediately if you miss a period

   c. Start the first pack of pills on the last day of your next period

   d. Sunday starters should use a backup method for the first week of the first pack of pills

77. The most commonly used method of determining bone density to establish a diagnosis of osteoporosis or the need for preventive treatment is:

   a. Dual energy X-ray absorptiometry

   b. Quantitative computerized tomography

   c. Quantitative ultrasound

   d. Single X-ray absorptiometry

78. Instructions for the use of nonoxynol-9 spermicide should include:

   a. Place spermicide close to the opening of the vagina for maximal effectiveness

   b. Remove excess spermicide from vagina within 6 hours to reduce vaginal irritation

   c. When used with a condom, spermicide will further decrease risk for STI

   d. Frequent use of spermicide may cause vaginal changes, making you more susceptible to HIV infection

79. According to CDC recommendations, which of the following is considered to be a category 4 condition for use of the indicated contraceptive method?

   a. Use of emergency contraceptive pills by a woman who has history of deep vein thrombosis

   b. Insertion of IUC in a woman with a history of PID

   c. Use of combination oral contraception by a 40-year-old woman who has migraine headaches without aura

   d. Use of progestin-only pills by a woman who has type 2 diabetes

80. Which of the following statements concerning coitus interruptus is *not* correct?

   a. It has a lower perfect use failure rate than the cervical cap

   b. It may result in a decreased risk for HIV transmission to the female partner

   c. Men are typically not able to predict the timing of ejaculation

   d. There is a decreased chance for the presence of pre-ejaculatory sperm with repeat acts of intercourse

Answers with Rationales

1. c. Increased FSH, increased LH, decreased estradiol

   During the menopause transition, there is a decreased production of estradiol as the number of responsive ovarian follicles decreases. This decrease in estradiol triggers the increased release of FSH and LH from the anterior pituitary gland.

2. b. Clinical breast examination

   ACOG and American Cancer Society recommend annual clinical breast examination for women age 40 and older. Routine Pap tests for women ages 40 to 65 is either every 5 years with HPV testing or every 3 years without HPV testing. Pelvic examinations other than during routine Pap tests are done if history or other physical examination findings indicate the need. Chlamydia testing in this age group is based on risk factors and symptoms of possible infection.

3. c. Sterilization

   The most prevalent contraceptive method among married women in the United States is sterilization (female and male).

4. c. Estrogen vaginal ring

   The menopausal woman who has symptoms related to vulvar/vaginal atrophy, no vasomotor symptoms, and normal bone density is best treated with local vaginal estrogen.

5. c. Lower cumulative dose of progestin

   Estrogen and progestin are taken every day with a continuous-combined HT regimen with lower cumulative dose of progestin than a continuous-cyclic HT regimen in which estrogen is taken every day and larger doses of progestin are added 10 to 14 days each month.

6. d. Woman on continuous-combined HT regimen with spotting that occurs after several months of amenorrhea

   Women using continuous-combined HT may initially have some unpredictable spotting and bleeding. After several months of use, the endometrium atrophies and amenorrhea usually results. If spotting or bleeding recurs after several months of amenorrhea, endometrial evaluation is warranted.

7. c. Montgomery's glands

   Montgomery's glands are the sebaceous glands that circle the nipple within the area of the areola.

8. a. Central nodes

   The pectoral, subscapular, and lateral axillary lymph nodes drain into the central nodes that are located high in the axilla between the anterior and posterior axillary nodes and are the most likely to be palpable. The central nodes drain into the infraclavicular and supraclavicular nodes.

9. a. In a healthy reproductive-age woman

   An acidic vagina pH (less than 4.5) is an expected finding in a healthy reproductive-age woman. This acidic pH is the result of the prevalence of *Lactobacilli* as a result of the influence of estrogen initiated during puberty. Vaginal infections such as trichomoniasis and bacterial vaginosis may alter the pH, making it alkaline. Women with atrophic vaginitis will also have a more alkaline pH as the result of decreased estrogen levels.

10. d. *Lactobacilli*
    Lactobacilli is the predominant vaginal organism responsible for an acidic pH in the reproductive-age woman.

11. d. Transformation zone
    Squamous metaplasia is the process whereby columnar cells of the endocervix are replaced by mature squamous epithelium. The transformation zone is the area around the junction of squamous and columnar cells (squamocolumnar junction) where squamous metaplasia occurs.

12. c. There is thickened cervical mucus
    The luteal phase of the menstrual cycle begins after ovulation occurs, lasts approximately 14 days (± 2 days), and ends with the first day of menses. Progesterone secreted from the corpus luteum causes thickened cervical mucus. The luteal phase corresponds with the uterine secretory phase.

13. a. FSH
    Follicle-stimulating hormone (FSH) is released by the anterior pituitary gland in response to GnRH from the hypothalamus. FSH stimulates ovarian follicular growth, resulting in increased levels of the estradiol.

14. c. Estrone
    The predominant estrogen after menopause is estrone. Estrone is converted from androstenedione produced by the adrenal gland and ovarian stroma.

15. d. Testosterone
    Testosterone is produced in the adrenal gland, ovarian stroma, and through conversion of androstenedione and DHA in peripheral tissues. Testosterone is aromatized to estradiol in peripheral tissues.

16. a. Follicular
    The follicular phase begins day 1 of menses and ends with ovulation. This phase is variable in time frame more so than the luteal phase, which is normally 14 days (± 2 days).

17. a. Estrogen
    Estrogen is the predominant hormone during the uterine proliferative phase of the menstrual cycle, which correlates with the ovarian follicular phase. Under the influence of estrogen, the endometrium grows/thickens in the proliferative phase.

18. c. She should start having a yearly combination mammogram and MRI
    ACOG recommends the combination of yearly mammogram and MRI in women with *BRCA* mutation beginning at age 25 or younger based on earliest age of onset of breast cancer in the family.

19. b. Ask about other menopausal symptoms such as hot flashes and night sweats
    Although more history and physical examination may be warranted, the best answer choice is to initially ask about other menopausal symptoms such as hot flashes and night sweats. These vasomotor symptoms can contribute to memory impairment and difficulty concentrating as a result of sleep disturbance. If she has vasomotor symptoms, short-term hormone therapy may be an option.

20. c. Transdermal estrogen patch
    The transdermal estrogen patch delivery method has no significant impact on HDL-C, LDL-C, triglycerides, or C-reactive protein. The estrogen agonist/antagonist (ospemifene) and vaginal estrogen cream are indicated for vulvar vaginal atrophy and related symptoms. Oral HT may increase HDL-C, triglycerides, and C-reactive protein and decrease LDL-C.

21. b. Estring vaginal ring
    Estring vaginal ring has little or no systemic absorption and does not require opposition by a progestogen.

22. b. Pseudohyphae
    The addition of potassium hydroxide (KOH) to the vaginal wet mount slide facilitates visualization of *Candida pseudohyphae* and buds.

23. a. Qualitative sensitive urine hCG test
    Sensitive urine hCG tests may detect pregnancy as early as 28 days from last menstrual period. Cross-reactions with other hormones are not a problem. A qualitative (positive/negative) test is the appropriate pregnancy test choice.

24. b. 40
    The American Cancer Society and ACOG recommend yearly mammograms for women starting at age 40.

25. d. She most likely was treated adequately for her syphilis and has not become reinfected
    Nontreponemal tests (VDRL, RPR) usually become nonreactive with time after treatment. Treponemal tests (FTA-ABS, TPI) usually remain positive indefinitely after treatment.

26. d. Elasticity
    Spinnbarkeit refers to the elasticity of cervical mucus (ability to be stretched between two fingers) seen at ovulation and under the influence of estrogen.

27. b. Combination oral contraceptives may potentiate the action of her bronchodilator
    Combination oral contraceptives may potentiate the action of some drugs to include benzodiazepines, tricyclic antidepressants, and theophylline.

28. d. Progestin-only contraceptive injections
    Some anticonvulsant medications, including phenytoin, induce cytochrome P-450 enzyme activity and can cause increased first-pass metabolism of combination oral contraceptives as well as progestin-only pills. Although there is no first-pass metabolism with transdermal contraceptive patch, the FDA applies the same warning about possible reduced efficacy. Depo medroxyprogesterone acetate injection effectiveness is not affected by anticonvulsant medications and may decrease the incidence of seizures in affected individuals.

29. d. She can use emergency contraception pills even if she has had other unprotected sex since her last period
    Emergency contraception pills should be taken as soon as possible after unprotected sex and within 120 hours for maximum effectiveness. If the woman has had previous unprotected sex since her last period and more than 120 hours ago, obtain a urine pregnancy test to rule out an existing pregnancy.

30. b. Has dysmenorrhea
    The levonorgestrel-releasing IUC may cause reduced menstrual bleeding or amenorrhea and reduce dysmenorrhea. The copper-releasing IUC may increase dysmenorrhea.

31. c. Keeping the IUC and repeating the Pap test in 3 years
    Actinomyces is a normal female genital tract organism. IUC users are more likely to have colonization. Pelvic infection from *Actinomyces* is a very rare although serious infection if it occurs.

The Pap test does not diagnose actinomycosis infection. The asymptomatic IUC user should be informed of the Pap test result and advised that the IUC does not need to be removed nor does she need any antibiotic treatment unless infection occurs.

32. c. Flat spring

The flat spring diaphragm has gentle spring strength and is good for a woman with very firm vaginal tone.

33. a. Diffuse sunburn-like rash

The risk of toxic shock is only 2 to 3/100,000 women per year, but theoretically may be increased in women who use the diaphragm or sponge. Symptoms of toxic shock include high fever, nausea/vomiting/diarrhea, syncope, joint/muscle aches, and a diffuse rash resembling sunburn.

34. c. It can remain in place for 48 hours

The diaphragm should not be left in place for more than 24 hours. The cervical cap may be left in place for up to 48 hours.

35. d. The patient needs to return for a hystosalpingogram 3 months after the procedure

The transcervical occlusion method of female sterilization (Essure) does not become effective immediately. The patient should use another method of contraception for 3 months after the procedure and then return for hystosalpingogram to confirm correct placement of the micro inserts and total tubal occlusion.

36. d. Stimulating uterine contractions

Misoprostol is commonly used in conjunction with mifepristone or methotrexate for medical abortions. Misoprostol is a prostaglandin analog. It softens the cervix and stimulates uterine contractions.

37. c. May cause irregular bleeding and spotting

Users of progestin-only implants may have irregular, prolonged, and more frequent bleeding especially in the first few months. Progestin-only implants do not cause any decrease in bone mineral density. Most users ovulate within 6 weeks after removal.

38. a. Nucleic acid amplification test (NAAT)

The CDC-recommended test for *Chlamydia* is NAAT. NAAT provides the option of testing with urine, vaginal (provider or patient obtained), or endocervical sample.

39. b. Estriol

Estriol is the least potent of the estrogens. It is derived from conversion of estrone and estradiol in the liver, uterus, placenta, and fetal adrenal gland.

40. d. Prostaglandin

Prostaglandins act at target sites near areas of secretion. They regulate contraction and relaxation of smooth muscle. Prostaglandins are produced by the endometrium with peak levels in the late secretory phase. They stimulate uterine myometrial contractions.

41. a. *Chlamydia* test

The 18-year-old female with one sexually transmitted infection is at risk for other sexually transmitted infections such as *Chlamydia*. Pap tests and HPV testing are not appropriate for this patient. Indications for a type-specific herpes serologic test would pertain to history of known exposure at least 4 weeks ago or previous herpes-type lesions with a negative culture.

42. a. Prevention of cardiovascular disease

The FDA-approved indications for the use of hormone therapy include relief of moderate to severe menopausal symptoms related to estrogen deficiency (vasomotor instability, vulvar/vaginal atrophy), and prevention of osteoporosis.

43. b. Has less adverse effects on coagulation factors

Estrogen delivered via a transdermal patch has no effect on cardiovascular markers (HDL-C, LDL-C, triglycerides, C-reactive protein). There is less effect on coagulation factors and a lower risk of venous thromboembolism with transdermal estrogen compared with oral estrogen in the menopausal woman.

44. d. Progestin-only contraceptive injections

Return to fertility after discontinuing progestin-only injections (DMPA) may take 6 to 12 months.

45. a. 9; 19

The woman who is going to use the calendar method for contraception should chart her menstrual cycles for several months. She should subtract 11 days from her longest recorded cycle and 18 days from her shortest cycle to estimate when she would be fertile and infertile. The woman with 27- to 30-day cycles should abstain from sexual intercourse from day 9 (27 minus 18) through day 19 (30 minus 11).

46. a. I should insert a new ring every 7 days

The contraceptive vaginal ring is worn in the vagina for 3 weeks followed by 1 week without the ring when the woman will have a withdrawal bleed. The exact position of the ring in the vagina is not important to effectiveness. The male condom can be used with the contraceptive vaginal ring.

47. c. Unexplained vaginal bleeding prior to evaluation

Unexplained vaginal bleeding prior to evaluation is a CDC category 3 for initiation of DMPA. Current and/or history of deep vein thrombosis or pulmonary emboli is category 2; drugs that alter liver enzymes do not influence effectiveness of DMPA and smoking at any age is category 1 for use of DMPA.

48. d. Another method of contraception should be considered when the infant starts sleeping through the night

Alternative contraception should be considered when any of the following occur—menses, regular supplementation, long periods without breastfeeding, baby is 6 months old.

49. d. Progestin-only pills

Progestin-only methods are CDC category 1 for lactating women 30 or more days postpartum. Combination hormonal contraceptives are CDC category 3 the first 42 days postpartum for women with other venous thromboembolism risk factors, which include obesity. Fertility awareness methods are not recommended until the woman has resumed regular menses. She is weaning her baby, so will not be able to rely on the lactational amenorrhea method for contraception.

50. b. 2:00 p.m. on Saturday

The diaphragm should be left in place for at least 6 hours after sexual intercourse and no longer than 24 hours.

51. a. Hepatitis B surface antigen

Hepatitis B surface antigen is present with both acute active infection and with a chronic active (carrier) state.

52. d. Sensitivity of both types of tests is the same

Both enzyme immunoassay (EIA) conventional tests with specimen sent to a lab and rapid tests with results available in the office detect HIV 1 and HIV 2 antibodies. With both tests, the antibodies are detectable in at least 95% of individuals within 3 months after infection.

53. c. She has bone loss that is at the level for diagnosis of osteopenia

Osteopenia is defined as a bone mineral density (BMD) between 1 and 2 standard deviations (SD) below that of a young normal adult. This is a T-score between −1 and −2.5.

54. d. She can have a blood test in 1 to 2 months to determine whether she has herpes antibodies

Type-specific serologic tests detect HSV-1 and HSV-2 antibodies. It may take 4 to 12 weeks for seroconversion.

55. c. Vestibule

The vestibule is enclosed by the labia minora. This area contains the urethral and vaginal openings, hymen, Skene's glands on each side of the urethral meatus, and Bartholin's glands with openings located posteriorly on either side of the vaginal orifice.

56. a. Normal uterus, normal ovaries

In a reproductive-age woman, the uterus is approximately 8 cm in length, 5 cm in width, and 2.5 cm in thickness with slightly larger dimensions in the multiparous woman than the nulliparous woman. Ovaries are approximately 3 cm × 2 cm × 1 cm.

57. a. Beginning breast development

Breast development begins with breast budding around age 9, the growth of pubic and axillary hair usually starts after breast development begins, and the peak growth spurt occurs around age 12 just prior to onset of menses.

58. b. Hypothalamus

Gonadotropin-releasing hormone (GnRH) is released from the hypothalamus in a pulsatile fashion. GnRH stimulates the anterior pituitary gland to release FSH and LH.

59. a. LH surge, ovulation, rise in BBT, thickened cervical mucus

The LH surge occurs in the follicular phase and peaks about 10 to 12 hours before ovulation occurs. There is an increase in basal body temperature (BBT) at the time of ovulation. After ovulation, the corpus luteum formed from the ruptured follicle secretes progesterone, which causes thickening of cervical mucus and sustained increase in BBT.

60. d. Vaginal contraceptive ring for woman older than 35 years of age who smokes 1 pack of cigarettes per day (ppd)

Smoking 15 or more cigarettes a day at age 35 years or older is a CDC category 4 for all of the combination hormonal contraceptives.

61. c. It may be used by individuals with latex allergy

The female vaginal condom is made of nitrile and previously polyurethane, so it may be used by individuals with latex allergy.

62. b. Decrease in risk for cervical cancer

Noncontraceptive benefits of combination oral contraceptives include decrease in benign breast disease, endometrial cancer, and ovarian cancer.

63. c. Intrauterine contraceptive

The perfect use and typical use failure rates are the same or very close to the same for both the levonorgestrel-releasing and copper-releasing intrauterine contraceptives. These methods do not require the woman to remember to do something each day or to have to have supplies available and use them at the time of sexual intercourse.

64. d. Transdermal contraceptive system

The transdermal contraceptive patch may be less effective in women who weigh 90 kg (198 lbs) or more.

65. c. Increase in first-pass metabolism in the liver

Drugs that increase production of the liver enzyme cytochrome P-450 may cause more rapid clearance of combination oral contraceptives during first-pass metabolism in the liver.

66. d. You should choose a site that ensures deep IM injection

The IM formulation of DMPA must be given as a deep injection in the deltoid or gluteal muscle. For obese women, the deltoid may be preferable.

67. a. If you are more than 3 hours late taking a pill, use a backup method for 48 hours

The major mechanism of action of progestin-only pills is the thickening of cervical mucus. Progestin-only pills must be taken at the same time each day to maintain adequate progestin for this effect. Progestin levels peak shortly after taking a pill and decline to nearly undetectable levels 24 hours later.

68. c. Refer her to a gynecologist for further evaluation

The ovaries atrophy after menopause and generally are not palpable.

69. b. Alveoli

Alveoli within the breast lobules are responsible for milk production.

70. d. Prolactin

Prolactin is released from the anterior pituitary gland in increasing amounts during pregnancy. Prolactin stimulates synthesis of milk proteins in mammary tissue.

71. a. Decreased vasocongestion and decreased vaginal expansion

With the decrease in estrogen after menopause, the vaginal walls thin and have decreased vascularization and elasticity. This may change genital sensations during sexual intercourse and may cause dyspareunia.

72. c. Fertility awareness methods

The perimenopausal woman who is having irregular menses may have unpredictable ovulation, so should not rely on fertility awareness methods for contraception.

73. d. Sexual orientation

Sexual orientation is the general term used to describe individuals' physical and/or romantic attractions to other people with the most common labels being heterosexual, homosexual (gay or lesbian), and bisexual. *Sexual identity* refers to one's self-label as heterosexual, homosexual, bisexual, or something else. Gender identity is the internal sense that one is female, male, or some variation of both.

74. b. I know that I am about to ovulate when my temperature rises at least 0.4 degrees Fahrenheit

The rise in basal body temperature (BBT) occurs at the time of ovulation. BBT cannot be used to predict ovulation but can be used to determine whether ovulation has occurred.

75. c. The IUC should be removed promptly regardless of her plans for the pregnancy

Removing the IUC reduces the risk for spontaneous abortion. There is no risk of congenital defects from copper exposure. If the IUC is left in place, she is at risk for spontaneous septic abortion as well as preterm delivery.

76. d. Sunday starters should use a backup method for the first week of the first pack of pills

First day of menses start does not require backup contraception. Quick start of combination oral contraceptives requires backup contraception for 7 days except if switching directly from one hormonal method to another. Sunday start requires 7 days of backup method unless it corresponds with first day of menses.

77. a. Dual energy X-ray absorptiometry
Dual energy X-ray absorptiometry is the most-used technique for bone density testing and has low radiation exposure.

78. d. Frequent use of spermicide may cause vaginal changes, making you more susceptible to HIV infection
Frequent spermicide use (2 or more times a day) may cause vulvovaginal epithelium disruption and a theoretical increase in susceptibility to HIV infection. Spermicide should be placed deep in the vagina close to the cervix and left there for at least 6 hours after sexual intercourse. When spermicide is used along with a condom, there is an increased contraceptive efficacy, but it will not further decrease risk for STI.

79. c. Use of combination oral contraception by a 40-year-old woman who has migraine headaches without aura
The use of combination oral contraception by a woman who is 35 years or older and who has migraine headaches with or without aura is a CDC category 4. The use of combination oral contraception by a woman of any age who has migraine headaches with aura is also a CDC category 4.

80. d. There is a decreased chance for the presence of pre-ejaculatory sperm with repeat acts of intercourse
This statement is incorrect. In itself, pre-ejaculatory fluid contains no sperm. However, with repeat acts of intercourse close together, subsequent pre-ejaculatory fluid may have "carryover" sperm from the previous ejaculation.

Bibliography

American Cancer Society. (2013). Breast awareness and self-exam. Retrieved from http://www.cancer.org/cancer/breastcancer/moreinformation/breastcancerearlydetection/breast-cancer-early-detection-acs-recs-bse

American College of Obstetricians and Gynecologists. (2009a). Cervical cytology screening. *ACOG Practice Bulletin, 109*, 1–12.

American College of Obstetricians and Gynecologists. (2009b). Practice bulletin # 103: Hereditary breast and ovarian cancer syndrome. *Obstetrics and Gynecology, 113*(4), 957–966.

American College of Obstetricians and Gynecologists. (2011). Practice bulletin # 122: Breast cancer screening. *Obstetrics and Gynecology, 118*(2), 372–382.

American College of Obstetricians and Gynecologists. (2013). *Well-woman care: Assessments and recommendations.* Washington, DC: Author.

Basson, R. (2001). Female sexual response: The role of drugs in the management of sexual dysfunction, *Obstetrics and Gynecology, 98*, 350–353.

Bickley, L. (2013). *Bates' guide to physical examination and history taking* (11th ed.). Philadelphia, PA: Lippincott Williams & Wilkins.

Carcio, H., & Secor, M. (2010). *Advanced health assessment of women: Clinical skills and procedures* (2nd ed.). New York, NY: Springer.

Centers for Disease Control and Prevention. (2010a). Sexually transmitted diseases treatment guidelines. *Morbidity and Mortality Weekly Report, 59*(RR12), 1–109.

Centers for Disease Control and Prevention. (2010b). U.S. medical eligibility criteria for contraceptive use. *Morbidity and Mortality Weekly Report, 59*(RR04), 1–6.

Centers for Disease Control and Prevention. (2011). Update to CDC's U.S. medical eligibility criteria for contraceptive use, 2010: Revised recommendations for the use of contraceptive methods during the postpartum period. *Morbidity and Mortality Weekly Report, 60*(RR26), 878–883.

Centers for Disease Control and Prevention. (2013). U.S. selected practice recommendations for contraceptive use, 2013: Adapted from the World Health Organization selected practice recommendations for contraceptive use, 2nd edition. *Morbidity and Mortality Weekly Report, 62*(RR05), 1–46.

Chernecky, C., & Berger, B. (2013). *Laboratory tests and diagnostic procedures* (6th ed.). St. Louis, MO: Saunders Elsevier.

Gibbs, R., Karlan, B., Haney, A., & Nygaard, I. (2008). *Danforth's obstetrics and gynecology* (10th ed.). Philadelphia, PA: Lippincott Williams & Wilkins.

Hatcher, R., Trussell, J., Nelson, A., Cates, W., Kowal, D., & Policar, M. (2011). *Contraceptive technology* (20th ed.). New York, NY: Ardent Media.

Hawkins, J., Roberto-Nichols, D., & Stanley-Haney, L. (2012). *Guidelines for nurse practitioners in gynecologic settings* (10th ed.). New York, NY: Springer.

Masters, W., & Johnson, V. (1966). *Human sexual response.* Boston, MA: Little Brown.

National Abortion Federation. (2005). *NAF protocol recommendations for use of methotrexate and misoprostol in early abortion.* Washington, DC: Author.

National Abortion Federation. (2013). *NAF protocol for mifepristone/misopristol in early abortion in the US.* Washington, DC: Author.

National Institute of Health (2014). *Breast cancer screening.* Retrieved from http://www.cancer.gov/cancertopics/pdq/screening/breast/HealthProfessional

National Osteoporosis Foundation. (2013). *Clinician's guide to prevention and treatment of osteoporosis.* Washington, DC: Author.

North American Menopause Society. (2010). *Menopause practice: A clinician's guide* (4th ed.). Mayfield Heights, OH: Author.

Rhoads, J., & Petersen, S. (2014). *Advanced health assessment and diagnostic reasoning* (2nd ed.). Burlington, MA: Jones & Bartlett Learning.

Seidel, H., Ball, J., Dains, J., Benedict, G., Flynn, J. A., Solomon, B. S., & Stewart, R. B. (2011). *Mosby's guide to physical examination* (7th ed.). St. Louis, MO: Mosby.

Saslow, D., Boetes, C., Burke, W., Harms, M., Leach, M. O., Lehman, C. D., . . . American Cancer Society Breast Cancer Advisory Group. (2007). American Cancer Society guidelines for breast cancer screening with MRI as an adjunct to mammography. *CA Cancer Journal for Clinicians, 57*, 75–89.

Saslow, D., Solomon, D., Lawson, H., Killackey, M., Kulasingam, S. L., Cain, J., . . . ACS-ASCCP-ASCP Cervical Cancer Guideline Committee. (2012). American Cancer Society, American Society for Colposcopy and Cervical Pathology, and American Society for Clinical Pathology screening guidelines for the prevention and early detection of cervical cancer. *CA Cancer Journal for Clinicians, 62*(3), 147–172.

Schuiling, K., & Likis, F. (2013). *Women's gynecologic health* (2nd ed.). Burlington, MA: Jones & Bartlett Learning.

Smith, R., Manassaram-Baptiste, D., Brooks, D., Cokkinides, V., Doroshenk, M., Saslow, D., Wender, R., & Brawley, O. (2014). Cancer screening in the United States, 2014: A review of current American Cancer Society guidelines and current issues in cancer screening. *CA: A Cancer Journal foe Clinicians, 64*(1), 30-51.

Speroff, L., & Darney, P. (2011). *A clinical guide for contraception* (5th ed.). Philadelphia, PA: Lippincott Williams & Wilkins.

Tharpe, N., Farley, C., & Jordan, R. (2013). *Clinical practice guidelines for midwifery and women's health* (4th ed.). Burlington, MA: Jones & Bartlett Learning.

5

Gynecological Disorders

Jamille Nagtalon-Ramos

© Kheng Guan Toh/ShutterStock, Inc.

Menstrual and Endocrine Disorders

Premenstrual Syndrome (PMS)

- Definition—the cyclic occurrence, in luteal phase, of a group of distressing physical and psychological symptoms, which begin 5–7 days before menses and resolve within 4 days after onset of menses and that disrupt normal activities and interpersonal relationships
- Etiology/incidence
  1. Unknown etiology; multifactorial and multiorgan disorder; suggested causes include metabolic and endocrine disorders, alterations in estrogen or progesterone levels, withdrawal of endogenous endorphins, fluid imbalance, vitamin and mineral deficiencies, and altered carbohydrate metabolism
  2. Prevalence may be greater than 50% with most women not requiring treatment; severe cases occur in 3–10% of women with PMS
- Signs and symptoms
  1. Symptoms recur cyclically in the luteal phase with symptom-free period in the follicular phase
  2. Range from mild to severe, resulting in interference with normal activities and personal relationships
     a. Physical
        (1) Headache
        (2) Breast changes
        (3) Fluid retention
        (4) Swelling
        (5) Abdominal bloating
        (6) Nausea/vomiting
        (7) Alterations in appetite
        (8) Food cravings
        (9) Lethargy/fatigue
        (10) Exacerbations of preexisting conditions, such as asthma
     b. Psychological
        (1) Irritability
        (2) Depression
        (3) Anxiety
        (4) Sleep alterations
        (5) Inability to concentrate
        (6) Anger
        (7) Violent behavior
        (8) Crying
        (9) Confusion
        (10) Changes in libido
- Physical findings—no specific physical findings
- Differential diagnosis
  1. A diagnosis of exclusion; all others must be ruled out
  2. Depression and/or anxiety
  3. Bipolar affective disorder
  4. Alcohol or substance abuse
  5. Personality disorders
  6. Chronic fatigue syndrome
  7. Fibromyalgia
  8. Diabetes
  9. Brain tumor
  10. Thyroid disease
  11. Hyperprolactinemia
  12. Perimenopause
- Diagnostic tests/findings
  1. Documentation of symptoms in a diary fashion for 2 to 3 months to evaluate for symptom consistency with ovulation and menses; retrospective recall is inaccurate
  2. Individualized testing, based upon symptoms, may include glucose tolerance test and thyroid profile; hormone levels of little value
- Management/treatment
  1. Nonmedical management
     a. No standard treatment; goal is to isolate symptom groups from history and diary and treat symptomatically
     b. Options for treatment
        (1) Self-help strategies recommended as first-line therapy; help client understand the possible causes of symptoms, reassuring her that no serious health threats exist, and there are no quick cures; patience and team effort are key

(2) Suggested dietary revisions are restriction of salt and refined sugar; limit caffeine, alcohol, and fat intake; hypoglycemic diet may be of value

(3) Vitamin and mineral supplementation as a treatment is poorly documented; magnesium or magnesium-rich foods, pyridoxine (no more than 100 to 300 mg a day), vitamin E (no more than 400 IU a day) may relieve some PMS symptoms; large doses of supplements may be toxic

(4) Calcium carbonate supplementation of 1200-1600 mg a day shown in randomized placebo-controlled trial to reduce PMS symptoms

(5) Chaste tree berry extract shown in placebo-controlled trial to reduce PMS symptoms

(6) Aerobic exercise 20 to 30 minutes at least 4 times a week

(7) Avoidance of known physical or emotional triggers

(8) Cognitive therapy, group therapy, relaxation therapy may improve physical and psychological symptoms

(9) Self-help, support groups, biofeedback, acupuncture/acupressure, light therapy may help some women

2. Medical management

a. Selection of medications based on type and intensity of symptoms

b. Spironolactone during luteal phase to reduce swelling and bloating

c. NSAIDS (antiprostaglandins) menstrually and premenstrually may reduce fluid retention and breast, lower back, abdominal, pelvic pain

d. Combined oral contraceptives (consider continuous or extended use regimens), other combination or progestin only contraceptive methods may be helpful in decreasing physical symptoms by suppressing ovulation and/or reducing menstrual bleeding and pain

e. Selective serotonin reuptake inhibitors (SSRIs) have been shown to alleviate severe PMS; may choose to take only in luteal phase each month

f. Danazol may improve PMS symptoms by suppressing ovulation; has significant androgen related side effects

g. Gonadotropin-releasing hormone (GnRH) agonists to inhibit cyclic gonadotropin release; has significant menopause like side effects; long-term therapy may predispose to heart disease or osteoporosis—limit use to 4 to 6 months unless combined with combination hormonal therapy

• Premenstrual dysphoric disorder (PMDD)

1. At least 5 PMS-type symptoms severe enough to markedly disrupt normal functioning in most if not all menstrual cycles

2. Occurs in luteal phase and resolves within 1 week after menses

3. Must include at least one of these symptoms—markedly depressed mood, marked anxiety, marked affective lability, persistent and marked anger

4. Prevalence, 3–10% of reproductive-age women

5. Treatment

a. Same therapeutic interventions as for PMS

b. Medications with FDA approval for treatment of PMDD include drospirenone containing combination hormonal contraceptives and the SSRIs fluoxetine, paroxetine, sertraline

c. Anxiolytic drugs (alprazolam, buspirone)—mixed results in PMDD treatment studies; high potential for drug dependence/abuse; use only short-term

Dysmenorrhea

• Definition

1. Painful menstruation—a sensation of cramping in lower abdomen during or just before menses; most severe on first day, usually lasts 2 days, may radiate to back and thighs

2. Primary—dysmenorrhea occurs unassociated with underlying pelvic pathology, rarely begins after age 20 years, associated with ovulatory cycles, is stimulated by prostaglandin release

3. Secondary—an underlying pelvic pathologic condition thought to be the cause

4. May occur at any age in menstruating women

• Etiology/incidence

1. Primary—seen in 50–75% of all menstruating women with 10–20% severe; prostaglandins stimulate contractile response on smooth muscles

2. Secondary—onset may be many years after menarche; most often in women older than age 20 years; organic disease is related

• Signs and symptoms

1. Primary

a. Pain begins shortly before the onset of menses and usually lasts no longer than 2 days

b. Described as colicky, crampy, and spasmodic pain in the lower abdomen, sometimes radiating to lower back and thighs

c. May interfere with work or school (15–29%)

2. Secondary

a. Pain may begin at any time during the cycle; may notice change in duration and amount of menstrual flow

b. Unlikely to be relieved by over-the-counter measures

c. Symptoms often persist longer then primary; related to organic pathology

• Physical findings

1. Primary—characterized by no abnormalities found on examination

2. Secondary—has findings consistent with pathologic condition

• Differential diagnosis

1. Imperforate hymen

2. Endometriosis

3. Cervical stenosis

4. Uterine abnormalities

5. Pelvic infection

6. Ovarian cysts

7. Pelvic congestion

8. Chronic pelvic pain

9. Adhesions

10. Sexually transmitted infections

11. Urinary tract infections

• Diagnostic tests/findings

1. Primary—no specific tests are ordered

2. Secondary

a. Analyze pain description to help determine etiology

b. Tests according to history and physical examination findings may include:
   (1) Vaginal ultrasound and hysterosalpingogram to evaluate pelvic structures
   (2) Laparoscopy to evaluate endometrial cavity
   (3) Cultures, smears to evaluate infections
   (4) Lower gastrointestinal (GI) evaluation
- Management/treatment
   1. Primary
      a. Prostaglandin synthetase inhibitors, nonsteroidal anti-inflammatory drugs (NSAIDs) are treatment of choice; best if begun at onset of menses, continuing for 48 to 72 hours; choices shown to be effective are mefenamic acid, naproxyn sodium, ibuprofen, and indomethacin
      b. Oral contraceptive pills (OCPs) are a good choice if contraception is needed; act by reducing prostaglandins and menstrual flow; may consider extended or continuous dosing regimens
      c. NSAIDs and OCPs may be used in combination
      d. Other hormonal contraceptives may also relieve symptoms by decreasing or eliminating menstrual bleeding—depot medroxyprogesterone acetate (DMPA), levonorgestrel-releasing intrauterine system (LNG-IUS)
      e. Self-help measures include exercise, warm heat, relaxation exercises
   2. Secondary treatment consistent with pathology

Amenorrhea

- Definition
   1. Absence of menses during reproductive years
   2. Primary—no menstruation previously; no menstruation by age 14 years in absence of development of secondary sex characteristics; no menstruation by age 16 years regardless of secondary sex characteristics
   3. Secondary—absence of menses in a previously menstruating woman; no menses for 6 months in a woman who usually has normal periods or for a length of time equivalent to three cycles
   4. A symptom, not a diagnosis
- Etiology/incidence
   1. Vaginal agenesis
   2. Imperforate hymen
   3. Atrophy
   4. Infection
   5. Irradiation and surgery resulting in destruction of endometrium (Asherman's syndrome)
   6. Stress
   7. Genetic anomalies
   8. Endocrine imbalances such as hyperthyroidism
   9. Weight abnormalities
   10. Medications
   11. Chronic illness
   12. Excessive exercise
   13. Malnutrition
   14. Incidence is approximately 5% in women who are not pregnant, lactating, or menopausal

- Signs and symptoms—absence of menses at the expected time
- Physical findings
   1. Abnormal vital signs may indicate chronic illness
   2. Abnormal visual fields may indicate a pituitary tumor
   3. Enlarged or nodular thyroid or breast discharge may indicate endocrine disorder
   4. Enlarged uterus may indicate pregnancy
   5. Delay in Tanner stage progression may indicate altered development of secondary sex characteristics, whereas hirsutism, clitoral enlargement, and acne may mean androgen excess
   6. Vaginal atrophy or clitoral hypertrophy
   7. Imperforate hymen
- Differential diagnosis
   1. Pregnancy
   2. Menopause
   3. Anorexia nervosa
   4. Disorders of ovary, anterior pituitary, and/or hypothalamus such as pituitary tumors, gonadotropin deficiency, polycystic ovarian syndrome, ovarian failure, Sheehan's syndrome
   5. Anatomic disorders such as genetic or congenital anomalies (Turner's syndrome, androgen insensitivity/resistance syndrome, congenital adrenal hyperplasia) and destructive changes such as Asherman's syndrome
   6. Chronic illness—hypothyroidism, hyperthyroidism, tuberculosis, alcohol abuse, type 1 diabetes mellitus, disorders of adrenal glands, obesity
   7. Medication effects—hormonal contraceptives, psychotrophic drugs (phenothiazines), reserpine, dilantin
- Diagnostic tests/findings
   1. Pregnancy test
   2. Serum prolactin level
   3. Serum T_4 and thyroid-stimulating hormone (TSH)
   4. If above tests are normal, may evaluate availability of estrogen with progestin challenge test
      a. Progesterone each day for 5 to 10 days—wait for bleeding, which should occur within 7 days; will indicate adequate estrogen production and stimulation as well as no problem with outflow tract
      b. Should withdrawal bleeding not occur, prime endometrium with estrogen to ensure proliferation; estrogen orally for 21 days, add progesterone orally for last 5 days
      c. Repeat challenge test; if bleeding occurs, order specific test to determine whether problem is in pituitary or ovary, or refer
   5. Determine karyotype
- Management/treatment
   1. Primary amenorrhea, refer to endocrinologist
   2. Treat thyroid abnormalities or refer
   3. If prolactin and TSH are normal and bleeding occurs after progestin challenge, initiate treatment for anovulation based on age, contraceptive needs, and lifestyle
   4. Treatment may include combination hormonal contraceptives or cyclic progestins
   5. Attain a normal weight/BMI and maintain
   6. Referral for ovulation induction if desires pregnancy

Infrequent Menstrual Bleeding

- Definition—infrequent uterine bleeding characterized by one or two bleeding episodes in a 90-day period; previously referred to as oligomenorrhea
- Etiology/incidence
  1. Occurs frequently in perimenopause
  2. Ovarian-pituitary-hypothalamus abnormalities
  3. Endocrine disorders such as thyroid or adrenal problems
  4. Systemic causes such as chronic illness, weight loss or gain, extreme stress, excessive exercise
  5. Drug use or abuse
- Signs and symptoms
  1. May alternate with episodes of amenorrhea or heavy vaginal bleeding
  2. May present as normal menstrual pattern during first year of menstruation or for several years prior to menopause
- Differential diagnosis
  1. Pregnancy
  2. Menopause
  3. Thyroid disorder
  4. Disturbance with hypothalamic-pituitary-ovarian axis
- Physical findings—consistent with pathology found in "Differential diagnosis" section
- Diagnostic tests/findings
  1. Pregnancy test
  2. Tests to evaluate function of thyroid, ovaries, pituitary, or hypothalamus (e.g., TSH, prolactin level, gonadotropin levels)
- Management/treatment
  1. If pregnant, discuss options
  2. Treat underlying cause (e.g., stress, weight—possibly refer to an endocrinologist)
  3. Prevent unopposed estrogen complications by giving progesterone therapy—medroxyprogesterone acetate 10 days of each month or combination hormonal contraceptives

Heavy and/or Prolonged Menstrual Bleeding

- Definition—heavy menstrual bleeding (HMB) is characterized by monthly blood loss volume of greater than 80 mL, prolonged menstrual bleeding is characterized by bleeding episodes lasting more than 8 days; heavy and/or prolonged menstrual bleeding previously referred to as menorrhagia
- Etiology/incidence
  1. Gynecologic causes—leiomyoma, adenomyosis, endometrial and endocervical polyps, endometrial hyperplasia, cervical and endometrial cancers
  2. Disturbances of hypothalamic-pituitary-ovarian axis causing continuous endometrial stimulation
  3. Imbalance of prostaglandins favoring those that cause vasodilation over those that cause vasoconstriction
  4. Inherited and acquired bleeding disorders—von Willebrand disease, idiopathic thrombocytopenia purpura, aplastic anemia, platelet dysfunction
  5. Systematic diseases—hepatic disease, early renal failure, adrenal hyperplasia, thyroid dysfunction

6. Medications—anticoagulants, some anticonvulsants, digitalis, nonhormonal intrauterine contraception, chronic aspirin or NSAID use
7. Other—physical trauma, extreme stress, obesity
- Signs and symptoms
  1. Often occurs at extremes of reproductive age—adolescence and perimenopause
  2. Women may have different definitions of what is excessive bleeding—it is relevant if it is disrupting her life
  3. Signs and symptoms will vary with cause of bleeding
- Physical findings—depend on cause of bleeding, see Etiology
- Differential diagnoses
  1. Pregnancy (ectopic or intrauterine)
  2. Gynecologic disorders
  3. Disturbances of hypothalamic-pituitary-ovarian axis
  4. Acquired or inherited bleeding disorders
  5. Systematic diseases
  6. Medication related
- Diagnostic tests/findings
  1. hCG for pregnancy
  2. Pap test for cervical cancer
  3. Complete blood count (CBC)
  4. FSH and LH to evaluate estrogen stimulation
  5. TSH
  6. Sexually transmitted infection testing as indicated
  7. Endometrial evaluation—biopsy, transvaginal ultrasound, saline infusion sonohysteroscopy
  8. Coagulation studies if indicated
- Management/treatment
  1. Hormonal
     a. Acute excessive bleeding—parenteral estrogen or high-dose oral estrogen gradually tapered, then medroxyprogesterone acetate (MPA) added last 10 days to initiate withdrawal bleeding; high-dose oral progestin therapy gradually tapered
     b. Moderate bleeding, not currently bleeding, and maintenance control—LNG-IUS is FDA approved for treatment of HMB; combination hormonal contraceptives cyclic, extended, or continuous regimens; DMPA; cyclic MPA
  2. Nonhormonal
     a. Treat anemia
     b. Nonsteroidal anti-inflammatory drugs (NSAIDS)—start at menses onset and continue for 5 days or until cessation of menstruation; increases ratio of vasoconstrictive prostaglandins to vasodilating prostaglandins
     c. Tranexamic acid—antifibrinolytic agent that blocks lysis of fibrin clots; take up to the first 5 days of menses; decrease blood loss in women who have increased endometrial plasminogen activity
  3. Surgical management
     a. Hysterectomy
     b. Endometrial ablation
     c. Dilatation and curettage (D & C) is diagnostic and therapeutic
  4. Complementary and alternative therapies
     a. Iron-rich food
     b. Stress management
     c. Acupuncture

Polycystic Ovarian Syndrome (PCOS)

- Definition—a symptom complex associated with menstrual irregularity due to oligo-ovulation or anovulation and clinical or biochemical signs of hyperandrogenism
- Etiology/incidence
  1. Etiology is unclear
  2. Primary hormonal abnormality is increased luteinizing hormone (LH) with low or normal follicle-stimulating hormone (FSH)—ratio is more than 3:1; results in dysregulation of androgen secretion with increased testosterone and androstenedione production
  3. Another cause may be hyperinsulinemia associated with insulin resistance; insulin has effects at both the ovarian stroma and the follicle; can have a significant impact on promoting or disrupting follicles
  4. Approximately 25% of normal women will demonstrate ultrasonographic evidence typical of polycystic ovaries
  5. Prevalence in reproductive women is approximately 6–7% (most common endocrine disorder in this population)
  6. Women are at risk for future development of endometrial cancer, diabetes mellitus, and heart disease; obesity increases risk of metabolic complications
- Signs and symptoms
  1. History of irregular menses (amenorrhea or infrequent menstrual bleeding)
  2. Gradual onset of hirsutism around puberty or in early 20s
  3. Signs of androgen excess—acne, hirsutism, deep voice, male pattern baldness
  4. May have acanthosis nigricans
  5. Obesity may be present (40%) or overweight
  6. Infertility
  7. Enlarged abdomen with striae
  8. Decreased vaginal rugae
  9. Possible visual impairment
- Differential diagnosis
  1. Obesity
  2. Hyperprolactinemia
  3. Thyroid dysfunction
  4. Cushing's disease
  5. Adrenal or ovarian tumors
- Physical findings
  1. Physical findings may be normal
  2. Ovaries may not always be palpable—50% will have enlarged ovaries
  3. Virilization—hirsutism, increased muscle mass, frontal balding, enlargement of clitoris, deepening of voice, and decreased breast size
  4. Abdominal obesity
  5. Acne
  6. Acanthosis nigricans and skin tags usually in neck area
- Diagnostic tests/findings
  1. Pregnancy test
  2. Progesterone challenge test resulting in bleeding
  3. LH elevated; FSH normal or low (3:1 ratio)
  4. Prolactin mildly elevated or normal

5. Serum total testosterone and free testosterone—mild to moderate elevation, which may mean androgen excess
6. Thyroid function tests—high or low TSH
7. Dehydroepiandrosterone sulfate (DHEAS)—normal to elevated
8. Endometrial biopsy—to rule out hyperplasia
9. Basal body temperature reading to indicate evidence of ovulation—use to schedule endometrial biopsy
10. Assess ovaries with ultrasonography
11. Laparoscopy to determine and manage fertility
12. Glucose and lipid levels
- Management/treatment
  1. Goal is to lower androgen levels, treat current clinical manifestations, and decrease risk for long-term effects of hyperandrogenism
  2. May be determined by desire for pregnancy and symptom patterns
  3. If pregnancy desired, refer to reproductive endocrinologist
  4. If pregnancy not desired, direct therapy on prevention of endometrial hyperplasia and pregnancy
     a. Endometrial biopsy may be indicated
     b. Medroxyprogesterone acetate for 10 days of month induces withdrawal bleeding
     c. Low-dose combined hormonal contraception with low androgenicity—inhibits LH secretion and LH-dependent ovarian androgen production, increases sex hormone binding globulin (SHBG) concentration binding free testosterone, regulates menstrual cycles, protects from endometrial cancer
  5. Be observant for signs of diabetes, heart disease, breast cancer, and endometrial cancer
  6. Weight loss if obese
  7. Insulin-sensitizing agents—metformin
  8. Excess hair removal—mechanical or eflornithine HCl topical cream for facial hair

Endometriosis

- Definition—the presence of endometrial stroma and glands outside uterus
- Etiology/incidence
  1. Etiology is not clearly understood
  2. Possible causes include:
     a. Retrograde menstruation (Sampson's theory)
     b. Immunologic factors
     c. Genetics
     d. Hormonal factors
  3. Found in 5–15% of surgeries performed on reproductive-age women and up to 30% of infertile women
  4. Typical patient is 20 to 30 years old, Caucasian, nulliparous (60–70%)
  5. Occurs in all races
  6. 7–10% of premenopausal women are affected; most common cause of chronic pelvic pain
  7. Endometriosis has been found in areas other than the pelvis, such as lungs, nose, and spinal column; most common sites are cul-de-sac, ovary, posterior uterus, and uterosacral ligaments
  8. Majority have a positive family history

- Signs and symptoms
  1. Wide range of clinical symptoms; severity does not correlate with extent of disease
  2. Most common complaints
     a. Dysmenorrhea
     b. Infertility
     c. Premenstrual spotting
     d. Menorrhagia
     e. Pelvic pain
     f. Dyspareunia
  3. Symptoms seen less often include:
     a. Low back pain
     b. Diarrhea
     c. Dysuria
     d. Hematuria
     e. Dyschezia
     f. Rectal bleeding
  4. Symptoms classically occur before or during menses
  5. Pain may be localized to involved area
  6. Infertility
- Physical findings
  1. Fixed, retroverted uterus
  2. Bilateral, fixed, tender adnexal masses
  3. Nodularity and tenderness of uterosacral ligaments and cul-de-sac
  4. Tenderness, thickening, and nodularity of rectal-vaginal septum
  5. Lesions may be visible on laparoscopy or laparotomy
  6. Cervical motion tenderness associated with menses
- Differential diagnosis
  1. Chronic pelvic inflammatory infection
  2. Acute salpingitis
  3. Adenomyosis
  4. Ectopic pregnancy
  5. Benign or malignant ovarian neoplasm
- Diagnostic tests/findings
  1. Direct visualization with laparoscopy or laparotomy may reveal classic implants; classified as Stage I—minimal, Stage II—mild, Stage III—moderate, Stage IV—severe
  2. CT and MRI provide only presumptive evidence
  3. CA-125 levels correlate with degree of disease and response to therapy, cannot be used for diagnosis because of low sensitivity and specificity
- Management/treatment
  1. No medical management provides universal cure; goal is to relieve pain, restore fertility, and prevent progression
  2. Medical management includes:
     a. Analgesics (NSAIDs are first choice)
     b. GnRH agonists and danazol induce regression of endometrial implants
     c. Progestins—Sub Q 104 DMPA is FDA approved for treatment; IM DMPA also effective
     d. Continuous use of combined oral contraceptive pills produces atrophy of implants and acyclic hormone environment
     e. Laser surgery may be employed
     f. Hysterectomy, bilateral salpingoophorectomy is curative
     g. May combine surgery and medication

  3. Key points
     a. May need long-term emotional support as a result of pain and infertility
     b. Delayed childbirth may lead to development of endometriosis
     c. Treatment is long term; may become a chronic illness
     d. Counsel regarding the risk of infertility

Adenomyosis

- Definition—benign condition in which ectopic endometrium is found within the myometrium; often is considered a type of endometriosis
- Etiology/incidence
  1. May be related to breakdown of the endometrium during labor and delivery; the cells of the endometrial basal layer grow downward, losing connection with the endometrium
  2. Incidence varies widely from 10–90% of hysterectomies revealing adenomyosis
  3. Diagnosis most common in parous women between ages 40 and 50 years
- Signs and symptoms
  1. Increasingly severe dysmenorrhea and heavy bleeding during menses are common
  2. Infertility
- Physical findings
  1. Boggy tender uterus
  2. Diffuse, globular enlargement—may be 8 to 10 weeks size
  3. May see evidence of anemia
- Differential diagnosis
  1. Endometriosis
  2. Leiomyomata
  3. Pregnancy
  4. Adhesions
- Diagnostic tests/findings
  1. Ultrasonography or MRI may rule out other pathology
  2. Endometrial biopsy for abnormal bleeding
- Management/treatment
  1. Symptomatic relief may be only requirement
  2. Hysterectomy may be indicated and is curative
  3. NSAIDs for pain
  4. Hormone suppression—symptoms usually subside after hormone production ceases

Hyperprolactinemia, Galactorrhea, and Pituitary Adenoma

- Definition
  1. Hyperprolactinemia—elevated levels of prolactin
  2. Galactorrhea—secretion of a nonphysiologic, milky fluid from the breast, unrelated to pregnancy
  3. Pituitary adenoma—benign tumor of pituitary; most common type secretes prolactin
- Etiology/incidence
  1. Etiology and incidence of pituitary adenoma is unknown; rarely malignant, can grow for years
  2. Prolactin-secreting adenomas account for 50% of all identified at autopsy

3. Most pituitary adenomas occur in women younger than 40 years of age
4. High prolactin level found in approximately one-third of women with amenorrhea of unknown origin; about one-third of women with secondary amenorrhea will have pituitary adenoma; one-third of women with high levels of prolactin will have galactorrhea
5. Galactorrhea should be evaluated in a nulliparous woman or in a parous woman if 12 months has passed since last pregnancy
- Signs and symptoms
  1. Hyperprolactinemia/galactorrhea
     a. Spontaneous clear or milky bilateral or unilateral breast secretions from multiple ducts
     b. Normal or irregular menses; secondary amenorrhea may occur
     c. Disturbances of vision and headaches may be present (if adenoma is cause)
  2. Pituitary adenoma
     a. Breast secretions
     b. Menstrual changes as described
     c. Severe vascular headaches and blurred vision
- Physical findings
  1. Normal funduscopic examination—if no adenoma
  2. Funduscopic examination may show papilledema if adenoma present
  3. Normal physical and gynecological examination
- Differential diagnosis
  1. Pregnancy/breastfeeding
  2. Breast cancer
  3. Hypothyroidism, hyperthyroidism
  4. Pituitary adenoma
  5. Excessive breast stimulation
  6. Disorders or injury of chest wall
  7. Medication effect (e.g., endogenous opiates, cannabis, heterocyclic antidepressants)
  8. Disturbances of ovarian function
  9. Benign and malignant brain neoplasm
- Diagnostic tests/findings
  1. Thyroid screening—e.g., TSH, T_4
  2. Serum prolactin—refer if more than 20 ng/mL; if in 100 to 300 ng/mL range—very suspicious for adenoma
  3. Pregnancy test
  4. Microscopy of breast secretions—milk indicated by fat globules
  5. CT or MRI of sella turcica to rule out adenoma
- Management/treatment
  1. Management may best be accomplished by referral to a reproductive endocrinologist
  2. If prolactin level is less than 20 ng/mL, may follow with yearly prolactin levels
  3. Pharmacologic
     a. Dopamine agonist (e.g., bromocriptine, which inhibits prolactin, provides symptomatic relief, decreases or stops galactorrhea); treatment of choice with highest cure
     b. Treat hypo-/hyperthyroidism

4. Surgical
   a. If medical management has failed to relieve symptoms of adenoma, transphenoid neurosurgery may be indicated
   b. Recurrence rate is 10–70%; requires close follow-up
5. Radiation
   a. Results are less satisfactory than surgery
   b. May take several years for prolactin level to fall
   c. Should be reserved for recurrences or those not responsive to medical management
6. Patient education
   a. Discontinue breast stimulation
   b. Disclose all drugs and medications being used

Benign and Malignant Tumors/Neoplasms

Cervical Polyps

- Definition—pedunculated growths arising from the mucosal surface of the endocervix
- Etiology/incidence
  1. Inflammation
  2. Trauma
  3. Pregnancy
  4. Abnormal local response to hypoestrogenic state
  5. Occurs in 4% of all gynecologic patients
  6. Most common benign neoplasm of the cervix; and most often seen in perimenopausal and multigravida women between ages 30 and 50 years
  7. Malignant changes are rare
- Signs and symptoms
  1. May be asymptomatic
  2. Leukorrhea
  3. Abnormal vaginal bleeding—intermenstrual, postcoital
- Physical findings
  1. Single or multiple, painless polypoid lesions at cervix
  2. Size ranges from a few millimeters to 2 to 3 cm
  3. Reddish-purple to cherry red in color; smooth and soft; bleeds easily
  4. Otherwise normal pelvic examination
- Differential diagnosis
  1. Adenocarcinoma
  2. Cervical carcinoma
  3. Prolapsed myoma
  4. Squamous papilloma
  5. Retained products of conception
  6. Sarcoma
- Diagnostic tests/findings
  1. Pap test to rule out premalignant cervical lesions or cancer
  2. Biopsy to rule out cancer
- Management/treatment
  1. Excisional polypoidectomy is usually curative
  2. Recur frequently

Leiomyomata Uteri (Fibroid, Myoma)

- Definition—nodular, discrete tumors varying in size from microscopic to large multiple, nodular masses; classified according to location
  1. Submucosal—protrude into the uterine cavity
  2. Subserosal—bulge through the outer uterine wall
  3. Intraligamentous—within the broad ligament
  4. Interstitial (intramural)—stays within the uterine wall as it grows; most common form of myoma
  5. Pedunculated—on a thin pedicle or stalk attached to the uterus
- Etiology/incidence
  1. Etiology unknown
  2. May arise from smooth muscle cells in the myometrium
  3. Most common benign gynecologic pelvic neoplasm
  4. Affects approximately 20% of women in their reproductive years
  5. Occurs more frequently in African American women than in Caucasian
  6. Asymptomatic fibroids may be seen in 40–50% of women older than age 40
  7. Increased family incidence
- Signs and symptoms
  1. Usually asymptomatic
  2. Menorrhagia—most common sign
  3. Pelvic pain is most often chronic—presents as dysmenorrhea, pelvic pressure, or dyspareunia; if pedunculated, twisted, and infarcted may cause acute pain
  4. Large fibroids may cause constipation; intestinal obstruction may result from compression; venous stasis may occur from pressure; pressure on bladder may result in urinary retention or overflow incontinence
- Physical findings
  1. Abdominal enlargement
  2. Enlarged, irregularly shaped, firm uterus; may be displaced
  3. Pedunculated tumor may protrude from cervix
  4. Tumors usually painless on palpation
  5. Wide variance in size (3 to 4 mm up to 15 lb)
  6. Potential complications
     a. Spontaneous abortion
     b. Premature labor
     c. Anemia
     d. Infertility
- Differential diagnosis
  1. Ovarian mass (benign or malignant)
  2. Pregnancy
  3. Leiomyosarcoma
  4. Uterine malignancy
  5. Adenomyosis
  6. Endometriosis
  7. Colon or rectal tumor (benign or malignant)
- Diagnostic tests/findings
  1. Pap test to rule out cervical cancer
  2. Pregnancy test to rule out pregnancy
  3. CBC if anemia suspected
  4. Occult blood test if rectal or colon symptoms or gastrointestinal problems
  5. Endometrial biopsy or D & C when abnormal bleeding present
  6. Ultrasound, sonohysterogram, CT, MRI confirm diagnosis
  7. Hysteroscopy to provide visualization of uterine cavity
- Management/treatment
  1. May require no treatment if asymptomatic
  2. Periodic observation and follow-up with bimanual examination may be indicated to ensure tumors are not growing or undergoing abnormal changes
  3. Pharmacologic
     a. GnRH agonist results in 40–60% reduction in volume; regrowth occurs about half the time; may be used to reduce volume preoperatively, before attempting pregnancy, when surgery is contraindicated, or in perimenopausal women to avoid surgery
     b. Progestational agents such as medroxyprogesterone acetate (MPA) may decrease fibroid size and bleeding
     c. Treat anemia if indicated
  4. Surgical
     a. Indications for surgery
        (1) Abnormal bleeding
        (2) Rapid growth
        (3) Definitive decision concerning mass if impossible without visualization
        (4) Encroachment of organs
     b. Hysterectomy when symptoms cannot be controlled
     c. Myomectomy through hysteroscopic resection can preserve fertility; up to 30% recurrence with this method

Ovarian Cysts

- Definition
  1. Functional—cysts of the ovary that occur secondary to hormonal stimulation
     a. Follicular—occur in the follicular phase of the menstrual cycle when continued hormonal stimulation prevents fluid resorption
     b. Corpus luteum—occur in the luteal phase, when corpus luteum fails to degenerate
  2. Dermoid (benign cystic teratoma)—most common ovarian germ cell tumor
- Etiology/incidence
  1. Follicular cysts
     a. Rare before menarche or after menopause
     b. Account for 20–50% of ovarian cysts; most common adnexal mass in reproductive years
     c. Often found incidentally during routine pelvic examination or ultrasound
     d. Usually resolves in 2 to 3 menstrual cycles, may rupture or undergo torsion causing pain
  2. Corpus luteum cysts
     a. Forms following the failure of the corpus luteum to degenerate after 14 days
     b. May hemorrhage into the cystic cavity
  3. Dermoid cysts (benign cystic teratoma)
     a. One of the most common neoplasms of the ovary (10–20%)

b. Occurs during the reproductive years

c. Composed usually of well-differentiated tissue from all three germ layers

d. Usually measures 5 to 10 cm in diameter; 10–15% are bilateral

- Signs and symptoms
  1. Functional cysts
     a. Usually asymptomatic
     b. May cause irregular menses, pelvic pressure, fullness (if mass is large), increase in abdominal girth/distention
     c. Acute pain if ruptures or if torsion occurs
     d. Large cysts may cause feeling of fullness, heaviness, and dull ache on affected side
  2. Dermoid (benign cystic teratoma)
     a. Usually asymptomatic
     b. Acute pain if twists or ruptures; may experience peritonitis
     c. May cause vague feelings of local pelvic pressure if large
     d. Abnormal uterine bleeding (rare)
  3. Signs of rupture include severe, sudden abdominal pain; mimics ruptured ectopic
- Physical findings
  1. Functional cysts are usually smaller than 8 cm, cystic to firm, mobile, sometimes tender, usually unilateral adnexal mass
  2. Dermoid cysts may measure 5 to 10 cm, usually unilateral, firm to cystic, often anterior to uterus
- Differential diagnosis
  1. Pregnancy; ectopic pregnancy
  2. Ovarian torsion
  3. Uterine fibroid; endometrioma
  4. Tubo-ovarian abscess
  5. Diverticulitis/abscess
  6. Distended bladder
  7. Congenital anomaly (pelvic kidney)
  8. Lymphadenopathy
  9. Malignant neoplasm (most often in older women)
- Diagnostic tests/findings
  1. Pregnancy test
  2. Ultrasound to evaluate mass—cystic or solid; septate, irregular, presence of papillations, bilateral or unilateral; rule out ectopic pregnancy
  3. CT scan with contrast or intravenous pyelogram (IVP) to evaluate kidney
- Management/treatment
  1. Functional cyst
     a. In reproductive years; cyst less than 6 cm in diameter, examine after next menses
     b. Combination hormonal contraceptives to suppress gonadotropin levels
     c. Mass between 6 and 8 cm, or is fixed or feels solid, pelvic ultrasound to ensure it is unilocular
     d. If painful, multilocular, or partially solid, surgery indicated
     e. Mass 8 cm, surgery indicated
     f. If 40 years old or older, use more caution and observe
  2. Dermoid cyst—determined by age, desire for pregnancy, and potential for malignancy; cystectomy or abdominal hysterectomy and bilateral salpingoophorectomy

Cervical Carcinoma

- Definition—slow penetration of the basement membrane and infiltration of malignant cells into the uterine cervix; characterized by histologically definable stages
- Etiology/incidence
  1. Approximately 14,500 new cases diagnosed annually with 4000 to 5000 deaths
  2. Highest incidence in Hispanics, then African Americans, then Caucasians
  3. Peak incidence between 45 and 55 years of age; increasing in young women
  4. Time between initial exposure to a carcinogen and subsequent development of carcinoma in situ considered to be 5 to 10 years
  5. Human papillomavirus (HPV) is the primary agent in the development of cervical intraepithelial neoplasia (CIN) and cervical cancer
  6. Risk factors
     a. Smoking
     b. Presence of HPV types with malignant potential (types 16, 18, and 31 most common)
     c. First coitus at early age (< 18 years)
     d. Multiple sexual partners or sexual partners with multiple partners
     e. Nonbarrier method of contraception
     f. Immunosuppression
     g. Long-term oral contraceptive use
     h. Never had Pap test or infrequent Pap tests
- Signs and symptoms
  1. May be asymptomatic
  2. Postcoital or irregular, painless bleeding
  3. Odorous bloody or purulent discharge
  4. Late symptoms
     a. Pelvic or epigastric pain
     b. Urinary or rectal symptoms
- Physical findings
  1. Appearance of cervix ranges from normal to severely ulcerated, necrotic, or large bulky lesion filling the vagina
  2. Cervix may be firm or "rock like" to soft and spongy
  3. Sanguineous or purulent, odorous vaginal discharge
  4. Anemia if bleeding heavy
- Differential diagnosis
  1. Metastasis from another primary site
  2. Cervicitis/sexually transmitted infections
  3. Cervical polyp
  4. Cervical ectopy
  5. Preinvasive lesion of cervix
  6. Condyloma acuminata
- Diagnostic tests/findings
  1. Pap test is gold standard for cost-effective screening
  2. Biopsy of gross lesions
  3. If malignancy is suspected, but no gross lesion visible, colposcopy is suggested with biopsy
  4. Colposcopic evaluation of vulva and vagina to rule out other lesions
  5. CT, MRI, cystoscopy, sigmoidoscopy, and barium enema may be indicated

▪ **Table 5-1   Gynecologic Cancer Symptoms**

Symptoms	Cervical Cancer	Ovarian Cancer	Uterine Cancer	Vaginal Cancer	Vulvar Cancer
Abnormal vaginal bleeding or discharge	●	●	●	●	
Pelvic pain or pressure		●	●		●
Abdominal or back pain		●			
Bloating		●			
Changes in bathroom habits		●		●	
Itching or burning or the vulva					●
Changes in vulvar color or skin, such as rash, sores, or warts					●

Source: Reproduced from Centers for Disease Control and Prevention, Gynecologic Cancers. Retrieved from http://www.cdc.gov/cancer/cervical/basic_info/symptoms.htm.

- Management/treatment
  1. Management should be by a gynecological oncologist involving staging, appropriate treatment, and follow-up
  2. Treatment may consist of surgery, radiation, chemotherapy, or a combination

Endometrial Carcinoma

- Definition—carcinoma of the body of the uterus; malignant transformation of endometrial glands and/or stroma
- Etiology/incidence
  1. Most common gynecologic malignancy—accounts for 90–95% of malignancies of the uterine corpus
  2. 30,000 new cases annually and 6000 deaths
  3. Median age is 63 years at onset—5% occurring in women younger than age 40
  4. Risk factors are linked to exposure to unopposed estrogen either endogenous or exogenous
     a. Diabetes, obesity, hypertension
     b. Family history
     c. Early menarche; late menopause
     d. Unopposed estrogen therapy
     e. Oligo-ovulation, anovulation
     f. Estrogen-secreting tumors (granulosa cell)
  5. Protective factors—multiparity, use of oral contraceptive pills, use of depot medroxyprogesterone acetate (DMPA)
- Signs and symptoms
  1. Painless vaginal bleeding is typically the first symptom
  2. Serous, odorous discharge (watery leukorrhea), soon replaced by bloody discharge, intermittent spotting, spotting-to-steady painless bleeding, then hemorrhage
  3. Lower abdominal pain (10%)
- Physical findings
  1. Blood may be present in the vaginal vault
  2. Advanced disease may have pelvic mass present, ascites
  3. Anemia may be present
  4. Uterus may be enlarged and soft
- Differential diagnosis
  1. Atrophic vaginitis

2. Cervical or endometrial polyps
3. Benign endometrial pathology (hyperplasia)
4. Dysfunctional uterine bleeding
5. Bleeding from hormone replacement therapy
6. Leiomyomas
7. Other genital/gynecologic cancers
- Diagnostic tests/findings
  1. Pap test may show glandular abnormalities
  2. Endometrial aspiration biopsy
  3. Ultrasound to measure endometrial stripe; if less than 5 mm thick, likelihood of endometrial cancer is rare
  4. Fractional dilatation and curettage is the gold standard for diagnosis
  5. Hysteroscopy may be useful in identifying lesions/polyps not found on biopsy
- Management/treatment
  1. Refer to gynecologist for early stage disease or oncologist
  2. Hysterectomy, bilateral salpingoophorectomy
  3. Surgical staging to determine treatment
  4. Radiation, chemotherapy, steroids (progesterone), or combination

Ovarian Carcinoma

- Definition—a malignant neoplasm of the ovary with the highest mortality rate of all cancers that are gynecologically related
- Etiology/incidence
  1. Malignancies of the ovary arise from any type of cell found in the ovary; epithelial carcinoma is the most common type (80–85%)
  2. Ovary may be site for metastasis from nonovarian cancers
  3. Etiology unknown
  4. Risk factors
     a. Family history in one first-degree relative—10% chance
     b. Family history in two first-degree relatives—50% chance
     c. Family susceptibility shown with the *BRCA1* gene
     d. Low parity
     e. Early menarche; late menopause
     f. Ovulation induction agents (possibly)

g. Postmenopausal hormonal estrogen therapy

h. High socioeconomic class

i. High dietary fat consumption

j. History of breast, colon, or endometrial cancer

5. Use of oral contraceptives reduces risk—protection lasts up to 2 decades after last use

6. Breastfeeding is associated with risk reduction

7. Fifth most common cancer in women

8. Second most common genital tract cancer

9. 25,000 new cases annually

10. Usual age of onset is near perimenopause or menopause—median age 61 years, peaks at 75 to 79 years

11. Mortality rate exceeds all other genital tract malignancies; presents in advanced stage

- Signs and symptoms

1. Early

a. Often asymptomatic; may be detected on routine pelvic examination

b. Symptoms are often mild, vague, and inconsistent

c. Abdominal discomfort or pain

d. Pressure sensation on the bladder or rectum

e. Pelvic fullness or bloating

f. Vague gastrointestinal symptoms

2. Late

a. Increasing abdominal girth

b. Abdominal pain

c. Abnormal vaginal bleeding

d. Gastrointestinal symptoms; nausea, loss of appetite, dyspepsia

- Physical findings

1. Palpation of fixed, irregular, nontender adnexal mass—usually bilateral (usually first diagnostic finding)

2. Ascites

3. Pleural effusion and subclavicular lymphadenopathy if advanced

4. Cachexia

- Differential diagnosis

1. Primary peritoneal cancer

2. Benign ovarian tumor

3. Endometriosis

4. Functional ovarian cyst

5. Ovarian torsion

6. Pelvic kidney

7. Pedunculated uterine fibroid

- Diagnostic tests/findings

1. Pelvic ultrasonography/CT/MRI

2. CA-125—elevated levels not diagnostic for ovarian cancers (elevations can occur with endometriosis, leiomyomata, pelvic inflammatory infection, hepatitis, and other malignancies); helpful to follow response to treatment with chemotherapy and subsequent follow-up

3. Definitive diagnosis is made with laparotomy

- Management/treatment

1. Surgical

a. Total abdominal hysterectomy, bilateral salpingoophorectomy, and omentectomy—establishes histologic staging and grading of tumor

b. Goal is removal of as much tumor as possible

2. Chemotherapy and/or radiation

3. Rule out metastasis with diagnostic evaluation of other organ systems

Vaginal Carcinoma

- Definition—abnormal proliferation of vaginal epithelium with malignant cells extending below the basement membrane

- Etiology/incidence

1. Comprises about 2% of malignancies—vaginal cancer is the rarest of gynecologic cancers

2. Mean age of diagnosis 65 years with a range of from 30 to 90 years of age

3. Etiology is multifactorial; risk factors include presence of HPV infection, other genital cancers, diethylstilbestrol (DES) exposure, prior radiation

4. Vaginal intraepithelial neoplasm is thought to be a precursor

5. Five-year survival ranges from 80% for stage I to 17% for stage V

- Signs and symptoms

1. May present with vaginal bleeding or odorous blood-tinged discharge—may cause pruritus

2. May have palpable or visible mass or lesion

3. Urinary problems if bladder involved

- Physical findings

1. Early lesions are raised, granular, and may be white

2. Late lesions are friable, granular, cauliflower-like, and may be palpable; ulceration may be superficial or deep

3. Most common site is upper one-third of vagina

4. If lesion darkly pigmented—suspect melanoma

- Differential diagnosis

1. Malignancy of another site extended or metastatic to the vagina

2. Vaginitis

3. Bleeding from uterus

4. Ulceration from foreign object (pessary, tampon)

- Diagnostic tests/findings

1. Pap test to evaluate for cervical cancer

2. Colposcopy and biopsy of lesions

3. For staging use cystoscopy, proctosigmoidoscopy, IV urography, chest radiography, barium enema

4. CT scan and MRI are used to evaluate metastasis

- Management/treatment

1. Treatment should be by a gynecological oncologist

2. Accurate diagnosis and stage are to be determined before treatment is planned

3. If lesion is precancerous (VAIN I, II, III), laser is appropriate

4. Local excision (partial vaginectomy) may be appropriate for early lesions

5. Radiation is mainstay of treatment

6. Radical surgery may be followed with radiation

Vulvar Carcinoma

- Definition—proliferation of malignant cells of vulva

- Etiology/incidence

1. Multifactorial

2. Increased risk in women with the human papillomavirus (HPV) (30–50%)

3. Risk factors
    a. History of abnormal Pap test
    b. Multiple sexual partners
    c. Cigarette smoking
    d. Chronic irritation
    e. Vulvar dermatoses
4. May be associated with other urogenital cancers
5. Accounts for 1–2% of all gynecologic cancer deaths per year
6. Vulvar malignancies arise from squamous cell carcinoma, melanoma, adenocarcinoma, basal cell carcinoma, and sarcomas
7. Mean age 65 years with a range from 30 to 90 years of age; incidence in young women is rising

- Signs and symptoms
    1. May be asymptomatic
    2. Lesions may be darkly or irregularly pigmented, white or red; multifocal or singular; flat, wart-like, or scaly
    3. Ulceration, erythema, irritation
    4. Pruritus (most common), pain, burning, bleeding
    5. Odorous discharge, may be blood-tinged
- Physical findings
    1. White, red, pigmented or ulcerated lesion
    2. Hyperkeratotic patches (leukoplakia)
    3. Excoriation and erythema
    4. Most common sites are labia majora and minora
    5. Bartholin's gland enlargement
    6. Inguinal lymphadenopathy
- Differential diagnosis
    1. Vulvar dermatoses
    2. Atrophy
    3. Condyloma acuminata
    4. Vulvar infection/inflammation
    5. Lymphogranuloma inguinale
    6. Paget's disease
- Diagnostic tests/findings
    1. Pap test, colposcopy to rule out other sites of disease
    2. Biopsy/wide resection to make definitive diagnosis
    3. CT and MRI, chest radiography to evaluate for metastasis
- Management/treatment
    1. Appropriate evaluation by a gynecological oncologist
    2. Local excision
    3. Simple or radical vulvectomy
    4. Topical treatment—immunologic agents, chemotherapy
    5. Careful follow-up—recurrence is common

Choriocarcinoma

- Definition—a frankly malignant form of gestational trophoblastic disease or may be primary in the ovary
- Etiology/incidence
    1. Gestational trophoblastic disease
        a. May follow any gestational event—intrauterine or ectopic pregnancy, abortion (50%); hydatidiform mole (50%)
        b. Malignant transformation occurs in the chorion
        c. One of the few metastatic tumors that is curable
    2. Nongestational—mixed germ cell tumor of ovary occurring in childhood or early adolescence; unusual in ages 20 to 30 years

3. Disseminates by blood to the lungs, vagina, brain, liver, kidneys, and gastrointestinal tract
- Signs and symptoms—often masquerades as other disease as a result of metastasis to other organs
    1. Irregular vaginal bleeding—intermittent to hemorrhage; continuing after immediate postpartum period; uterine subinvolution
    2. Amenorrhea (from gonadotropin secretion)
    3. Hemoptysis, cough, dyspnea with lung metastasis
    4. Evidence of central nervous system metastasis—headache, dizziness, fainting
    5. Gastrointestinal—rectal bleeding/tarry stools
    6. Abdominal pain
    7. Hematuria from renal metastasis
- Physical findings
    1. Abdominal mass/ascites
    2. Blood in vaginal vault
    3. Vaginal or vulvar lesion may indicate metastasis
    4. Enlarged, soft uterus
    5. Abnormalities of multiple organs if metastatic
- Differential diagnosis
    1. May imitate other diseases—suspect strongly if follows a pregnancy event
    2. Intrauterine pregnancy
    3. Invasive mole
    4. Benign ovarian tumor
    5. Other gynecologic malignancies
- Diagnostic tests/findings
    1. Quantitative hCG
    2. Abnormal beta hCG regression titers following molar pregnancy
    3. CT scan abdomen, pelvis, and head
    4. Lumbar puncture may be necessary
    5. Chest radiography
- Management/treatment
    1. Should be managed by a gynecological oncologist
    2. Treatment is usually with surgery and chemotherapy or chemotherapy alone
    3. Appropriate follow-up to monitor side effects, disease improvement, and recurrence
    4. Nonmetastatic—good prognosis; metastatic—good to poor prognosis

Vaginal Infections

Bacterial Vaginosis (BV)

- Definition—an alteration of the normal flora of the vagina with dominance of anaerobic bacteria
- Etiology/incidence
    1. Loss of lactobacilli (hydrogen-peroxide-producing strains) results in elevated pH and subsequent overgrowth of bacteria—bacteria concentrations are 100- to 1000-fold
    2. No single offending organism—*Gardnerella vaginalis*, *Mycoplasma hominis*, *Bacteroides* species, *Haemophilus*, *Mobiluncus*, *Corynebacterium* are among the anaerobes

3. Although BV is not a "vaginitis" and is not sexually transmitted (increased bacteria numbers without inflammation [no increase in white blood cells, WBCs]; succinic acid produced by organisms alter migration of WBC to bacteria at elevated pH), women with BV are at an increased risk for acquiring sexually transmitted infections (STIs) such as HIV and herpes simplex virus 2 (HSV-2)
4. Risk factors include multiple male or female sexual partners, new sex partner, shared sex toys, and douching
5. May be associated with intra-amniotic infection, postpartum and postoperative infection, complications after gynecologic surgery, endometritis, pelvic inflammatory disease (PID)
6. Most common vaginal infection in the United States in women ages 15–44
- Signs and symptoms
  1. Most often asymptomatic
  2. Pruritus occasionally
  3. Heavy grayish, yellowish, whitish, odorous, homogenous vaginal discharge; may coat the vulva
  4. Rancid or fishy odor during menses and postcoitally
- Physical findings
  1. Copious amount of homogenous, whitish-gray vaginal discharge
  2. Normal-appearing vulva and vaginal mucosa
  3. Discharge may coat vulva
  4. Presence of foul odor
- Differential diagnosis
  1. Trichomoniasis
  2. Candidiasis
- Diagnostic tests/findings
  1. Wet mount of vaginal secretions
  2. Presence of three of the following Amsel criteria is diagnostic:
     a. Vaginal pH greater than or equal to 4.5
     b. Clue cells on saline wet mount (epithelial cells with borders obscured as a result of stippling with bacteria)
     c. Homogeneous discharge, white, noninflammatory discharge smoothly coating vaginal wall
     d. Positive "whiff test"—fishy odor of vaginal discharge before and after addition of 10% KOH (caused when anaerobic bacteria combined with potassium hydroxide); may also have positive whiff test in the presence of blood, semen, and *Trichomonas*
  3. Commercially available card tests for detection of elevated pH, presence of amine
  4. Gram stain reveals true clue cells, numerous abnormal bacteria
  5. Cultures for anaerobes are unnecessary
- Management/treatment
  1. Metronidazole 500 mg orally for 7 days
  2. Metronidazole gel 0.75% one full applicator (5 g) intravaginally at bedtime for 5 days
  3. Clindamycin cream 2%, one full applicator (5 g) intravaginally at bedtime for 7 days
  4. Alternative regimens
     a. Clindamycin orally for 7 days
     b. Clindamycin ovules intravaginally at bedtime for 3 days

5. Treatment of male sex partner will not change course of disease or prevent recurrences
6. BV may be transferred between female sex partners
   a. May cause a disulfiram effect (flushing, vomiting) if metronidazole is taken when alcohol is consumed; counsel patient to avoid alcohol use for 24 hours after completion of metronidazole
   b. Side effects—metallic taste, nausea, headache, dry mouth, dark-colored urine
   c. May cause disturbance in depth perception
   d. Not to be taken with anticoagulants—may prolong prothrombin time
7. Clindamycin cream is oil-based and might weaken latex condoms and diaphragms for 5 days after use; if using these methods for contraception, counsel to refrain from sexual intercourse until the conclusion of the treatment regimen
8. Avoid douching because this may increase risk for relapse
9. Treatment in pregnancy—discussed elsewhere in this text

Trichomoniasis

- Definition—vaginal infection caused by an anaerobic flagellated protozoan parasite
- Etiology/incidence
  1. Pathogenesis unknown; humans are the only host
  2. Caused by the *Trichomonas* organism; survives best in a pH of 5.6 to 7.5
  3. Sexually transmitted; theoretically possible fomite spread, but unlikely
  4. Responsible for 25% of vaginal infections—females symptomatic (25%); men rarely symptomatic
  5. Risk factors include multiple sexual partners, presence of another STI, non condom use; women who exchange sex for payment and use injectable drugs are at a higher risk
  6. Use of barrier contraceptive methods may decrease prevalence
  7. May be associated with premature rupture of the membranes and preterm labor
- Signs and symptoms
  1. Symptoms variable; most men and women infected with trichomoniasis are asymptomatic
  2. Any combination of the following symptoms may be seen; copious, homogeneous, malodorous, yellowish-green discharge; vulva irritation; pruritus and edema; and occasionally dysuria, urgency, frequency of urination, postcoital and intermenstrual bleeding
  3. Erythema of vulva and vagina with excoriation may be seen
  4. Onset of symptoms often occurs after menses
- Physical findings
  1. Erythema, edema, excoriation of vulva may be seen
  2. Red speckles—"strawberry spots"—on vagina and cervix (punctate lesions called colpitis macularis)
  3. Infection may be found in endocervix, vagina, bladder, Bartholin's glands, and periurethral glands
  4. Homogeneous, watery, yellowish-green, grayish, frothy vaginal discharge
  5. pH greater than or equal to 5.0
  6. Cervix may bleed easily when touched

- Differential diagnosis
  1. Bacterial vaginosis
  2. Candidiasis
  3. Trauma from foreign body
- Diagnostic tests/findings
  1. Saline wet mount (60–70% sensitive), higher sensitivity with immediate evaluation of wet preparation slide of vaginal secretions—motile trichomonads; increased WBC
  2. Gram stain—no advantage over wet mount
  3. Definitive test—culture
  4. Urine microscopic examination may reveal live trichomonads
  5. Detection on Pap test 40% positive predictive value
  6. Rapid tests (results in 10–45 minutes) on vaginal secretions (> 82% sensitive, > 97% specific)
- Management/treatment
  1. Metronidazole 2 g orally in a single dose
  2. Tinidazole 2 g orally in single dose
  3. Alternative regimen—metronidazole 500 mg orally twice daily for 7 days
  4. May cause a disulfiram effect (flushing, vomiting) if metronidazole or tinidazole is taken when alcohol is consumed; counsel patient to avoid alcohol use for 24 hours after completion of metronidazole or 72 hours after completion of tinidazole
  5. For treatment failures—exclude reinfection; retreat with metronidazole orally twice a day for 7 days or tinidazole orally in a single dose
  6. All sexual partners should be treated
  7. Pregnancy—discussed elsewhere in this text
  8. Screen for other sexually transmitted infections as indicated
  9. Encourage "safer sex practices" to reduce reinfection and chance of other STI

Vulvovaginal Candidiasis (VVC)

- Definition—inflammatory vulvovaginal process caused by the yeast organism, *Candida* species, which superficially invades the epithelium cells
- Etiology/incidence
  1. Second most common vulvovaginal infection—caused by *Candida*, a dimorphic fungus
  2. 75% of women will have at least one episode in their reproductive years; 45% will have a second episode; 5% or less will have recurrent intractable episodes; up to 20% of women in their childbearing years will have yeast isolated; 20–30% will have dual or multiple pathogens
  3. *C. albicans* species is responsible 85–90% of the time; *C. glabrata* and *C. tropicalis* are responsible for majority of remaining infections and more resistant to therapy
  4. Predisposing factors to candidal overgrowth include pregnancy, reproductive age group, uncontrolled diabetes, immunosuppressive disorders, frequent intercourse, antibiotic use, high-dose corticosteroids
- Signs and symptoms
  1. May have a combination of the following:
     a. Irritation of vulva, pruritus, soreness, external dysuria, excoriation
     b. Edema
     c. Erythema
     d. Discharge may be thick, curdy, thin, or watery, with yeast odor
     e. Dyspareunia (upon penetration)
- Physical findings
  1. Discharge is usually adherent to the vaginal wall
  2. Erythema of vulva and vagina
  3. Cervix appears normal on speculum examination
- Differential diagnosis
  1. Trichomoniasis
  2. Bacterial vaginosis
  3. Vulvar dermatoses
  4. Allergic reaction
  5. Urethritis/cystitis
- Diagnostic tests/findings
  1. Wet mount of vaginal secretions with 10% potassium hydroxide (KOH) will reveal mycelia, spores, and pseudohyphae
  2. Vaginal pH usually normal (< 4.5); amine test negative
  3. Increased WBC on wet mount
  4. Fungal culture confirms diagnosis
  5. Gram stain may be positive
  6. Pap test 50% sensitive
  7. Routine cultures may detect asymptomatic colonization; not performed routinely—may be used in recurrences
- Management/treatment
  1. Treatment indicated if:
     a. Symptomatic
     b. Patient desires
     c. Is immunosuppressed
  2. Azole family of antifungals is usual treatment and more effective than nystatin
  3. Single dose or 3-day topical azole regimens effective for uncomplicated VVC
  4. Fluconazole 150 mg orally in a single dose
  5. Treatment for recurrent VVC—if four or more symptomatic episodes in 1 year; usually no apparent predisposing factor; culture to determine if non-*albicans Candida* species; consider longer duration therapy and maintenance regimens (several regimens suggested with both topical azoles and oral fluconazole); consider use of intravaginal probiotics
  6. Key points
     a. Azole creams and suppositories are oil-based and may weaken latex condoms and diaphragms
     b. Treatment of partner is not recommended unless male has balanitis
     c. Severe VVC (extensive erythema, edema, fissure formation) usually requires 7- to 14-day topical azole regimen or repeat dose of fluconazole 72 hours after initial dose
     d. Women with uncontrolled diabetes or receiving corticosteroid therapy who have VVC may require 7- to 14-day treatment regimen
     e. Encourage use of cotton underwear
     f. Pregnancy—discussed elsewhere in this text

Sexually Transmitted Infections (STIs)

Chlamydia

- Definition—infection of epithelial cells of the genital tract of men and women; may cause pneumonia and/or conjunctivitis in neonates
- Etiology/incidence
  1. Caused by an intracellular organism, *Chlamydia trachomatis*, which replicates in the host, causing inclusions in stained cells
  2. Most common STI in the United States—approximately 4 million acquired infections annually (reporting not required in all states)
  3. Chlamydia infection may be the etiology of 50% of pelvic infections
  4. May be transmitted vertically to the neonate in up to 70% of untreated women (conjunctival or pneumonic infection)
  5. Sequelae of chlamydia include cervicitis, endometritis, PID, ectopic pregnancy, infertility, acute urethral syndrome, postpartum infections, premature labor and delivery, premature rupture of the membranes, and perinatal morbidity
  6. Risk factors
     a. Sexually active women younger than age 25
     b. Multiple partners or partners with multiple sexual partners
     c. Nonuse of barrier methods of contraception
- Signs and symptoms
  1. May be asymptomatic
  2. Postcoital bleeding; intermenstrual bleeding or spotting
  3. Symptoms of urinary tract infection—dysuria, frequency
  4. Vaginal discharge
  5. Abdominal pain
  6. Males—usually asymptomatic; may have dysuria, urethral discharge, pruritus
- Physical findings
  1. Mucopurulent endocervical discharge; edematous, tender cervix with easily induced bleeding
  2. Suprapubic pain or slight tenderness upon palpation
  3. Males—mucoid to mucopurulent urethral discharge
- Differential diagnosis
  1. Gonococcal infection
  2. Urethritis or urinary tract infection
  3. Salpingitis
- Diagnostic tests/findings—presence of organism in various laboratory tests is basis for diagnosis
  1. Culture—expensive
  2. Nonculture methods—nucleic acid amplification test (NAAT) recommended by Centers for Disease Control and Prevention (CDC, 2010)
  3. Gonococcal (GC) culture or nonculture test to rule out concomitant gonorrhea
  4. Serologic testing for syphilis, wet mount testing for vaginal infection, consider HIV screen
- Management/treatment
  1. CDC (2010) recommendations
     a. Azithromycin 1 g orally, single dose
     b. Doxycycline 100 mg orally for 7 days
  2. Alternative regimens
     a. Erythromycin base 500 mg orally for 7 days
     b. Erythromycin ethylsuccinate 800 mg orally 7 days
     c. Ofloxacin 300 mg orally 7 days
     d. Levofloxacin 500 mg orally for 7 days
  3. Treatment in pregnancy—discussed elsewhere in this text
  4. Doxycycline should not be used in pregnancy; may cause discoloration of teeth in children
  5. Erythromycin estolate is contraindicated in pregnancy because of drug-related hepatotoxicity
  6. Quinolones (ofloxacin, levofloxacin) are contraindicated in pregnancy
  7. Sex partners should be evaluated, tested, and treated if they had sexual contact with patient during the 60 days preceding onset of symptoms in the patient or diagnosis of chlamydia
  8. The most recent sex partner should be evaluated and treated even if the time of the last sexual contact was more than 60 days before symptom onset or diagnosis (CDC, 2010)
  9. Intercourse should be avoided for 7 days after single-dose treatment, or until 7-day regimen is completed
  10. Partner treatment is essential for decreasing risk for reinfection of patient
  11. Test of cure
     a. Not recommended if treated with CDC-recommended or alternative regimens and not pregnant
     b. Consider test of cure if suspect noncompliance with treatment or if symptoms persist
     c. Wait at least 3 weeks after treatment to do test of cure—prior to 3 weeks may get false negative
     d. Majority of posttreatment infections are reinfection—retest at 3 months post treatment or next office visit

Condyloma Acuminata, Venereal Warts

- Definition—a sexually transmitted, viral disease affecting the vulva, vagina, cervix, and perianal area
- Etiology/incidence
  1. Caused by human papillomavirus (HPV)
  2. Approximately 100 species of HPV; more than 30 types infect anogenital mucosal surfaces; potential for malignancy is variable (low-risk and high-risk HPV types); may be infected with multiple types simultaneously
  3. Sexually transmitted by skin-to-skin contact through viral shedding; fomite spread is possible but rare
  4. Highly contagious—25–65% of partners develop HPV
  5. Incubation period 4 to 6 weeks
  6. The most common viral, sexually transmitted infection in the United States
  7. Genital warts most commonly associated with low-risk types of HPV (6, 11)
  8. Persistent infection with high-risk types of HPV is associated with almost all cervical cancers and many vulvar, vaginal, and anal cancers
  9. About 10% of women infected with HPV develop persistent HPV infections

10. Risk factors
    a. Previous or current other STI
    b. First intercourse at an early age (< 16 years); multiple sexual partners
    c. Male partner who has (or has had) multiple partners
    d. Factors that suppress the immune system—diabetes, pregnancy, steroid hormones, folate deficiencies, immunosuppressive diseases

- Signs and symptoms
    1. Wart-like lesions—pedunculated conical or cauliflower appearance; granular, rough texture to skin
    2. Lesions may be singular, multiple, or in clusters on perineum, vulva, vagina, cervix, under the foreskin of the uncircumcised penis, on the shaft of the circumcised penis, and perianal area
    3. Perianal area may bleed easily, be painful, odorous, and pruritic
    4. Color usually whitish to pinkish gray
    5. May have associated heavy, malodorous discharge (BV)

- Physical findings
    1. Wart-like lesions—conical, cauliflower appearance; may be multiple anywhere on perineum, perianal area, vagina, cervix, or penis
    2. May appear granular, macular, or cobblestone; may be subclinical or microscopic
    3. Color varies pink to gray; darkly pigmented—have high suspicion for malignancy
    4. Many times will have concomitant BV

- Differential diagnosis
    1. Verrucous carcinoma
    2. Normal variants of skin tags
    3. *Molluscum contagiosum*
    4. Condyloma lata
    5. Seborrheic keratosis or other benign skin disorders

- Diagnostic tests/findings
    1. Diagnosis is made by visual inspection
    2. Biopsy if diagnosis uncertain; no response to or worsening during standard therapy; patient immunocompromised; warts pigmented, indurated, bleeding, ulcerated
    3. Serologic testing for syphilis; testing for other STIs; wet mount testing for vaginal infections; consider HIV testing

- Management/treatment
    1. Goal of treatment is to eliminate present visible disease and improve symptoms
    2. If untreated, may resolve on own, persist, remain unchanged, or increase in size or number
    3. As no treatment has been proven to be better than another, treatment depends on patient preference, availability of resources, and provider experience
    4. Keep area dry and clean
    5. Advise condom use
    6. Physical agents
        a. Cryotherapy with liquid nitrogen; repeat every 1 to 2 weeks for 6 weeks
        b. Excision with tangential shave excision, curettage, electrocautery, or scissors or excision with laser
    7. Chemical or keratolytic agents
        a. Trichloracetic or bichloracetic acid (80–90% solution); apply small amount carefully to wart, allow to dry; will turn white; apply sodium bicarbonate or talc to neutralize or remove unreacted acid; may reapply weekly; safe in pregnancy
        b. Podophyllin resin (10–25%) in compound tincture of benzoin—CDC recommends application of small amount to each wart, wash off in 1 to 4 hours; repeat weekly up to 6 weeks; pregnancy risk Category C; contraindicated when breastfeeding
        c. If lesions are not resolved at the end of 6 weeks of treatment, reevaluate, change treatment, or refer
    8. Patient-applied treatment
        a. Imiquimod 5% cream applied sparingly at bedtime three times a week; area washed with mild soap 6 to 10 hours after application; safety in pregnancy is unknown
        b. Podophilox 0.5% gel or solution; applied sparingly to visible warts; safety in pregnancy is unknown
        c. Use only on external warts
    9. Immunotherapy—interferon
    10. Combination therapy may be useful, especially in single-treatment failures
    11. Refer if treatment fails or if lesions are darkly pigmented, indurated, ulcerated, suspicious, or biopsy positive for HPV type with malignant potential
    12. Rule out high-grade squamous intraepithelial lesion (HGSIL) before treating cervical condyloma
    13. Emphasize importance of regular Pap test
    14. HPV vaccination of all young girls and women (recommended for ages 11–26 years), boys and young men (recommended for ages 9–26 years)

Gonorrhea

- Definition—a sexually transmitted bacterial infection with an affinity for columnar and transitional epithelium
- Etiology/incidence
    1. *Neisseria gonorrhoeae*—Gram-negative, intracellular diplococcus requiring carbon dioxide environment to survive
    2. Sites for uncomplicated GC may be urethra, endocervix (most common), Skene's glands, Bartholin's glands, and/or anus
    3. Most commonly sexually transmitted; neonate may become infected during birth
    4. Incubation period 3 to 5 days
    5. More than 1 million cases reported annually, may be as many as 2 million
    6. Occurs in individuals younger than age 30 approximately 80% of the time
    7. Male-to-female transmission estimated at 50–90%; female-to-male transmission 20–25%
    8. Since 1976 penicillinase-producing strains have been present—some are now resistant to tetracycline, spectinomycin, or quinolones
    9. Risk factors
        a. Sexually active women younger than age 25
        b. Multiple sexual partners or partners with multiple partners
        c. History of STI
        d. Inconsistent condom use
        e. Commercial sex work
        f. Illicit drug use

- Signs and symptoms
  1. May be asymptomatic or symptomatic at several sites—anal, vaginal, penis, pharynx, joints
  2. Anal bleeding
  3. Pharyngeal erythema and exudate
  4. Pelvic discomfort; dysuria
  5. Vulvar pain (Skene's, Bartholin's glands, testicular pain and/or swelling)
  6. Joint pain; erythema and inflammation of joints
  7. Potential complications
     a. Septic arthritis and bacteremia
     b. Skin lesions, pharyngitis; proctitis
     c. PID; perihepatitis
     d. Infections of glands (Skene's, Bartholin's)
     e. Gonorrhea ophthalmia neonatorum (in neonates)
     f. Premature rupture of the membranes, chorioamnionitis, and prematurity
- Physical findings
  1. May have purulent vaginal discharge; white, yellow, or green penile discharge; inflamed Skene's; or Bartholin's glands
  2. 20% invade uterus after menses with symptoms of endometritis, salpingitis, or pelvic peritonitis
- Differential diagnosis
  1. Nongonococcal mucopurulent cervicitis (MPC)
  2. Chlamydia
  3. Vaginitis
  4. Males—nongonococcal urethritis (NGU)
- Diagnostic tests/findings
  1. Gram stain of no value in women (60–70% false negative)
  2. Culture on Thayer-Martin medium
  3. Nonculture methods—nucleic acid amplification test (NAAT) recommended by CDC (2006)
  4. Serologic testing for syphilis; chlamydia testing; consider HIV screen
- Management/treatment
  1. CDC recommendations for uncomplicated infections of cervix, urethra, and rectum
     a. Ceftriaxone 250 mg intramuscularly AND either azithromycin 1 g orally as a single dose or doxycycline 100 mg orally twice daily for 7 days (CDC, 2012)
     b. A coinfection with *C. trachomatis* is usually found with *N. gonorrhoeae*. Recommendation by CDC is for patients to be routinely treated for uncomplicated genital *C. trachomatis* infection when treating for *N. gonorrhoeae*
  2. Treatment in pregnancy—discussed elsewhere in this text
  3. Key points
     a. A test of cure is not needed if uncomplicated gonorrhea was treated with the recommended regimen
     b. Avoid sexual intercourse until all partners are treated and no longer have symptoms
     c. Patient's sexual partner or partners within 60 days before onset of symptoms or diagnosis of infection should be evaluated and treated
     d. If the patient's last sexual encounter was > 60 days, treatment for the patient's most recent sexual partner is recommended

Herpes Simplex (Genital Herpes Simplex, HSV)

- Definition—a common, incurable, chronic, recurrent, viral disease
- Etiology/incidence
  1. Causative organism—two serotypes of the herpes simplex virus
     a. Type I (HSV-1) commonly found in the mouth, accounts for 15% of genital infections
     b. Type II (HSV-2) causes 85% of genital infections
  2. Approximately 50 million people infected; 1 million new cases each year
  3. 80–90% of people with HSV-2 infection report no history of signs/symptoms
  4. Asymptomatic shedding of virus accounts for the majority of transmission
  5. Usually transmitted by skin-to-skin contact; rarely spread by fomite transmission
  6. 80–90% chance a female will develop herpes following sexual contact with an infected male
  7. Risk factors
     a. Previous or present infection with an STI
     b. Trauma to skin (port of entry of virus)
     c. Immunosuppressed individual
     d. Multiple sexual partners
  8. Complications
     a. Herpes encephalitis
     b. Herpes meningitis
     c. Diffuse infection in immunocompromised individuals
     d. Perinatal infection
  9. Genital herpes and pregnancy
     a. Most women who infect their neonates have no known history of HSV
     b. Infection is transmitted during labor and delivery
- Signs and symptoms—three HSV syndromes (primary infection, nonprimary first episode infection, and recurrent infection)
  1. Primary infection
     a. Systemic symptoms—two-thirds will have systemic symptoms; fever, malaise, headache; symptoms usually begin within 1 week of exposure, peak within 4 days and subside over the next week
     b. Localized genital pain
     c. Course of genital lesions
        (1) Local prodrome; pruritus, erythema about 1 to 2 days before appearance of lesions
        (2) Formation of small, painful vesicles over labia majora, minora, mons pubis, and occasionally vagina (4 to 10 days)
        (3) Vesicles rupture, forming shallow, painful, wet ulcerations lasting 1 to 2 weeks
        (4) Lesions heal without scarring
     d. Tender inguinal lymphadenopathy may be the last symptom to resolve
     e. 75% will have a discharge
     f. 90% will have cervical involvement characterized by vesiculation and tendency to bleed easily
  2. First episode nonprimary—initial clinical episode in patients with previously circulating antibodies to HSV-1 or HSV-2
     a. Symptoms same as primary
     b. Few constitutional symptoms
     c. Shorter, milder course

3. Recurrent genital herpes infection
   a. Symptoms same as primary—usually milder (resolve 7 to 10 days)
   b. Usually no constitutional symptoms
   c. Shorter durations of symptoms
      (1) Prodrome—1–2 days
      (2) Vesicles—3–5 days
      (3) Dry-out days—2–3 days
- Physical findings
  1. Small, painful vesicles and ulceration at varying stages of progression
  2. Exquisite pain at site of lesion
  3. Inguinal lymphadenopathy
- Diagnostic tests/findings
  1. Gold standard is an HSV culture properly collected from the base of the vesicle or ulcer and properly transported to a high-quality laboratory
  2. Pap test—low sensitivity, high specificity
  3. Nonculture methods—PCR assay for HSV DNA
  4. Type-specific serologic tests (TSSTs) are available to identify HSV-1 and HSV-2 antibodies; sensitivity 91–100%, specificity 92–98% at 6–12 weeks after initial infection
  5. Serologic testing for syphilis; tests for other STIs; consider HIV testing
- Management/treatment
  1. HSV-1 and HSV-2 have no cure; systemic antiviral drugs partially control symptoms; do not eradicate the latent virus nor affect the risk, recurrence, frequency, or severity of the symptoms once drug is discontinued; suppressive therapy may reduce viral shedding
  2. Medical management
     a. First clinical episode
        (1) Acyclovir 400 mg orally three times a day or 200 mg orally five times a day for 7 to 10 days
        (2) Famciclovir 250 mg orally three times a day for 7 to 10 days
        (3) Valacyclovir 1 g orally twice a day for 7 to 10 days
     b. Episodic treatment for recurrent genital herpes initiate within 1 day of lesion onset or during prodrome
        (1) Acyclovir 400 mg orally three times a day or 800 mg orally twice a day for 5 days
        (2) Acyclovir 800 mg orally three times a day for 2 days
        (3) Famciclovir 125 mg orally twice a day for 5 days
        (4) Famciclovir 1000 mg orally twice a day for 1 day
        (5) Famciclovir 500 mg once, followed by 250 mg twice a day for 2 days
        (6) Valacyclovir 500 mg orally twice a day for 3 days
        (7) Valacyclovir 1 g orally once a day for 5 days
     c. Suppressive treatment of recurrent genital herpes—reduces frequency of recurrences, decreases rate of transmission of HSV-2 to sexual partners
        (1) Acyclovir 400 mg orally twice a day
        (2) Famiciclovir 250 mg orally twice a day
        (3) Valacyclovir 500 mg or 1.0 g orally one a day.
     d. Sexual partners
        (1) Asymptomatic—counsel, encourage self-examination; condoms

       (2) Symptomatic—use same treatment regimen
     e. Pregnancy—discussed elsewhere in this text
     f. Special considerations
        (1) Allergy, intolerance, and adverse reaction; rare—desensitization may be necessary
        (2) HIV infection
           (a) Episodes may be prolonged or more severe in persons infected with HIV
           (b) Episodic or suppressive therapy is often beneficial
           (c) Acyclovir, famciclovir, and valacyclovir are safe for use in immunocompromised individuals in recommended doses
        (3) Severe infection—hospitalize for IV acyclovir therapy
  3. Nonpharmacologic symptom relief
     a. Cool, topical compresses with Burow's solution as needed; will reduce swelling and inflammation
     b. Local hygiene; topical anesthetics; cool air with fan or hair dryer

Molluscum Contagiosum

- Definition—a mildly contagious viral epithelium proliferation of the skin
- Etiology/incidence
  1. Caused by the virus *Molluscum contagiosum*, an unassigned pox virus containing double-stranded DNA
  2. Occurs worldwide—more common in tropical and subtropical regions
  3. Most common in children and young adults
  4. Transmitted by skin to skin, fomite, and autoinoculation
  5. Incubation period 2 to 7 weeks
- Signs and symptoms
  1. Reddish to yellow, waxy, smooth, firm, spherical papules; umbilicated apex contains central plug; usually less than 20 lesions ranging from pinhead size to 2–5 millimeters in diameter
  2. Presents on trunk and lower extremities in children
  3. Presents on lower abdominal wall, inner thigh, pubic area, genitalia in adults
  4. Usually asymptomatic; may have pain, pruritus, and inflammation
- Physical findings
  1. Lesions are multiple, but usually number less than 20
  2. Characteristic light-colored papules with an umbilicated center
  3. Lesions found on face, neck, trunk, lower extremities, abdomen, inner thigh, genital area
- Differential diagnosis
  1. Varicella
  2. Lichen planus
  3. Warts/condyloma
  4. Keratoacanthomas
  5. Subepidermal fibrosis
  6. Epidermal cysts
- Diagnostic tests/findings
  1. Biopsy usually not indicated—cytoplasmic inclusions—molluscum bodies
  2. Test for other STIs in young adults

- Management/treatment
  1. Usually resolve spontaneously without scarring
  2. Superficial incision; express contents with comedo extractor
  3. Curettage with cautery
  4. For multiple lesions, cryotherapy with liquid nitrogen, silver nitrate
  5. Treatment may cause scarring

Syphilis

- Definition—a chronic infectious, sexually transmitted process that progresses predictably through distinct stages
- Etiology/incidence
  1. Caused by *Treponema pallidum*
  2. Organism enters skin through microscopic breaks in the skin during sexual contact
  3. Incubation period 10 to 90 days, average 21 days
  4. Occurs worldwide, primarily involving adults 20 to 35 years of age; has become epidemic in the United States; includes syphilis in pregnancy and congenital syphilis
  5. Increased incidence associated with greater use of illicit drugs and high-risk behavior associated with drug use
  6. Racial differences in incidence are associated with social factors; higher incidence in urban areas
  7. Approximately 90,000 cases annually in the United States
- Signs and symptoms
  1. Four stages of syphilis
     a. Primary
        (1) May be asymptomatic
        (2) Primary lesion (chancre) arises at the point of entry—evident 10 to 90 days following contact
        (3) Painless, ulcerated lesion with raised border and indurated base, rolled edges—spontaneously disappears in 3 to 6 weeks
        (4) May appear anywhere the organism enters, primary genitals, mouth, or anus
        (5) Painless lymphadenopathy may occur
     b. Secondary
        (1) Follows resolution of the primary stage, symptoms become systemic
        (2) Localized or diffuse mucocutaneous lesions (palms, soles, mucous patches, and condylomata lata) with generalized lymphadenopathy along with flu-like symptoms (low-grade fever, headache, sore throat, malaise, arthralgias)
        (3) May begin 4 to 6 weeks after appearance of primary lesion and resolve in 1 week to 2 months
     c. Latent
        (1) Begins after spontaneous resolution of secondary stage
        (2) No clinical manifestation
        (3) Detected by serologic testing
        (4) If no treatment, patient goes into early latent phase for less than 1 year duration (asymptomatic)
        (5) Early latent phase—within 1 year of acquiring disease
        (6) Late latent phase—after 1 year duration
        (7) Late latent phase of unknown duration
        (8) May remain in this stage or progress to tertiary stage

  (9) All patients diagnosed with syphilis should also be tested for HIV infection
     d. Tertiary
        (1) Characterized by gummas (nodular lesions) involving skin, mucous membranes, skeletal system, and viscera
        (2) Cardiac symptoms, aortitis, aneurysm, or aortic regurgitation
        (3) Neurosyphilis may present without symptoms or with nerve dysfunction, acute or chronic meningitis, stroke, tabes dorsalis, meningovascular syphilis, general paralysis, insanity, iritis, chorioretinitis, and leukoplakia
        (4) Not infectious
- Physical findings
  1. Chancre on vulva, vagina, cervix, penis, or at site of entry of organism—begins primary stage
  2. Secondary stage manifestations may be generalized maculopapular rash, mucocutaneous lesion, adenopathy
  3. Condyloma lata—wart-like lesions on vulva, penis, perianal region, and upper thighs
  4. Tertiary may be manifested by multiple organ involvement
  5. Gummas—tertiary manifestation; appear as nodules that enlarge, ulcerate, and become necrotic
- Differential diagnosis
  1. Other genitoulcerative diseases; herpes, chancroid, lymphogranuloma venereum, granuloma inguinale
  2. Genital carcinoma
  3. Trauma
- Diagnostic tests/findings
  1. Dark field microscopy of fluid from lesions reveals *Treponema*
  2. Serologic testing
     a. Nontreponemal—Venereal Disease Research Laboratory (VDRL), rapid plasma reagin (RPR); 80–90% accurate in making a diagnosis
     b. Treponemal—fluorescent treponemal antibody absorption test (FTA-ABS), *T. pallidum* particle agglutination (TP-PA)
     c. A positive RPR or VDRL must be confirmed with a FTA-ABS or TP-PA
     d. Nontreponemal test titers usually correlate with disease activity, and results should be reported quantitatively; a fourfold change in titer is equal to two dilutions (e.g., 1:16 to 1:4 or 1:8 to 1:32)
  3. Lumbar puncture—late or tertiary
  4. False positives for serologic testing (1%); caused by viral infections, IV drug use, pregnancy
  5. Tests for other STIs, consider HIV testing
- Management/treatment
  1. Who must be treated
     a. Pregnant women
     b. Individuals with positive dark field examination or positive treponemal antibody test
     c. People treated previously who have a fourfold rise in quantitative nontreponemal test
     d. Patients with uncertain diagnosis
     e. Persons who were exposed within the 90 days preceding the diagnosis of primary, secondary, or early latent syphilis in a sexual partner—treat presumptively even if seronegative

f. Persons who were exposed more than 90 days before the diagnosis of any stage of syphilis in a sexual partner—treat presumptively if test results not immediately available and opportunity for follow-up is uncertain

2. Treatment (CDC, 2010)
   a. Primary or secondary
      (1) Benzathine penicillin G 2.4 million IM in a single dose
      (2) Doxycycline 100 mg orally bid for 2 weeks or tetracycline 500 mg orally qid for 2 weeks, for nonpregnant penicillin allergic
   b. Latent
      (1) Early latent—benzathine penicillin G 50,000 units/kg IM, up to the adult dose of 2.4 million units in a single dose
      (1) Late latent or latent of unknown duration—benzathine penicillin G 50,000 units/kg IM, up to the adult dose of 2.4 million units given IM as three doses at 1-week intervals (total 150,000 units/kg up to the adult dose of 7.2 million units)
   c. Pregnancy—discussed elsewhere in this text
   d. HIV-positive individuals
      (1) May have a higher incidence of neurologic involvement and higher rate of treatment failure—careful follow-up is important
      (2) Serologic test results may be atypical
      (3) When clinical picture is positive and serologic test is negative, biopsy, dark field, or direct fluorescent antibody staining is done

3. Follow-up
   a. Quantitative nontreponemal serologic tests are repeated at 6, 12, and 24 months
   b. Titers should decline at least fourfold within 12 to 24 months
   c. A fourfold increase indicates inadequate treatment or a new infection
   d. Pregnant women without a fourfold drop in titer in a 3-month period need repeat treatment
   e. Treponemal tests remain positive for lifetime in most individuals regardless of treatment or disease activity
   f. Report all cases to proper agency for follow-up of sexual contacts

Chancroid

- Definition—an acute, contagious, ulcerative, bacterial infection that is sexually transmitted
- Etiology/incidence
  1. *Haemophilus ducreyi* is a short, nonmotile, Gram-negative rod (anaerobe) that grows in chains known as "school of fish" pattern
  2. Incubation period 4 to 5 days
  3. Occurs only in a few areas of the United States in discrete outbreaks; prevalence has decreased in the United States
  4. Most often seen in tropical and subtropical climates; in regions of Africa and the Caribbean

5. Known cofactor is heterosexual transmission of HIV—strongly associated with increase in incidence of HIV rates in the United States and other countries
6. 10% will be coinfected with syphilis and HSV
7. Recent increases in the United States associated with drug use, urban poverty, prostitution, and those acquiring chancroid outside the United States

- Signs and symptoms
  1. May be asymptomatic
  2. Papules or painful ulcerations on labia, anogenital skin, vagina, cervix in women; around the prepuce, frenulum, on coronal sulcus in men
  3. May be foul odor
  4. One week after onset, bilateral, tender, suppurant inguinal lymphadenopathy (bubo) develops (30–60%)
  5. Lesions resolve in 1 to 2 weeks if treated; 1 to 3 months if untreated

- Physical findings
  1. Deep ulcerations with irregular, scalloped borders
  2. Bilateral, tender, suppurant inguinal lymphadenopathy
  3. Lesions found on labia, vagina, anogenital skin, and cervix
  4. May have foul odor

- Differential diagnosis
  1. Genital herpes
  2. Syphilis
  3. Malignancy of vulva
  4. Trauma
  5. Donovanosis

- Diagnostic tests/findings
  1. Gram stain reveals Gram-negative rods or chains
  2. Definitive test is culture to identify *H. ducreyi*—collect from lesion or bubo; difficult to isolate on culture; use specific medium (sensitivity < 80%)
  3. Clinical signs pathognomonic
     a. Genital ulcers with typical characteristics
     b. Regional lymphadenopathy
     c. Negative test for HSV
     d. Suppurant inguinal adenopathy
  4. Serologic testing for syphilis and HIV

- Management/treatment
  1. Cured with treatment; may leave scarring in severe cases
  2. CDC recommendations
     a. Azithromycin 1 g orally in a single dose
     b. Ceftriaxone 250 mg IM in a single dose
     c. Ciprofloxacin 500 mg orally twice a day for 3 days
     d. Erythromycin base 500 mg three twice a day orally for 7 days
  3. Ciprofloxacin is contraindicated for pregnant and lactating women and for persons younger than 18 years
  4. Follow-up—reexamine in 3 to 7 days; if ulcerations have not improved, reevaluate
  5. Management of sexual partners—if sexual contact occurred during 10 days preceding onset of patient's symptoms, evaluate and treat
  6. HIV testing needed at the time for chancroid diagnosis

Lymphogranuloma Venereum (LGV)

- Definition—an ulcerative, bacterial, sexually transmitted disease
- Etiology/incidence
  1. Caused by serotypes L1, L2, and L3 of *Chlamydia trachomatis*, a bacterium, an obligate, intracellular parasite that infects columnar epithelium
  2. Occurs infrequently in the United States
  3. Endemic in tropical areas and travelers to endemic areas
  4. Incubation period 5 to 21 days or longer
  5. Infects men more than women (5:1)
- Signs and symptoms
  1. May be asymptomatic
  2. May report painless ulcerations that may go unnoticed and heal within days (50%)
  3. Tender adenopathy usually occurs 1 to 4 weeks after ulcer; may have fever, malaise, headache, myalgia
  4. Painful bowel movements; blood or pus from the rectum
- Physical findings
  1. Painless genital ulcer at site of inoculation; disappears in a few days
  2. Tender inguinal and/or femoral lymphadenopathy; most commonly unilateral
  3. Rectal exposure in women or men who have sex with men (MSM) may result in proctocolitis or inflammatory involvement of perirectal or perianal lymphatic tissues resulting in fistulas and strictures
- Differential diagnosis
  1. Inguinal or suppurant adenitis
  2. Chancroid
  3. HSV
  4. Syphilis
  5. Vulvar cancer
- Diagnostic tests/findings
  1. Aspiration and culture of material from fluctuant lymph nodes—50% of cases will show chlamydia
  2. Serologic testing—titer of more than 1:64 shows active disease
  3. Complete blood count will show mild leukocytosis or monocytosis
  4. Elevated sedimentation rate
  5. Screening for other STIs
  6. Encourage HIV screen
- Management/treatment
  1. CDC recommends:
     a. Doxycycline 100 mg orally twice a day for 21 days OR
     b. Erythromycin base 500 mg orally four times a day for 21 days
  2. Follow-up—follow clinically until signs and symptoms have resolved
  3. Management of sexual partner
     a. Examine and test those who had sexual contact with the patient during the 60 days prior to onset of symptoms and treat with a chlamydia regimen (azithromycin 1 g orally single dose or doxycycline 100 mg orally twice a day for 7 days)
     b. Evaluate for other STIs

Pelvic Inflammatory Disease (PID)

- Definition—comprises a spectrum of inflammatory disorders of the upper female genital tract, including any combination of salpingitis, endometritis, tubo-ovarian abscess, and pelvic peritonitis
- Etiology/incidence
  1. Causative organisms include *Chlamydia trachomatis*, *Neisseria gonorrhea*, polymicrobial infection (*Escherichia coli*, *G. vaginalis*, *Haemophilus influenzae*, Mycoplasma *hominis*)
  2. 1 million cases are diagnosed annually
  3. 200,000 hospitalizations at a cost of $5 billion
  4. 25% of cases result in infertility, ectopic pregnancy, chronic pelvic pain and are at risk for major abdominal surgery
  5. One-third of women with gonorrhea or chlamydia cervicitis will progress to PID if untreated
  6. Teenagers account for one-fifth of total cases
  7. Risk factors
     a. Sexually active females younger than 20 years
     b. Multiple sexual partners
     c. Previous episode of PID
     d. Presence of chlamydia, gonorrhea, and/or bacterial vaginosis
     e. Vaginal douching
  8. Oral contraceptive pill use is protective
- Signs and symptoms
  1. May be acute or mild
  2. Abdominal pain
  3. Vaginal discharge
  4. Fever
  5. Dysuria
  6. Dyspareunia
  7. Nausea/vomiting
  8. Vaginal spotting or bleeding (30%)
- Physical findings
  1. Lower abdominal tenderness, adnexal tenderness, and cervical motion tenderness of varying degrees—minimum criterion for empiric treatment of PID in sexually active young women and other women at risk for STI with complaint of pelvic or lower abdominal pain is presence of one or more of these three findings on pelvic examination
  2. Adnexal mass
  3. Fever of more than 101°F (> 38.4°C)
  4. Mucopurulent cervical or vaginal discharge
  5. WBCs on microscopic wet mount evaluation of vaginal fluid
- Differential diagnosis
  1. Ectopic pregnancy
  2. Appendicitis
  3. Ruptured ovarian cyst
  4. Torsion of adnexal mass
  5. Ulcerative colitis
  6. Degenerative leiomyoma
  7. Renal calculus
- Diagnostic tests/findings
  1. Testing to provide laboratory documentation of cervical infection with *C. trachomatis* or *N. gonorrhoeae*
  2. Sedimentation rate elevation and/or C-reactive protein

3. Criteria for definitive diagnosis (in case of unsure diagnosis or poor response to treatment)
   a. Histologic evidence of endometritis on endometrial biopsy
   b. Sonography or other radiographic tests revealing tubo-ovarian abscess
   c. Laparoscopy—abnormalities consistent with PID
- Management/treatment
  1. Oral Regimen A—ceftriaxone 250 mg IM once plus doxycycline 100 mg orally bid for 14 days, with or without metronidazole 500 mg orally bid for 14 days
  2. Regimen B—cefoxitin 2 g IM once with probenecid 1 g orally administered concurrently in a single dose plus doxycycline 100 mg orally bid for 14 days, with or without metro-nidazole 500 mg orally twice a day for 14 days
  3. Regimen C—other third-generation cephalosporin IM once plus doxycycline orally bid for 14 days, with or without metro-nidazole orally bid for 14 days
  4. Criteria for hospitalization
     a. Patient is pregnant
     b. Pelvic abscess is suspected
     c. When surgical emergency cannot be ruled out (ectopic pregnancy, appendicitis)
     d. Severe illness, high fever, nausea, and vomiting
     e. Failure of outpatient therapy
  5. Follow-up, reexamine within 72 hours—if not significantly improved, review diagnosis and treatment; may need hospitalization
     a. Criteria for improvement—defervescence, reduction in direct or rebound abdominal tenderness; reduction in adnexal, uterine, and cervical motion tenderness
     b. Counsel on safer sexual practices
  6. Partner treatment—treat if contact occurred with patient during the 60 days prior to onset of symptoms

Urinary Tract Disorders

Urinary Tract Infections (UTIs)

- Definition—a term that encompasses a broad range of clinical conditions affecting the urinary tract
  1. Cystitis—infection of the bladder
  2. Urethritis—infection of the distal urethra
  3. Acute pyelonephritis—infection of the kidney
- Etiology/incidence
  1. *Escherichia coli* most common organism (80%), also *Staphylococcus saprophyticus* (15%), *Proteus mirabilis*, *Klebsiella pneumoniae* (all reside in the GI tract)
  2. Colonization of bacteria in the vagina due to alterations in pH increase the risk of bladder colonization
  3. More common in women than in men (ratio 1:8), with a 1–3% prevalence in nonpregnant women
  4. There are four major pathways of infection
     a. Ascending from urethra (> 90%)
     b. Hematogenous
     c. Lymphatic
     d. Direct extension from another organ

5. Risk factors
   a. Neurologic disease
   b. Renal failure
   c. Diabetes
   d. Anatomic abnormalities
   e. Pregnancy
   f. Stones
   g. Instrumentation
   h. Poor success with medical regimen
   i. Poor hygiene
   j. Infrequent voiding
   k. Diaphragm, tampon, and spermicide use
   l. Sexual activity—coital frequency, new sexual partner
   m. Immunosuppression
   n. Sickle cell disease or trait
   o. Douching
   p. Catheterization
   q. Estrogen deficiency
- Signs and symptoms
  1. Range from mild to severe
     a. Acute cystitis
        (1) Abrupt onset
        (2) Dysuria
        (3) Frequency of urination
        (4) Urgency of urination
        (5) Suprapubic pain
        (6) Nocturia
        (7) Painful bladder spasms
        (8) Pyuria
        (9) Hematuria (gross)
     b. Pyelonephritis
        (1) Chills, fever
        (2) Dysuria
        (3) Frequency of urination
        (4) Urgency of urination
        (5) Cloudy malodorous urine
        (6) Nausea, vomiting
     c. Urethritis
        (1) Gradual onset
        (2) Frequency of urination
        (3) Malodorous vaginal discharge
- Physical findings
  1. UTI presentation inconsistent
  2. Pyelonephritis
     a. Unilateral or bilateral costovertebral angle tenderness
     b. Fever
     c. Flank or abdominal pain
     d. Vomiting
- Differential diagnosis
  1. Vaginitis
  2. Sexually transmitted infection
  3. Fungal infections of urethra or bladder
  4. Interstitial cystitis
  5. Infected calculus
  6. Fistula
  7. Obstructive uropathy
  8. Tuberculosis of bladder

9. Malignancy
10. Side effects of chemotherapy or radiation
- Diagnostic tests/findings
    1. Urine microscopy on clean catch—test shows more than 5 WBC per high-powered field (HPF) and the presence of bacteria with few squamous cells
    2. Urine culture and sensitivity
        a. Traditional criterion for infection—a colony count of more than 100,000 organisms per milliliter
        b. As few as 10,000 colonies have been known to produce symptoms
        c. Evaluated for sensitivity to medications
    3. Enzymatic (dipstick) testing—less reliable (75% sensitivity)
        a. Indicates hematuria; nitrites indicate presence of bacteria; leukocyte esterase indicates presence of WBC
        b. Send urine for urinalysis and/or culture and sensitivity if dipstick is negative in symptomatic woman
    4. Test for vaginitis, and STIs if indicated
    5. Cystoscopy if indicated
- Management/treatment
    1. Uncomplicated UTI
        a. Treat even before tests results are available
        b. Use 3-day regimens—single-dose treatment is less effective
        c. Suggested medical regimens for nonpregnant women:
            (1) Nitrofurantoin orally
            (2) Ciprofloxacin orally
            (3) Ofloxacin orally
            (4) Norfloxacin orally
            (5) Sulfamethoxazole-trimethoprim orally
    2. Recurrent infections—use above regimens for 7 days
    3. Pyelonephritis—use above regimens for 10 days
    4. Recurrent infection—retest and retreat
    5. Prevention/prophylaxis
        a. Void after intercourse
        b. Discontinue use of spermicides and diaphragm
        c. Intravaginal/topical estrogen in women with atrophy of genitalia
        d. Avoid delay in emptying bladder
    6. Referral
        a. Patients with possible pyelonephritis
        b. Patients who experience relapse after complete course of antibiotics
        c. Pregnant women
        d. Women with history of pyelonephritis
        e. Chronic disease such as diabetes
        f. Suspected renal calculus, interstitial cystitis
        g. Women who frequently use catheters

Urinary Incontinence

- Definition—involuntary loss of urine
- Etiology/incidence
    1. Etiologies alone or in combination
        a. Age-related genitourinary anatomic changes
        b. Medications (e.g., diuretics, antidepressants, antihistamines, sedatives)
        c. Nerve damage from stroke, demyelinating disorders
        d. Infections, tumors, diabetes, herniated disc
        e. Bladder neoplasm, fistulas, damage to urogenital structures, atrophy (decrease in estrogen)
        f. Restricted mobility, cognitive and functional impairment
        g. Multiparity, obesity, smoking, constipation, and family history in first-degree relative are risk factors
        h. Urge incontinence—most often associated with uninhibited detrusor contractions
    2. 10–25% of women between 15 and 64 years will suffer from incontinence
    3. 50% of nursing home population experience incontinence
    4. Fewer than 50% of individuals seek help; most are silent sufferers
- Signs and symptoms
    1. Stress incontinence
        a. Loss of urine, usually in small amounts, with coughing, laughing, sneezing
        b. Vaginal dryness if atrophy present
    2. Urge incontinence
        a. Involuntary loss of urine preceded by a sudden, strong urge to urinate
        b. Usually voids large amounts
        c. Difficulty in controlling once flow begins
        d. Occurs without warning—cold weather, physical activity, laughing, sexual intercourse, or placing a key in a door lock
        e. Patient will often complain of frequent voiding, urgency, nocturnal enuresis (10–30%)—overactive bladder
    3. Mixed urinary incontinence—presents with both symptoms of stress and urge incontinence
- Physical findings
    1. Urinary leakage with increased abdominal pressure
    2. Relaxed pelvic floor muscles—cystocele
    3. Vaginal atrophy, perineal irritation
- Differential diagnosis
    1. Urinary tract infection
    2. Prolapse of bladder
    3. Tumor compressing bladder
    4. Vaginal atrophy
    5. Stool impaction
- Diagnostic tests/findings
    1. Review prescription and nonprescription drugs for etiologic factors
    2. Voiding diary
    3. Urinary stress test to assess loss of urine when coughing and straining
    4. Postvoid residual measurement using catheter or scan
    5. Urinalysis/culture to evaluate for infection
    6. Cystometry, urethroscopy, and cystoscopy may be useful
    7. Urodynamic testing is confirmatory
- Management/treatment
    1. Transient incontinence can usually be treated with identification and treatment of underlying medical problems, behavior therapy such as habit training and timed voiding
    2. Stress incontinence—pelvic muscle exercises/pelvic floor training with Kegel exercises and biofeedback, weight loss if obese, treatment for constipation, pessaries

3. Urge incontinence—bladder retraining with scheduled voiding, biofeedback, Kegel exercises, avoiding bladder irritants, surgical removal of obstruction, anticholinergic agents (oxybutynin chloride, tolterodine tartrate)
4. Mixed incontinence—combine measures for urge and stress incontinence
5. Surgery according to diagnosis
6. Referral to a urogynecologist

Breast Disorders

Fibrocystic Breast Changes

- Definition—"nondisease" that includes nonproliferative microcysts, macrocysts, and fibrosis; and proliferative changes such as hyperplasia and adenosis; hyperplasia with atypia is associated with a moderate risk for breast cancer
  1. Cystic changes—refers to dilatation of ducts; may regress with menses, may persist, or may disappear and reappear
  2. Fibrous change—mass develops following an inflammatory response to ductal irritation
  3. Hyperplasia—a layering of cells; has malignant potential if atypical
  4. Adenosis—related to changes in the acini in the distal mammary lobule; ducts become surrounded by a firm, hard, plaque-like material
- Etiology/incidence
  1. Etiology not understood; occurs in response to endogenous hormone stimulation, primarily estrogen
  2. Conflicting studies on association with ingestion of foods or beverages containing methylxanthines
  3. Most common benign breast condition in women
  4. Palpable nodular changes observed in more than half of adult women 20 to 50 years of age; common ages 35 to 50 years
  5. Detectable on radiography in 90% of women age 40 or older
  6. Usually a regression of the signs after menopause
- Signs and symptoms
  1. Breast pain and nodularity; usually bilateral
  2. Frequently occurs or increases 1 to 2 weeks before menses
  3. May have clear or white nipple discharge
- Physical findings
  1. Multiple, usually cystic masses that are well defined, mobile, and often tender
  2. Absence of breast skin changes
  3. Most common sites—upper outer quadrant and axillary tail
  4. May have clear to white nipple discharge
- Differential diagnosis
  1. Carcinoma
  2. Galactorrhea
  3. Mastitis
  4. Costochondritis
- Diagnostic tests/findings
  1. Mammography to identify and characterize masses
  2. Ultrasound to determine whether mass is cystic

3. Fine needle aspiration (FNA) if dominant mass; cytologic evaluation
4. Biopsy or excision if dominant mass or following findings are present:
   a. Bloody fluid on aspiration
   b. Failure of mass to disappear after aspiration
   c. Recurrence of a cyst after two aspirations
   d. Solid mass not diagnosed as fibroma
   e. Bloody nipple discharge
   f. Nipple ulceration; presence of skin edema or erythema
- Management/treatment
  1. Treatment not necessary
  2. Aspiration of palpable cysts may be curative
  3. Patients with symptomatic nodularity or with mastalgia are best treated medically
     a. Oral contraceptive pills; good first choice (improvement seen in 70–90% of women)
     b. Danazol
     c. Tamoxifen
     d. Bromocriptine
     e. Restriction of methylxanthines (caffeine, tea, cola, chocolate)
     f. Vitamin E to control breast pain (controversial; no more than 50 to 600 IU a day)
     g. Mild analgesics; supportive brassiere

Fibroadenoma

- Definition—benign breast mass derived from fibrous and glandular tissue
- Etiology/incidence
  1. Etiology unknown; development soon after menarche—appears to be hormone related
  2. Most common benign, dominant mass in younger women
  3. Occurs most often in women 15 to 25 years of age
  4. Pregnancy may stimulate growth; may regress with menopause
- Signs and symptoms
  1. Painless, single, rubbery mass
  2. Round to lobular in shape
  3. May be from 2 to 4 cm in size to 15-cm tumors
  4. No nipple discharge
  5. Does not change with menstrual cycle
- Physical findings
  1. Firm, well-delineated, freely movable, smooth, rubbery, round, typically marble-sized, nontender mass; usually unilateral
  2. No nipple discharge
- Differential diagnosis
  1. Carcinoma of the breast
  2. Cystosarcoma phyllodes
  3. Benign cyst
- Diagnostic tests/findings
  1. Fine needle aspiration (FNA) to determine whether cystic or solid
  2. Excisional biopsy
  3. Ultrasonography and/or mammography will help distinguish singular from multiple nonpalpable masses (ultrasound best choice for young women)

- Management/treatment
  1. Observation, if diagnosis is confirmed and younger than 25 years
  2. May be removed to alleviate patient anxiety or if diagnosis is uncertain
  3. Follow up with monthly self-breast examinations and annual breast examination by clinician; annual mammograms if criteria of age and risk factors met
  4. Key points
     a. No mass is obviously benign—each should be carefully evaluated to rule out carcinoma
     b. Nipple discharge is seldom associated with carcinoma of the breast; when there is spontaneous clear, serous, or bloody discharge or postmenopausal discharge present cancer should be ruled out with a thorough evaluation
     c. Breast discomfort is usually associated with fibrocystic changes

Intraductal Papilloma

- Definition—benign lesion of the lactiferous duct, most common in the perimenopausal age group, 35–50 years old
- Etiology/incidence
  1. Proliferation and overgrowth of epithelial tissue of the subareolar collection duct
  2. Most common cause of pathologic nipple discharge
- Signs and symptoms
  1. Bloody, serous, or turbid discharge (not milk)—which may occur spontaneously
  2. Mass not usually palpable
  3. Feeling of fullness or pain beneath areola (possible)
- Physical findings
  1. Expression of serosanguinous nipple discharge from a single duct when pressure applied to affected duct
  2. Poorly delineated, soft mass may be palpated
  3. Papilloma are usually singular
- Differential diagnosis
  1. Intraductal carcinoma
  2. Multiple papillomatosis
  3. Galactorrhea
- Diagnostic tests/findings
  1. Microscopy of breast fluid to visualize fat globules
  2. Cytology of fluid—false-negative rates of 20% for cancer
  3. Mammography
  4. Radiologic ductogram—use is controversial
  5. Excisional biopsy of duct
- Management
  1. Refer for surgical excision
  2. Excisional biopsy is curative

Breast Carcinoma

- Definition—malignant neoplasm of the breast
- Etiology/incidence
  1. Possible interaction of ovarian estrogen and nonovarian estrogen; estrogen of exogenous origin with susceptible breast tissue
  2. Most common female malignancy—second to lung cancer as leading cause of cancer-related death; incidence is steadily increasing in United States
  3. Incidence increases with age (75% are > 40 years of age)
  4. Cumulative lifetime risk is 10.2% or 1 in 9; increase in numbers may indicate better detection and larger numbers of women in their 40s and 50s
  5. Risk factors
     a. Women with *BRCA1* and *BRCA2*
     b. Advancing age
     c. Mother and/or sister with breast cancer
     d. Previous breast cancer
     e. Perimenopausal status
     f. Previous endometrial or colon cancer
     g. Previous breast biopsy with atypical hyperplasia, lobular neoplasm
     h. Menarche before age 12; menopause after age 55
     i. Nulliparity, first pregnancy after 30
     j. Hormone replacement therapy, oral contraceptive pills (questionable)
     k. Obesity, environmental factors; exposure to radiation or pesticides
     l. Heavy alcohol use; fat in diet
- Signs and symptoms
  1. Breast mass—most often upper-outer quadrant
  2. May have spontaneous clear, serous, or bloody nipple discharge
  3. May have retraction, dimpling, skin edema, erythema
  4. Axillary, supraclavicular, or infraclavicular lymphadenopathy may be present
- Physical findings
  1. Mass fixed, poorly defined, irregular, usually nontender; palpable at 1 cm
  2. May have nipple discharge, irritation, retraction, edema
  3. Enlarged lymph nodes
- Differential diagnosis
  1. Fibroadenoma
  2. Fibrocystic breast changes
  3. Trauma
  4. Mastitis
- Diagnostic tests/findings
  1. Mammogram detects 30–50% of cancers
  2. Ultrasound to distinguish solid from cystic mass
  3. Histology for definitive diagnosis—specimen obtained through open biopsy, needle biopsy, fine needle aspiration (FNA), or stereotactic core needle biopsy
  4. CT scan of liver, lungs, bone to rule out metastasis
  5. Presence of estrogen receptors determined by assay
  6. Sentinel node biopsy
  7. Negative mammogram and negative aspiration cytology does not exclude malignancy
- Management/treatment
  1. Referral to oncologist if malignancy is suspected; staging will determine appropriate treatment options
  2. Early breast cancer—surgery or surgery and radiation; 60–70% choose lumpectomy, axillary node dissection, and breast radiation

3. Medical therapy for hormone receptor positive tumors—tamoxifen, aromatase inhibitors

4. Radiotherapy and cytotoxic chemotherapy are adjuvant therapy in late disease

Congenital and Chromosomal Abnormalities

Müllerian Abnormalities

- Definition—congenital anomalies involving the uterus, fallopian tubes, and upper vagina resulting from absence of anti-Müllerian hormone (AMH)
- Etiology/incidence
  1. Possible causes include teratogenesis, genetic inheritance, and multifactorial expression
  2. Occurs in up to 15% of women with recurrent spontaneous abortion and in 5–19% of infertile women
- Signs and symptoms
  1. History of pregnancy loss or infertility
  2. Amenorrhea, dysmenorrhea
  3. Dyspareunia
- Physical findings
  1. Many variations may occur
     a. Lack of development (agenesis); e.g., no vagina, uterus, tubes, uterine cavity
     b. Incomplete development (hypoplasia); e.g., partial vagina, bicornate uterus, partial uterine cavity
     c. Incomplete canalization (atresia); e.g., imperforate hymen, cervical atresia
     d. One-third have urinary tract abnormalities (e.g., ectopic kidney, renal agenesis, horseshoe-shaped kidney, abnormal collecting ducts)
  2. Ovaries may be developed, resulting in well-developed secondary sexual characteristics
- Differential diagnosis
  1. Various congenital anomalies
  2. Anomalies of urinary tract
  3. Primary amenorrhea
- Diagnostic tests/findings
  1. Structural abnormalities detected by ultrasonography, MRI, hysterosalpingogram, laparoscopy
  2. Chromosomal abnormalities ruled out with karyotyping (46XX)
- Management/treatment
  1. Referral to reproductive endocrinologist
  2. Surgical intervention

Androgen Insensitivity/Resistance Syndrome

- Definition—genetically transmitted androgen receptor defect; individual is genotypic male (46XY) but phenotypic female or has both female and male characteristics; previously called testicular feminization

- Etiology/incidence
  1. Individual has testes and a 46XY karyotype
  2. Transmitted by maternal X-linked recessive gene; a defect in androgen receptors; 25% risk of affected child, 25% risk of carrier
  3. Third most common cause of primary amenorrhea; represents 10% of all cases
  4. Risk of malignant transformation of gonads (5%); incidence of malignancy is rare before puberty
- Signs and symptoms
  1. Often not detected until puberty
  2. Primary amenorrhea
  3. Infertility
- Physical findings
  1. Uterus and ovaries are absent and a blind pouch vagina is present; labia underdeveloped; absent or scant pubic hair
  2. Normally developed breast with small nipples and pale areola
  3. Inguinal hernias (50%) or labial masses in infant child due to partially descended testes; testes may be intra-abdominal
  4. Scant body hair
  5. Growth and development are normal; overall height usually greater than average
  6. May have horseshoe kidneys
- Differential diagnosis
  1. Müllerian anomalies (agenesis)
  2. Incomplete androgen insensitivity
- Diagnostic tests/findings
  1. Karyotype reveals 46XY; phenotypically female or has both female and male characteristics
  2. Testosterone greater than 3 ng/mL and LH levels normal to slightly elevated
- Management/treatment
  1. Once full development is attained (after puberty), gonads should be removed at about age 16 to 18 years
  2. Estrogen replacement therapy after gonads removed
  3. Evaluate other family members; sensitive counseling

Turner's Syndrome

- Definition—gonadal dysgenesis; an abnormality in or an absence of one of the X chromosomes; phenotypically female; described by Henry H. Turner in 1938
- Etiology/incidence
  1. Usually a deficiency of paternal contribution of sex chromosomes reflecting paternal nondisjunction
  2. Occurs in 1 out of 2500 to 5000 liveborn girls
  3. Most common chromosomal abnormality found on spontaneous abortuses (45X)
  4. 60% of Turner's patients have a total loss of one X chromosome; 40% are mosaics or have structural aberrations in the X or Y chromosome
- Signs and symptoms
  1. Turner phenotype recognizable at any time of development
     a. Short stature, webbed neck, shield chest with widely spaced nipples, increased carrying angle of elbow, arched palate, low neck hairline, short fourth metacarpal bones, disproportionately short legs, swollen hands and feet, lack of breast development, scant pubic hair

b. Amenorrhea; lack of sexual development
c. Autoimmune disorders; Hashimoto's thyroiditis (hypothyroidism [10%] with goiter formation), Addison's disease (adrenal insufficiency), alopecia, and vitiligo
d. Hearing loss
e. Normal intelligence; may have difficulty with mathematical ability, visual–motor coordination, and spatial–temporal processing

- Physical findings
  1. No secondary sex characteristics
  2. Uterus present; absent or streak ovaries; infertile
  3. Congenital anomalies as described under signs and symptoms
  4. Renal (horseshoe kidney) and cardiac anomalies (coarctation of aorta, bicuspid aortic valves, mitral valve prolapse, aortic aneurysm)
  5. Hearing loss
  6. Hypothyroidism, adrenal insufficiency
  7. Alopecia, vitiligo
- Differential diagnosis—other forms of gonadal dysgenesis
- Diagnostic tests/findings
  1. Genetic karyotyping
  2. Ultrasonography or MRI scan
  3. Renal ultrasonography, cardiology consultation
- Management/treatment
  1. Recognition of multisystem involvement and involvement of multiple medical specialists
  2. Refer to endocrinologist
  3. Estrogen and progesterone replacement
  4. Human growth hormone
  5. Participation in a genetic support group

Additional Gynecologic Disorders

Chronic Pelvic Pain

- Definition—a nonspecific term associated with actual or potential tissue damage; noncyclic or cyclic pelvic pain that lasts longer than 6 months, is not relieved by nonnarcotic analgesics, and is of sufficient severity to cause functional disability and/or lead to seeking medical care
- Etiology/incidence
  1. Gynecologic, musculoskeletal, gastrointestinal, urologic, neurologic, and psychosomatic origin
  2. Relationship between pelvic pain and the underlying gynecologic pathology is often inexplicable
  3. Gynecologic causes
     a. Endometriosis
     b. Salpingo-oophoritis (PID)
     c. Adhesions
     d. Pelvic congestion syndrome
     e. Ovarian remnant syndrome
     f. Myomata uteri
     g. Endometritis
     h. Adenomyosis
     i. Gynecologic malignancies (especially late stage)

4. 48% associated with prior psychosexual trauma, including molestation, incest, and rape
5. Accounts for up to 10% of gynecologic consultations, 10% of laparoscopies, and 12% of hysterectomies in the United States, costing $2 billion annually
6. Mean age is 28.6 years
7. 20% have coexistent psychological pathology
8. No significant differences by race, education, mean age of menarche, menstrual cycle, or gravidity and parity
9. Diagnosis is difficult and patients are often referred to many specialists while becoming frustrated, angry, and/or defensive

- Signs and symptoms
  1. Paroxysms of sharp, stabbing, sometimes crampy, or dull continuous pain, usually severe
  2. Dysmenorrhea, dysuria, or vaginal pain
  3. Pain may or may not be reproducible by manipulation of pelvic organs on bimanual examination
  4. Feeling of pelvic pressure or heaviness
- Physical findings
  1. Physical and gynecologic examination may be normal
  2. Findings consistent with specific medical, musculoskeletal, neurologic, gastrointestinal disorder
  3. Findings consistent with specific gynecologic disorder
- Differential diagnosis
  1. Pregnancy, ectopic, spontaneous abortion, trophoblastic disease
  2. Gynecologic disease—endometriosis, PID, cancer or torsion of ovaries, rupture of ovarian cyst
  3. Nongynecologic disease—renal calculi, irritable bowel, appendicitis, urinary tract diseases, including interstitial cystitis; musculoskeletal, neurologic, gastrointestinal disorders
- Diagnostic tests/findings
  1. Laboratory studies are of little value in the diagnosis of chronic pelvic pain
  2. Pregnancy test, CBC, erythrocyte sedimentation rate (ESR), urinalysis
  3. Pelvic ultrasonography, hysteroscopy
  4. If bowel or urinary symptoms; barium enema, upper GI series, IV pyelogram
  5. If musculoskeletal disease suspected; lumbosacral radiography and orthopaedic consultation
  6. Diagnostic laparoscopy—ultimate method of diagnosis
- Management/treatment
  1. Appropriate referral for treatment of organic pathology
  2. Referral for psychiatric evaluation if no physical causes found; counseling for prior sexual trauma or domestic violence
  3. May need both medical and psychological management
  4. Supplemental therapies may include biofeedback, acupuncture, transcutaneous nerve stimulation (TENS)

Pelvic Relaxation

- Definition—a nonspecific term denoting a condition occurring chiefly as weakness and defect in supportive muscles and ligaments of the pelvis that includes:
  1. Cystocele—herniation of the bladder into the vaginal lumen
  2. Urethrocele—herniation of the urethra into the vagina

3. Cystourethrocele—both urethra and bladder are herniated
4. Rectocele—bulging or herniation of the anterior rectal wall and posterior vaginal wall into the opening of the vagina
5. Enterocele—a portion of the large or small intestine herniates into the upper vagina or dissects into the rectovaginal space
6. Vaginal prolapse—loss of support of the vaginal apex resulting in eversion toward the introitus
7. Uterine prolapse—descent of the uterus and cervix into the vagina toward the introitus

- Etiology/incidence
  1. Weakness in supporting structures include the pelvic diaphragm, ligaments, and fascia—commonly related to neuromuscular injury at childbirth, resulting in denervation injury of muscular floor
  2. Other causes include conditions that cause chronic increase in abdominal pressure—obesity, straining, chronic lung disease (coughing); nerve function altered by diabetes, pelvic surgery, neurologic disorders, and hypoestrogenism

- Signs and symptoms
  1. May be asymptomatic and discovered during routine examination
  2. Pelvic, vaginal, and low back pain and pressure
  3. Bulging or mass in vagina; difficulty in walking
  4. Urinary incontinence, incomplete bladder emptying, difficulty in evacuation of feces
  5. Exposed vagina may become dry and ulcerated; purulent discharge

- Physical findings
  1. Descent of the anterior or posterior vaginal walls; various degrees of descent of the cervix into the vagina indicating uterine prolapse
  2. Poor muscle strength in pubococcygeal muscles
  3. Complete prolapse of uterus (prodentia); ulceration, purulent discharge, bleeding

- Differential diagnosis
  1. Tumors of pelvis or abdomen involving any abdominal structure
  2. Diverticulum of urethra

- Diagnostic tests/findings
  1. Rule out tumors with appropriate evaluation as indicated
  2. Valsalva to assess full extent of prolapse

- Management/treatment
  1. Nonsurgical treatment—usually pessary
  2. Surgical treatment to correct vaginal anatomy (if severe)
  3. Kegel exercise to help improve muscle tone
  4. To avoid straining with bowel movements—use of stool softeners, dietary intervention (e.g., increase fluid intake, raw fruits and vegetables with skin, dried fruits, high-fiber breakfast foods)
  5. Use of biofeedback modalities

Toxic Shock Syndrome

- Definition—rare, potentially fatal, febrile condition affecting multiple systems
- Etiology/incidence
  1. Associated with toxins produced by strains of *Staphylococcus aureus*
  2. Occurs most often in Caucasian women younger than 30 years of age using tampons during menstruation; rarely associated with other articles placed in the vagina, such as diaphragms, sponges, and cervical caps
  3. Incidence is 1 to 2 per 100,000 per year in women using tampons
  4. 10% of population lacks sufficient antitoxin antibodies to *S. aureus*
  5. Nonmenstruating associated cases (55%) are caused by puerperal sepsis, post-Cesarean endometritis, mastitis, PID, wound infection, insects

- Signs and symptoms
  1. Sudden-onset fever, 102°F or greater
  2. Diffuse macular sunburn-like rash over face, trunk, and extremities that desquamates 1 to 2 weeks after onset
  3. Hyperemia of conjunctiva, oropharynx, tongue, vagina
  4. GI symptoms—nausea, vomiting, diarrhea, abdominal tenderness, dysphagia
  5. Genitourinary—vaginal discharge, adnexal tenderness
  6. Flu-like symptoms—headache, sore throat, myalgia, rigors, photophobia, arthralgia
  7. Cardiorespiratory—symptoms of pulmonary edema, disseminated intravascular coagulation (DIC), endocarditis, acute respiratory distress syndrome (ARDS)
  8. Organ failure symptoms—renal, hepatic

- Physical findings
  1. Fever
  2. Diffuse macular erythematous rash and desquamation
  3. Hyperemia of conjunctiva, oropharynx, tongue, vagina
  4. Orthostatic hypotension
  5. Abdominal tenderness
  6. Vaginal discharge, adnexal tenderness
  7. Physical signs of pulmonary edema, disseminated intravascular coagulation, endocarditis, acute respiratory distress syndrome (ARDS)
  8. Altered sensorium

- Differential diagnosis
  1. Septic shock
  2. Rocky Mountain spotted fever
  3. Scarlet fever
  4. Staph food poisoning
  5. Meningococcemia (meningitis)
  6. Legionnaires disease
  7. PID

- Diagnostic tests/findings
  1. Cultures to determine source of infection (e.g., throat, vagina, cervix, blood)
  2. Serologic tests to rule out Rocky Mountain spotted fever, syphilis, rubeola
  3. Urinalysis
  4. Evaluation for presence of multiorgan involvement—serum multichemical analysis, clotting profile, blood gases, CBC with differential (platelets # 100,000/mm³)
  5. Diagnostic criteria includes involvement of three or more organs or systems that include—cardiopulmonary, central nervous system (CNS), hematologic, liver, renal, mucous membranes, musculoskeletal, gastrointestinal

- Management/treatment
  1. Refer immediately to hospital for emergency treatment in intensive care setting
  2. Prevention
     a. Avoidance of tampons or leave in place no longer than 4 hours; alternate with pads
     b. Educate regarding signs and symptoms and prompt treatment
     c. History of TSS—avoid tampons, cervical caps, diaphragms

Diethylstilbestrol (DES) In Utero

- Definition—a synthetic nonsteroidal estrogen approved by the FDA for use from 1940 to 1971 to prevent miscarriage and premature labor; prenatal DES exposure increased risk for developing breast cancer and clear cell adenocarcinoma of the cervix and vagina
- Etiology/incidence
  1. Vagina originally lined with columnar epithelium, which is eventually replaced with squamous epithelium; if DES is introduced, that transformation is not completed; one-third of exposed patients will have columnar epithelium in the vagina (adenosis)
  2. Structural changes of the cervix and vagina occur in 25% of females exposed in utero to DES; transverse vaginal septum, cervical collar, uterine constriction band
  3. Occurrence of these abnormalities is related to the dose of medication and the first time exposed; risk is significant if administration was begun after the 18th week of gestation
  4. Increased incidence of preterm delivery, spontaneous abortion, and ectopic pregnancy
  5. Clear cell carcinoma of the vagina occurs rarely, a 1/1000 risk
  6. Columnar epithelium of vagina is especially susceptible to HPV
  7. 25% of male offspring may be affected with cryptorchidism, small testes, epididymal cysts
- Signs and symptoms
  1. May have discharge, postcoital bleeding, dyspareunia
  2. May report infertility; poor pregnancy outcomes
- Physical findings
  1. Vaginal adenosis (most common)
  2. Nodularity of cervix or vagina
  3. Visible cervical abnormalities (e.g., ridges, cockscomb, collar, hood on anterior cervix, pseudopolyps, hypoplasia)
  4. Colposcopically resembles dysplasia; mosaic pattern, punctation
  5. Transverse or longitudinal vaginal septum
  6. Uterine abnormalities; T-shaped uterus, bicornate or didelphis uterus, septate uterus
- Differential diagnosis
  1. Congenital anomalies
  2. Genetic disorders
- Diagnostic tests/findings
  1. Pap test of squamocolumnar junction to rule out cancer
  2. Colposcopy and biopsy of suspicious areas
  3. Hysterosalpingogram or ultrasonography to evaluate structural anomalies

- Management/treatment
  1. No current therapy
  2. Follow annually with Pap test/colposcopy
  3. Thorough palpation of vagina, cervix, and vaginal wall for masses
  4. Refer if abnormality suspected

Vulvar Dermatoses

- Definition—nonneoplastic disorders of vulvar epithelium growth and nutrition producing a number of gross changes; three major vulvar dermatoses: lichen sclerosus; lichen planus (other names include erosive lichen planus, erosive vaginitis, desquamative vaginitis); lichen simplex chronicus (previously known as "nonneoplastic epithelial disorders"); may be seen on other parts of the body
- Etiology/incidence
  1. Lichen sclerosus—chronic skin condition primarily affecting the vulvar area, the trunk, forearms, and breasts; most common in postmenopausal women
  2. Lichen planus—inflammatory skin condition manifested in the vulva, vagina, and other mucous membranes; typically seen in peri- and postmenopausal women
  3. Lichen simplex chronicus—thickening of skin in response to chronic rubbing or scratching; more common in people with hay fever or chronic inflammation; chronic *Candida* often the initiating factor
- Signs and symptoms
  1. Lichen sclerosus
     a. Skin easily traumatized; bruises and purpura common; blisters, ulceration
     b. Severe itching and burning; lesions do not correlate with discomfort
     c. Skin of vulva thin and wrinkled
     d. Obliteration of clitoris
  2. Lichen planus
     a. May affect gingival and oral mucosa
     b. Untreated may cause vaginal adhesions
     c. Flares and remits spontaneously
     d. Secondary infection may occur
     e. May be accompanied with vaginal discharge
  3. Lichen simplex chronicus
     a. Characterized by the chronic itch–scratch cycle
     b. Can appear on any body surface
     c. Severe itching
     d. Thickening of vulvar skin
- Physical findings
  1. May be found on other parts of the body
  2. Lichen sclerosus
     a. Loss of pigmentation, symmetry of distribution, and loss of vulvar architecture with obliteration of the clitoris
     b. Thickened dermis; white, thin, wrinkled, and scaly
     c. Bruises or purpura, blisters, ulcers
     d. Does not affect the vagina
     e. Confetti pattern of small dots can be confluent

3. Lichen planus
   a. Shiny, smooth, flat-topped papules, plaques on the skin and white patches of erosions on mucous membranes; may be widespread on vaginal mucosa
   b. Papules are purplish and range from pinpoint size to more than 1 cm in diameter; may scatter, coalesce into plaques, or become annular or linear along scars or scratch marks
   c. May be found on wrists, shins, and buccal mucosa; occasional scarring and alopecia on scalp; nails—ridging, nail loss
   d. Superficial vaginal adhesions
   e. Flares and remits spontaneously—lasts from weeks to several years
4. Sometimes, autoimmune diseases are associated with lichen sclerosus and lichen planus—vitiligo, alopecia areata, ulcerative colitis, myasthenia gravis, and hypogammaglobulinemia
5. Lichen simplex chronicus
   a. Thickened, leathery, lichenified plaques on labia majora
   b. Other locations—nape of neck, ankle, forearm, antecubital and popliteal fossae; hair and scalp (excoriated papules)
   c. Pruritus especially with stress; scratching is sometimes violent, patient stops only when skin becomes eroded and painful
- Differential diagnosis
  1. Vitiligo
  2. Vulvar carcinoma
  3. Seborrheic dermatitis
  4. Psoriasis
  5. Tinea
  6. Vaginitis
  7. Sexually transmitted infection
  8. Parasitic infection
- Diagnostic tests/findings
  1. Colposcopy
  2. Biopsy is the gold standard for diagnosis
  3. Saline and KOH wet mount to rule out vaginitis
  4. STI testing if indicated
- Management/treatment
  1. Lichen simplex chronicus—antifungal cream as directed (terconazole first choice)
  2. Superpotent topical steroids found to be best treatment for vulvar dermatoses that have thickened skin; clobetasol
  3. Apply sparingly
  4. Treatment may not be necessary in the absence of active disease—flares require initiation of topical steroid with a tapering regimen
  5. High-potency steroids should not be used for long periods of time (cause thinning of the skin and "rebound" dermatitis when discontinued)
  6. Should not be used when change in skin texture or thickness is absent
  7. Skin redness alone should not be treated with anything more potent than 1% hydrocortisone cream
  8. Testosterone ointment of no value
  9. Advise gentle soaps and cotton underwear

10. Long-term/chronic conditions require patience on part of clinician and patient; counseling may be necessary; no overnight cure
11. May try Burow's solution soaks for relief of local irritation

Vestibulitis

- Definition—marked inflammation of the minor vestibular glands; reasons unclear
- Etiology/incidence—may be bacterial, fungal, or viral agents; or unknown etiology
- Signs and symptoms
  1. Introital discomfort and dyspareunia of varying degrees; may be severe and incapacitating; dysuria
  2. Pain described as burning (most common)
- Physical findings
  1. Gross examination may be unremarkable
  2. Colposcopy or careful examination with a magnifying glass reveals tiny erythematous foci with mild edema around gland openings
  3. Hymen constricted, firm, and tender to palpation
- Differential diagnosis
  1. Vaginitis
  2. Sexually transmitted infection
  3. Lichen planus, sclerosus, or simplex chronicus
  4. Contact dermatitis
  5. Trauma
- Diagnostic tests/findings
  1. Colposcopy reveals classic inflammation of gland openings
  2. Pain can be reproduced by vestibule contact with a cotton-tipped applicator
  3. Wet mount and saline microscopic assessment; rule out vaginitis
  4. Testing for STI as indicated
- Management/treatment
  1. Treat inflammation if cause is determined; frequently candidiasis
  2. Gabapentin or amitriptyline
  3. Surgery (laser) or excision may be useful; frequent recurrences
  4. Counseling or psychological support including antidepressants are useful to assist with chronic pain
  5. Expect long-term chronic therapy

Vulvodynia

- Definition—chronic vulvar discomfort, especially burning sensation
- Etiology/incidence
  1. Constant pain usually means neurologic dysfunction of some kind (pudendal neuralgia, dyesethetic vulvodynia, "essential" vulvodynia, peripheral neuropathy, chronic local pain syndrome [CLPS], and others)
  2. May be related to urethral syndrome or interstitial cystitis
- Signs and symptoms
  1. Severe burning, stinging, irritation, or "rawness"
  2. No visible dermatoses or intermittent symptoms
  3. Two major presentations
     a. Constant pain
     b. Pain with intercourse (dyspareunia)

- Physical findings—no visible lesions or dermatoses
- Differential diagnosis
  1. Vaginal infection
  2. Allergy/sensitivity
  3. Psychogenic disorder—history of sexual abuse, rape, incest
- Diagnostic tests/findings
  1. Colposcopy/biopsy to rule out dermatoses, pathology
  2. Testing to evaluate bladder—infection or other pathology
  3. Evaluate vaginal secretions as indicated
- Management/treatment
  1. Treat infections as appropriate
  2. Amitriptyline, gabapentin, and/or clonazepam often helpful

Infertility

- Definition—inability to conceive after 1 year of unprotected coitus
- Etiology/incidence
  1. Ovulatory dysfunction (15%)—poorly receptive cervical mucus due to estrogen levels, polycystic ovarian syndrome (PCOS), primary ovarian failure
  2. Tubal and pelvic pathology (35–40%)—fibroids, neoplasm, congenital anomalies, salpingitis, adhesions, endometritis, cervicitis, endometriosis
  3. Male factor (35–40%)
     a. Abnormal semen analysis, oligospermia, abnormal sperm penetration and sperm antibodies
     b. Sperm exposure to heat, radiation, environmental toxins
     c. Coital frequency, cannabis, cocaine, DES exposure
     d. Anatomic abnormalities such as hypospadias, retrograde ejaculation (obstruction), varicocele
  4. Aging women—increased incidence when oocytes are of advanced age
  5. Cigarette and cannabis smoking (inhibits GnRH); greatest risk with smoking at an early age
  6. Thyroid disease
  7. Diethlystilbestrol exposure; also increases risk for spontaneous abortion and stillbirth
  8. Infrequent intercourse; possible sexual dysfunction
- Signs and symptoms—none specifically
- Physical findings—none specifically
- Differential diagnosis—none
- Diagnostic tests/findings
  1. Hysterosalpingogram
     a. Fluoroscopic radiography of the uterus and fallopian tubes to determine tubal patency and intrauterine/fallopian tube abnormalities; used to evaluate patients with history of infertility, spontaneous abortion, preterm delivery; contraindicated in patients allergic to radiopaque dye, pregnant, or with abnormal bleeding
     b. Dye is instilled in the uterus through the cervix; it then spreads through fallopian tubes; followed by radiographic assessment
  2. Hysteroscopy
     a. Minor operative procedure allows for inspection of endocervix and endometrial cavity; useful in the evaluation of infertility, abnormal bleeding, and endometrial cancer

     b. Under anesthesia, lighted hysteroscope is inserted through the cervix into the uterine cavity
  3. Postcoital testing (Huhner's test)
     a. Microscopic evaluation of sperm count and variability in cervical mucus following intercourse
     b. Instructions
        (1) No intercourse 48 hours prior to test
        (2) Intercourse during frame of ovulation
        (3) Evaluation within 6 to 24 hours
        (4) Specimen of mucus collected from cervix
        (5) Sperm evaluation for normal characteristics
  4. Basal body temperature
     a. Basal body temperature detects increase in body temperature in response to progesterone; indicates ovulation/anovulation; times ovulation for purpose of conception/contraception
     b. Procedure
        (1) Temperature reading each morning prior to arising/drinking/eating/activity
        (2) Recorded on graph
        (3) Normal value in follicular phase less than or equal to 98°F
        (4) Rises in luteal phase 0.4° to 0.6°F
        (5) Increase maintained until the next menses begins
        (6) This sustained increase indicates biphasic/ovulatory cycle
  5. Ovulation prediction testing
     a. Urine test for LH
     b. Predicts ovulation within 24 to 26 hours
- Management/treatment
  1. Female factors, ovulatory dysfunction—ovulation induction therapy
  2. Luteal phase defect—progesterone
  3. Infections/endometriosis—appropriate therapy
  4. Tubal occlusion/obstruction—surgery
  5. Male factor—antisperm antibodies treated by washing sperm or immunosuppressive drug therapy, varicocele repair, vasectomy reversal (50–60% success rate), nonreversible procedures require assisted reproductive technology
  6. Assisted reproductive technology (ART)—all the techniques used to achieve pregnancy that involve direct retrieval of oocytes from the ovary
     a. In vitro fertilization (IVF)—oocytes are extracted, fertilized in the laboratory, then transferred through the cervix into the uterus (most common procedure, success rate 15–20%)
     b. Gamete intrafallopian transfer (GIFT)—placement of oocytes into the fallopian tube (25% success rate)
     c. Zygote intrafallopian transfer (ZIFT)—placement of fertilized oocytes into the fallopian tube (18–20% successful)
     d. Tubal embryo transfer (TET)—placement of cleaving embryos into the fallopian tubes (not often used)
     e. Peritoneal oocyte and sperm transfer (POST)—placement of oocytes and sperm in the pelvic cavity (play minimal role in treatment)
     f. Subzonal insertion of sperm by microinjection (SUZI)—used for male factor
  7. Sensitive counseling; infertility support groups

Cervical Cancer Screening Abnormalities

- Definition—collection and microscopic evaluation of epithelial cells of the cervix and endocervix suggestive of future cervical cancer; results may range in degree from normal to atypical, mild, moderate, and severe abnormalities to invasive cancer
- Cervical cancer screening (as per joint recommendations of the American Cancer Society, the American Society of Colposcopy and Cervical Pathology, and the American Society for Clinical Pathology, 2013)
  1. Women younger than 21 years of age—no screening recommended regardless of sexual debut
  2. Women between 21 and 29 years of age—Pap test every 3 years
  3. Women between 30 and 65 years of age—screening with Pap test and HPV testing every 5 years
  4. Women > 65 years of age—no screening recommended if adequate prior negative results
- Abnormalities may be reported in one or more of three synonymous terms
  1. Cervical dysplasia
  2. Cervical intraepithelial neoplasia (CIN)
  3. Squamous intraepithelial lesion (SIL)
  4. The most common nomenclature in use today is the Bethesda System (1988, revised 1991 and 2002)
- The 2001 Bethesda System for reporting results of cervical cytology includes:
  1. Specimen adequacy
     a. Satisfactory for evaluation; will note presence/absence of endocervical/transformation zone component
     b. Unsatisfactory for evaluation—specimen obscured by blood or inflammation, inadequate number of squamous cells, air dried slide, not processed because unlabeled
  2. Interpretation/results
     a. General categorization
        (1) Negative for intraepithelial lesion or malignancy
        (2) Epithelial cell abnormality
        (3) Other
     b. Negative for intraepithelial lesion or malignancy
        (1) No epithelial abnormality
        (2) Will report presence of organisms
           (a) *Trichomonas*
           (b) Fungal organisms consistent morphologically with *Candida* species
           (c) Shift in vaginal flora suggestive of bacterial vaginosis
           (d) Bacteria morphologically consistent with *Actinomyces* species
           (e) Cellular changes consistent with herpes simplex virus
        (3) May report other nonneoplastic findings
           (a) Reactive cellular changes associated with inflammation, radiation, intrauterine device
           (b) Glandular cells status posthysterectomy
           (c) Atrophy
     c. Epithelial cell abnormalities
        (1) Squamous cell abnormalities
           (a) Atypical squamous cells of undetermined significance (ASC-US)
           (b) Atypical squamous cells cannot exclude HSIL (ASC-H)
           (c) Low-grade squamous intraepithelial lesion (LSIL); encompasses human papillomavirus/mild dysplasia/cervical intraepithelial neoplasia 1 (CIN 1)
           (d) High-grade squamous intraepithelial lesion (HSIL); encompasses moderate dysplasia/carcinoma in situ CIN 2 and CIN 3
           (e) Squamous cell carcinoma
        (2) Glandular cell abnormalities
           (a) Atypical glandular cells (AGC) specified as endocervical, endometrial, or glandular cells
           (b) Atypical glandular cells, favor neoplastic some features of neoplasm but not sufficient to reach interpretation of adenocarcinoma in situ
           (c) Endocervical adenocarcinoma in situ (AIS)
        d. Other—endometrial cells in women 40 years of age or older
- Management/treatment
  1. Specimen adequacy
     a. Satisfactory for evaluation—no action needed
     b. Unsatisfactory for evaluation—assess and treat as needed if inflammation is cause; repeat Pap test in 4–6 months; may defer to annual repeat if adequate history of normal Pap tests
  2. Organisms
     a. *Trichomonas vaginalis*—highly predictive, but not 100%; treat if indicated
     b. *Candida* species—most are asymptomatic colonization and require no treatment; if symptomatic, treat
     c. Bacterial vaginosis—correlate with clinical findings; treat if indicated
     d. *Actinomyces*—evaluate for signs/symptoms of pelvic infection if intrauterine contraceptive (IUC) present; if has pelvic infection, remove IUC and treat with antibiotics; otherwise, no treatment or IUC removal needed
     e. Herpes simplex virus—high predictive value; counsel client
  3. Reactive changes associated with inflammation
     a. Examine—microscopy, STI tests as indicated
     b. Treat any identified cause
     c. It is of no value to treat empirically with topical sulfa cream
     d. Repeat Pap test if indicated
  4. Endometrial cells in premenopausal woman with normal menstrual pattern—insignificant; must be evaluated with endometrial biopsy in postmenopausal woman or in premenopausal woman with abnormal bleeding
  5. Atrophy—treat if symptomatic
  6. Epithelial cell abnormalities (ASCCP 2013)
     a. ASC-US—see Figure 5-1.
     b. ASC-US or LSIL in women ages 21–24 years—see Figure 5-2.
     c. LSIL—see Figure 5-3.
     d. LSIL in pregnant women—see Figure 5-4.
     e. ASC-H—see Figure 5-5.
     f. HSIL in women ages 21–24 years—see Figure 5-6.
     g. HSIL—see Figure 5-7.
     h. AGC—see Figures 5-8 and 5-9.

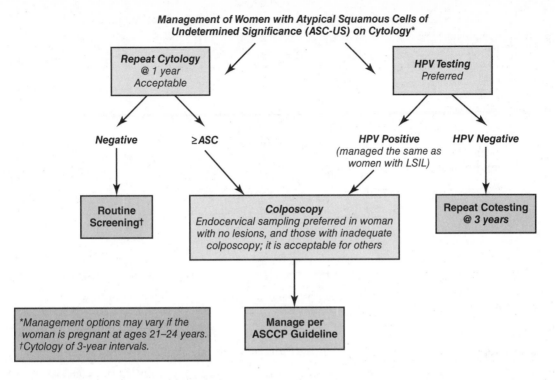

- **Figure 5-1 Management of Women with Atypical Squamous Cells of Undetermined Significance (ASC-US) on Cytology**

Reprinted from The Journal of Lower Genital Tract Disease Volume 17, Number 5, with the permission of ASCCP © American Society for Colposcopy and Cervical Pathology 2013. No copies of the algorithms may be made without the prior consent of ASCCP.

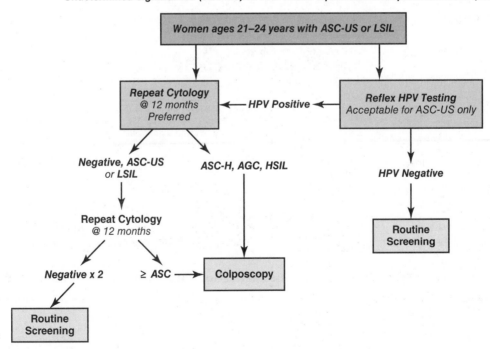

- **Figure 5-2 Management of Women Ages 21–24 years with either Atypical Squamous Cells of Undetermined Significance (ASC-US) or Low-Grade Squamous Intraepithelial Lesion (LSIL)**

Reprinted from The Journal of Lower Genital Tract Disease Volume 17, Number 5, with the permission of ASCCP © American Society for Colposcopy and Cervical Pathology 2013. No copies of the algorithms may be made without the prior consent of ASCCP.

Management of Women with Low-Grade Squamous Intraepithelial Lesions (LSIL)‡

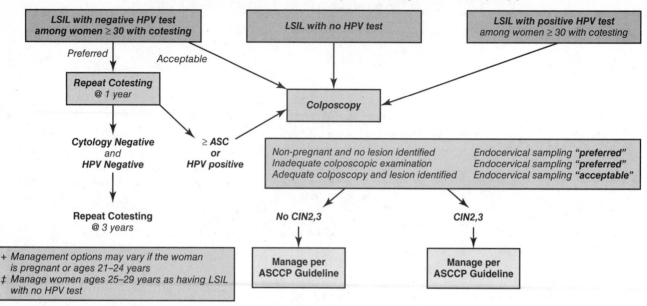

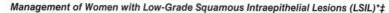

- **Figure 5-3 Management of Women with Low-Grade Squamous Intraepithelial Lesions (LSIL)**

Reprinted from The Journal of Lower Genital Tract Disease Volume 17, Number 5, with the permission of ASCCP © American Society for Colposcopy and Cervical Pathology 2013. No copies of the algorithms may be made without the prior consent of ASCCP.

Management of Pregnant Women with Low-Grade Squamous Intraepithelial Lesions (LSIL)

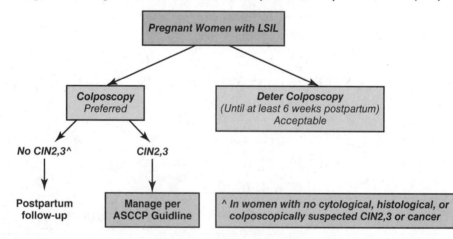

- **Figure 5-4 Management of Pregnant Women with Low-Grade Squamous Intraepithelial Lesions (LSIL)**

Reprinted from The Journal of Lower Genital Tract Disease Volume 17, Number 5, with the permission of ASCCP © American Society for Colposcopy and Cervical Pathology 2013. No copies of the algorithms may be made without the prior consent of ASCCP.

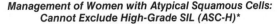

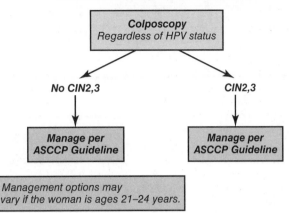

- **Figure 5-5 Management of Women with Atypical Squamous Cells: Cannot Exclude High-Grade SIL (ASC-H)**

Reprinted from The Journal of Lower Genital Tract Disease Volume 17, Number 5, with the permission of ASCCP © American Society for Colposcopy and Cervical Pathology 2013. No copies of the algorithms may be made without the prior consent of ASCCP.

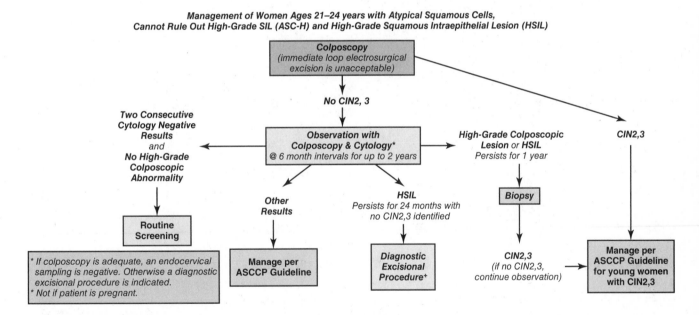

- **Figure 5-6 Management of Women Ages 21–24 years with Atypical Squamous Cells, Cannot Rule Out High-Grade SIL (ASC-H) and High-Grade Squamous Intraepithelial Lesion (HSIL)**

Reprinted from The Journal of Lower Genital Tract Disease Volume 17, Number 5, with the permission of ASCCP © American Society for Colposcopy and Cervical Pathology 2013. No copies of the algorithms may be made without the prior consent of ASCCP.

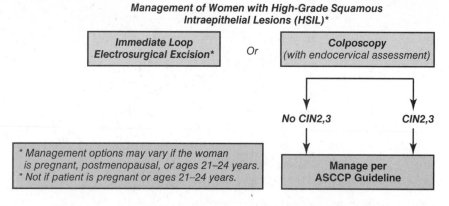

Figure 5-7 Management of Women with High-Grade Squamous Intraepithelial Lesions (HSIL)

Reprinted from The Journal of Lower Genital Tract Disease Volume 17, Number 5, with the permission of ASCCP © American Society for Colposcopy and Cervical Pathology 2013. No copies of the algorithms may be made without the prior consent of ASCCP.

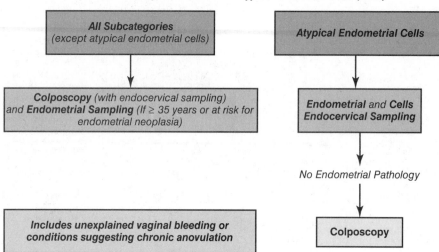

Figure 5-8 Initial Workup of Women with Atypical Glandular Cells (AGC)

Reprinted from The Journal of Lower Genital Tract Disease Volume 17, Number 5, with the permission of ASCCP © American Society for Colposcopy and Cervical Pathology 2013. No copies of the algorithms may be made without the prior consent of ASCCP.

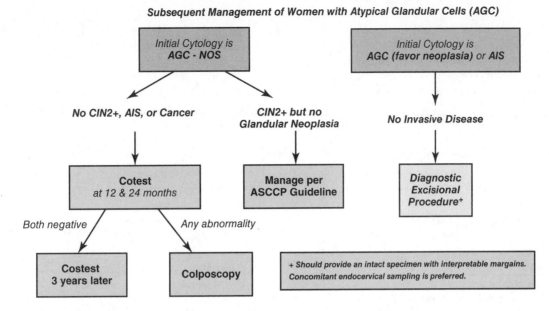

Subsequent Management of Women with Atypical Glandular Cells (AGC)

- **Figure 5-9 Subsequent Management of Women with Atypical Glandular Cells (AGC)**

Reprinted from The Journal of Lower Genital Tract Disease Volume 17, Number 5, with the permission of ASCCP © American Society for Colposcopy and Cervical Pathology 2013. No copies of the algorithms may be made without the prior consent of ASCCP.

Questions

Select the best answer.

1. Premenstrual syndrome is suspected when a woman experiences symptoms only during:
   a. Ovulation
   b. The luteal phase
   c. The LH surge
   d. The follicular phase

2. Primary dysmenorrhea can best be treated with:
   a. Dopamine agonists
   b. GnRH agonists
   c. Prostaglandin inhibitors
   d. Tricyclic antidepressants

3. The most common cause for chronic pelvic pain in reproductive-age women is:
   a. Adenomyosis
   b. Endometriosis
   c. Pelvic inflammatory infection
   d. Uterine fibroids

4. Which of the following contraceptive methods has also been FDA approved for treatment of endometriosis?
   a. Combination oral contraceptive pills
   b. Levonorgestrel IUS
   c. Progestin-only contraceptive pills
   d. Sub Q 104 DMPA

5. A complication of pelvic inflammatory disease is:
   a. Adenomyosis
   b. Endometriosis
   c. Infertility
   d. Irritable bowel syndrome

6. The most common cause of urge urinary incontinence is:
   a. Detrusor irritability
   b. Neuromuscular injury
   c. Pelvic organ prolapse
   d. Sphincter incompetence

7. During a vaginal examination, you observe bulging of the anterior wall when you ask the patient to bear down. This is most likely a:
   a. Congenital abnormality
   b. Cystocele
   c. Rectocele
   d. Uterine prolapse

8. The definitive diagnosis of endometriosis is made with:
   a. CT scan
   b. Laparoscopy
   c. Serum CA-125
   d. Transvaginal ultrasound

9. Adenomyosis can be suspected when a woman has a/an:
   a. Boggy, tender uterus
   b. Enlarged irregularly shaped uterus
   c. Fixed retroverted uterus
   d. Prolapsed uterus

10. The most common benign neoplasm of the cervix is:
    a. Bartholin's gland cyst
    b. Squamous papilloma

c. Pedunculated myoma

d. Polyp

11. A 22-year-old female presents with complaint of malodorous vaginal discharge and vulvar itching. On examination, a watery, yellowish-green vaginal discharge is noted along with vulvar and vaginal erythema. The most likely findings on a wet mount examination will be:

a. Clue cells

b. *Lactobacilli*

c. Pseudohyphae

d. Trichomonads

12. Characteristics of Turner's syndrome include:

a. Uterus absent, ovaries absent

b. Uterus absent, ovaries present

c. Uterus present, ovaries absent

d. Uterus present, ovaries present

13. A 58-year-old woman complains of severe vulvar pruritus. On genital examination you note thin skin and purpura on the vulva. You suspect the diagnosis may be:

a. Lichen sclerosus

b. Local allergic reaction

c. Lichen simplex chronicus

d. Vulvodynia

14. Treatment of molluscum contagiosum includes:

a. Azithromycin 1 g orally in a single dose

b. Erythromycin base 500 mg orally four times a day for 21 days

c. Trichloracetic or bichloracetic acid (80–90% solution)

d. Cryotherapy with liquid nitrogen

15. Which of the following best describes the mechanism of action of tranexamic acid in the treatment of heavy menstrual bleeding?

a. Acts as an antifibrinolytic to block lysis of fibrin clots

b. Causes rapid growth of endometrium to control acute, heavy bleeding episode

c. Increases the ratio of vasoconstricting prostaglandins to vasodilating prostaglandins

d. Suppresses endometrial proliferation to manage chronic heavy menstrual bleeding

16. Hirsutism is most commonly seen with:

a. Androgen insensitivity syndrome

b. Asherman's syndrome

c. Polycystic ovarian syndrome

d. Turner's syndrome

17. A 22-year-old experiences 6 months of amenorrhea. Laboratory test results include normal prolactin and thyroid-stimulating hormone and negative pregnancy test. The next action will be to:

a. Administer progestin challenge test

b. Measure testosterone

c. Order hysterosalpingogram

d. Order MRI or CT scan of pituitary gland

18. The most common cause of menstrual abnormality in a reproductive-age woman is:

a. Adenomyosis

b. Anovulation

c. Coagulopathy

d. Ectopic pregnancy

19. The pain of primary dysmenorrhea is

a. Always associated with pathology such as endometriosis

b. Colicky, spasmodic, sometimes radiating up the back to the shoulders

c. Colicky, spasmodic, sometimes radiating to the thighs and low back

d. A dull ache associated with underlying pathology

20. A 16-year-old woman has not yet begun menstruating but does have pubic hair. She is best described as having:

a. Asherman's syndrome

b. Oligomenorrhea

c. Primary amenorrhea

d. Secondary amenorrhea

21. Which of the following is the most accurate method to predict the occurrence of ovulation?

a. Huhner's test

b. Evaluation of cervical mucus

c. LH surge test

d. Basal body temperature

22. Toxic shock syndrome should be suspected in a woman presenting with sudden-onset fever, flu-like symptoms, recent tampon use, and:

a. Dysuria

b. Heavy vaginal bleeding

c. Pale conjunctiva and vaginal walls

d. Macular rash on face and trunk

23. A known risk factor for cancer of the vulva is:

a. Cigarette smoking

b. Early menarche

c. Multiparity

d. Uncircumcised partner

24. Polycystic ovarian syndrome predisposes to an increased incidence of:

a. Adrenal tumors

b. Endometriosis

c. Endometrial cancer

d. Ovarian cancer

25. In which of the following conditions would you expect to have a positive progestin challenge test?

a. Androgen insensitivity syndrome

b. Asherman's syndrome

c. Polycystic ovarian syndrome

d. Turner's syndrome

26. The most common presenting symptom of vulvar cancer is:

a. Bleeding

b. Pruritus

c. Vaginal discharge

d. Vaginal odor

27. This treatment for chlamydia should not be used in pregnancy because it may lead to the discoloration of teeth in children.

a. Ciprofloxacin

b. Doxycycline

c. Penicillin

d. Trimethoprim

28. A 26-year-old female has a Pap test report of ASC-US. This is her first abnormal Pap test. HPV-DNA testing is negative for high-risk HPV types. Recommended follow-up would include:
    a. Colposcopy in 6 months
    b. Repeat Pap smear in 4 to 6 months
    c. Repeat HPV-DNA testing in 1 year
    d. Repeat cotesting in 3 years

29. A treatment for atrophic vaginitis with the goal of prevention of recurrence is:
    a. Antifungal cream
    b. Low-potency topical steroids
    c. Oral progestin therapy
    d. Topical estrogen cream

30. A 24-year-old woman presents with complaint of nontender mass in her left breast that does not change with menstrual cycle. On examination, you note a freely movable, 0.5 cm × 1 cm, firm, rubbery nontender mass. The most likely diagnosis is:
    a. Fibroadenoma
    b. Fibrocystic breast changes
    c. Intraductal papilloma
    d. Cystosarcoma phyllodes

31. The Bethesda System equivalent for moderate dysplasia or CIN III on a Pap test is:
    a. Atypical glandular cells of undetermined significance (AGS-US)
    b. Carcinoma in situ
    c. High-grade squamous epithelial lesion
    d. Low-grade squamous intraepithelial lesion

32. Potential causes for galactorrhea include all of the following *except*:
    a. Heavy tobacco use
    b. Hypothyroidism
    c. Opiate use
    d. Pituitary adenoma

33. Leiomyomata arising from tissue within the uterine wall are:
    a. Interstitial
    b. Pedunculated
    c. Subserosal
    d. Submucosal

34. The most common presenting symptom of leiomyomata uteri is:
    a. Infertility
    b. Menorrhagia
    c. GI symptoms
    d. Urinary frequency

35. Another name for a dermoid cyst is:
    a. Benign cystic teratoma
    b. Follicular cyst
    c. Hyperplastic endometroma
    d. Müllerian cyst

36. Your examination of a female patient indicates that she has external genital warts. You will want to explain to her that:
    a. Her partner needs a blood test to see if he has subclinical infection
    b. She should have Pap tests every 6 months
    c. There is no therapy that will eliminate the HPV virus
    d. You cannot start treatment until you have her Pap test results

37. A 36-year-old is seen in your office on day 18 of her cycle for her routine annual examination. She has no complaints. Pelvic exam reveals a 9-cm firm pelvic mass anterior to the uterus. The most likely diagnosis is:
    a. Benign cystic teratoma
    b. Ectopic pregnancy
    c. Endometrioma
    d. Follicular cyst

38. Unopposed estrogen may predispose a 52-year-old woman to:
    a. Endometrial hyperplasia
    b. Fibrocystic breast changes
    c. Follicular cysts
    d. Ovarian carcinoma

39. A diagnosis of stress urinary incontinence is confirmed on the basis of:
    a. Probable etiology
    b. Pelvic muscle tone evaluation
    c. Urodynamic testing
    d. Symptom profile

40. The most common presenting symptom of cervical cancer is:
    a. Dyspareunia
    b. Lower abdominal pain
    c. Irregular bleeding
    d. Yellow vaginal discharge

41. The first step in the evaluation of a HSIL Pap test result is:
    a. HPV DNA testing
    b. Immediate loop electrosurgical excision or colposcopy with endocervical assessment
    c. Endometrial biopsy
    d. Repeat Pap test at 6 and 12 months

42. Persistent vague abdominal pain or discomfort in a 65-year-old woman may be an early sign of:
    a. Choriocarcinoma
    b. Benign cystic teratoma
    c. Endometrial cancer
    d. Ovarian cancer

43. A risk factor for endometrial cancer is:
    a. DES exposure
    b. Early menopause
    c. Obesity
    d. Multiparity

44. The most lethal gynecologic malignancy is:
    a. Cervical carcinoma
    b. Choriocarcinoma
    c. Endometrial carcinoma
    d. Ovarian carcinoma

45. A positive "whiff" or amine test is suggestive of:
    a. Atrophic vaginitis
    b. Bacterial vaginosis
    c. Chronic lichen sclerosus
    d. Recurrent candidiasis

46. An indicator of loss of lactobacilli in the vagina is:
    a. Elevated pH
    b. Increased WBCs on wet mount
    c. Malodorous vaginal discharge
    d. Vaginal itching

47. Trichomoniasis is best treated with:
    a. Oral fluconazole
    b. Oral metronidazole
    c. Topical clindamycin cream
    d. Topical metronidazole cream

48. Which of the following treatments for genital warts may be used during pregnancy?
    a. Imiquimod cream
    b. Podophyllin resin
    c. Podofilox gel
    d. Trichloracetic acid

49. A sexually active 18-year-old presents with postcoital spotting, dysuria, and a yellow discharge. On exam you find her cervix is erythematous and bleeds with contact. The most likely diagnosis is:
    a. Cervical cancer
    b. Chlamydia
    c. Primary syphilis
    d. Tampon injury

50. Risk factors for ovarian cancer include:
    a. Diabetes
    b. Late menopause
    c. History of human papillomavirus
    d. Oral contraceptive pill use for more than 5 years

51. Recommendations for repeat testing after treatment for chlamydia with doxycycline include:
    a. Test of cure 1 to 2 weeks after treatment if suspect noncompliance
    b. Test of cure 3 to 4 weeks after treatment for all patients
    c. Test for possible reinfection 1 month after treatment
    d. Test for possible reinfection 3 months after treatment

52. Effective treatment for the symptomatic relief of herpes genitalis is:
    a. Ceftriaxone
    b. Famciclovir
    c. Silver nitrate
    d. Tetracycline

53. A lesion of secondary syphilis is:
    a. Condyloma acuminata
    b. Condyloma lata
    c. Molluscum contagiosum
    d. Inguinal bubo

54. Primary syphilis may be suspected when the patient presents with:
    a. A maculopapular rash
    b. An indurated, painless ulcer on the cervix
    c. Enlarged, tender inguinal lymph nodes
    d. Tender vesicles and papules on the vulva

55. Herniation of the bladder into the vagina is called:
    a. Cystocele
    b. Enterocele
    c. Urethrocele
    d. Vaginal prolapse

56. A 66-year-old woman with a history of pruritus presents with an ulceration of the vulva. The most likely diagnosis is:
    a. Chancroid
    b. Secondary trauma
    c. Syphilis
    d. Vulvar carcinoma

57. A 26-year-old woman presents with multiple, painless, umbilicated papules on her mons pubis. The most likely diagnosis is:
    a. Condyloma acuminata
    b. Condyloma lata
    c. Lymphogranuloma venereum
    d. Molluscum contagiosum

58. Which of the following statements concerning herpes genitalis is true?
    a. Suppressive therapy does not reduce viral shedding
    b. Systemic symptoms are uncommon during recurrences
    c. Topical acyclovir is as effective as oral acyclovir for recurrences
    d. Transmission of the virus is unlikely to occur during the prodromal phase

59. Disorders of pelvic support may be associated with all of the following *except*:
    a. Obesity
    b. Neuromuscular injury during childbirth
    c. Pelvic surgery
    d. Frequent urinary tract infections

60. A 58-year-old woman complains that she feels like she is "sitting on a ball." She has significant constipation and rectal pressure. On examination you will most likely find:
    a. Cystocele
    b. Hemorrhoid
    c. Rectocele
    d. Urethrocele

61. Vaginal cancer is most commonly found in which part of the vagina?
    a. The hymenal ring
    b. Midway of the vagina
    c. The posterior fourchette
    d. The upper one-third of the vagina

62. Females exposed to DES in utero are at increased risk for:
    a. Breast cancer
    b. Ovarian cancer
    c. Vaginal cancer
    d. Vulvar cancer

63. Anticholinergic agents may be used in the treatment of:
    a. Stress incontinence
    b. Urge incontinence
    c. Vestibulitis
    d. Vulvodynia

64. Neoplasm with the highest mortality rate of all cancers that are gynecologically related is:
    a. Leiomyoma
    b. Endometrial carcinoma
    c. Choriocarcinoma
    d. Ovarian carcinoma

65. The most common cause of pathologic nipple discharge in perimenopausal women is:
    a. Breast cancer
    b. Fibroadenoma
    c. Intraductal papilloma
    d. Prolactin-secreting pituitary adenoma
66. The most common germ cell tumor is:
    a. Benign cystic teratoma
    b. Choriocarcinoma
    c. Embryonal carcinoma
    d. Vaginal agenesis
67. An examination finding that is considered a minimum criterion for empirical treatment of PID in a sexually active young woman presenting with lower abdominal or pelvic pain is:
    a. Adnexal mass
    b. Cervical motion tenderness
    c. Fever higher than 101°F (> 38.4°C)
    d. Vaginal discharge
68. A 16-year-old patient comes to the office because she has never had a menstrual period. She has normal breast development, scant pubic hair, and a blind vaginal pouch with no palpable uterus or ovaries. The most likely diagnosis is:
    a. Androgen insensitivity/resistance syndrome
    b. Mullerian agenesis
    c. Sheehan's syndrome
    d. Turner's syndrome
69. The gonads should be removed after puberty in a person with androgen insensitivity/resistance syndrome to prevent:
    a. Endometrial hyperplasia
    b. Gonadal malignancies
    c. Increased risk for breast cancer
    d. Psychological trauma
70. The most common method of assisted reproductive technology is:
    a. Gamete intrafallopian transfer (GIFT)
    b. Intracytoplasmic sperm injection (ICZI)
    c. In vitro fertilization (IVF)
    d. Zygote intrafallopian transfer (ZIFT)
71. Turner's syndrome can be suspected when the patient has primary amenorrhea and:
    a. Blind vaginal pouch with imperforate hymen
    b. Low IQ and visual disturbances
    c. Normal breast development but lack of pubic and axillary hair growth
    d. Short stature and webbed neck
72. The most common chromosomal abnormality in spontaneously aborted fetuses is:
    a. Fitz-Hugh-Curtis syndrome
    b. Fragile X syndrome

c. Müllerian duct abnormalities
d. Turner's syndrome
73. Reactive cellular changes on a Pap test report are most likely the result of:
    a. Inflammation
    b. Low-grade epithelial lesion
    c. Glandular cell abnormalities
    d. Oral contraceptive use
74. A patient with latent syphilis may present with:
    a. A maculopapular rash
    b. An indurated painless ulcer
    c. Condyloma lata
    d. No signs of infection
75. The CDC recommendation for follow-up of a female treated for PID with a recommended outpatient regimen is:
    a. Advise patient to return if pain and/or fever persists more than 5 days
    b. Reexamine patient within 72 hours after initiation of treatment
    c. Retest for chlamydia and gonorrhea in 2 weeks
    d. See patient in 1 week for second dose of ceftriaxone IM
76. Which of the following medications is most likely to cause a metallic taste?
    a. Acyclovir
    b. Azithromycin
    c. Fluconazole
    d. Metronidazole
77. A patient-applied treatment for human papillomavirus (HPV) is:
    a. Bichloracetic acid
    b. Clindamycin cream
    c. Imiquimod
    d. Podophyllin resin
78. Risk factors for breast carcinoma include:
    a. Early menopause
    b. History of endometrial cancer
    c. Multiparity
    d. History of intraductal papilloma
79. Characteristic "strawberry spots" on the cervix may be seen with:
    a. Bacterial vaginosis
    b. Chlamydia
    c. Herpes genitalis
    d. Trichomoniasis
80. Typical characteristics of vulvodynia include:
    a. Constant vulvar burning and discomfort
    b. Inflammation of the vestibular glands
    c. Thickened plaques on vulva
    d. Vulvovaginal edema and erythema

Answers with Rationales

1. b. The luteal phase
   Premenstrual syndrome is the cyclic occurrence of a group of distressing physical and psychological symptoms in luteal phase, which begin 5–7 days before menses, and which resolve within 4 days after onset of menses.

2. c. Prostaglandin inhibitors
   Prostaglandin synthetase inhibitors, nonsteroidal anti-inflammatory drugs (NSAIDs), are the treatment of choice for primary dysmenorrhea. They work best if begun at onset of menses and continue for 48 to 72 hours. Choices shown to be effective are mefenamic acid, naproxyn sodium, ibuprofen, and indomethacin.

3. b. Endometriosis
   Seven percent to 10% of premenopausal women are affected by endometriosis; it is the most common cause of chronic pelvic pain.

4. d. Sub Q 104 DMPA
   Sub Q 104 DMPA is FDA approved for treatment of endometriosis. Other medical management includes analgesics (nonsteroidal anti-inflammatory drugs are first choice), gonadotropin-releasing hormone (GnRH) agonists, and danazol to induce regression of endometrial implants; IM DMPA also has been found to be effective.

5. c. Infertility
   Twenty-five percent of cases result in infertility, ectopic pregnancy, or chronic pelvic pain and are at risk for major abdominal surgery.

6. a. Detrusor irritability
   Urge urinary incontinence is most often associated with uninhibited detrusor contractions. Patients often complain of frequent voiding, urgency, nocturnal enuresis (10–30%)—overactive bladder.

7. b. Cystocele
   Cystole is the herniation of the bladder into the vaginal lumen.

8. b. Laparosccopy
   Direct visualization with laparoscopy or laparotomy may reveal classic implants; classified as Stage I—minimal, Stage II—mild, Stage III—moderate, and Stage IV—severe.

9. a. Boggy, tender uterus
   Physical findings for a patient with adenomyosis are as follows: boggy, tender uterus; diffuse, globular enlargement—may be 8 to 10 weeks size and may see evidence of anemia.

10. d. Polyp
    Polyps are the most common benign neoplasm of the cervix. They are most often seen in perimenopausal and multigravida women between the ages of 30 and 50 years.

11. d. Trichomonads
    Physical findings for someone infected with trichomoniasis are as follows: copious, homogeneous, malodorous, yellowish-green discharge; vulva irritation; pruritus and edema; and occasionally dysuria, urgency, frequency of urination, postcoital and intermenstrual bleeding, and erythema of vulva and vagina with excoriation. Onset of symptoms often occurs after menses.

12. c. Uterus present, ovaries absent
    Characteristics found in persons with Turner's syndrome: no secondary sex characteristics, uterus present; absent or streak ovaries; infertile, congenital anomalies as described under signs and symptoms; renal (horseshoe kidney) and cardiac anomalies (coarctation of aorta, bicuspid aortic valves, mitral valve prolapse, aortic aneurysm), and hearing loss.

13. a. Lichen sclerosus
    Physical findings in women with lichen sclerosus include skin that is easily traumatized; bruises and purpura; blisters, ulceration, severe itching and burning; lesions that do not correlate with discomfort; skin of vulva that is thin and wrinkled; and obliteration of the clitoris.

14. d. Cryotherapy with liquid nitrogen
    Molluscum contagiosum usually resolves spontaneously without scarring. Treatment includes superficial incision, express contents with comedo extractor, and curettage with cautery. For multiple lesions, use cryotherapy with liquid nitrogen or silver nitrate.

15. a. Acts as an antifibrinolytic agent to block lysis of fibrin clots
    Tranexamic acid is effective in blocking lysis of fibrin clots and when taken up to the first 5 days of menses reduces bleeding in women who have increased endometrial plasminogen activity.

16. c. Polycystic ovarian syndrome
    In polycystic ovarian syndrome (PCOS), there is a gradual onset of hirsutism around puberty or in the early 20s.

17. a. Administer progestin challenge test
    To evaluate an amenorrheic patient, obtain a pregnancy test, serum prolactin level, serum T_4, and thyroid-stimulating hormone (TSH) tests. If all these tests are negative or normal, evaluate the availability of estrogen with a progestin challenge test.

18. b. Anovulation
    Dysfunctional uterine bleeding (DUB) is a variety of bleeding manifestations secondary to chronic anovulation.

19. c. Colicky, spasmodic, sometimes radiating to the thighs and low back
    Primary dysmenorrhea is characterized by pain that begins shortly before the onset of menses and usually lasts no longer than 2 days. The pain is described as colicky, crampy, and spasmodic in the lower abdomen that sometimes radiates to the lower back and thighs.

20. c. Primary amenorrhea
    Primary amenorrhea is characterized by no menstruation by age 16 regardless of secondary sex characteristics.

21. c. LH surge test
    A surge of the luteinizing hormone precedes ovulation. This extra burst of luteinizing hormone affects the ovary and prompts the release of an egg. LH can be detected in the urine a few hours after the surge.

22. d. Macular rash on face and trunk
    Toxic shock syndrome (TSS) is characterized by sudden-onset fever of 102°F or greater and diffuse macular sunburn-like rash over face, trunk, and extremities that desquamates 1 to 2 weeks after onset.

23. a. Cigarette smoking

Risk factors for developing vulvar carcinoma are history of abnormal Pap test, multiple sexual partners, cigarette smoking, chronic irritation, and vulvar dermatoses.

24. c. Endometrial cancer

Women with polycystic ovarian syndrome (PCOS) are at risk for future development of endometrial cancer, diabetes mellitus, and heart disease; obesity increases risk of metabolic complications.

25. c. Polycystic ovarian syndrome

A positive progestin challenge test with anovulation, and an LH/FSH ratio > 2.0, with or without ultrasonography confirmation of polycystic ovaries is associated with polycystic ovarian syndrome (PCOS).

26. b. Pruritus

Symptoms associated with vulvar cancer include vulvar pruritus (most common), pain, burning, bleeding, odorous discharge that be blood tinged, and lesions.

27. b. Doxycycline

Doxycycline should not be used in pregnancy because it may cause discoloration of teeth in children.

28. d. Repeat cotesting in 3 years

As per the 2013 ASCCP guidelines, for women with atypical squamous cells of undetermined significance (ASC-US) on cytology and negative for high-risk HPV types, the recommendation is for repeat cotesting in 3 years.

29. d. Topical estrogen cream

Application of topical estrogen to the affected area is recommended for women with atrophy of genitalia.

30. a. Fibroadenoma

Fibroadenoma are firm, well delineated, freely movable, smooth, rubbery, round, typically marble-sized, nontender masses and they are usually unilateral.

31. c. High-grade squamous epithelial lesion

As per the Bethesda System, the equivalent of CIN III on a Pap test is high-grade squamous intraepithelial lesion (HSIL).

32. a. Heavy tobacco use

Potential causes for galactorrhea include hypo-/hyperthyroidism, use of illicit drugs such as opiates and cannabis, excessive breast stimulation, breast cancer, and pituitary adenoma.

33. a. Interstitial

Leiomyomata can be found in different areas within and around the uterine cavity and surrounding ligaments. Submucosal myomas protrude into the uterine cavity. Subserosal myomas bulge through the outer uterine wall. Intraligamentous myomas are found within the broad ligament. Interstitial (intramural) myomas stay within the uterine wall as it grows; they are the most common form of myoma. Pedunculated myomas are on a thin pedicle or stalk attached to the uterus.

34. b. Menorrhagia

Patients with a leiomyata are usually asymptomatic. If they do present with symptoms, menorrhagia is the most common presentation.

35. a. Benign cystic teratoma

A dermoid cyst is also known as a benign cystic teratoma. It is the most common ovarian germ cell tumor.

36. c. There is no therapy that will eliminate the HPV virus

Goal of treatment is to eliminate present visible disease and improve symptoms; however, there is no therapy that will completely eliminate the HPV virus.

37. a. Benign cystic teratoma

Benign cystic teratomas usually measure between 5 and 10 cm in diameter and they are composed of well-differentiated tissue from all three germ layers. Patients are usually asymptomatic but may experience acute pain if the teratoma twists or ruptures.

38. a. Endometrial hyperplasia

Unopposed estrogen may predispose a woman to endometrial hyperplasia, which is the thickening of the uterine lining caused by excess estrogen. Although this is not a form of cancer, it can lead to uterine cancer.

39. c. Urodynamic testing

Incontinence is diagnosed by urodynamic testing. The following methods are also used to guide making the proper diagnosis: review of prescription and nonprescription drugs for etiologic factors, analysis of voiding diary, urinary stress test to assess loss of urine when coughing and straining, postvoid residual measurement using catheter or scan, and urinalysis/culture to evaluate for infection. Cystometry, urethroscopy, and cystoscopy may be useful, and urodynamic testing is confirmatory.

40. c. Irregular bleeding

Early in the disease process, women with cervical carcinoma may be asymptomatic. The most common presenting symptom of advanced cervical cancer is irregular, painless bleeding or odorous bloody or purulent discharge. Late symptoms include pelvic or epigastric pain and urinary or rectal symptoms.

41. b. Immediate loop electrosurgical excision or colposcopy with endocervical assessment

As per the ASCCP (2013) guidelines, the next step to managing a HSIL Pap test result is immediate loop electrosurgical excision or colposcopy with endocervical assessment.

42. d. Ovarian cancer

Early signs of ovarian carcinoma include abdominal discomfort or pain, pressure sensation on the bladder or rectum, pelvic fullness or bloating, and vague gastrointestinal symptoms.

43. c. Obesity

Risk factors for endometrial carcinoma include diabetes, obesity, hypertension, family history, early menarche, late menopause, unopposed estrogen therapy, oligo-ovulation, anovulation, and estrogen-secreting tumors (granulosa cell).

44. d. Ovarian cancer

Mortality rate from ovarian carcinoma exceeds all other genital tract malignancies because of the fact that it presents in advanced stage.

45. b. Bacterial vaginosis

A positive "whiff" test is the fishy odor that may be found when 10% KOH is added to a vaginal discharge sample of a patient with bacterial vaginosis. The whiff test is part of Amsel's criteria for diagnosing bacterial vaginosis along with vaginal pH ≥ 4.5, clue cells on saline wet mount, and homogeneous white discharge coating the vaginal wall.

46. a. Elevated pH

Loss of lactobacilli (hydrogen–peroxide-producing strains) results in elevated pH and subsequent overgrowth of bacteria—bacteria concentrations are 100- to 1000-fold.

47. b. Oral metronidazole

For the treatment of trichomoniasis, the Centers for Disease Control and Prevention recommends metronidazole 2 g orally in a single dose (CDC 2010).

48. d. Trichloracetic acid

For the treatment of genital warts in pregnancy, the Centers for Disease Control and Prevention recommends trichloracetic or bichloracetic acid (80–90% solution): apply a small amount carefully to wart and allow it to dry. It will turn white. Then, apply sodium bicarbonate or talc to neutralize or remove unreacted acid. May reapply weekly (CDC 2010).

49. b. Chlamydia

Signs and symptoms of chlamydia include postcoital bleeding; intermenstrual bleeding or spotting; symptoms of urinary tract infection—dysuria, frequency; vaginal discharge; and abdominal pain. Physical findings include mucopurulent endocervical discharge; edematous, tender cervix with easily induced bleeding; suprapubic pain; or slight tenderness upon palpation.

50. b. Late menopause

Risk factors for ovarian carcinoma include low parity, early menarche, late menopause, high socioeconomic class, high dietary fat consumption, and history of breast, colon, or endometrial cancer.

51. d. Test for possible reinfection 3 months after treatment

Because doxycycline is one of the recommended treatment regimens, a test of cure is not recommended for nonpregnant women. However, because a majority of posttreatment infections are reinfection, retest the patient at 3 months post treatment or at the next office visit.

52. b. Famciclovir

According to the Centers for Disease Control and Prevention, the recommended treatment regimen for herpes genitalis is:

- Acyclovir 400 mg orally three times a day or 200 mg orally five times a day for 7 to 10 days
  OR
- Famciclovir 250 mg orally three times a day for 7 to 10 days
  OR
- Valacyclovir 1 g orally twice a day for 7 to 10 days

53. b. Condyloma lata

Patients with secondary syphilis present with localized or diffused mucocutaneous lesions in the palms, soles, mucous patches, and condyloma lata, and with generalized lymphadenopathy along with flu-like symptoms (low-grade fever, headache, sore throat, malaise, arthralgias).

54. b. An indurated, painless ulcer on the cervix

Primary syphilis is suspected if a person presents with a painless, ulcerated lesion with raised border and indurated base, rolled edges that spontaneously disappears in 1 to 6 weeks.

55. a. Cystocele

A cystocele is the herniation of the bladder into the vaginal lumen.

56. d. Vulvar carcinoma

The most common signs and symptoms of vulvar carcinoma include pruritus (most common); pain; burning; bleeding lesions that may be darkly or irregularly pigmented, white or red, multifocal or singular, and flat, wart-like, or scaly; erythematous irritated ulceration; and odorous discharge that may be blood-tinged.

57. d. Molluscum contagiosum

Molluscum contagiosum has characteristic light-colored papules with an umbilicated center that can be found on the trunk, lower extremities, abdomen, inner thigh, or genital area.

58. b. Systemic symptoms are uncommon during recurrences

A recurrent genital herpes infection usually takes on a milder course and does not present with systemic symptoms such as fever, malaise, and headache.

59. d. Frequent urinary tract infections

Weakness in supporting structures include the pelvic diaphragm, ligaments, and fascia—commonly related to neuromuscular injury at childbirth, resulting in denervation injury of muscular floor. Other causes include conditions that cause chronic increase in abdominal pressure—obesity, straining, chronic lung disease (coughing), nerve function altered by diabetes, pelvic surgery, neurologic disorders, and hypoestrogenism.

60. c. Rectocele

A rectocele typically presents as a bulging or herniation of the anterior rectal wall and posterior vaginal wall into the opening of the vagina.

61. d. The upper one-third of the vagina

The most common site of vaginal carcinoma is the upper one-third of the vagina.

62. c. Vaginal cancer

Females exposed to diethylstilbestrol (DES) in utero are at increased risk for clear cell carcinoma of the vagina (although rarely, a 1/1000 risk).

63. b. Urge incontinence

Management/treatment of urge incontinence includes bladder retraining with scheduled voiding, biofeedback, Kegel exercises, avoidance of bladder irritants, surgical removal of obstruction, and use of anticholinergic agents (oxybutynin chloride, tolterodine tartrate).

64. d. Ovarian carcinoma

Ovarian carcinoma is a malignant neoplasm of the ovary with the highest mortality rate of all cancers that are gynecologically related.

65. c. Intraductal papilloma

Intraductal papilloma is a benign lesion of the lactiferous duct found commonly in the perimenopausal age group, 35–50 years old, and is the most common cause of pathologic nipple discharge.

66. a. Benign cystic teratoma

Benign cystic teratoma is the most common ovarian germ cell tumor and one of the most common neoplasms of the ovary (10–20%).

67. b. Cervical motion tenderness

Lower abdominal tenderness, adnexal tenderness, and cervical motion tenderness of varying degrees are minimum criteria for empirical treatment of pelvic inflammatory disease (PID) in sexually active young women.

68. a. Androgen insensitivity/resistance syndrome

Androgen insensitivity/resistance syndrome is a genetically transmitted androgen receptor defect. The individual is genotypic male (46XY) but phenotypic female or has both female and male characteristics. The individual has normally developed breasts with small nipples and areola, scanty or absent pubic hair, a blind vaginal pouch, and no uterus or ovaries. Testes are present and may be partially descended or intra-abdominal.

69. b. Gonadal malignancies
Once full development is attained (after puberty) in a person with androgen insensitivity syndrome, gonads should be removed at about age 16 to 18 years to reduce risk of malignant transformation of the gonads (5%). Incidence of malignancy is rare before puberty.

70. c. In vitro fertilization (IVF)
In vitro fertilization is the most common assisted reproductive technology with a success rate of 15–20%. IVF is a series of complex procedures wherein the oocytes are extracted, fertilized in the laboratory, and then transferred through the cervix into the uterus.

71. d. Short stature and webbed neck
People with Turner's syndrome phenotypically present with short stature, webbed neck, shield chest with widely spaced nipples, increased carrying angle of elbow, arched palate, low neck hairline, short fourth metacarpal bones, disproportionately short legs, swollen hands and feet, lack of breast development, and scant pubic hair.

72. d. Turner's syndrome
Turner's syndrome (45X) is the most common chromosomal abnormality found on spontaneous abortuses.

73. a. Inflammation
According to the 2001 Bethesda System for reporting results of cervical cytology, results may include reactive cellular changes, which are typically associated with inflammation, radiation, or an intrauterine device.

74. d. No signs of infection
Patients with latent syphilis show no signs of infection; detection is through serologic testing.

75. b. Reexamine patient within 72 hours after initiation of treatment

After treatment for pelvic inflammatory disease (PID), follow-up and reexamination within 72 hours post treatment are recommended. If the patient is not significantly improved, review the diagnosis and treatment; the patient may need hospitalization.

76. d. Metronidazole
Side effects of metronidazole include metallic taste, nausea, headache, dry mouth, and dark-colored urine.

77. c. Imiquimod
Patient-applied treatments for HPV include the following:
- Imiquimod 5% cream applied sparingly at bedtime three times a week; area washed with mild soap 6 to 10 hours after application; safety in pregnancy is unknown
- Podophilox 0.5% gel or solution applied sparingly to visible warts; safety in pregnancy is unknown

78. b. History of endometrial cancer
Risk factors for breast carcinoma include the following:
- The *BRCA1* and *BRCA2* genes
- Advancing age
- Mother and/or sister with breast cancer
- Previous breast cancer
- Perimenopausal status
- Previous endometrial or colon cancer
- Previous breast biopsy with atypical hyperplasia, lobular neoplasm
- Menarche before age 12; menopause after age 55
- Nulliparity, first pregnancy after 30
- Hormone replacement therapy, oral contraceptive pills (questionable)
- Obesity, environmental factors; exposure to radiation or pesticides
- Heavy alcohol use; fat in diet

79. d. Trichomoniasis
Red speckles—"strawberry spots"—on the vagina and cervix (punctate lesions called colpitis macularis) are classic findings in trichomoniasis. Erythema, edema, and excoriation of vulva may also be seen.

80. a. Constant vulvar burning and discomfort
Vulvodynia usually presents as severe burning, stinging, irritation, or "rawness" with no visible dermatoses or intermittent symptoms; dyspareunia; and constant pain.

Bibliography

American College of Obstetricians and Gynecologists. (2011). Chronic pelvic pain. *Frequently Asked Questions, FAQ099.* Retrieved from https://www.acog.org/~/media/For%20Patients/faq099.pdf?dmc=1&ts=20140225T2014159365

American College of Obstetricians and Gynecologists. (2012a). Endometrial hyperplasia. *Frequently Asked Questions, FAQ147.* Retrieved from http://www.acog.org/~/media/For%20Patients/faq147.pdf?dmc=1&ts=20140225T1741226436

American College of Obstetricians and Gynecologists. (2012b). Practice Bulletin 91: Treatment of urinary tract infections in nonpregnant women. *Obstetrics and Gynecology, 111*(3), 785–794. doi:10.1097/AOG.0b013e318169f6ef.

American College of Obstetricians and Gynecologists. (2012c). Practice Bulletin 131: Screening for cervical cancer. *Obstetrics and Gynecology, 120*(5), 1222–1238. doi:http://10.1097/AOG.0b013e318277c92a.

American College of Obstetricians and Gynecologists. (2013a). Practice Bulletin 63: Urinary incontinence in women. *Obstetrics and Gynecology, 105,* 1533–1545.

American College of Obstetricians and Gynecologists. (2013b). Practice Bulletin 140: Management of abnormal cervical cancer screening test results and cervical cancer precursors. *Obstetrics and Gynecology, 122*(6), 1338–1367. doi:10.1097/01.AOG.0000438960.31355.9e.

American Society for Colposcopy and Cervical Pathology. (2013). ASCCP Algorithms: Updated consensus guidelines for managing abnormal cervical cancer screening tests and cancer precursors. Retrieved from http://www.asccp.org/portals/9/docs /algorithms%207.30.13.pdf

Centers for Disease Control and Prevention. (2010). Sexually transmitted diseases treatment guidelines, 2010. *Morbidity and Mortality Weekly Report, 59*(RR-12). Retrieved from http://www.cdc.gov /sTD/treatment/2010/STD-Treatment-2010-RR5912.pdf

Centers for Disease Control and Prevention. (2012). Update to CDC's *Sexually Transmitted Diseases Treatment Guidelines, 2010*: Oral cephalosporins no longer a recommended treatment for gonococcal infections. *Morbidity and Mortality Weekly Report, 61*(31), 590–594.

Fraser, I., Critchley, J., Broder, M., & Munro, M. (2011). The FIGO recommendations on terminologies and definitions for normal and abnormal uterine bleeding. *Seminars in Reproductive Medicine, 29*(5), 383–390.

Gibbs, R., Karlan, B., Haney, A., & Nygaard, I. (2008). *Danforth's obstetrics and gynecology* (10th ed.). Philadelphia, PA: Lippincott Williams & Wilkins.

North American Menopause Society. (2010). *Menopause practice: A clinician's guide* (4th ed.). Cleveland, OH: Author.

Schuiling, K. D., & Likis, F. E. (2011). *Women's gynecologic health* (2nd ed.). Burlington, MA: Jones & Bartlett Learning.

Solomon, D., Davey, D., Kurman, R., Moriarty, A., O'Connor, D., Prey, M., … Bethesda 2001 Workshop. (2002). Consensus statement: The 2001 Bethesda System—terminology for reporting results of cervical cytology. *Journal of the American Medical Association, 287*(16), 2114–2119.

Speroff, L., Glass, R. H., & Kase, N. G. (2010). *Clinical gynecologic endocrinology and infertility* (7th ed.). Baltimore, MD: Williams and Wilkins.

Tharpe, N., & Farley, C. (2012). *Clinical practice guidelines for midwifery and women's health* (4th ed.). Burlington, MA: Jones & Bartlett Learning.

6

Prenatal Care and Fetal Assessment

Jamille Nagtalon-Ramos

Human Reproduction and Fertilization

- Process of gametogenesis
  1. Definition—development of gametes; oogenesis or spermatogenesis
  2. Essential concepts
     a. Oogenesis—developmental process by which the mature human ovum is formed; haploid number of chromosomes
     b. Spermatogenesis—formation of mature functional spermatozoa; haploid number of chromosomes
     c. Meiosis—a process of two successive cell divisions, producing cells, egg, or sperm, that contain half the number of chromosomes found in somatic cells
     d. Mitosis—type of cell division of somatic cells in which each daughter cell contains the same number of chromosomes as the parent cell
     e. Haploid number of chromosomes 23—possessing half the diploid or normal number of chromosomes, that is, 46, as found in somatic or body cells
- Process of fertilization
  1. Definition—union of ovum and spermatozoan; usually occurs in fallopian tubes within minutes or no more than a few hours of ovulation; most pregnancies occur when intercourse occurs within 2 days of ovulation
  2. Stages of development
     a. Zygote—a diploid cell with 46 chromosomes that results from the fertilization of the ovum by a spermatozoan
     b. Blastomeres—mitotic division of the zygote (cleavage) yields daughter cells called blastomeres
     c. Morula—the solid ball of cells formed by 16 or so blastomeres; mulberry-like ball of cells that enters the uterine cavity 3 days after fertilization
     d. Blastocyst—after the morula reaches the uterus, a fluid accumulates between blastomeres, converting the morula to a blastocyst; inner cell mass at one pole to become embryo; outer cell mass will be trophoblast

     e. Embryo—stage in prenatal development between the fertilized ovum and the fetus (i.e., between 2nd and 8th weeks inclusive)
     f. Fetus—the developing conceptus after the embryonic stage
     g. Conceptus—all tissue products of conception: embryo (fetus), fetal membranes, and placenta
- Physiology of implantation of the blastocyst
  1. Definition—blastocyst adheres to the endometrial epithelium by gently eroding between the epithelial cells of the surface endometrium; invading trophoblasts burrow into the endometrium; the blastocyst becomes encased and covered over by the endometrium
  2. Implantation occurs 6–7 days after fertilization and usually in the upper, posterior wall of the uterus
  3. Provides physiologic exchange between the maternal and embryonic environment prior to full placental function

Development of the Placenta, Membranes, and Amniotic Fluid

- Essential concepts
  1. Chorion—an extra-embryonic membrane that, in early development, forms the outer wall of the blastocyst; from it develop the chorionic villi, which establish an intimate connection with the endometrium, giving rise to the placenta
  2. Chorion frondosum—the outer surface of the chorion whose villi contact the decidua basalis; the placental portion of the chorion
  3. Chorion laeve—the smooth, nonvillous portion of the chorion
  4. Syncytiotrophoblast—outer layer of cells covering the chorionic villi of the placenta that are in contact with the maternal blood or decidua
  5. Cytotrophoblast—thin inner layer of the trophoblast composed of cuboidal cell
  6. Decidua capsularias—the part of the decidua that surrounds the chorionic sac

7. Decidua basalis—the part of the uterine decidua that unites with the chorion to form the placenta
8. Decidua parientalis (vera)—the endometrium during pregnancy except at the site of the implanted blastocyst
9. Amnion—the innermost fetal membrane; a thin, transparent sac that holds the fetus suspended in the liquor amnii or amniotic fluid; it grows rapidly at the expense of the extra-embryonic coelom, and by the end of the third month it fuses with the chorion, forming the amniochorionic sac, commonly called the bag of waters

- Placenta—serves as fetal lungs, liver, and kidneys until birth while growing and maintaining the conceptus in a balanced, healthy environment
  1. Anatomy
     a. Trophoblasts
     b. Chorionic villi
     c. Intervillous spaces
     d. Chorion
     e. Amnion
     f. Decidual plate
  2. Steroid and protein hormones—human trophoblasts produce more diverse steroid and protein hormones and in greater amounts than any endocrine tissue in all of mammalian physiology
     a. Steroid hormones
        (1) Estradiol-17B—responsible for the growth of the uterus, fallopian tubes, vagina, and breast development
        (2) Estriol—an estrogen metabolite excreted by the placenta during pregnancy that is found in the urine of pregnant women
        (3) Progesterone—secreted by the corpus luteum; essential in preparing the uterus for implantation of the fertilized ovum and maintaining the pregnancy
        (4) Aldosterone—responsible for regulation of the body's salt and water balance
        (5) Cortisol—plays a role in the metabolism of fats, glucose, and proteins
     b. Protein and peptide hormones
        (1) Placental lactogen (hPL/HPL)—placental hormone that inhibits maternal insulin activity during pregnancy; decreases to undetectable levels soon after delivery of the placenta
        (2) Chorionic gonadatropin (hCG)—hormone secreted by the placenta to help maintain corpus luteum function and production of progesterone; levels found in serum and urine assays of pregnant women as early as a week after conception
        (3) Placental adrenocorticotropin hormone (ACTH)—the role of this hormone is related to the regulation of the secretion of glucocorticoids
        (4) Pro-opiomelanocortin—a precursor polypeptide
        (5) Chorionic thyrotropin—a type of hormone similar to thyroid-stimulating hormone that has the ability to increase metabolism
        (6) Growth hormone variant—hormone plays a vital role in growth control

        (7) Parathyroid hormone-related protein (PTH-rP)—essential bone differentiation and formation and development of mammary gland
        (8) Calcitonin—hormone responsible for calcium balance
        (9) Relaxin—produced in placenta and corpus luteum and believed to help with relaxing the uterine myometrium during pregnancy
     c. Hypothalamic-like releasing and inhibiting hormones
        (1) Thyrotropin-releasing hormone (TRH)—responsible for the regulation of thyroid-stimulating hormone (TSH)
        (2) Gonadotropin-releasing hormone (GnRH)—essential in controlling the secretion of luteinizing hormone (LH) and follicle-stimulating hormone (FSH)
        (3) Corticotropin-releasing hormone (CRH)—works with vasopressin hormone to regulate the release of adrenocorticotropic hormone (ACTH)
        (4) Somatostatin—responsible for inhibiting the release of growth hormone, prolactin, and thyrotropin
     d. Regulation of blood flow in the placenta; maternal blood traverses the placenta randomly without preformed channels and enters the intervillous spaces in spurts propelled by the maternal arterial pressure
     e. The placental "barrier"—the placenta does not maintain absolute integrity between maternal and fetal circulations as indicated by the presence of fetal blood cells in maternal circulation and the development of erythroblastosis fetalis
     f. Oxygen and glucose are transported across the placenta via facilitated diffusion
- Umbilical cord
  1. Anatomy
     a. Vessels—two arteries that carry fetal deoxygenated blood to the placenta; smaller in diameter than the vein, and one vein carrying oxygenated blood from the placenta to the fetus characterized by twisting or spiraling to minimize snarling
     b. Measurements—0.8–2 cm in diameter; average length of 55 cm with range of 30–100 cm
     c. Wharton's jelly—extracellular matrix consisting of specialized connective tissue that serves as protection for the umbilical cord
  2. Abnormalities of length—positively influenced by amniotic fluid volume and fetal mobility
     a. Extremely short cord—associated with abruptio placentae or uterine inversion; the latter is rare
     b. Abnormally long cord—associated with vascular occlusion by thrombi and true knots
- Amniotic fluid
  1. Production—produced by amniotic epithelium; water transfers across amnion and through fetal skin; in second trimester fetus starts to swallow, urinate, and inspire amniotic fluid
  2. Volume maintenance—fetal swallowing seems to be a critical mechanism affecting fluid volume because polyhydramnios is consistently present when fetal swallowing is inhibited, but other factors, such as tracheoesophageal atresia, contribute to volume balance

3. Polyhydramnios—an excess of amniotic fluid; Amniotic Fluid Index greater than or equal to 24 cm or a maximum deepest vertical pocket of equal to or greater than 8 cm
   a. Incidence—about 1% of all pregnancies
   b. Significance—two-thirds are idiopathic; one-third is associated with fetal anomalies, maternal diabetes, or multiple gestation
   c. Etiology—central nervous system or gastrointestinal tract fetal anomalies (e.g., anencephaly, tracheoesophageal atresia)
   d. Signs and symptoms—uterine size larger than expected for gestational age (GA), difficulty auscultating fetal heart rate (FHR) and palpating fetal parts, mechanical pressure exerted by the large uterus (i.e., dyspnea, edema, heartburn, nausea)
   e. Diagnosis
      (1) Physical findings—a fundal height measurement that is 3–4 cm greater than the normal height warrants an ultrasound to determine reason for enlarged uterus; palpation of fetal parts and auscultation of fetal heart beat may be difficult
      (2) Ultrasonography (USG)—an Amniotic Fluid Index (AFI) measurement of > 24 cm confirms polyhydramnios diagnosis; USG may also identify associated fetal anomaly
   f. Pregnancy outcome—the greater the polyhydramnios, the higher the perinatal mortality; preterm labor increases; risk for postpartum hemorrhage is higher given that the uterus was enlarged; increased risk for cord prolapse with rupture of membranes; also associated with erythroblastosis
   g. Management—treat only if symptomatic and if benefits outweigh risks
      (1) Amniocentesis—to reduce fluid volume if polyhydramnios is severe (AFI > 35 cm); amniotic fluid can be tested for fetal lung maturity and also be sent for chromosomal studies
      (2) Indomethacin—impairs production of lung liquid, increases fluid movement through fetal membranes, or decreases fetal urine production
4. Oligohydramnios—decreased amniotic fluid volume, defined as an Amniotic Fluid Index of 5 cm or less
   a. Conditions associated with oligohydramnios
      (1) Fetal—almost always present with fetal urinary tract obstruction or renal agenesis
         (a) Chromosomal abnormalities
         (b) Congenital anomalies
         (c) Growth restriction
         (d) Demise
         (e) Postterm pregnancy
         (f) Ruptured membranes
      (2) Placental
         (a) Abruption
         (b) Twin-to-twin transfusion syndrome
      (3) Maternal
         (a) Uteroplacental insufficiency
         (b) Hypertension
         (c) Preeclampsia
         (d) Diabetes

      (4) Drugs
         (a) Prostaglandin synthesis inhibitors
         (b) Angiotensin-converting enzyme inhibitors
      (5) Idiopathic
   b. Prognosis
      (1) Early onset has poor outcome and risk of pulmonary hypoplasia greatly increased; if due to early premature rupture of membranes, risk of stillbirth increased
      (2) Late pregnancy onset leads to more Cesarean sections for fetal distress
   c. Management
      (1) Sonographic evaluation for fetal anomalies and growth restriction
      (2) Amnioinfusion in the intrapartum period for the treatment of repetitive variable decelerations

Embryonic and Fetal Development

- Embryonic development—the period of organogenesis, which begins in the third week after fertilization and spans for 8 weeks; this is around the time a woman may miss her next menstrual period and when pregnancy tests would turn positive by detecting human chorionic gonodatropin (hCG). However, serum and urine assays can detect hCG as early as a week after conception
  1. Fourth week—partitioning of heart begins; arm and leg buds form; amnion begins to unsheathe the body stalk that becomes the umbilical cord
  2. Sixth week—head is much larger than body; heart is completely formed; fingers and toes present
  3. All major organ systems are formed except for lungs
- Fetal development—begins 8 weeks after fertilization; 10 weeks after onset of last menstrual period (LMP)
  1. 12 weeks—uterus palpable at the symphysis; fetus begins to make spontaneous movements
  2. 16 weeks—experienced observers can determine sex on ultrasound
  3. 20 weeks—weighs 300 g; weight now begins to increase in a linear manner
  4. 24 weeks—weighs 630 g; fat deposition begins; terminal sacs in the lungs still not completely formed
  5. 28 weeks—weighs 1100 g; papillary membrane has just disappeared from the eyes; has 90% chance of survival if otherwise normal
  6. 32–36 weeks—continues to increase weight as more subcutaneous fat accumulates

Diagnosis and Dating of Pregnancy

- Diagnosis
  1. Signs of pregnancy
     a. Presumptive—subjective (what the woman reports)
        (1) Amenorrhea
        (2) Nausea and/or vomiting
        (3) Urinary frequency, nocturia
        (4) Fatigue

(5) Breast tenderness, tingling, enlargement, and changes in color

(6) Vasomotor symptoms

(7) Skin changes

(8) Congestion of vaginal mucus

(9) Maternal belief that she is pregnant

  b. Presumptive—objective (physical examination)

(1) Continuation of elevated basal body temperature

(2) Chadwick's sign

(3) Appearance of Montgomery's tubercles or follicles

(4) Expression of colostrum

(5) Breast changes

  c. Probable

(1) Enlargement of the abdomen

(2) Enlargement of the uterus

(3) Palpation of the fetal outline

(4) Ballottement

(5) Change in the shape of the uterus

(6) Piskacek's sign

(7) Hegar's sign

(8) Goodell's sign

(9) Palpation of Braxton Hicks contractions

(10) Positive pregnancy test

  d. Positive

(1) Fetal heart tones—heard with a fetoscope at approximately 18–20 weeks, and by Doppler ultrasound as early as 10 weeks' gestation

(2) Sonographic evidence of pregnancy

(3) Palpation of fetal movement

2. Differential diagnosis

  a. Pregnancy

  b. Leiomyoma

  c. Ovarian cyst

  d. Pseudocyesis

- Dating of pregnancy—determining estimated date of confinement or delivery or birth (EDC or EDD or EDB)

1. Average duration of human pregnancy—280 days, 10 lunar months, 9 calendar months

2. Methods to determine EDC, EDD, EDB

  a. Naegele's rule—subtract 3 months, add 7 days to the first day of the last menstrual period (LMP), then add 1 year *or* add 9 months and 7 days to the first day of the LMP

  b. Additional information is needed to more precisely set EDB, which can include:

(1) Complete menstrual history

(2) Contraceptive history

(3) Sexual history

(4) Physical examination for signs and symptoms of pregnancy

(5) Quickening—maternal perception of fetal movement, which usually occurs between 18 and 20 weeks for primiparas; earlier for multigravidas at about 14–18 weeks

3. USG for gestational age determination

  a. Combination of measurements is more accurate than any one of the following measurements:

(1) Crown rump length (CRL)

(2) Biparietal diameter

(3) Head circumference

(4) Abdominal circumference

(5) Femur length

  b. Accuracy by trimester

(1) First trimester—CRL is accurate to 3–5 days

(2) Second trimester—biparietal diameter and femur length are most accurate to within 7–10 days

(3) Third trimester—after 26 weeks all measurements are less accurate; variation in biparietal diameter and femur length is 14–21 days

Maternal Physiologic Adaptations to Pregnancy

- Effects of pregnancy on the organs of reproduction and implications for clinical practice

1. Uterus

  a. Nonpregnant uterus is about 70 g with a 10-mL cavity

  b. First trimester—at 6 weeks the uterus is soft, globular, and asymmetric (Piskacek's sign); at 12 weeks it is 8–10 cm and is rising out of the pelvis

  c. Early second trimester—at 14 weeks, the uterus is one-quarter of the way to umbilicus; at 16 weeks it is halfway to the umbilicus; at 20 weeks the fundus is approximately at the umbilicus

  d. After 20 weeks, number of centimeters with tape measure equals number of weeks of gestation within 2 cm

  e. By term, the uterus weighs about 1100 g with a 5-liter volume

2. Cervix

  a. Develops increased vascularity

  b. Hegar's sign is softening of the isthmus

  c. Chadwick's sign is bluish color of the cervix

  d. Goodell's sign is softening of the cervix

  e. A thick mucus plug forms secondary to glandular proliferation

3. Ovaries—corpus luteum

  a. Anovulation secondary to hormonal interruption of the feedback loop

  b. Corpus luteum persists under the influence of the hormone hCG until about 12 weeks

  c. Corpus luteum is responsible for the secretion of progesterone to maintain the endometrium and pregnancy until the placenta takes over production

  d. Ovaries also thought responsible for production of relaxin

4. Vagina

  a. Chadwick's sign—bluish color

  b. Thickening of vaginal mucosa

  c. Increase in vaginal secretions

  d. Some loosening of connective tissue in preparation for birth

5. Breasts

  a. Increase in size secondary to mammary hyperplasia

  b. Areola becomes more deeply pigmented and increases in size

  c. Colostrum may be expressed after the first several months

    d. Montgomery's follicles

    e. Vascularity increases

6. Pelvis—four pelvic types

    a. Anthropoid

      (1) 23.5% of white women and 50% of nonwhite women

      (2) Shape favors a posterior position of the fetus

      (3) Adequate for a vaginal birth due to large size

    b. Android

      (1) Commonly known as a "male" pelvis

      (2) 32.5% of white women and 15.7% of nonwhite women

      (3) Heavy, heart-shaped pelvis leads to increased posterior positions, dystocia, operative births

    c. Gynecoid

      (1) Commonly known as the "female" pelvis

      (2) 41–42% of women's pelvis shapes

      (3) Good prognosis for vaginal birth

    d. Platypelloid

      (1) Rare pelvic type

      (2) Occurs in less than 3% of women

      (3) Prognosis of vaginal delivery is poor secondary to short Anterior-Posterior (AP) diameter

- Effect of pregnancy on major body systems, with related clinical implications and patient education needs

1. Gastrointestinal

    a. Mouth and pharynx

      (1) Gingivitis is common and may result in bleeding of gums

      (2) Increased salivation

      (3) Epulis (a focal swelling of gums) may develop and resolves after the birth

      (4) Pregnancy does not increase tooth decay

    b. Esophagus

      (1) Decreased lower esophageal sphincter pressure and tone

      (2) Widening of hiatus with decreased tone

      (3) Heartburn is common

    c. Stomach

      (1) Decreased gastric emptying time

      (2) Incompetence of pyloric sphincter

      (3) Decreased gastric acidity and histamine output

    d. Large and small intestines

      (1) Decreased tone and motility

      (2) Altered enzymatic transport across villi resulting in increased absorption of vitamins

      (3) Displacement of intestines, cecum, and appendix by the enlarging uterus

    e. Gallbladder

      (1) Decreased tone

      (2) Decreased motility

    f. Liver

      (1) Altered production of liver enzymes

      (2) Altered production of plasma proteins and serum lipids

2. Genitourinary/renal

    a. Dilation of renal calyces, pelvis, and ureters resulting in increased risk of urinary tract infection

    b. Decreased bladder tone

    c. Renal blood flow increases 35–60%

    d. Decreased renal threshold for glucose, protein, water-soluble vitamins, calcium, and hydrogen ions

    e. Glomerular filtration rate increases 40–50%

    f. All components of the renal-angiotensin-aldosterone system increase, resulting in retention of sodium and water, resistance of pressor effect of angiotensin II, and maintenance of normal blood pressure

3. Musculoskeletal

    a. Relaxin and progesterone affect cartilage and connective tissue

      (1) Results in a loosening of the sacroiliac joint and symphysis pubis

      (2) Encourages the development of the characteristic gait of pregnancy

    b. Lordosis

4. Respiratory

    a. Level of diaphragm rises about 4 cm because of the increase in uterine size

    b. Thoracic circumference increases by 5–6 cm and residual volume is decreased

    c. A mild respiratory alkalosis occurs because of decreased PCO_2

    d. Congestion of nasal tissues occurs

    e. Respiratory rate changes very little, but the tidal volume, minute ventilatory, and minute oxygen uptake all appreciably increase

    f. Some women experience a physiologic dyspnea due to the increased tidal volume and lower PCO_2

5. Hematologic changes

    a. Blood volume increases 30–50% from nonpregnant levels

    b. Plasma volume expands, which results in a physiologic anemia

    c. Hemoglobin averages 12.5 g/dL

    d. Some require an additional gram of iron during pregnancy

    e. Pregnancy can be considered a hypercoagulable state because fibrinogen (Factor I), and Factors VII–X all increase during pregnancy

6. Cardiovascular system

    a. Cardiac volume increases by about 10% and peaks at about 20 weeks

    b. Resting pulse increases by 10–15 beats per minute with the peak at 28 weeks

    c. Slight cardiac shift (up and to the left) due to the enlarging uterus

    d. 90% of pregnant women develop a physiologic systolic heart murmur

    e. May have exaggerated splitting of S1, audible third sound, or soft transient diastolic murmur

    f. Cardiac output is increased

    g. Diastolic blood pressure is lower in first two trimesters because of the development of new vascular beds and relaxation of peripheral tone by progesterone that result in decreased flow resistance

7. Integumentary system

    a. Vascular changes

      (1) Palmar erythema

      (2) Spider angiomas

(3) Varicose veins and hemorrhoids

(4) Hyperpigmentation is believed to be related to estrogens and progesterone, which have a melanocyte-stimulating effect

(5) Chloasma, freckles, nevi, and recent scars may darken

(6) Linea nigra

(7) Increase in sweat/sebaceous activity

(8) Change in connective tissues resulting in striae gravidarum

b. Hair growth

(1) Estrogen increases the length of the anagen (growth) phase of the hair follicles

(2) Mild hirsutism may develop in early pregnancy

8. Endocrine

a. Pituitary

(1) Prolactin levels are 10 times higher at term than in the nonpregnant state

(2) Enlarges by more than 100%

b. Thyroid

(1) Increases in size (about 13%)

(2) Normal pregnant woman is euthyroid because of estrogen-induced increase in thyroxin-binding globulin (TBG)

(3) Thyroid-stimulating hormone (TSH) does not cross the placenta

(4) Thyroid-stimulating immunoglobulins and thyrotropin-releasing hormone (TRH) cross the placenta

c. Adrenal glands

(1) Remain the same size; however, there is an increase in the zona fasciculata that produces glucocorticoid

(2) Twofold increase in serum cortisol

d. Pancreas

(1) Hypertrophy and hyperplasia of the B cells

(2) Insulin resistance as a result of the placental hormones, especially hPL

9. Metabolism

e. Weight gain during pregnancy

(1) Recommended weight gain is 11–40 lb depending on prepregnancy body mass index (BMI)

(2) Average weight gain is 28 lb—1.5 lb for placenta, 2 lb for amniotic fluid, 2.5 lb for uterine growth, 3 lb for increased blood volume, 1 lb for increased breast tissue, 7.5 lb for the fetus, and the remainder for maternal fat deposits

(3) Protein metabolism is increased

(4) Fat deposit and storage are increased to prepare for breastfeeding

(5) Carbohydrate metabolism is altered; blood glucose levels are 10–20% lower than prepregnant states

Maternal Psychological/Social Changes in Pregnancy

- Pregnancy is a time of many transitions, a woman is vulnerable, and maternal moods may be labile

- First trimester (1–13 weeks)—focus on physical changes and feelings

1. Psychological responses

a. Ambivalence

b. Adjustment

2. Prenatal anticipatory guidance

a. Normal changes of pregnancy

(1) Increased pigmentation

(2) Linea nigra

(3) Striae gravidarum

(4) Breast fullness

(5) Urinary frequency

(6) Nausea/vomiting

(7) Fatigue

b. Calculate and explain EDD and comparison with uterine size

c. Client's and healthcare provider's expectations for visits

d. Importance of ongoing care in pregnancy to promote well-being and prevent and recognize problems

e. Rationale for vitamins and iron supplements

f. Resources available for education, emergency care, etc.

g. Discuss/review danger signs and symptoms

- Second trimester (14–26 weeks)—more aware of the fetus as a person

1. Psychological responses

a. Acceptance

b. Period of radiant health

2. Prenatal anticipatory guidance

a. Fetal growth, movement, and fetal heart tones (FHT)

b. Personal hygiene, brassieres, vaginal discharge, etc.

c. Infant feeding—breast and/or bottle

d. Avoidance and alleviation of—backache, constipation, hemorrhoids, leg aches, varicosities, edema, and round ligament pain

e. Nutritional needs, diet, and weight gain

f. Discuss/review danger signs and symptoms

- Third trimester

3. First part (27–36 weeks)—concerned with baby's needs

a. Psychological responses

(1) Introversion

(2) Period of watchful waiting

b. Prenatal anticipatory guidance

(1) Fetal growth and well-being

(2) Review hygiene, clothing, body mechanics and posture, positions of comfort

(3) Physical and emotional changes

(4) Sexual needs/intercourse

(5) Alleviation of backache, Braxton Hicks contractions, dyspnea, round ligament pain, leg aches, or edema

(6) Confirm infant feeding plans and discuss preparation for breastfeeding

(7) Preparation for baby supplies and help at home

(8) Prenatal classes/approach

(9) Involvement of significant other

(10) Review danger signs at each visit

(11) Provide contraceptive counseling

(12) If planning tubal ligation, prepare papers if required

c. Women anticipate birth and infant care
  (1) Discuss fetal movement
  (2) Personal hygiene needs/concerns, alleviation of discomforts of pregnancy
  (3) Discuss recognition of Braxton Hicks and prodromal contractions and differentiation from true labor
  (4) Discuss labor, contractions, and labor progress and expectations of labor
  (5) Breathing and relaxation techniques; labor support options
  (6) Provisions for needs of other children, sibling issues, and care of children during hospital stay
  (7) Review signs of labor
  (8) Continue discussion of relaxation and breathing techniques; latent labor coping skills
  (9) Final home preparations
  (10) Discuss procedures particular to home/birthing center (BC), hospital—analgesia, IVs, examinations, labor care, birthing plans, postpartum care, and supplies needed
  (11) Confirm plans for transport to the hospital, who to call, and where to go; hospitalization and process of admission
  (12) Consider birth control/family planning needs
  (13) Discuss emergency arrangements in the event of danger signs, premature rupture of membranes (PROM), bleeding, severe headache, pain, etc.

- Risk factors for psychological well-being
  1. Limited support network
  2. High levels of stress
  3. Psych/mental health issues
  4. Problem pregnancies

Overview of Antepartum Care

- Purpose and objectives of antepartum care—to differentiate normal and pathologic maternal-fetal alterations throughout pregnancy by employing maternal-fetal assessment methods, techniques, and parameters appropriate to the antepartum period, specifically:
  1. Application of the management process, including components of history and physical examination at initial and interval visits
  2. Critical evaluation of indications and techniques for the application of therapeutics during the antepartum period
  3. Incorporation of current evidence and research in the care of women and families during the antepartum period
- Definition of the essential concepts (Centers for Disease Control and Prevention, 2013)
  1. Fertility rate—number of live births/1000 females 15–44 years of age
  2. Birth rate—number of births divided by total population in the given year(s)
  3. Live birth—birth of an infant, no matter the age of gestation, showing any signs of life (e.g., spontaneous breathing, beating of the heart, pulsation of the cord, movement of voluntary muscles)

4. Fetal death—spontaneous intrauterine death of a fetus at any time during the pregnancy; also referred to as "stillbirth" if it occurs after 20 weeks or more
5. Neonatal period—28 completed days after birth
6. Perinatal period—from 28 weeks gestational age up to 7 days after birth; also defined as births weighing 500 g or more and ending at 28 completed days after birth
7. Stillbirth rate (fetal death rate)—the ratio of fetal deaths divided by the sum of births (including live births and fetal deaths) in any given year
8. Neonatal death—early neonatal death is death during the first 7 days after birth; late neonatal death is death between 7 and 28 days
9. Neonatal mortality rate—the number of neonates dying before reaching 28 days of age per 1000 live births in a given year
10. Perinatal mortality rate—the number of perinatal deaths per 1000 total births
11. Infant mortality rate—number of infant deaths (first 12 months of life) per 1000 live births
12. Maternal morbidity—illness or disease associated with childbearing
13. Maternal mortality ratio—number of maternal deaths that result from the reproductive process/100,000 live births
14. Abortus—fetus or embryo removed or expelled from the uterus during the first half of gestation (20 weeks or less), weighing less than 500 g
15. Preterm infant—infant born before 37 completed weeks (259th day)
16. Term infant—infant born after 37 completed weeks of gestation up until 42 completed weeks of gestations (260–294 days)
17. Postterm infant—infant born any time after completion of the 42nd week beginning with day 295
18. Direct maternal death—death of the mother resulting from obstetric complications of pregnancy, labor, or the puerperium; and from interventions, omissions, incorrect treatment, or a chain of events resulting from any of these factors

Antepartum Visit

- Terminology that describes women and their pregnancies (King, Brucker, & Kriebs, 2013)
  1. Gravida—the number of times a woman has been pregnant
  2. Para—refers to the number of pregnancies carried to the 20th week of gestation or the delivery of an infant weighing more than 500 g, no matter the outcome
  3. Nulligravida—a woman who has never been pregnant
  4. Nullipara—a woman who has not carried a baby to 500 g or 20 weeks
  5. Primigravida—a woman who is pregnant for the first time
  6. Primipara—a woman who has carried a pregnancy past the 20th week of gestation or who is currently pregnant for the first time and is carrying past the 20th week
  7. Multigravida—a woman pregnant two or more times
  8. Multipara—a woman who has carried two or more pregnancies past the 20th week of gestation or who has delivered an infant weighing more than 500 g more than once

9. Grand multipara—has given birth seven times or more
10. GTPAL numerical description of parity—five-digit system that counts all fetuses/babies born rather than pregnancies carried to viability: G = gravida; number of pregnancies (regardless of outcome). T = term babies (37 weeks or 2500 g). P = premature babies (20–36 weeks; 500–2499 g). A = abortions (any fetus born < 20 weeks and 500 g). L = current living children
- Components of the antepartum visit (initial and return)
  1. The Pregnant Patient's Bill of Rights
  2. Complete history
     a. Menstrual history
     b. Contraceptive history
     c. Obstetric history including quickening
     d. Medical-surgical history
     e. Sexual history
     f. History or current physical, sexual, emotional abuse
     g. Medicines and/or complementary alternative medicines and therapies
     h. Family history
     i. Genetic risk
     j. Health habits
     k. Environmental exposures
     l. Social history
     m. Exercise and nutrition history
     n. Immunizations
  3. Physical examination
     a. Height, weight, and vital signs
     b. Complete physical examination
     c. Abdominal examination
        (1) Fundal height—measured in centimeters, from pubic symphysis to the fundus of the uterus
        (2) Leopold's maneuvers—four abdominal palpation maneuvers used to determine the following fetal characteristics:
           (a) Lie
           (b) Presentation
           (c) Position
           (d) Attitude
           (e) Variety
           (f) Estimated fetal weight
        (3) Fetal heart tones—auscultation of presence and pattern of fetal heart rate
        (4) Bimanual examination—performed in the first trimester to determine uterine size to estimate gestational age
        (5) Clinical pelvimetry—measurement of the features of the bony pelvis with the examiner's hand
     d. The pelvis (only the true pelvis is of significance)—true pelvis is bony canal through which the fetus passes and that lies below the pelvic brim (linea terminalis)
        (1) Three planes of obstetric significance—inlet, midplane, and outlet
        (2) Critical diameters for evaluation of pelvic adequacy
           (a) Inlet—AP, transverse
           (b) Midplane—AP, transverse, posterior sagittal
           (c) Outlet—AP, transverse, posterior sagittal
        (3) Assessing and measuring the pelvis—clinical pelvimetry

(a) Diagonal conjugate—extends from middle of sacral promontory to middle of lower margin of symphysis pubis; only AP diameter that can be measured clinically; should be more than 11.5 cm
(b) Pubic arch—formed by the descending rami of pubic bones and inferior margin of symphysis pubis; angle should be at least 90 degrees
(c) Interspinous diameter—distance between the ischial spines, normally measures 10 cm, is smallest diameter of the pelvis and defines the midplane
(d) Ischial spines—may be prominent, encroaching, or blunt; assess the sidewalls and the sacrum; best if blunt
(e) Sacrosciatic notch—note shape and width in fingerbreadths
(f) Sidewalls—sidewalls extend from the upper anterior angle of the sacrosciatic notch to the ischial tuberosities and are assessed as straight, convergent, or divergent; should be straight
(g) Sacrum—assess the inclination of the sacrum, the length, and the curvature; curved is best
(h) Intertuberous diameter—distance between the ischial tuberosities, about 11 cm

4. Laboratory studies used in the provision of antepartum care
   a. Initial visit
      (1) Blood type, Rh factor, antibody screen, complete blood count (CBC), rapid plasma reagin (RPR) or venereal disease research laboratory (VDRL), rubella titer, hepatitis B surface antigen (HB$_s$Ag), urine culture/screen
      (2) HIV testing should be recommended to all pregnant women with option to decline testing
      (3) Gonorrhea (GC), chlamydia (CT), and wet prep tests, as indicated by history and physical examination findings
      (4) Pap test per routine recommendations
      (5) Positive purified protein derivative (PPD) skin test, hemoglobin (Hgb) electrophoresis, genetic screening tests as indicated by history and risk factors
   b. Genetic screening
      (1) First-trimester screening—performed between 11 and 14 weeks; combining serologic testing for pregnancy-associated plasma protein (PAPP-A) and human chorionic gonadotropin (hCG), an ultrasound exam to measure nuchal translucency, along with the mother's age, a risk for trisomy 18 and 21 is calculated
      (2) Second-trimester screening (also known as "multiple marker screening")—performed between 15 and 20 weeks to detect neural tube defects and trisomy 18 and 21; serologic testing measuring maternal serum alphafetoprotein (MSAFP), estriol, and hCG is called "triple screen," and with the addition of inhibin A, this becomes a "quad screen"
      (3) Combined first- and second-trimester screening—results of first- and second-trimester screening are combined to increase accuracy of detecting trisomy 21
   c. Ultrasound
      (1) Fetal cardiac activity
      (2) Fetal presentation

(3) Placental position

(4) Fetal number

(5) Fetal biometry

(6) Fetal number

(7) Anatomic survey

(8) Specialized examination, as indicated

    (a) Targeted/detailed anatomic survey

    (b) Doppler flow

    (c) Biophysical profile

    (d) Fetal echocardiography

(9) As an adjunct to diagnostic testing

  d. Gestational diabetes screening at 24–28 weeks—see the section on diabetes in "Medical Complications" later in this chapter

  e. Repeat antibody screen at 26–28 weeks for Rh-negative mother

  f. Repeat CBC/hematocrit (Hct), VDRL/RPR, chlamydia, GC, HIV, HBsAg as indicated by history, physical examination findings, and risk factors in third trimester

  g. Group B streptococcus (GBS) screening at 35–37 weeks—vaginal introitus and rectal specimens

  h. Some other laboratory studies that might be indicated include:

(1) Amniocentesis or chorionic villus sampling (CVS)

(2) Tay-Sachs screening

(3) Maternal/paternal chromosomal studies

(4) Chest radiographs

(5) Blood chemistry (Basic or comprehensive metabolic panel)

(6) Thyroid studies

(7) Toxoplasmosis testing

(8) Cytomegalovirus (CMV)

(9) Herpes simplex virus (HSV) cultures or antibody testing

(10) Antinuclear antibody (ANA)

(11) Antiphospholipid antibodies

(12) Serum iron studies

(13) Blood glucose studies (3-hour glucose tolerance test [GTT], fasting blood sugar [FBS], 2-hour postprandial, and hemoglobin A1c)

5. Subsequent (interval) prenatal visits—frequency of

  a. Every 4 weeks to 28 or 32 weeks

  b. From 28 or 32 weeks to 36 weeks every 2 weeks

  c. Weekly visits from 36 weeks to 41 weeks

  d. Some prefer biweekly visits 41 weeks to delivery

  e. Schedule more frequent visits as appropriate; some providers recommend fewer prenatal visits if there are no problems

6. Content of prenatal revisits

  a. History

  b. Physical examination—blood pressure, urine dipstick, weight, FHT, fundal height

  c. Anticipatory management

  d. Anticipatory guidance

  e. Health education and counseling

  f. Appropriate screening

- Prenatal risk factors

1. History

  a. Genetic factors

(1) Maternal age at or older than 35 years

(2) Previous child with a chromosome abnormality

(3) Family history of birth defects or mental retardation

(4) Ethnic/racial origins

    (a) African—sickle cell disease

    (b) Mediterranean or East Asian—B thalassemia

    (c) Jewish—Tay-Sachs disease

  b. Multiple pregnancy losses/previous stillbirth

  c. Psychological/mental health disorders

  d. History of intrauterine growth restriction (IUGR)

  e. Preterm birth(s)

2. Current pregnancy

  a. Abnormal multiple marker screening

  b. Exposure to possible teratogens

(1) Radiation

(2) Alcohol/medications/other substances

(3) Occupational exposures

(4) Infections

    (a) Toxoplasmosis

    (b) Rubella

    (c) CMV

    (d) Syphilis

  c. Intrauterine growth restriction (IUGR)

  d. Oligohydramnios/polyhydramnios

  e. Diabetes

(1) Pregestational

(2) Gestational

(3) Insulin dependent

  f. Hypertension

(1) Chronic

(2) Gestational

  g. Preeclampsia/eclampsia

  h. Multiple gestation

  i. PROM

  j. Post dates

  k. Decreased fetal movement

  l. Rh isoimmunization

Common Discomforts of Pregnancy and Comfort Measures

- Nausea and vomiting of pregnancy (most common in first trimester)

1. Small, frequent meals, no restriction on the kind of food nor how often

2. Discontinue prenatal vitamins with iron until nausea and vomiting resolved; continue folic acid

3. Raspberry tea or peppermint tea, carbonated beverages, hard candy

4. Acupressure, including sea bands for wrists

5. Ginger 1 g per day in divided doses

6. Pyridoxine (vitamin B_6) 25 mg bid or tid orally

7. Doxylamine 12.5 mg bid or qid with pyridoxine orally

8. Metoclopramide 5 to 10 mg g q6–8h orally

9. Promethazine 25 mg q4h per rectal suppository

- Breast tenderness
  1. Good support brassiere
  2. Careful lovemaking
  3. Reassurance that it will soon pass
- Backache
  1. Consider other differential diagnoses for musculoskeletal strain, sciatica, sacroiliac joint problem, preterm labor, urinary tract infection
  2. Nonpathologic—related to normal changes in pregnancy
     a. Massage
     b. Application of ice or heat
     c. Hydrotherapy
     d. Pelvic rock
     e. Good body mechanics
     f. Pillow in lumbar area when sitting or between legs when lying on side
     g. Pregnancy support harness or girdle
     h. Good support brassiere
     i. Supportive low-heeled shoes
  3. Sacroiliac joint problems
     a. Teach appropriate exercises
     b. Nonelastic sacroiliac belt
     c. Trochanteric belt worn below the abdomen at the femoral heads to increase joint stability
- Fatigue
  1. Reassurance that this is a normal first-trimester problem and will pass
  2. Mild exercise and good nutrition
  3. Decrease activities and plan rest periods
  4. Decrease fluid intake in evening to decrease nocturia
- Heartburn
  1. Small, frequent meals
  2. Decrease amount of fluids taken with meals; drink fluids between meals
  3. Papaya (may recommend fresh, dried, juice, or enzymes)
  4. Elevate head of bed 10–30 degrees
  5. Slippery elm bark throat lozenges
  6. Antacids
  7. Proton pump inhibitors and H_2 blockers—Pregnancy Category B
- Constipation
  1. Increased fluids, fiber
  2. Prune juice or warm beverage in the morning
  3. Encourage exercise
  4. Stool softeners
- Hemorrhoids
  1. Avoid constipation or straining with a bowel movement
  2. Elevate hips with pillow or knee–chest position
  3. Sitz baths
  4. Witch hazel or Epsom salt compresses
  5. Reinsert hemorrhoid with lubricated finger
  6. Kegel exercises
  7. Topical anesthetics; Pregnancy Category C if combined with steroid
- Varicosities
  1. Support stockings; apply before getting out of bed
  2. Avoid wearing restrictive clothing
  3. Perineal pad if vaginal varicosities
  4. Rest periods with legs elevated; avoid crossing legs
- Leg cramps
  1. Decrease phosphate in diet; no more than two glasses of milk per day
  2. Massage affected leg
  3. Do not point toes, flex ankle to stretch calf
  4. Keep legs warm
  5. Walk, exercise
  6. Calcium tablets
  7. Magnesium tablets
- Presyncopal episodes
  1. Change positions slowly
  2. Push fluids; regular caloric/glucose intake
  3. Avoid lying flat on back; avoid prolonged standing or sitting
- Headaches
  1. Rule out migraines, pathologic causes of headache
  2. Head, shoulder, and/or neck massage
  3. Acupressure
  4. Hot or cold compresses
  5. Rest
  6. Follow a regular sleep schedule
  7. Warm baths
  8. Meditation and biofeedback
  9. Aromatherapy
  10. Eat smaller, more frequent meals
  11. Mild analgesic such as acetaminophen 325 mg 1–3 tablets every 4 hours as needed
- Leukorrhea
  1. Rule out vaginitis and sexually transmitted infection (STI)
  2. Good perineal hygiene
  3. Wear cotton-crotch panties; change panties as often as necessary
  4. Unscented pantiliners
  5. Instructions to avoid douching and use of feminine sprays
- Urinary frequency
  1. Decrease fluids in evening to avoid nocturia
  2. Avoid caffeine
  3. Rule out urinary tract infection
- Insomnia
  1. Warm bath
  2. Hot drink—warm milk, chamomile tea
  3. Quiet, relaxing, minimally stimulating activities
  4. Avoid daytime napping
- Round ligament pain
  1. Rule out other causes of abdominal pain, such as appendicitis, ovarian cyst, placental separation, inguinal hernia
  2. Warm compresses, ice compresses
  3. Hydrotherapy
  4. Avoid sudden movement or twisting movements
  5. Flex knees to abdomen, pelvic tilt
  6. Support uterus with a pillow when lying down
  7. Maternity abdominal support or girdle
- Skin rash
  1. Ice
  2. Oatmeal bath

3. Diphenhydramine—25 mg orally every 4 hours as needed for itching
4. Dermatology referral as needed
- Carpal tunnel syndrome (tingling and numbness of fingers)
  1. Good posture
  2. Lying down
  3. Rest and elevate affected hands
  4. Ice, wrist splints
  5. Mild analgesic such as acetaminophen 325 mg 1–3 tabs every 4 hours as needed

Nutrition During Pregnancy

- Recommended daily allowances
  1. Calories—2500 kcal
  2. Protein—average of 60 g/day throughout pregnancy
- Weight gain in pregnancy
  1. Body mass index (BMI) (weight/height^2)—only anthropometric measurements with documented clinical value for assessment of gestational weight gain
  2. Weight-for-height categories
     a. Underweight—BMI less than 18.5
     b. Normal weight—BMI 18.5–24.9
     c. Overweight—BMI 25.0–29.9
     d. Obese—BMI 30.0 or higher
  3. Determinants of gestational weight gain
     a. Prepregnant weight—if overweight at conception, more likely to gain less weight than normal-weight woman
     b. Low gestational weight gain associated with
        (1) Low family income
        (2) Black race
        (3) Young age
        (4) Unmarried status
        (5) Low educational level
     c. Multiple gestation
     d. Developing pathology—toxemia
  4. Consequences of gestational weight gain
     a. Low gestational weight gain is associated with
        (1) Growth-restricted infants
        (2) Fetal and infant mortality
     b. High gestational weight gain is associated with
        (1) Greater rate of large infant weight, may increase risk for
           (a) Fetopelvic disproportion
           (b) Operative delivery (forceps, vacuum, or Cesarean)
           (c) Birth trauma
           (d) Asphyxia
           (e) Postpartum hemorrhage
           (f) Mortality
        (2) Above associations are more pronounced in short women (< 157 cm or 62 in.)
  5. Recommended patterns and quantity of weight gain
     a. Normal prepregnant weight—0.8–1.0 lb per week during second and third trimesters for total of 25–35 lb
     b. Underweight before pregnancy—1.0–1.3 lb per week in second and third trimesters for total of 28–40 lb
     c. Overweight before pregnancy—0.5–0.7 lb per week in second and third trimesters for total of 15–25 lb
     d. Obese before pregnancy—0.4–0.6 lb per week in second and third trimesters for total of 11–20 lb
- Diet history—recall of fluid and solid food intake in the last 24 hours with the purpose of evaluating adequacy of nutrition and formulating a plan for nutrition counseling
  1. Components of diet history
     a. Qualitative components of the intake
     b. Quantitative, but only if weight is an issue
     c. Ascertain how typical the last 24-hour intake was to usual intake
  2. Components of diet counseling
     a. Diet assessment
     b. Set a weight gain goal with the woman for the pregnancy
     c. Discuss food preferences and relationship to goal
     d. Review generally or specifically at each visit, depending on results
     e. Include fetal growth as part of parameters
  3. Cultural and personal beliefs about nutrition that may modify a diet plan include:
     a. Pica—ingestion of nonfood substances (i.e., starch, clay)
     b. Vegetarianism
     c. Hot and cold foods and when they can be eaten
     d. Discern eating patterns and beliefs pertinent to pregnancy in the woman's culture

The Woman and Her Family and Their Role in Pregnancy

- Family
  1. Assessment of family size, structure, and relationships
  2. Significant individuals involved in pregnancy
  3. Family roles and their relationship to family function
     a. Occupations
     b. Income levels
     c. Education levels
     d. Nationality and ethnic background
     e. Relationship status and intensity
  4. Feelings and thoughts about this pregnancy and any past pregnancies and births
- Pregnancy as essential, permanent family and life change
  1. The significance of change in relation to pregnancy
  2. Role adaptation needed to successfully cope with pregnancy
  3. Family resources to be mobilized to enable the family to cope
     a. Clear and continuous communication of information
     b. Decision making by the woman and family as indicated
     c. Family's development of an appropriate birth plan
        (1) Childbirth preparation
        (2) Breastfeeding
        (3) Child-rearing classes
     d. Information regarding critical resources in birth site
        (1) Labor and birth procedures and expectations
        (2) Rooming-in
        (3) Breastfeeding support

(4) Sibling visitation and/or presence at birth

(5) Family visitation

(6) Possibility of early discharge

- Perinatal loss and associated grief stages and process
    1. Factors associated with the concept of loss and grieving
        a. Perception of the individual(s) experiencing the loss and its severity
        b. Support and assistance in doing grief work
    2. Types of maternity losses
        a. Infertility
        b. Loss of a baby
            (1) Miscarriage
            (2) Abortion
            (3) Stillbirth
            (4) Adoption
        c. Loss of expectations
            (1) Premature infant
            (2) Congenital deformities
            (3) "Damaged" infant
            (4) Exclusive wife/husband relationship
    3. Stages of grief
        a. Shock, manifested by
            (1) Denial
            (2) Disbelief
            (3) Fear
            (4) Isolation
            (5) Crying
            (6) Hostility
            (7) Bitterness
            (8) Introversion
            (9) Sadness
            (10) Numbness
        b. Physical signs and symptoms
            (1) Weight loss
            (2) Insomnia
            (3) Fatigue
            (4) Restlessness
            (5) Shortness of breath
            (6) Chest pain
        c. Suffering—the reality stage
            (1) Acceptance of the reality
            (2) Adaptation
            (3) Preoccupation with lost person
            (4) Questioning of what happened and why
            (5) Feelings of fear, guilt, and anger persist
        d. Resolution—acceptance and adaptation is complete
            (1) Reinvests in other significant relationships
            (2) Moves on but remembers lost person
    4. Maladaptive grief reactions
        a. Avoidance or distortion of normal grief expression
        b. Agitated depression; psychosomatic conditions
        c. Morbid attachment to possessions of deceased
        d. Persistent loss of self-esteem
    5. Healthcare provider's role in helping the normal grieving process
        a. Listen
        b. Facilitate woman's expression of feelings

c. Provide nonjudgmental environment

d. Accept behaviors of grief

Teaching and Counseling

- Principles of learning that apply to women/families during pregnancy
    1. Factors that facilitate or impede learning
        a. Readiness of the learner; time to discuss
        b. Healthcare provider's knowledge of woman's and family's learning needs
        c. Group teaching—enhances and enriches learning
    2. Factors that critically influence teaching/learning
        a. Alternative lifestyles; different cultures
        b. Disadvantaged social milieus
        c. Age and maturity—adolescents, educational level, life experience
- Principles of teaching for role of parent educator
    1. Individual teaching and counseling—topic and quantity of information need to fit the client
    2. Prioritize information provision
        a. Respond to questions or experiences of the woman
        b. Anticipatory guidance of pregnancy realities
        c. Danger signs of critical complications; drug dangers, both over-the-counter (OTC) and illegal drugs; and any other information needed for health and well-being of woman and fetus
- Childbirth education
    1. Preparation for childbearing—ultimately aids in reducing need for analgesics/anesthetics during labor
        a. Formal or informal
        b. Content to be included:
            (1) Bodily changes in pregnancy with associated reproduction anatomy
            (2) Exercises for activities of daily living (ADL) during pregnancy and for labor
            (3) Nutrition
            (4) Fetal growth and development
            (5) Substance abuse
            (6) Signs of beginning labor
            (7) Information for infant feeding decision making
            (8) Preparation for breastfeeding
            (9) Postpartal course and care
            (10) Preparation of siblings for birth
            (11) Pain coping strategies in labor
            (12) Vaginal birth after Cesarean (VBAC) versus elective repeat Cesarean section (ERCS) if previous C-section
    2. Learning needs of the breastfeeding woman
        a. Anticipatory guidance for woman with inverted nipples
        b. Principles of milk production
            (1) Caloric needs of mother
            (2) Liquid needs of mother
            (3) Mechanics of proper infant positioning and latching on
            (4) Factors that affect milk supply
    3. Learning needs for parenthood
        a. Plans for the baby's health care

b. Needs and adaptation for the home

c. Identification of family/social supports

- Family planning
  1. Pregnancy learning needs for postpartum contraceptive options
  2. Learning needs when considering postpartum bilateral tubal ligation
     a. Expert counseling
     b. Signing consent papers
- Human sexuality and pregnancy
  1. The effects of pregnancy on female and male sexual response
  2. Changes in sexual desire throughout pregnancy—influenced by hormones, energy level, relationship, body image, fears of hurting baby, cultural beliefs and practices
  3. Concept of body image—may feel awkward, clumsy, ugly, especially in late pregnancy
  4. Factors during pregnancy that may alter this image—support or lack thereof for her feelings; responses, either positive or negative, from people of importance
  5. Variations in sexual practice and their use during pregnancy
     a. Positions for intercourse—alternate positions may enhance comfort with increase in abdominal size
     b. Cunnilingus
     c. Fellatio
     d. Anal intercourse
  6. Sexual activity may be continued throughout a healthy pregnancy
  7. The potential relationship between orgasm and uterine contractions
     a. Contraindicated if preterm labor threatens
     b. May help initiate labor

Pharmacologic Considerations in the Antepartum Period

- Teratogens (derived from Greek word meaning "monster")—any agent that acts during embryonic or fetal development to produce a permanent alteration of form or function
- FDA risk factor categories for prescription drugs in pregnancy
  1. Category A—adequate, well-controlled studies in pregnant women have not shown an increased risk of fetal abnormalities
  2. Category B—animal studies have revealed no evidence of harm to the fetus; however, there are no adequate and well-controlled studies in pregnant women OR animal studies have shown an adverse effect, but adequate and well-controlled studies in pregnant women have failed to demonstrate a risk to the fetus
  3. Category C—animal studies have shown an adverse effect, and there are no adequate and well-controlled studies in pregnant women OR no animal studies have been conducted, and there are no adequate and well-controlled studies in pregnant women
  4. Category D—studies, adequate and well-controlled or observational, in pregnant women have demonstrated a risk to the fetus; however, the benefits of therapy may outweigh the potential risk

  5. Category X—studies, adequate and well-controlled or observational, in animals or pregnant women have demonstrated positive evidence of fetal abnormalities. The use of the product is contraindicated in women who are or may become pregnant (Demian, & Rizk, 2011)
- Indications and contraindications for the use of vaccinations during pregnancy
  1. Tdap – the Advisory Committee on Immunization Practices (ACIP) recommends Tdap vaccination during each pregnancy whether or not the patient has received Tdap (or Td) in the past (CDC, 2012)
  2. Hepatitis B—high-risk women who are antigen and antibody negative can be vaccinated during pregnancy
  3. Tetanus—vaccination during pregnancy can protect at-risk newborns against neonatal tetanus; in maternal trauma, may be indicated
  4. Rubella (German measles)—attenuated live-virus vaccine contraindicated immediately before or during pregnancy; offer vaccination postpartum
  5. Varicella—attenuated live-virus vaccine (Varivax) contraindicated in pregnancy; offer vaccination postpartum
  6. Influenza—trivalent inactivated influenza vaccine (TIV) recommended for all pregnant women during influenza season; live attenuated nasal influenza vaccine contraindicated during pregnancy

Techniques Used to Assess Fetal Health

- Ultrasound (USG, US)
  1. Definition—method in which intermittent high-frequency sound waves are transmitted through tissues by way of a transducer placed on the abdomen or in the vagina and are then reflected off the underlying structures so that tissues, fluid, bones, fetal activity, and vessel pulsations are discernible
  2. Types of ultrasound
     a. Abdominal ultrasound is the most commonly used method
     b. Transvaginal ultrasound may be used in early pregnancy
  3. Some uses for ultrasound in obstetrics
     a. Assessment of bleeding in the first trimester
     b. Rule out (R/O) suspected ectopic pregnancy or hydatidiform mole
     c. Estimated gestational age for patients with uncertain LMP
     d. Evaluation of size/dates discrepancy
     e. R/O suspected multiple gestations or fetal anomalies
     f. Adjunct to special procedures—reproductive endocrinology procedures, CVS, amniocentesis, fetoscopy
     g. Sex identification
     h. Evaluation of second- and third-trimester bleeding
     i. Evaluation of pelvic mass or uterine abnormality
     j. Evaluation of placental problems, location, grade
     k. Evaluation of fetal growth—macrosomia, intrauterine growth restriction (IUGR), AFI
     l. Biophysical profile—AFI, fetal movements, respiratory movements, fetal tone
     m. Estimation of fetal size and/or presentation
     n. R/O suspected fetal demise

- Doppler velocimetry blood flow assessment
  1. Used in tertiary settings only if uteroplacental insufficiency resulting in IUGR is suspected or is present
  2. Detects velocity of blood flow through the fetal umbilical artery to the placenta and is displayed in a waveform
  3. Normal waveforms produced when the ratio of systolic to diastolic blood flow (S/D ratio) is around 3; abnormal ratio is more than 3
- Amniocentesis
  1. Amniotic fluid is aspirated from the amniotic sac and evaluated for genetic well-being or disorders, and fetal lung maturity
  2. Usually performed between 14 and 16 weeks for genetic evaluation or assessment of neural tube defects
  3. Used later in pregnancy—assessment of lung maturity; R/O amnionitis or fetal hemolytic disease (Rh or anti-D)
  4. Risks—infection, bleeding, preterm labor, PROM, fetal loss
  5. Benefits
     a. Provides early diagnosis and may decrease morbidity and mortality if elective abortion (AB) is sought
     b. May decrease psychological stress; support systems can be established prior to delivery
     c. If a lethal anomaly is diagnosed and pregnancy continues, allows parents/care providers to plan (i.e., avoid a C-section)
  6. Special precaution—if mother is Rh negative and at risk for isoimmunization, administer RhoGAM with amniocentesis
- Chorionic villus sampling (CVS)/chorionic villus biopsy (CVB)
  1. A sample of chorionic villi from placenta is aspirated either transabdominally or transcervically; outer trophoblastic layer is obtained because these tissues have same genetic makeup as the fetus; tissue is examined for genetic information
  2. Used for prenatal diagnosis; performed between 10 and 13 weeks
  3. Benefits
     a. Performed 3–4 weeks earlier than amniocentesis
     b. Cultures grow rapidly, resulting in early diagnosis
  4. Risks
     a. Infection, bleeding, miscarriage
     b. Risk of limb deformities (if performed before 9 weeks)
     c. Technically more difficult
     d. Contraindicated when there is a maternal blood group sensitization
- Fetal movement counting/Fetal kick counts—maternal self-report of fetal movement to assess fetal wellness
  1. Fetal movement counting (FMC)
     a. Most women are aware of fetal movement between 16 and 22 weeks' gestation; multiparas are generally aware of movement sooner than nulliparas are
     b. The fetus has periods of sleep and wakefulness that change according to gestation
     c. Fetal movement is strongest between 29 and 38 weeks
     d. Fetal movement counting is a safe, simple, no-cost, noninvasive fetal assessment technique
     e. Research has demonstrated that fetal activity is a good predictor of well-being
     f. Dramatic decrease or cessation of movement is cause for concern

  2. Methods for performing FMC—adjusted to client's abilities with instructions to count fetal movements starting at 28 weeks (identifiable risk present) or 34–36 weeks (low risk for uteroplacental insufficiency)
     a. Sanovsky's protocol
        (1) Count FM 30 minutes three times daily; four or more movements in a 30-minute period is reassuring
        (2) If fewer than four movements in a 30-minute period, then continue for 1 hour
        (3) Contact care provider if fewer than 10 movements or if movements become weak
     b. Cardiff "Count to 10" method
        (1) A chart to check off 10 fetal movements in one counting session
        (2) Start at approximately the same time daily
        (3) Chart how long it took to count 10 movements
        (4) If fewer than 10 movements in 10 hours or amount of time to reach 10 movements increases, a nonstress test (NST) should be performed
- Nonstress test (NST)
  1. Method to assess fetal well-being by observing the fetal heart rate response to fetal movement
  2. 75% of fetuses at 28 weeks will experience heart rate accelerations in association with fetal movement
  3. External electronic fetal monitoring is used to record fetal heart rate accelerations in response to fetal movement
  4. Accelerations may be spontaneous or may be induced by vibroacoustic stimulation (VAS)
  5. Fetal hypoxia depresses the medullary center in the brain that controls fetal heart rate response, resulting in depression of frequency or amplitude of the fetal heart rate
  6. Indications for assessment of fetal well-being with NST include:
     a. Decreased fetal movement
     b. Postdates
     c. Diabetes, hypertension, IUGR
  7. Interpretation of results
     a. Reactive—2 or more accelerations in fetal heart rate of 15 or more beats per minute, lasting for 15 seconds or more, within a 15- to 20-minute period
     b. Nonreactive—FHR fails to demonstrate the required accelerations within a 40-minute period, requiring further evaluation
     c. Unsatisfactory or inconclusive—fetal heart rate tracing that is uninterpretable or of poor quality, sometimes caused by a vigorous infant; test should be repeated (individual site protocols vary)
     d. NSTs may be affected by any of the following:
        (1) Fetal sleep
        (2) Smoking within 30 minutes of testing
        (3) Maternal intake of medications
        (4) Fetal central nervous system (CNS) anomalies
        (5) Fetal hypoxia and/or acidosis
     e. A nonreactive NST may be followed by a biophysical profile (BPP), a contraction stress test, or a repeat NST
     f. If indicated, NSTs should be repeated either weekly or biweekly

- Contraction stress test (CST)/oxytocin challenge test (OCT)—assessment of fetal well-being by observing fetal heart rate response to uterine contractions
  1. Physiology
     a. During uterine contractions, placental vessels are compressed and intervillous blood flow to the fetus is decreased
     b. A fetus who is compromised or hypoxic does not have reserves
  2. Method
     a. Test is conducted in hospital
     b. Electronic fetal monitoring (EFM); monitor the FHR response to uterine contractions
     c. Contractions may be spontaneous, the result of administration of exogenous oxytocin, or from nipple stimulation
     d. An acceptable test is one with 3 contractions lasting 40–60 seconds that are palpable
  3. Results
     a. Negative—no late or variable decelerations
     b. Equivocal or suspicious—presence of nonrepetitive or nonpersistent decelerations, or long-term variability is absent
     c. Positive—persistent late decelerations with 50% or more of the contractions
  4. Contraindications to CST
     a. Absolute—previous classical C-section or myomectomy, placenta previa, at risk for preterm labor
     b. Relative—gestational age less than 37 weeks, multiple gestation
- Biophysical profile (BPP)—procedure utilizing ultrasound to evaluate five fetal variables to assess fetal risk; prospective studies have demonstrated that BPP is superior to CST as a predictor of fetal well-being or distress
  1. Method
     a. Test is composed of five observable variables—NST, muscle tone, breathing movements, gross body movements, and amniotic fluid volume
     b. In addition to NST, the fetus is evaluated via USG for a 30-minute time period to observe the remaining four variables
  2. BPP scoring—each of the five variables is scored from 0 (abnormal) to 2 (normal); the scores for each are totaled
     a. Breathing movements—one or more episodes in 30 minutes; none = 0, present = 2
     b. Body movement—three or more discrete body or limb movements in 30 minutes; none = 0, present = 2
     c. Tone—one or more episodes of extension with return to flexion; none = 0, present = 2
     d. Qualitative amniotic fluid volume (AFV)—at least one pocket of amniotic fluid that measures at least 2 cm in 2 perpendicular planes; none = 0, present = 2
     e. Reactivity—reactive NST; nonreactive scored as 0, reactive = 2
  3. Scoring interpretation criteria
     a. 8–10 is normal (in absence of oligohydramnios)
     b. 6 is equivocal, repeat testing
     c. 4 or less is considered abnormal
  4. Modified BBP, NST, and amniotic fluid index—(see the section on postterm pregnancy later in this chapter)

- Percutaneous umbilical blood sampling (PUBS or cordocentesis)
  1. Definition—process in which a needle is introduced under real-time ultrasound through the maternal abdomen and then into the umbilical cord; blood is then aspirated or blood and/or medications are introduced into the fetus
  2. Usually performed after 20 weeks
  3. Used for prenatal diagnosis—Rh (anti-D) disease, fetal infections, blood factor abnormalities, chromosomal or genetic disease, fetal hypoxia assessment
  4. Used to treat the fetus—fetal transfusion, administer drug therapy
  5. Concerns
     a. Similar to amniocentesis and CVS procedures
     b. Must be performed by a skilled individual able to secure immediate delivery and appropriate level of neonatal care
- Methods to assess fetal lung maturity
  1. Respiratory distress (RDS) is a major problem associated with preterm birth
  2. Assessment of fetal lung maturity is accomplished by assessing the amniotic fluid
  3. Different tests may be used to assess the factors that help prevent atelectasis
  4. Prior to 39 weeks' gestation, there should be an evaluation of fetal lung maturity if labor induction or Cesarean delivery is electively scheduled to help prevent iatrogenic prematurity and respiratory distress syndrome
     a. Lecithin/sphingomyelin ratio (L/S)
        (1) Lecithin is elevated after 35 weeks
        (2) Sphingomyelin remains fairly constant
        (3) Ratio of 2:1 or greater is indicative of fetal lung maturity except in diabetes
        (4) L/S ratio may also not be accurate in hydrops fetalis and nonhypertensive glomerulonephritis
     b. Phosphatidylglycerol (PG)
        (1) Appears after 35 weeks when lungs are mature
        (2) If PG present, in combination with a favorable L/S ratio, confirms lung maturity
     c. Shake test
        (1) Amniotic fluid is shaken in a tube with saline and 95% ethanol for 15 seconds
        (2) A complete ring of bubbles on the surface is indicative of fetal lung maturity
        (3) Advantage of this procedure is it can be conducted at the bedside
        (4) Has a low false-positive rate
        (5) Has a high false-negative rate
     d. Foam stability test
        (1) Similar to the shake test but amniotic fluid is shaken with various amounts of 95% ethanol only
        (2) Foam formation is indicative of lung maturity
        (3) Collection of amniotic fluid
        (4) With intact membranes, fluid is obtained by amniocentesis
        (5) With rupture of membranes (ROM), fluid can be aspirated with a sterile syringe and sent for evaluation

e. Lamellar body counts
   (1) Lamellar bodies increase in number as pregnancy progresses and are secreted into fetal alveoli and eventually into amniotic fluid
   (2) Lamellar body particles in amniotic fluid obtained by amniocentesis has a precision of 5–10%; amniotic fluid from vaginal pool may contain mucus that can affect results
f. Fluorescent polarization test
   (1) Fluorescent polarization used to measure the ratio of surfactant to albumin
   (2) High values indicate high levels of surfactant
   (3) Blood and meconium may have erroneous results

Selected Obstetric Complications

- Abuse
1. Substance abuse
   a. Substances with known potential for abuse/addiction
      (1) Alcohol—17 million (6.9% of U.S. population) report heavy drinking (5 or more drinks/occasion on 5 or more days in last 30 days)
      (2) Nicotine—71 million (28.6% of U.S. population) currently use tobacco products
      (3) Illegal drugs—prevalence in 2007 was 19.9 million in United States (8.0%) reporting use in past month
         (a) Cocaine
         (b) Hallucinogens
         (c) Heroin
         (d) Marijuana
         (e) Nonmedical use of prescription psychotherapeutics and pain relievers
   b. Historical evolution of the concept of alcohol use in the United States
      (1) After World War II, dominant view linked excessive use of prescription drugs, alcohol, and use of illicit drugs with emotional instability, weak will, and poor character
      (2) Jellinek's 1960 disease model for alcoholism made it a chronic, relapsing disease with a genetic component
      (3) Major definition shift paved the way for the Alcoholics Anonymous approach to treatment
   c. Substance abuse in pregnancy
      (1) Prevalence—according to the Substance Abuse and Mental Health Services Administration National Survey on Drug Use and Health (Substance Abuse and Mental Health Services Administration, 2010)
         (a) 16.3% smoked cigarettes in the past month
         (b) 10.8% reported current alcohol use
         (c) 3.7% engaged in binge drinking
         (d) 4.4% were current illicit drug users
   d. Factors associated with increased risk for substance abuse in pregnancy include:
      (1) Lack of education
      (2) Low self-esteem
      (3) Depression
      (4) Family problems and/or family history of substance abuse
      (5) Financial problems and poverty
      (6) Abusive relationships
      (7) Feelings of hopelessness
      (8) Drug-abusing partner
   e. Maternal medical and obstetric complications of substance abuse include:
      (1) Smoking
         (a) Maternal effects—preeclampsia, abruption placentae, placenta previa, spontaneous abortion, ectopic pregnancy, and premature rupture of membranes
         (b) Infant effects—IUGR, premature birth, and small for gestational age
      (2) Alcohol
         (a) Maternal effects—spontaneous abortion and possibly some subtle neurologic problems in school-age child
         (b) Infant effects—fetal alcohol syndrome (FAS), fetal alcohol effects (FAE), or alcohol-related birth defects (ARBD)
      (3) Illicit drugs
         (a) Effects less well known, and knowledge of long-term implications is limited
         (b) Research findings confounded by social and economic factors
         (c) Polydrug use further confounds the reality
         (d) Maternal effects of heroin and methadone—eclampsia, placental abruption, IUGR, intrauterine death, postpartum hemorrhage, preterm labor, premature rupture of membranes
         (e) Infant effects—jitteriness, hyperreflexia, restlessness, sleeplessness, poor feeding pattern, vomiting, diarrhea, shrill cry
   f. Screening
      (1) Toxicology screen; most commonly done on maternal urine; more recently, meconium, infant hair sample, amniotic fluid, cord tissue
      (2) History—more information gathered regarding length of time and quantity of use
      (3) Combination of both
   g. Screening tools for alcohol use
      (1) CAGE
         C—have you felt the need to cut down on your drinking?
         A—have people annoyed you by criticizing your drinking?
         G—have you ever felt bad or guilty about your drinking?
         E—have you ever had a drink first thing in the morning to steady your nerves or get rid of a hangover (eye-opener)
      (2) TWEAK
         Tolerance—how many drinks can you hold?
         Worried—have close friends or relatives worried or complained about your drinking in the past year?
         Eye-openers—do you sometimes take a drink in the morning when you first get up?

Amnesia—has a friend or family member ever told you about things you said or did while you were drinking that you could not remember?

Cut down—do you sometimes feel the need to cut down on your drinking?

  h. Management
    (1) Ideal—stop using harmful substances
    (2) Reduce quantity and types of substances used
    (3) Mobilize resources to support and encourage
    (4) Drug rehabilitation
  i. Ethical considerations—who should be screened?
    (1) Universal and mandatory versus none for anyone
    (2) Screening of those with positive history or who exhibit signs of use
  j. Legal implications
    (1) Mandatory reporting to child protective services
    (2) Possible loss of infant
    (3) Criminal prosecution of woman
2. Intimate partner abuse/violence against women (VAW)
  a. Incidence of VAW—more than half of all women experience some form of abuse at some point in their lives
  b. Screening techniques for ascertaining the presence of VAW; essential questions asked during history taking include:
    (1) Have you ever been emotionally or physically abused by your partner or someone important to you?
    (2) Within the past year, have you been hit, slapped, kicked, shoved, or otherwise hurt by anyone?
    (3) Have you ever been hit, slapped, kicked, or otherwise physically hurt while you were pregnant?
  c. Definitions of VAW
    (1) Physical
      (a) Pushes, slaps, punches
      (b) Locks woman in or out of the house
      (c) Refuses to buy food
      (d) Refuses access to medical care
      (e) Destroys property or pets
      (f) Abuses children
    (2) Emotional
      (a) Engages in name calling or insults
      (b) Isolates from family and friends
      (c) Publicly humiliates
      (d) Makes all decisions
      (e) Withholds affection
    (3) Sexual
      (a) Treats women as sex objects
      (b) Forces sexual acts with self or others
      (c) Jealous anger with accusations
      (d) Withholds sex and affection
      (e) Engages in sadistic sexual acts
    (4) Financial
      (a) Withholds money
      (b) Runs up bills woman must pay
      (c) Makes all monetary decisions
      (d) Manipulates relationship through money
  d. Diagnosis of abuse
    (1) History
      (a) Depression or suicide attempts
      (b) Substance abuse
      (c) Childhood abuse (sexual or physical)
      (d) Multiple injuries
      (e) Complaints of chronic pain
      (f) Repeated spontaneous abortions (SAB), threatened abortions (TAB)
      (g) STI
    (2) Physical
      (a) Assessing for injuries—multiple bruises in various stages of recovery; proximal versus distal—proximal tends to be intentional; hidden injuries—breasts, abdomen, back, etc.
      (b) Treatment delays—old scars or bruises visible
      (c) Patterned injuries—with reasonable certainty can determine what kind of object caused injury (e.g., bite marks)
      (d) Physical findings inconsistent with history
      (e) Genital trauma, vaginismus
      (f) Poor weight gain in pregnancy
    (3) Others
      (a) Partner appears "overprotective"
      (b) Missed appointments
  e. Effect of pregnancy on VAW
  f. Risks in pregnancy in the situation of violence/abuse, to the woman and fetus
  g. Management
    (1) Data collection
    (2) Forensic examination
    (3) Safety
    (4) Counseling
    (5) Acute intervention
    (6) Long-term aid
    (7) Referral
  h. Community resources for victims of violence/abuse
  i. Legal and emergency issues related to domestic violence
- First-trimester bleeding
  1. Definition—bleeding occurring within the first 12 weeks of pregnancy
    a. 40% of women have some bleeding in the first trimester
    b. 80% of spontaneous abortions occur in the first 12 weeks
    c. 90% of pregnancies with bleeding will continue to term after FHT observed
  2. Differential diagnosis
    a. Implantation bleeding
    b. Threatened abortion
    c. Ectopic pregnancy
    d. Cervicitis
    e. Cervical polyps
    f. Vaginitis
    g. Trauma/intercourse
    h. Disappearing twin
    i. Autoantibody/autoimmune disorder
  3. Diagnosis
    j. Pelvic examination
      (1) Speculum examination to visualize the cervix
      (2) Bimanual examination to assess uterus and adnexa for size and tenderness

(3) Laboratory diagnosis
   (a) Serum hCG is positive 8–9 days after fertilization
   (b) b-hCG doubles every 48 hours with normal intrauterine pregnancy (IUP)
   (c) b-hCG increases by only one-third when an ectopic pregnancy exists

(4) Rule of 10
   (a) b-hCG equals 100 at time of missed menses
   (b) b-hCG is 100,000 at 10 weeks (peak)
   (c) b-hCG 10,000 at term
   (d) b-hCG elimination half-life about 24 hours
   (e) 90% of ectopics have b-hCG less than 6500

4. Treatment—depends on etiology

- Spontaneous abortion
  1. Types of abortion
     a. Spontaneous abortion—occurring without apparent cause
     b. Threatened abortion—appearance of signs and symptoms of possible loss of the fetus (i.e., vaginal bleeding with or without intermittent pain)
     c. Inevitable abortion—cervix is dilating, uterus will be emptied
     d. Incomplete abortion—an abortion in which part of the products of conception has been retained in the uterus
     e. Complete abortion—all the products of conception have been expelled
     f. Missed abortion—the fetus died before completion of 20 weeks' gestation, but products of conception are retained for a prolonged period of time (2 or more weeks)
     g. Habitual abortion—three or more consecutive abortions
  2. Etiology—fetal factors
     a. Abnormal development of zygote such as from chromosomal abnormalities is responsible for about 60%
     b. Autosomal trisomy is the most frequently identified chromosomal anomaly, followed by Turner's syndrome
  3. Etiology—maternal factors
     a. Incidence increases with parity and/or short interconceptional period
     b. Incidence increases with maternal and paternal age
  4. Common causes of spontaneous abortion
     a. Anatomic anomalies
     b. Infections
     c. Immune factors, including autoimmune clotting disorders
     d. Endocrine effects
     e. Recreational drugs/EtOH/environmental toxins
        (1) Smoking
        (2) Ethanol (EtOH)
        (3) Caffeine
        (4) Radiation
        (5) Cocaine
        (6) Anesthetic gasses/surgery
     f. Severe malnutrition
     g. Age of gametes
  5. Management
     a. Obtain blood type if not known
     b. Draw baseline serum b-hCG
     c. Repeat b-hCG in 48 hours
     d. Ultrasound

e. Should be able to visualize transabdominally an IUP at hCG of 6500
f. Should be able to visualize transvaginally an IUP at hCG of 2000
g. RhoGAM for unsensitized Rh-negative women

- Inevitable or incomplete abortion
  1. Surgical dilation and curettage (D&C)
  2. Chemical D&C
  3. Observant management
  4. Emotional support and anticipatory guidance
- Threatened abortion or disappearing twin
  1. Pelvic rest
  2. Emotional support and anticipatory guidance
- Ectopic pregnancy
  1. Definition—implantation of the blastocyst anywhere other than the endometrium
  2. 95% of ectopic pregnancies occur in the fallopian tube
  3. Second leading cause of maternal death in United States
  4. Occurs in about 1 per 85 pregnancies; rate is highest in the 35- to 44-year age group
  5. Etiology
     a. STI—especially chlamydia and gonorrhea
     b. Therapeutic abortion followed by infection
     c. Endometriosis
     d. Previous pelvic surgery
     e. Failed bilateral tubal ligation
     f. Mechanical—problems with tubes such as scarring
     g. Functional—menstrual reflux, hormonal alteration of tubal motility
  6. Sites for ectopic
     a. Ampulla—78% of ectopics
     b. Isthmus—12% of ectopics
     c. Interstitial—2% of ectopics
     d. Fimbria—less than 1% of ectopics
     e. Other sites—abdominal, ovarian, and broad ligament
  7. Symptoms
     a. Amenorrhea but frequently has some vaginal spotting
     b. Lower pelvic and/or abdominal pain, which is unilateral
     c. Unilateral tender adnexal mass
     d. Some have no symptoms
  8. Clinical picture
     a. Severe abdominal pain
     b. Cervical motion tenderness
     c. Free fluid on ultrasound
     d. Cul-de-sac fullness
     e. Shoulder pain second to diaphragmatic irritation
     f. Vertigo or fainting
  9. Diagnosis
     a. Physical examination
     b. Serum b-hCG (90% of ectopics have b-hCG less than 6500; abnormal interval increases)
     c. Ultrasound
     d. Culdocentesis
     e. Laparoscopy
  10. Differential diagnosis
     a. Pelvic inflammatory disease (PID)
     b. Ovarian cyst
     c. Appendicitis

11. Management
    a. Consult and transfer to medical management
    b. Tubal preservation is the goal
    c. Salpingectomy/salpingostomy/tubal resection
    d. Methotrexate
    e. RhoGAM for Rh-negative women
- Hydatidiform mole
  1. Incidence—1:1500 to 1:2000
  2. Highest incidence at beginning and end of reproductive years with greatest incidence after age 45
  3. Symptoms
     a. Abnormal uterine bleeding
     b. Size/dates discrepancy
     c. Lack of fetal activity
     d. Hyperemesis gravidarum
     e. Gestational hypertension before 20 weeks
     f. Passage of vesicular tissue
  4. Diagnosis
     a. Ultrasound
     b. Serum b-hCG
  5. Management
     a. Uterine evacuation by suction curettage
     b. Close surveillance for persistent trophoblastic proliferation or malignant changes
     c. Recommend avoidance of pregnancy for 1 year
     d. Serial b-hCG levels every 2 weeks until normal, then once a month for 6 months, then every 2 months for 1 year
     e. Chest radiograph
- Second-trimester bleeding—bleeding is less common
  1. Midtrimester spontaneous abortion
     a. Etiology
        (1) May be associated with autoimmune disorders
        (2) May be related to cocaine use
        (3) May be related to anatomic or physiologic factors
  2. Incompetent cervix
     a. Symptoms
        (1) Painless dilation
        (2) Bloody show
        (3) Spontaneous rupture of membranes
        (4) Vaginal/pelvic pressure
     b. Risk factors
        (1) Previous midtrimester loss
        (2) Cervical surgery
        (3) Diethylstilbestrol (DES)
     c. Treatment
        (1) Consult
        (2) Cervical cerclage after 12–14 weeks
        (3) Success rate of 80–90%
        (4) Risk of ruptured membranes or infection
        (5) Monitor cervical length via transvaginal ultrasound
  3. Placental anomalies
     a. Low-lying placenta
        (1) One-third of women have low-lying placenta in first trimester
        (2) Only 1% have previa in the third trimester
     b. Partial abruption
        (1) May resolve
        (2) May reabsorb

c. Diagnosis
   (1) Ultrasound
   (2) Consult as needed
- Third-trimester bleeding
  1. Incidence—4% of all pregnancies
  2. Never perform a digital vaginal examination on a woman's cervix in the presence of third-trimester bleeding unless certain there is no previa!
  3. Placenta previa (responsible for 20% of third-trimester bleeds)
     a. Definition—placenta is located over or next to the internal cervical os; may be partial (not totally covering the os), marginal (palpable at margin of os), or complete (completely covering the os)
     b. Incidence
        (1) From 0.4% to 0.6%
        (2) Occurs in 1 of 300 pregnancies
     c. Risk factors
        (1) Multiparity
        (2) Previous C-section or other uterine surgery
        (3) Smoking
     d. Signs and symptoms
        (1) Primary—associated with painless vaginal bleeding
        (2) Secondary—unengaged fetal presentation and/or malpresentation
        (3) Sometimes bleeding is associated with contractions
     e. Diagnosis
        (1) History
        (2) Ultrasound
     f. Management
        (1) Consult, in some practices may co-manage
        (2) Observant management until delivery
        (3) If bleeding, hospitalize
        (4) Tocolytic therapy may be considered
        (5) May be able to deliver vaginally if bleeding is not severe and os is not completely covered
        (6) If vaginal birth is considered, will need double setup for birth
        (7) If complete previa, medical management and Cesarean birth
  4. Placental abruption (cause of 30% of third-trimester bleeds)
     a. Definition—premature separation of the placenta from the uterus that may be partial or complete
     b. Risk factors
        (1) Hypertension—chronic or gestational
        (2) Trauma
        (3) Smoking
        (4) Cocaine use
        (5) Multiparity
        (6) Uterine anomalies or tumors
     c. Signs and symptoms
        (1) Vaginal bleeding
        (2) Uterine tenderness and rigidity
        (3) Contractions or uterine irritability and/or tone
        (4) Fetal tachycardia or bradycardia
     d. Complications
        (1) Shock
        (2) Fetal compromise or death
        (3) Disseminated intravascular coagulation (DIC)

e. Diagnosis
(1) Clinical evaluation
(2) Fetal monitoring
(3) Ultrasound
f. Management
(1) "Get help"
(2) Monitor clotting studies and Hgb/Hct, platelets
(3) Stabilize mother
(4) Effect delivery as indicated by fetal or maternal condition

- Selected problems during pregnancy
  1. Birth defects or anomalies—common terms and definitions
     a. Malformation—the fetus or structure is genetically abnormal (e.g., limb contracture resulting from diastrophic dysplasia)
     b. Deformation—a genetically normal fetus develops in an abnormal uterine environment causing structural changes (e.g., oligohydramnios causing limb contractures)
     c. Disruption—a genetically normal fetus suffers an insult resulting in disruption of normal development (e.g., early amnion rupture causing limb deformities)
     d. Syndrome—multiple abnormalities have the same cause (e.g., trisomy 18)
     e. Sequence—abnormalities occurred sequentially as result of one insult (e.g., oligohydramnios leading to pulmonary hypertension, limb contractures, and facial deformities)
     f. Association—set of abnormalities that frequently occur together but have no linked etiology
  2. Genetic abnormalities
     a. Critical concept definitions
        (1) Phenotype—the expression of genes present in an individual (e.g., eye color, blood type)
        (2) Genotype—the total hereditary information present in an individual; the pair of genes for each characteristic
     b. Definitions of critical patterns of inheritance
        (1) Single-gene (Mendelian) disorders
           (a) A mutation in a single locus or gene, in one or both members of a gene pair
           (b) Incidence—0.4% by age 25; 2% during lifetime
        (2) Autosomal dominant—when only one member of a gene pair determines the phenotype (e.g., *BRCA1* and *BRCA2* breast cancer)
        (3) Autosomal recessive—trait is expressed only when both copies of the gene are the same (e.g., cystic fibrosis, sickle cell anemia)
        (4) Sex-linked
           (a) X-linked diseases are usually recessive (e.g., color blindness, hemophilia)
           (b) Y-linked diseases relate to sexual determination, cellular functions, and bone development
     c. Inborn errors of metabolism—autosomal recessive disease resulting from absence of an essential enzyme causing incomplete metabolism of proteins, fats, or sugars (e.g., phenylketonuria [PKU])
     d. Definition of essential terms
        (1) Autosome—any chromosome other than sex (X or Y) chromosomes

(2) Genome—the complete set of chromosomes or the entire genetic information present in a cell
(3) Euploidy—state of complete sets of chromosomes
(4) Aneuploidy—state of having an abnormal number of chromosomes
(5) Polyploidy—abnormal number of haploid chromosome complements
(6) Deletion—portion of a chromosome that is missing
(7) Ring chromosome—when deletions occur at both ends of the chromosome, the ends may untie to form a ring
(8) Isochromosomes—composed of either two short arms or two long arms of the chromosome fused together
e. Trisomy 21—Down syndrome, the most common, nonlethal trisomy
(1) Incidence—1 in 800–1000 newborns
(2) Etiology—almost 95% due to nondisjunction of maternal chromosome 21
(3) Signs and symptoms
   (a) Marked hypotonia
   (b) Tongue protrusion
   (c) Small head
   (d) Flattened occiput
   (e) Flat nasal bridge
   (f) Epicanthal folds and slanting palperbral fissures
   (g) Nuchal skin fold
   (h) Short, stubby fingers
   (i) Single palmar crease
   (j) Fifth fingers are curved inward
   (k) IQ range—25–50
(4) Recurrence risk—1% until age-related risk status reached after age 35
f. Genetic counseling
(1) Goals for first step—to educate the woman and her family about testing options, indications for and implications of results
(2) Goals after abnormal screen—to inform woman of options to address the results
(3) Indications for genetic studies
   (a) General screening for anomalies (e.g., neural tube defect, trisomy 21)
   (b) History of birth defects or mental retardation
   (c) Family history of genetic disorders
   (d) Exposure to teratogens
   (e) Ingestion of medications in early pregnancy known to be teratogenic (i.e., seizure prevention drugs)
   (f) Has increased likelihood because of age or ethnic roots
3. Sexually transmitted infections (STIs) (Centers for Disease Control and Prevention [CDC], 2010, 2013)
a. Definition—transmission of pathogens through sexual activities and behaviors
b. Incidence—more than a total of 110 million new and existing STI cases in the United States (Satterwhite, et al., 2013)
c. Diseases characterized by genital ulcers
(1) Syphilis
   (a) Incidence—114,000 new and existing cases in the United States (2008)

(b) Clinical manifestations—primary syphilis

    i. Incubation—10–90 days, usually less than 6 weeks

    ii. Primary genital lesion difficult to see, goes unnoticed—cervical chancre more common in pregnancy

    iii. Painless firm ulcer with raised edges

    iv. Heals after 2–6 weeks; may have nontender enlarged inguinal lymph nodes

(c) Clinical manifestations—secondary syphilis

    i. Variable skin rash appears 4–10 weeks after chancre heals

    ii. Not noticed in 25%—may be limited to genitalia

    iii. Condylomata lata—elevated areas that may cause vulvar ulcerations

    iv. Alopecia sometimes occurs

(d) Etiology

    i. Chronic infection—spirochetes cause lesions in major organs

    ii. Recent infection more likely to affect fetus

    iii. Placental changes—large, pale

(e) Diagnosis

    i. VDRL or RPR—first prenatal visit

    ii. Fluorescent treponemal antibody absorption test (FTA-ABS) or microhemagglutination assay for antibodies to *Treponema pallidum* (MHA-TP) confirms nonspecific VDRL/RPR

    iii. Repeat, or do a nontreponemal screening at time of delivery

(f) Treatment—98% effective

    i. Penicillin—dual purpose in pregnancy; eradicate maternal infection and prevent infection in the newborn

    ii. Early syphilis—benzathine penicillin G 2.4 million units IM; some recommend a second dose in 1 week, particularly for secondary stage or in third trimester

    iii. Syphilis of more than 1 year duration—benzathine penicillin G 2.4 million units IM weekly x 3 doses

(g) Penicillin allergy

    i. Skin test to confirm allergy

    ii. Desensitize, then treat as above

(h) Congenital syphilis or stillbirth—may be only sign of maternal infection

    i. Incidence—historically accounted for 30% of all stillbirths

    ii. United States 1998—30 per 100,000 births

(i) Jarisch-Herxheimer reaction

    i. Acute febrile reaction often with headache and myalgia occurring within first 24 hours of treatment initiation; not an allergic reaction; most common in early syphilis treatment

    ii. Might induce early labor or cause fetal distress; should not prevent or delay therapy

    iii. Advise pregnant women of this possible reaction

    iv. May use antipyretics for symptoms; resolves in 24 hours

(2) Herpes simplex virus (HSV)

(a) Incidence—24 million new and existing cases in the United States (2008)

(b) Signs and symptoms—primary infection

    i. Incubation—3–6 days

    ii. Pruritic papular eruption that becomes painful and vesicular, multiple lesions

    iii. Inguinal adenopathy

    iv. Transient flu-like symptoms

    v. By 2–6 weeks all signs and symptoms are gone

(c) Signs and symptoms—recurrent infection

    i. Reactivation results in virus shedding

    ii. Signs and symptoms are less intense but occur at same site

(d) Diagnosis

    i. Viral culture or polymerase chain reaction (PCR) detection

    ii. Type-specific serologic tests

(e) Treatment

    i. Antivirals—acyclovir, valacyclovir—primary or first episode infection, symptomatic recurrent episode; daily suppression from 36 weeks' gestation until delivery

    ii. Analgesics and topical anesthetics

(f) Management of birth—Cesarean delivery indicated only if woman has active genital lesions or prodromal symptoms

(3) Human papillomavirus (HPV)

(a) Incidence—79 million new and existing cases in the United States (2008)

(b) HPV type and associated conditions

    i. HPV-16—cervical, vaginal, and vulvar neoplasia

    ii. HPV-6, 11, also 16, 18, 30s, 40s, 50s, 60s—condylomata acuminata

    iii. HPV-16, 18, 45, 56, 31, 33, 35, 39, 51, 52, 58, 66—cervical intraepithelial neoplasia and cancer

(c) Treatment

    i. Imiquimod, podophyllin, podofilox are contraindicated in pregnancy

    ii. Cryotherapy, trichloracetic acid (TCA), surgical removal if indicated

(d) Management of birth—Cesarean delivery should not be used solely to prevent transmission to newborn; Cesarean delivery may be indicated if genital warts obstruct pelvic outlet or if vaginal delivery would result in excessive bleeding

d. Diseases characterized by urethritis/cervicitis

(1) Gonorrhea

(a) Incidence—107.5 cases per 100,000 population; highest in 20- to 24-year age group (CDC, 2012)

(b) Prevalence in pregnancy—varies with high at 7%

(c) Risk factors—single, adolescence, poverty, drug abuse, prostitution, concomitant STI, lack of antepartal care

(d) GC is marker for chlamydia

(e) Diagnosis—screen at first visit; repeat at 28 weeks in high-risk groups

(f) Clinical significance in pregnancy—associated with septic spontaneous or induced abortion

(g) Treatment

  i. Recommended:

    Ceftriaxone 250 mg IM × 1

    PLUS

    Azithromycin 1 g PO × 1

    Alternative regimen, if ceftriaxone not available:

    Cefixime 400 mg PO × 1

    PLUS

    Azithromycin 1 g PO × 1

    PLUS

    Test of cure in 1 week

    If the patient has severe cephalosporin allergy:

    Azithromycin 2 g PO × 1

    PLUS

    Test of cure in 1 week

  ii. Concomitant treatment for chlamydia if infection is not ruled out

(2) *Chlamydia trachomatis* (CT)

(a) Incidence—584 cases per 100,000 population (CDC, 2008); most common reportable STI

(b) Risk factors—age younger than 25, presence or history of STI, multiple partners, new sexual partner in last 3 months

(c) Signs and symptoms—urethritis, mucopurulent cervicitis, acute salpingitis

(d) Differential diagnosis—normal pregnancy, cervical mucus

(e) Diagnosis—nucleic acid amplification test (NAAT) is most specific and sensitive test available

(f) Treatment

  i. Tetracyclines and quinolones are contraindicated in pregnancy

  ii. Recommended:

    Azithromycin 1 g PO × 1

    OR

    Amoxicillin 500 mg orally TID × 7 days

  iii. Alternative regimens:

    Erythromycin base 500 mg PO QID × 7 days

    OR

    Erythromycin base 250 mg PO QID × 14 days

    OR

    Erythromycin ethylsuccinate 800 mg PO QID × 7 days

    OR

    Erythromycin ethylsuccinate 400 mg PO QID × 14 days

  iv. Repeat testing 3 weeks after completion of treatment

e. Diseases characterized by vaginal discharge

(1) Bacterial vaginosis (BV)

(a) Associated with premature rupture of membranes, chorioamnionitis, preterm labor and birth, intra-amniotic infection, postpartum endometritis, post-Cesarean wound infection

(b) Treatment in pregnancy

  i. Treatment recommended for all pregnant women with symptoms

  ii. Recommended regimens:

    Metronidazole 500 mg PO BID × 7 days

    OR

    Metronidazole 250 mg PO TID × 7 days

    OR

    Clindamycin 300 mg PO BID × 7 days

  iii. Avoid alcohol during use of metronidazole and for 24 hours thereafter

(2) Trichomoniasis

(a) Associated with premature rupture of membranes, preterm delivery, low birth weight

(b) Treatment in pregnancy

  i. No data to support treatment reduces perinatal morbidity

  ii. Metronidazole 2 g PO × 1 at any stage of pregnancy

(3) Vulvovaginal candidiasis (VVC)

(a) Treatment of uncomplicated VVC in pregnancy—topical treatment with azoles for 7 days—butoconazole, clotrimazole, miconazole, terconazole, nystatin

(b) Treatment of recurrent or severe VVC in pregnancy—may require longer duration of therapy with topical azoles

4. Small for gestational age (SGA) and intrauterine growth restriction (IUGR)

a. Definitions—small for gestational age (SGA), intrauterine growth restriction (IUGR), or fetal growth restriction are terms used interchangeably to describe a fetus or newborn whose size is smaller than the norm. SGA is a neonatal diagnosis and describes an infant who falls below the 10th percentile. IUGR is used to describe impaired or restricted intrauterine growth and is considered a pathologic process. The majority of SGA babies are IUGR

b. Differentiation

(1) The genetic design of a constitutionally small infant (parents are also small)

(2) Low birth weight secondary to poor nutrition

c. Incidence—3–8%; leads to 18% mortality rate

d. Symmetric growth restriction

(1) Appears around 18–20 weeks

(2) Caused by

(a) Congenital infections

(b) Chromosomal abnormalities

(c) Maternal drug use—tobacco, alcohol, Dilantin (phenytoin), cocaine, heroin

(3) Increased risk of adverse long-term sequelae

e. Asymmetric growth restriction

(1) Appears later in the pregnancy

(2) Asymmetry is caused by a reduction in cell size, not number of cells, resulting in "head-sparing"

(3) Due to abnormalities in uteroplacental perfusion

(4) Caused by

    (a) Maternal factors

        i. Hypertension

        ii. Anemia

        iii. Collagen disease

        iv. Insulin-dependent diabetes mellitus (IDDM)

    (b) Placental factors

        i. Previa

        ii. Abruption

        iii. Malformations

        iv. Infarctions

    (c) Fetal factors

        i. Multiple gestation

        ii. Anomalies

(5) Diagnosis

    (a) Review history

    (b) Physical examination

        i. Fundal height

        ii. Estimation of fetal weight (EFW)

    (c) Ultrasound to confirm diagnosis

        i. Anomalies

        ii. Serial studies for growth

        iii. AFI

        iv. Doppler flow studies

        v. Placenta grading and assessment

(6) Fetal effects

    (a) Fetus adjusts to conditions by conserving energy and decreasing metabolic requirements

    (b) Fetus stops growing

    (c) Risk of intrauterine fetal demise

(7) Management

    (a) Consult

    (b) If you are able to identify a cause, counsel and make adjustments

        i. Decrease smoking

        ii. Nutrition evaluation

        iii. Maternal positions that facilitate uteroplacental blood flow, left lateral or sitting

        iv. Emotional support and anticipatory guidance

    (c) Serial ultrasounds for growth

    (d) Serial NSTs and AFI or BPPs (weekly or biweekly)

    (e) TORCH titer

    (f) Amniocentesis, chromosome evaluation of parents

    (g) If lungs are mature, consider delivery

5. Large for gestational age (LGA)/macrosomia

  a. Definition—in United States, babies weighing more than 4000 g at birth (macrosomia) or over the 90th percentile in weight for gestational age

  b. Risk factors

    (1) Ethnic/racial origins

    (2) Obesity

    (3) Previous LGA/macrosomic neonate

    (4) Previous shoulder dystocia

    (5) Size of the father

    (6) Birth weight of both the mother and the father

    (7) Diabetes or history of gestational diabetes

    (8) Previous uterine myomata

    (9) Multiparity

  c. Physical examination

    (1) Fundal height

    (2) EFW and palpation of fetal parts

    (3) Maternal body habitus

  d. Differential diagnosis

    (1) Inaccurate dating

    (2) Polyhydramnios

    (3) Multiple gestation

    (4) Diabetes

    (5) Uterine fibroids

  e. Management

    (1) Discuss risks/challenges

    (2) Diet counseling

    (3) Ultrasound for EFW

    (4) Carefully assess clinical pelvimetry

    (5) Consult

    (6) Monitor for shoulder dystocia

6. Preterm birth

  a. Definition—a combination of prematurity, expressed as a birth at 37 weeks' gestation or earlier, and low birth weight, indicated by infant weight of 2500 g or less; with improved neonatal care, the greatest contribution to mortality and serious morbidity comes from infants of less than 34 weeks' gestation

  b. Incidence of preterm birth by gestational age—11.99% of births are 37 weeks or less (CDC, 2010)

  c. Factors associated with preterm birth

    (1) Largely unknown

    (2) Previous history of preterm labor and birth

    (3) Number of prior preterm births

    (4) Cervical incompetence

    (5) Uterine overdistention—multiple gestation, polyhydramnios

    (6) Acute inflammatory response

    (7) Bacterial infections—urinary tract or genital tract

    (8) Poor nutritional status

    (9) Prepregnancy underweight and inadequate gain during pregnancy

    (10) Abruptio placenta

    (11) Preterm premature rupture of membranes

    (12) Substance abuse—cocaine, alcohol, cigarettes

    (13) Chorioamnionitis

    (14) Placenta previa

    (15) Fetal death

    (16) Short interval between pregnancies

    (17) Preeclampsia

  d. Risk scoring systems to identify women at risk for preterm birth have not been successful

  e. Signs and symptoms

    (1) Painful or painless uterine contractions

    (2) Pelvic pressure

    (3) Menstrual-like cramps

    (4) Watery or bloody vaginal discharge

    (5) Low back pain

f. Markers for predicting preterm birth
  (1) Fetal fibronectin (fFN) screening
    (a) Use only in women at high risk for preterm birth
    (b) fFN normally present in cervical secretions until 16–20 weeks' gestation and then again late in pregnancy
    (c) Negative test results useful in ruling out imminent (within 14 days) preterm birth before 37 weeks' gestation (predictive value up to 94%)
    (d) Positive test at 24–34 weeks may predict imminent preterm birth (predictive value 46%)
  (2) Home uterine activity monitoring—data insufficient to support use in preventing preterm birth
  (3) Endocervical length
    (a) Cervical shortening determined with ultrasound associated with preterm birth
    (b) Usefulness limited by lack of proven treatments to affect outcomes
g. Diagnosis—American College of Obstetricians and Gynecologists (ACOG) and American Academy of Pediatrics (AAP) criteria for 20–37 weeks' gestation
  (1) Contractions—4 in 20 minutes or 8 in 60 minutes plus progressive change in the cervix
  (2) Cervical dilatation greater than 2 cm
  (3) Cervical effacement of 80% or more
h. Management—goal is to delay preterm birth (prior to 34 weeks) and enhance infant's resources to cope with life outside the uterus
  (1) Premature rupture of membranes—two approaches
    (a) Expectant management/nonintervention until spontaneous labor begins
    (b) Intervention with corticosteroids in conjunction with or without tocolytics to advance fetal maturation
    (c) Birth is inevitable, but delaying the birth seems to decrease infant mortality
    (d) Hospitalize
    (e) Corticosteroids
    (f) Antimicrobials
  (2) With intact membranes
    (a) Corticosteroids—clear benefits for birth at 24–34 weeks, but unclear for 34 weeks or longer; treatment is most effective when time interval from rupture to birth is a minimum of 24 hours and a maximum of 7 days
    (b) Bed rest—ineffective to stop labor; associated with increased risk of thromboembolic problems
    (c) Hydration and sedation—ineffective
    (d) Tocolytic drugs
      i. Beta-adrenergic receptor agonists—ritodrine and terbutaline—relatively little effect with serious maternal side effects (i.e., pulmonary edema, cardiac insufficiency, hyperglycemia, death)
      ii. Magnesium sulfate—evidence shows no effect for stopping labor, and hypermagnesemia may have toxic effect on mother and fetus

      iii. Prostaglandin inhibitors—indomethacin; adversely affects fetus (i.e., necrotizing enterocolitis, intracranial hemorrhage)
      iv. Calcium-channel blockers—nifedipine; shows promise but not adequately researched yet
      v. Oxytocin analog—atosiban; research to date shows it did not improve infant outcomes
7. Multiple gestation—identify as early as possible
  a. Incidence
    (1) Monozygotic—4/1000 worldwide
    (2) Dizygotic—8/1000 worldwide
    (3) Accounts for fewer than 1% of births but more than 10% of perinatal mortality
    (4) Incidence varies with race and increases with age, parity, and heredity
  b. Dizygotic (DZ) (fraternal)—fertilization of two separate ova by two separate sperm
    (1) Use of fertility drugs increases chance
    (2) Clomid—1/10 risk
    (3) Gonadotropins—1/5 risk
    (4) In vitro fertilization (IVF) increases risk
  c. Monozygotic (MZ) (identical)—division of a single egg fertilized by a single sperm
    (1) Risk factors are unknown
    (2) Time of ovum division determines membrane development
      (a) Day 0–3—dichorionic, diamniotic (30%)
      (b) Day 4–8—monochorionic, diamniotic (68%)
      (c) After day 8—monochorionic, monoamniotic (2%)
      (d) After day 13—conjoined twins (< 1%)
  d. Family history increases risk
  e. Clinical skills are important to identify multiple pregnancies
  f. Signs and symptoms
    (1) Fundal height greater than dates
    (2) Earlier or exaggerated discomforts of pregnancy
    (3) Two distinct heartbeats
    (4) Outline of more than one fetus
    (5) Palpation of multiple small parts
    (6) Ultrasound of two or more fetuses
  g. Differential diagnosis
    (1) Macrosomia
    (2) Uterine, ovarian, or pelvic mass
    (3) Distended bladder
    (4) Polyhydramnios
    (5) Hydatidiform mole
    (6) Inaccurate dates
  h. Potential complications
    (1) Hyperemesis
    (2) Preterm labor, PROM, preterm birth
      (a) 36% deliver before 36 weeks' gestation
      (b) 50% deliver before 37 weeks' gestation
    (3) Low birth weight—55% are less than 5 lb
    (4) Twin-to-twin transfusion
    (5) Oligohydramnios
    (6) Perinatal asphyxia
    (7) Preeclampsia
    (8) Postpartum hemorrhage

(9) Pyelonephritis

(10) Maternal anemia

(11) Placental problems

    (a) Previa

    (b) Abruption

(12) Fetal anomalies

i. Antepartum management

  (1) Consult

  (2) Discuss risks and benefits of management, serial ultrasounds, and regular fetal surveillance

  (3) Counsel about maternal nutrition, rest, exercise, and stress

    (a) Increased nutritional needs

    (b) Increased iron

    (c) Small frequent meals

    (d) Exercise limitations and bed rest are both controversial

  (4) Provide emotional support

  (5) Evaluate weekly for weight, fetal growth, signs/symptoms of preterm labor, and elevated BP

  (6) Preterm labor monitoring

    (a) Possible administration of glucocorticoids for lung maturity

    (b) Tocolytic therapy

    (c) Birth plan should include availability of physician consultant for birth

8. Malpresentations of significance during the prenatal period—breech and shoulder (transverse lie)

  a. Concept—the presentation determines the presenting part

  b. Breech—longitudinal lie with buttocks in the lower pole

    (1) Incidence

      (a) 14% between 29 and 32 weeks

      (b) 3.5% at term

    (2) Variations

      (a) Frank—legs are extended up over the fetal abdomen and chest

      (b) Complete—legs are flexed at the hips and knees

      (c) Footling or incomplete—one or both feet or knees are lowermost

    (3) Etiology—some situation that distorts the shape of the fetus or the uterus

      (a) Uterine septum

      (b) Fetal anomaly (e.g., hydrocephaly)

      (c) Fetal attitude (e.g., extension of spinal column or neck)

      (d) Placenta previa

      (e) Conditions resulting in abnormal fetal movement or muscle tone

    (4) Diagnosis

      (a) Abdominal examination—Leopold's maneuvers findings (four maneuvers)

        i. Fetal part in the fundus is round, hard, freely moveable, and ballotable

        ii. Find back and small parts

        iii. Part in lower pole is large, nodular body

        iv. Determine degree of engagement and reaffirm previous findings by confirming lack of cephalic prominence in lower pole

      (b) Vaginal findings compared to vertex findings

        i. No fetal skull sutures or fontanels

        ii. Round indentation (anus)

        iii. Tissue texture is softer than head, if complete breech; toes, feet, or knees may be palpated if footling

    (5) Treatment

      (a) External cephalic version

      (b) Moxibustion

      (c) Anticipatory guidance regarding plan for version as well as plans for persistent breech

  c. Shoulder—transverse lie in which the shoulder or arm is found in the lower pole

    (1) Incidence—0.4%

    (2) Etiology

      (a) Multiparity

      (b) Placenta previa

      (c) Polyhydramnios

      (d) Uterine anomalies

9. Hypertensive disorders of pregnancy (American College of Obstetricians and Gynecologists, 2013)

  a. Definitions

    (1) Chronic hypertension—BP 140/90 mm Hg or higher diagnosed before pregnancy, before 20 weeks' gestation, or after 12 weeks postpartum

    (2) Chronic hypertension with superimposed preeclampsia—chronic hypertension with new-onset proteinuria at greater than 300 mg in 24 hours, but no proteinuria before 20 weeks' gestation; or sudden increase in proteinuria or blood pressure or platelet count of less than 100,000/mm³ in women with hypertension (HTN) and proteinuria before 20 weeks' gestation

    (3) Preeclampsia—associated with symptoms such as headaches, visual disturbances, epigastric pain, and rapid edema development. The diagnosis of preeclampsia include the development of blood pressure greater than or equal to 140/90 mm Hg on two occasions at least 4 hours apart after 20 weeks of gestation or a blood pressure > 160/100 (confirmed within a few minutes) in a woman who was previously normotensive and proteinuria greater than or equal to 300 mg per 24-hour urine collection or protein/creatinine ratio greater than or equal to 0.3 or, if other quantitative methods are unavailable, a dipstick result of 1+ OR in the absence of proteinuria, new-onset hypertension with the new onset of the following:

      • Thrombocytopenia—platelet count < 100,000/microliter

      • Renal insufficiency—serum creatinine > 1.1 mg/dL or doubling of serum creatinine concentration without renal disease

      • Impaired liver function—doubling of normal levels of liver transaminases

- Pulmonary edema
- Cerebral or visual symptoms

    (4) HELLP syndrome—*H*emolytic anemia, *E*levated *L*iver enzymes, and *L*ow *P*latelet count

    (5) Eclampsia—seizures that cannot be attributed to other causes in a woman with preeclampsia

b. Management of hypertension in pregnancy

    (1) Consult—will need to co-manage and/or transfer care

    (2) For pregnant women with chronic hypertension being treated with antihypertensive medications, it is suggested that BP levels be maintained between 120/80 and 160/105 mm Hg

    (3) For women with chronic hypertension who are at a great risk for adverse pregnancy outcomes, it is recommended to place these women on low-dose aspirin (60–80 mg) PO daily starting in the late first trimester

    (4) For women with chronic hypertension, without other maternal or fetal complications, delivery before 38 weeks is not recommended

    (5) Recommended first choice of antihypertensives for women who require pharmacologic therapy includes labetalol, nifedipine, and methyldopa

    (6) Close surveillance of women with preeclampsia without severe features, include assessment of maternal symptoms, daily fetal movement counts, twice-weekly blood pressure monitoring, weekly serologic assessment of platelets and liver enzymes

    (7) For women with severe preeclampsia, magnesium sulfate for the prevention of eclampsia is recommended in the intrapartum-postpartum period

    (8) Fetal surveillance may include

       (a) Monitor for IUGR

       (b) NSTs

       (c) AFI/BPP

c. Risk factors

    (1) Nulliparity

    (2) Adolescent or advanced maternal age (> 35 years)

    (3) Multiple gestation

    (4) Family history of preeclampsia or eclampsia

    (5) Obesity and insulin resistance

    (6) Chronic hypertension

    (7) Limited exposure to father of baby's sperm—new partner, donor insemination

    (8) Antiphospholipid antibody syndrome and thrombophilia

d. Theory of causes

    (1) Abnormal trophoblast invasion

    (2) Coagulation abnormalities

    (3) Vascular endothelial damage

    (4) Cardiovascular maladaptation

    (5) Immunologic phenomena

    (6) Genetic predisposition

    (7) Dietary deficiencies or excesses

e. Antepartum management of preeclampsia

    (1) Consult diet assessment

    (2) Adequate fluids

    (3) Restricted activities (some experts advise)

    (4) Monitor BP, proteinuria, edema, weight, intake and output, deep tendon reflexes (DTRs), subjective symptoms

f. Laboratory tests

    (1) Creatinine

    (2) Hgb/Hct

    (3) Platelets

    (4) Liver function tests (LFTs)

    (5) 24-hour urine for protein

    (6) Creatinine clearance

g. Assessment of fetus

    (1) Daily fetal movement assessment

    (2) NST

    (3) AFI/BPP

    (4) USG for growth

h. Intrapartum management

    (1) Goal to prevent seizures

    (2) Magnesium sulfate

       (a) Given IV

       (b) Used as an anticonvulsant

       (c) Side effects—flushing, somnolence

       (d) Overdosage signs and symptoms

          i. Loss of patellar reflex

          ii. Muscular paralysis

          iii. Respiratory arrest

          iv. Aggravated by decreased urine output ($MgSO_4$ is excreted by kidneys)

    (3) Antidote is calcium gluconate

    (4) Valium (diazepam) as anticonvulsant rarely used

    (5) Antihypertensives

       (a) Hydralazine IV is antihypertensive of choice in severe preeclampsia

       (b) Others—labetalol (beta blocker), nifedipine

    (6) Diuretics are *not* recommended—woman is already volume depleted

i. HELLP syndrome—affects 10% of patients with severe preeclampsia

    (1) Diagnosis

       (a) Hemolysis

       (b) Abnormal peripheral blood smear

       (c) Increased bilirubin at 1.2 mg/dL or greater

       (d) Elevated liver enzymes—AST, ALT, LDH

       (e) Platelet count at less than 100,000

    (2) Treatment

       (a) Plasma volume expansion

       (b) Bed rest

       (c) Crystalloids

       (d) Albumin 5–25%

       (e) Delivery as indicated

       (f) Magnesium sulfate

j. Eclampsia

    (1) Signs and symptoms—same as pre-eclampsia with seizures

    (2) Management—medical management

       (a) Magnesium sulfate

       (b) Administer oxygen

       (c) Safety—prevent injuries and minimize aspiration during seizures

       (d) Stabilize and deliver

k. Prevention of pregnancy-induced hypertension
  (1) Calcium and vitamin D supplementation if at risk and have low dietary intake
  (2) Low-dose aspirin—consider in high-risk pregnancies

10. Postterm pregnancy
  a. Definition—pregnancy continuing beyond 42 completed weeks' gestation
  b. Incidence
    (1) 6–12% of pregnancies go beyond 42 weeks
    (2) 25% of postterm pregnancies result with babies who have postmaturity syndrome
    (3) Associated with increased morbidity and mortality
  c. Diagnosis
    (1) Based on careful gestational age assessment
      (a) Certain last known menstrual period (LNMP)
      (b) Early examination
      (c) Sizing by bimanual examination
      (d) Fundal height
      (e) Fetal heart tones by Doppler and fetoscope
    (2) Report of sexual history
    (3) Report of quickening
    (4) Early USG gestational dating
      (a) Crown rump length (CRL) best (between 6 and 14 weeks)
      (b) Or dating using femur length (FL), abdominal circumference (AC), head circumference (HC), and biparietal diameter (BPD) before 26 weeks
  d. Potential complications
    (1) Shoulder dystocia—if fetus macrosomic
    (2) Problems related to oligohydramnios
    (3) Problems related to uteroplacental insufficiency
    (4) Neonatal meconium aspiration
    (5) Stillbirth
  e. Management
    (1) Fetal movement counts between 40 and 41 weeks
      (a) At 41 weeks begin biweekly NST/AFI or BPP
      (b) BPP if abnormal NST (CST used less frequently)
      (c) Doppler velocimetry
      (d) Consult
      (e) Expectant management and delivery
        i. Consider induction when cervix is ripe
        ii. Prostaglandins may be used to promote cervical ripening
        iii. Methods of labor induction—oxytocin, membrane stripping, amniotomy, nipple stimulation
        iv. Deliver if any indication of fetal compromise or oligohydramnios
        v. Be prepared for possible meconium staining of fluid

Medical Complications

- Urinary tract infection (UTI)
  1. Risk factors
    a. History of UTI
    b. Sickle cell trait
    c. Diabetes
    d. Pregnancy
      (1) The increased progesterone of pregnancy causes relaxation of the smooth muscles of the genitourinary (GU) tract
      (2) Decreased ureteral peristalsis and ureteral dilation present
      (3) Physical pressure on bladder
      (4) Urinary stasis
      (5) Incidence
        (a) Occurs in 2–7% of all pregnancies
        (b) 25–30% will progress on to pyelonephritis if left untreated
  2. Cystitis; infection of the bladder
    a. May be asymptomatic (asymptomatic bacteriuria)
    b. Usual signs of UTI (although acute cystitis is relatively rare in pregnancy)
    c. Uterine contractions
    d. Suprapubic discomfort
    e. Urgency and frequency
  3. Pyelonephritis—infection of the kidneys
    a. Fever and chills
    b. Nausea and vomiting
    c. Costovertebral angle (CVA) tenderness
    d. Dysuria
    e. Flu-like symptoms
  4. Bacterial causes of UTIs
    a. *E. coli* (most common)
    b. Klebsiella
    c. Proteus
    d. *Neisseria gonorrhoeae*
    e. Pseudomonas
  5. Diagnosis
    a. Symptoms
    b. Urinalysis
    c. Culture and sensitivity of more than 100,000 colonies of pathogenic bacteria
    d. If protein and white blood cells (WBCs) are present on urine dipstick, consider culture
    e. Screen every 4 weeks in sickle cell trait, diabetes, and previous pyelonephritis in this pregnancy
  6. Management
    a. Asymptomatic bacteriuria and UTI
      (1) Treat with antibiotic even if no symptoms
      (2) Adequate fluids
      (3) Cranberry juice
      (4) Antimicrobial therapy—Single-dose treatment does not seem to be effective in pregnant women; however a 3-day course for initial infection has been proven to be as effective as a 7–10 day course. Recurrent infections may require longer treatment regimens
        (a) Cephalosporins—Cephalexin (Keflex) 250 mg PO QID or 500 mg BID
        (b) Ampicillin—250–500 mg PO QID
        (c) Amoxicillin-calvulanic acid (Augmentin)—875 mg PO BID

(d) Nitrofurantoin (contraindicated in late third trimester and in women with G-6-PD)—100 mg PO BID

(e) Trimethoprim/sulfamethoxazole (Bactrim-DS) (contraindicated in third trimester or if have G-6-PD)—1 (800/160 mg) PO BID

(5) Follow up 2 weeks later with a test of cure

(6) Screen for symptoms in subsequent prenatal visits, and if symptomatic, proceed with urinalysis. A urine culture should be obtained if dipstick is positive for leukocyte esterase and nitrites

(7) If recurrent infection, consider suppressive therapy for the remainder of the pregnancy

(a) Nitrofurantoin 100 mg PO QHS

(b) Cephalexin (Keflex) 250 mg PO QHS

(8) Patient education

b. Pyelonephritis

(1) Hospitalization

(2) IV antibiotics

(3) IV hydration

(4) Antipyretics

(5) Pain control

(6) Monitor for preterm labor

- Human immunodeficiency virus (HIV/AIDS)

1. Etiology—DNA retroviruses termed human immunodeficiency viruses, HIV-1 and HIV-2; most cases worldwide are HIV-1; retroviruses have genomes that encode reverse transcriptase, allowing the virus to make DNA copies of itself in the host cells

2. Incidence—approximately 25% of HIV-positive adults in United States are women; HIV/AIDS is number one cause of death for black women 25 to 34 years of age; 40% of HIV-infected infants born to women unaware of HIV status until after delivery

3. Transmission

a. Sexual intercourse (80%)

b. IV drug use (19%)

c. Other (1%)

d. Mother to infant

(1) 15–25% if woman does not receive antiretroviral (ARV) therapy during pregnancy

(2) Less than 1% if woman receives multiagent ARV and if has undetectable viral load at delivery

4. Diagnosis

a. Risk assessment—drug use/sexual histories

b. Universal screening of pregnant women for HIV as part of routine prenatal tests with option to decline (opt-out screening) recommended

c. Repeat screening in third trimester if high risk, high incidence of HIV in reproductive-age women in geographic area, signs or symptoms of acute HIV infection

d. Rapid HIV testing at labor and delivery if status unknown (CDC, 2010)

e. HIV testing

(1) Antibody testing

(a) Screening tests—enzyme immunoassay (EIA) or rapid test

(b) Confirmatory tests if screening test is positive—Western blot or immunofluorescence assay (IFA)

(2) Direct viral screens

(a) Nucleic acid testing if suspect acute retroviral syndrome or recent infection

(b) Confirm with subsequent antibody testing to document seroconversion

5. Signs and symptoms of initial HIV infection

a. Incubation period from exposure to clinical disease—days to weeks

b. Acute viral illness syndrome—lasts 10 days or less

c. Fever

d. Night sweats

e. Fatigue

f. Rash

g. Headache

h. Lymphadenopathy

i. Pharyngitis

j. Myalgias

k. Arthralgias

l. Nausea

m. Vomiting

n. Diarrhea

o. Becomes asymptomatic and chronic viremia begins

p. Time to immunodeficiency syndrome is 10 years

6. Signs and symptoms of AIDS

a. Generalized lymphadenopathy

b. Oral hairy leukoplakia

c. Aphthous ulcers

d. Thrombocytopenia

e. Opportunistic infections

f. Esophageal or pulmonary candidiasis

g. Persistent herpes

h. Cytomegalovirus

i. Molluscum contagiosum

j. Pneumocystis

k. Toxoplamosis

l. Neurologic disease—50%

m. CD4$^+$ count of less than 200 is definitive diagnosis

7. Management of HIV-positive women

a. Infection control

b. Initial evaluation

c. Complete review of systems (ROS)

d. Physical examination

e. Initial labs—HIV antibody, CD4$^+$ count, viral load

f. Follow-up by team of experts; interdisciplinary approach is most effective

g. Prevention of vertical transmission

(1) Viral load is strongest predictor for vertical transmission

(2) Multiagent ARV therapy during pregnancy—start after first trimester if mother does not need treatment

(3) Intravenous zidovudine therapy during labor and delivery

(4) Avoid artificial rupture of membranes if delivery is not imminent

(5) Consider C-section at 38 weeks if viral load is greater than 1000 copies/mL

(6) Treat infant with ARV therapy—usual regimen is 6 weeks

h. Prevention of opportunistic infections

i. Standard precautions for all blood and body fluid-borne pathogens to include blood, all body fluid secretions and excretions, nonintact skin, and mucous membranes

8. Treatment—antepartum
   a. Goals are treatment of maternal infection and reduction of risk for perinatal transmission
   b. Highly active antiretroviral therapy (HAART) that includes:
      (1) Two nucleoside analogs—zidovudine, didanosine, zalcitabine, lamivudine and
      (2) Protease inhibitor—indinavir, ritonavir, saquinavir, or nonnucleoside analogue—nevirapine, delavirdine, efavirenz
      (3) Start after first trimester unless mother needs treatment

9. Treatment—intrapartum
   a. Zidovudine IV throughout labor and delivery for vaginal birth
   b. Zidovudine IV starting 3 hours before C-section and through delivery

10. Counseling
    a. Pretest counseling is important
    b. Informed consent
    c. Posttest counseling is also important

11. Legal issues
    a. Confidentiality
    b. Reporting
    c. Partner notification
    d. Discrimination

12. Concurrent disease concerns for HIV-infected women
    a. Syphilis
    b. TB
    c. HPV
    d. Hepatitis B
    e. Pneumococcal infection

13. Possible effects on pregnancy outcome
    a. PROM
    b. Preterm labor and birth
    c. Low birth weight
    d. Fetal demise
    e. HIV transmission to fetus

14. Fetal assessment as clinically indicated
    a. US
    b. FMC
    c. Serial US as needed
    d. NST with AFI, BPP

15. Intrapartum care
    a. Avoid invasive procedures
    b. Maintain universal body fluid precautions for all births
    c. Cleanse maternal secretions from baby as soon as possible
    d. Drain umbilical cord for cord blood/avoid needles
    e. Breastfeeding is *not* recommended—16% probability of transmission of HIV infection to infant
    f. Give emotional support

- Toxoplasmosis
  1. Incidence—15–40% of pregnant women have antibodies to toxoplasmosis
     a. Primary infection in pregnancy is 1/1000
     b. Most infections are asymptomatic
     c. Of those infected
        (1) 10% will have damage resulting in lower IQ and deafness
        (2) Severe congenital infection occurs 1/10,000
        (3) Infection can also cause abortion, prematurity, and IUGR
  2. Diagnosis
     a. Laboratory data
     b. Testing does not allow diagnosis between primary and secondary infection
     c. Testing for antitoxoplasma IgG antibody is difficult to interpret, so not a practical test to perform
  3. Prevention
     a. Fully cook meat
     b. Do not drink unpasteurized milk or cheese
     c. Avoid kitty litter
     d. Good hand washing following gardening or wear gloves

- Rubella
  1. Incidence (World Health Organization, 2013)
     a. Rare in United States
     b. Only 9 new cases of rubella in 2012
     c. One-half of new cases have occurred in persons born outside United States
     d. 10–20% of reproductive women are susceptible to rubella
     e. Eleven cases of congenital rubella syndrome from 2002–2012 in the United States
     f. Risk of long-term complications from congenital rubella syndrome (CRS) highest if mother infected in first trimester
     g. Most common complications are deafness, IUGR, cataracts, retinopathy, patent ductus arteriosus
  2. Pathophysiology
     a. Rubella is a single-stranded RNA virus
     b. Acquired respiratory disease
     c. Occurs 2–3 weeks following exposure
     d. Infectious virus is present in respiratory tract 1 week prior to symptom development
  3. Symptoms—rash
     a. Discrete pink-red maculopapular rash
     b. Appears first on face, then trunk and extremities
     c. May also have lymphadenopathy, fever, arthralgias
     d. Symptoms last 3 days
     e. Up to 50% of all infections are subclinical
  4. Laboratory testing
     a. Demonstrate serologic conversion
     b. Recent rubella infection will result in specific IgM in the fetal blood
     c. Can use CVS to recover virus
  5. Treatment—prevention
     a. No available antiviral therapy
     b. Vaccination of susceptible reproductive-age women preconception or postpartum

c. No documented cases of CRS from vaccine, but recommend giving at least 4 weeks prior to attempting a pregnancy or postpartum; may give while breastfeeding
- Varicella-zoster (VZV)
  1. Herpes virus causing two common infections
     a. Varicella—chicken pox
        (1) Primary infection is rare in pregnancy
        (2) Greatest risk for congenital varicella syndrome is when mother is infected in first 20 weeks
        (3) Maternal infection occurring from 6 days before to 2 days after delivery can be passed to newborn, causing serious infection—5% mortality
        (4) Varicella infection causes varicella pneumonia in 10–30% of adults
     b. Herpes zoster—shingles
        (1) Secondary infection
        (2) Poses little risk to mother or baby
  2. Incidence
     a. Among pregnant women, 5/1000
     b. VZV is highly contagious and peaks in winter and spring
  3. Pathophysiology
     a. Respiratory inhalation of virus particles
     b. Results in a viremia
     c. Incubation period is 10–21 days, usually 14 days
     d. Virus may be transmitted up to 2 days prior to rash
  4. Diagnosis
     a. Prior to rash, adults experience fever, malaise, myalgias, and headache
     b. Rash—maculopapular rash that becomes vesicles
     c. New vesicles continue for 3–4 days
     d. Crusted by 1 week
  5. Complications
     a. Pneumonia
     b. Increased risk of preterm labor and birth
  6. Treatment
     a. Antiviral agent—IV acyclovir for severe infection in woman
     b. Infection in mother 6 days before delivery—give varicella-zoster immunoglobulin (VZIG), prepare for tocolysis to delay delivery, give VZIG to infant
     c. Infection in mother within 3 days postpartum—give infant VZIG
  7. Prevention
     a. Varicella vaccination for all susceptible reproductive-age women preconception (at least 4 weeks before attempting pregnancy) or postpartum
     b. Varicella-zoster immunoglobulin (VZIG) as early as possible if pregnant woman exposed and susceptible
- Tuberculosis (TB)
  1. Definition—infection, mostly in the lung, by *Mycobacterium tuberculosis*; clinical disease occurs in 10% of those infected
  2. Populations at risk for tuberculosis
     a. HIV-infected women
     b. Foreign-born women from countries with high TB prevalence
     c. Medically underserved low-income populations
     d. Close contacts of persons with active infection
     e. Alcoholics and IV drug users
  3. Incidence (CDC, 2012)
     a. 9945 new cases in United States (2012); 3.2 per 100,000 persons
     b. In 2011, nearly 9 million cases of TB worldwide; and around 1.4 million TB-related deaths in the world
  4. Screening tests for tuberculosis
     a. Purified protein derivative (PPD) intradermally
        (1) If negative (i.e., no induration) no further assessment is needed
        (2) Positive test interpreted by risk factors
           (a) 5 mm is positive for very high risk—HIV positive, with abnormal chest radiograph, recent contact with active case
           (b) 10 mm is positive for high risk (i.e., foreign born, HIV-negative IV drug user, low-income populations, associated medical problems)
           (c) 15 mm is positive for those with none of these risks
        (3) Vaccination with bacillus Calmette–Guérin (BCG) requires special guidance for interpretation
  5. Signs and symptoms
     a. Cough with minimal sputum production
     b. Low-grade fever
     c. Hemoptysis
     d. Weight loss
  6. Diagnosis
     a. Chest radiograph
     b. Sputum for acid fast bacillus
     c. Extrapulmonary disease occurs in any organ; disseminated disease exists in 40% of HIV-positive patients
  7. Treatment (CDC, 2012)
     a. In the absence of risk factors, wait until after delivery to avoid unnecessary medications during pregnancy
     b. Isoniazid (INH) daily or twice weekly using directly observed therapy
     c. Supplementation with 10–25 mg/day of pyridoxine (vitamin B_6) recommended
     d. 12-dose regimen not recommended for pregnant women or women expecting to become pregnant during the treatment period
     e. Potential for increased risk for hepatotoxicity during pregnancy and the first 2–3 months postpartum
     f. Breastfeeding is not contraindicated with TB treatment
     g. Precautions
        (1) Liver toxicity
        (2) Drug resistance
- Diabetes
  1. Definition—endocrine disorder of abnormal carbohydrate metabolism resulting in inadequate production and/or utilization of insulin
  2. Gestational diabetes
     a. Occurs in 2–12% of pregnancies
     b. Results from the diabetogenic effect of pregnancy
     c. hPL (human placental lactogen) acts as an insulin antagonist
     d. Estrogen and progesterone may also act as insulin antagonists

3. Diagnosis
   a. Risk assessment at initial prenatal visit
   b. High risk (USDHHS, 2013)
      (1) Overweight or obese
      (2) Prior history of gestational diabetes mellitus (GDM)
      (3) Prior large for gestational age infant weighing more than 9 lb
      (4) > 25 years old
      (5) Strong family history of type 2 diabetes
      (6) Are African American, Hispanic, American Indian, Alaska Native, Native Hawaiian, or Pacific Islander
      (7) Are being treated for HIV
   c. Low risk (CDC, 2010)
      (1) < 25 years old
      (2) Normal weight before pregnancy
      (3) Member of ethnic group with low prevalence of diabetes
      (4) No known diabetes in first-degree relatives
      (5) No history of abnormal glucose tolerance
      (6) No history of poor obstetric outcome
4. Screening (American Diabetes Association, 2012; American College of Obstetricians and Gynecologists [ACOG], 2013c)
   a. High risk—screen as soon as possible using standard diagnostic testing
   b. All women not considered low risk—screen at 24–28 weeks
      (1) Two-step approach
         (a) Screen with a 1-hour 50-g glucose challenge test (GCT)
         (b) If 130 mg/dL (90% sensitivity) or more, or greater than 140 mg/dL (80% sensitivity), perform diagnostic 100-g 3-hour diagnostic oral glucose tolerance test (OGTT) on another day after an overnight 8-hour fast
         (c) Diagnosis of GDM can be made if 2 of the following results from the 3-hour testing are abnormal utilizing either the Carpenter and Coustan or the National Diabetes Data Group criteria:

Status	Plasma or Serum Glucose Level – Carpenter and Coustan Conversion		Plasma Level – National Diabetes Data Group Conversion	
	mg/dL	mmol/L	mg/dL	mmol/L
Fasting	95	5.3	105	5.8
One hour	180	10.0	190	10.6
Two hours	155	8.6	165	9.2
Three hours	140	7.8	145	8.0

      (2) One-step approach
         (a) Perform a 75-g 2-hour oral glucose tolerance test (OGTT) after an overnight 8-hour fast
         (b) Measure fasting plasma glucose and at 1 and 2 hours post-OGTT
         (c) Diagnostic criteria for one-step approach for GDM—presence of any abnormal number of the following plasma glucose values
            • Fasting 92 mg/dL or greater
            • 1 hour 180 mg/dL or greater
            • 2 hours 153 mg/dL or greater
5. Presence of three or more of the following risk factors increases the chance of perinatal mortality:
   a. Uncontrolled hyperglycemia
   b. Ketonuria, nausea, vomiting
   c. Pregnancy-induced hypertension (PIH), edema, proteinuria
   d. Pyelonephritis
   e. Lack of compliance with care
   f. Maternal age older than 35 years
6. Management—objective is to maintain strict levels of maternal glucose for optimum perinatal outcomes
   a. Co-manage or transfer to perinatal center
   b. Diet
      (1) 30 kcal/kg of actual or ideal body weight
      (2) 25% at breakfast
      (3) 30% at lunch
      (4) 30% at dinner
      (5) 15% at snack
   c. Distribution of calories
      (1) Protein 20% of calories
      (2) Fat 30–35% of calories
      (3) Carbohydrates 45–50% of calories
   d. Medications
      (1) Oral hypoglycemics—glyburide and acarbose are pregnancy Category B; others are Category C
      (2) Insulin
   e. Maternal monitoring
      (1) PIH
      (2) Changing insulin requirements
      (3) Decreased need in first trimester because of low hPL levels
      (4) Increases in second trimester because of increasing hPL levels
      (5) HgbA$_{1c}$/fasting plasma
   f. Fetal monitoring
      (1) Increased risk of neural tube defects and cardiac anomalies in nongestational diabetics
      (2) Ultrasound for IUGR, macrosomia, polyhydramnios
      (3) FMCs beginning at 28 weeks
      (4) NSTs with AFI or CST beginning at 36 weeks
      (5) May consider amniocentesis for L/S ratio (maturity is 3:1 with positive PG)
   g. Immediate postpartum—monitor insulin requirements (usually decrease 24–48 hours after delivery of the placenta)
   h. 75-g 2-hour OGTT at 6–12 weeks postpartum—screen for diabetes and then follow with subsequent screening for diabetes or prediabetes
• Thyroid disease
   1. Definition—most common thyroid diseases in pregnancy are nontoxic goiter, hyperthyroidism, hypothyroidism, and thyroiditis
   2. Impact of pregnancy on maternal thyroid physiology is great; structural and functional changes related to pregnancy can cause confusion in defining abnormalities

3. Thyroid enlarges somewhat because of hyperplasia and increased vascularity but does not cause serious thyromegaly
4. Thyroid hormones in pregnancy—total serum thyroxine (TT_4) and triiodothyronine (TT_3) concentrations increase; TSH and free thyroxine (FT_4) levels are not affected
5. Thyrotoxicosis or hyperthyroidism
   a. Incidence—1/2000 pregnancies
   b. Signs and symptoms
      (1) Tachycardia, more than normal in pregnancy
      (2) Elevated sleeping pulse rate
      (3) Thyromegaly
      (4) Exophthalmos
      (5) Failure to gain weight with normal or increased food consumption
   c. Diagnosis
      (1) Elevated serum free thyroxine (FT_4) or free thyroxine index (FTI) levels
      (2) Suppressed TSH levels
   d. Treatment
      (1) Control with thioamide drugs; propylthiouracil or methimazole
      (2) Thyroidectomy if medical approach unsuccessful but easier done outside of pregnancy because of increased vascularity
   e. Maternal and fetal outcomes
      (1) Good if treatment successful
      (2) If not, higher incidence of preeclampsia and heart failure as well as preterm birth, IUGR, and stillbirth
- Blood incompatibilities—D(Rh) isoimmunization
  1. Incidence (Rh2)
     a. Highest incidence found in Basques of France and Spain (25–40%)
     b. White Americans approximately 15%
     c. African Americans approximately 5–8%
     d. American Hispanics approximately 5–10%
  2. Types
     a. ABO incompatibility
        (1) 20–25% of pregnancies are ABO incompatible
        (2) Isoimmunization causes 60% of fetal hemolytic disease
     b. Maternal serum contains anti-A or anti-B
        (1) Rarely causes more than fetal anemia with mild to moderate hyperbilirubinemia in the first 24 hours of life
        (2) Due to the fact that the IgM anti-B or IgM anti-A crosses the placenta poorly
     c. Sensitization caused by minor antigens
        (1) Some cause hemolytic disease, some do not
        (2) Believed to be the result of incompatible transfusion, although may be seen in multiparas
     d. Kell—may have mild to severe with hydrops (K-kills)
     e. Duffy—Fy^a may have mild to severe with hydrops; Fy^b—not associated with problems
  3. Pathogenesis for Rh isoimmunization
     a. Three requirements
        (1) Fetus must be D+ and mother D–
        (2) Mother must be able to be sensitized
        (3) Fetal cells must gain access into the mother's blood stream in sufficient quantities

   b. Occurs when
      (1) There is a transfusion of incompatible blood to the mother, usually before pregnancy
      (2) A fetomaternal exchange of blood during
         (a) Delivery
         (b) Spontaneous or induced abortion (woman may not realize she is pregnant)
         (c) Amniocentesis
         (d) Ectopic
         (e) Placental separation
         (f) Unknown cause
  4. Implications
     a. Maternal
        (1) No significant maternal complications
        (2) Fetal loss
     b. Fetal
        (1) Mother produces anti-D antibodies (IgG), which cross the placenta
        (2) Hemolysis of fetal red blood cells (RBCs) then occurs
        (3) Fetal anemia results with hematopoiesis in liver and spleen
        (4) Fetal liver and spleen enlarge
        (5) Liver and spleen show degenerative changes
        (6) Erythroblastosis fetalis results (ascites, cardiac failure, hydrothorax)
        (7) Hydrops fetalis with generalized edema
     c. Newborn
        (1) Maternal IgG is still present and attacking RBCs
        (2) Further RBC breakdown occurs
        (3) Fetal liver is immature and unable to clear RBCs
        (4) Hyperbilirubinemia results
        (5) Bilirubin causes kernicterus with CNS damage and possible death
  5. Management
     a. Unsensitized pregnancy—mother Rh negative with negative antibody titer
        (1) ABO/D group and antibody titer at first visit
        (2) Repeat antibody screen at 28 weeks and give RhoGAM if remains unsensitized
        (3) RhoGAM is protective for 12 weeks
        (4) If infant is Rh positive, give mother RhoGAM again after delivery
     b. Sensitized pregnancy—mother Rh negative with positive antibody titer (> 1:4)
        (1) Consult—co-manage or transfer care
        (2) Follow fetus with serial ultrasounds to assess for signs of ascites
        (3) Follow titers to assess need for amniocentesis
- Acquired anemias
  1. Iron-deficiency anemia
     a. Definition—hemoglobin less than 11.0 g/dL first trimester, 10.5 g/dL second trimester, 11.0 mg/dL third trimester and postpartum
     b. Etiology—related to poor nutrition resulting in inadequate iron stores; consequence of expansion of blood volume with inadequate expansion of maternal hemoglobin mass
     c. Signs and symptoms—not apparent unless severely anemic

d. Differential diagnosis
   (1) Anemia associated with chronic disease
   (2) Blood loss effect
e. Diagnostic tests
   (1) Serum ferritin levels lower than normal
   (2) Microcytic, hypochromic erythrocytes
   (3) Serum iron-binding capacity elevated (but not a significant finding since it is elevated in pregnancy in absence of iron deficiency)
f. Associated with low birth weight, premature delivery, perinatal mortality
g. Management and treatment—correct the hemoglobin mass deficit and rebuild iron stores
   (1) Iron replacement therapy
   (2) Ferrous sulfate, ferrous gluconate, ferrous fumarate
   (3) Include vitamin C and folic acid
   (4) Intramuscular therapy if unable to take orally or if severely anemic
   (5) Iron therapy for 3 months after anemia corrected

2. Anemia from acute blood loss
   a. Definition—drop in hemoglobin due to moderate-to-severe blood loss, which can occur at any time in pregnancy
   b. Etiology—abortion, ectopic pregnancy, hydatidiform mole, placenta previa, abruptio placenta, placenta implantation anomalies, etc.
   c. Management and treatment
      (1) Massive hemorrhage requires restoration of volume and cells to maintain perfusion of vital organs
      (2) Treat residual iron depletion (Hb 7 g/dL or greater) with oral iron for 3 months as long as woman is afebrile and able to ambulate

3. Megaloblastic anemia
   a. Definition—group of hematologic disorders characterized by blood and bone marrow abnormalities caused by impaired DNA synthesis
   b. Prevalence—rare in the United States
   c. Etiology—in the United States, during pregnancy, most always results from folic acid deficiency due to lack of consumption of green leafy vegetables, legumes, and animal protein
   d. Signs and symptoms—nausea, vomiting, and anorexia, which worsen as deficiency increases
   e. Diagnosis—laboratory tests showing hypersegmentation of neutrophils, macrocytic erythrocytes, bone marrow megaloblastic erythropoiesis
   f. Risks to fetus—neural tube defects
   g. Prevention—folic acid (0.4 mg daily for childbearing-aged women; 4 mg daily prior to and during pregnancy for women with history of previous neural tube defect infant), nutritious diet, and iron

- Inherited anemias—hemoglobinopathies
  1. Sickle cell hemoglobinopathies
     a. Sickle cell anemia (SS disease)
     b. Sickle cell–hemoglobin C disease (SC disease)
     c. Sickle cell–b-thalassemia disease (S–b-thalassemia disease)

2. Etiology—individual inherits a gene for S hemoglobin from each parent, or an S and a C gene from each, or an S and b-thalassemia gene from each
3. Incidence
   a. SS disease—1 in 12 African Americans has sickle cell trait—SA hemoglobin; incidence is 1 in 576 theoretically but is, in fact, less common
   b. SC disease—1 in 40 African Americans has hemoglobin C gene; incidence of SC disease in African American pregnant women is 1 in 2000
   c. Sickle cell–b-thalassemia disease—1 in 2000 African American women
4. Signs and symptoms—SS is worst of hemoglobinopathies in pregnancy
   a. Sickle cell crisis occurs more frequently in pregnancy
   b. Infections and pulmonary complications more common
   c. Contributes to maternal mortality
5. Differential diagnosis
   a. Thalassemia
   b. G-6-PD deficiency
6. Physical findings
   a. Hb 7 g/dL or less
   b. Intense pain of crisis particularly in third trimester, in labor, and in puerperium
   c. Fever due to dehydration or infection
   d. Acute chest syndrome—pleuritic pain, cough, fever, lung infiltrate, and hypoxia
7. Management and treatment
   a. Consult and co-manage
   b. Weekly fetal surveillance after 32–34 weeks
   c. Pain medication
   d. Follow-up (including possible need for paternal blood screening and genetic counseling)
   e. Counseling for current and future pregnancies

- Appendicitis
  1. Incidence—suspected in 1/1000; found in 1/1500 pregnant woman; most common reason for surgical exploration during pregnancy
  2. Pregnancy confounds signs and symptoms of appendicitis
     a. Nausea, vomiting, and anorexia of pregnancy versus appendicitis
     b. Displacement of the appendix by the growing uterus moves the point of pain and tenderness associated with appendicitis
     c. Leukocytosis, to some extent, occurs in pregnancy
     d. Confounding diagnoses, especially in pregnancy; pyelonephritis, renal colic, placental abruption, and degeneration of a myoma
     e. In late pregnancy, symptoms may be very atypical
  3. Diagnosis and management
     a. Persistent abdominal pain and tenderness is most critical symptom
     b. Immediate surgical exploration indicated if suspected
     c. Diagnosis correct in 50–65% of cases; verify to prevent peritonitis

- Neoplastic disease
  1. Incidence of cancer in pregnancy—uncommon; second leading cause of death in women ages 15–44 in United States
  2. Most frequent types of cancers in pregnancy—genital tract, breast, and malignant melanoma
  3. Principle of treatment—the woman should not be penalized for being pregnant
  4. Approach to the pregnant woman with cancer
     a. Surgical intervention for diagnosis, staging, or therapeutic purposes is well tolerated; oophorectomy may be done after 8 weeks of gestation since placental hormone production is sufficient
     b. Radiation of 15–20 rads may cause microcephaly and mental retardation in the fetus
     c. Chemotherapy risk for the fetus depends on GA, but avoid at 5–10 weeks if possible
  5. Breast cancer
     a. Incidence—most common malignancy at all ages; estimated at 10–30/100,000 pregnancies
     b. Effects of pregnancy on breast cancer—none of note; stage of the disease at time of diagnosis and treatment more important to survival
     c. Diagnosis—same as for nonpregnant women; any suspicious breast mass should be diagnosed immediately using one or more of the following methods:
        (1) Needle aspiration can differentiate a cyst or galactocele from solid tumor
        (2) Tissue biopsy if needle biopsy results are not diagnostic
        (3) Mammography—but more difficult because of denser tissue; requires adequate shielding; radiation is less than 100 mrad
        (4) Once cancer diagnosis made, limited metastatic search and chest radiogram done; computed tomography (CT) bone and liver scans are contraindicated because of ionizing radiation
     d. Treatment
        (1) Surgery as soon as the diagnosis is confirmed
        (2) Radiotherapy not recommended
        (3) Chemotherapy can be given in pregnancy
     e. Recommendations for future pregnancies—little evidence exists to say that survival is adversely affected by pregnancy after mastectomy for breast cancer
  6. Malignant melanoma
     a. Incidence—estimated at 0.14 to 2.8 per 1000 live births
     b. Skin changes to watch and report—pigmented lesion that changes
        (1) Contour
        (2) Surface elevation
        (3) Discoloration
        (4) Itching
        (5) Bleeding
        (6) Ulceration
     c. Clinical stages
        (1) Stage I—no positive lymph nodes (85%); tumor thickness is single most important factor in predicting survival at this stage
        (2) Stage II—nodes are positive
        (3) Stage III—distant metastases
     d. Effect of pregnancy—usually have thicker tumors when diagnosed in pregnancy
     e. Treatment—surgery and chemotherapy if indicated
  7. Cervical cancer
     a. Incidence—most common form of cancer in pregnancy—carcinoma in situ 1.3/1000; invasive carcinoma 1/2200 pregnancies
     b. Abnormal Pap tests equal 3% during pregnancy
     c. Colposcopy to confirm and identify lesions
     d. Treatment—varies with stage of cancer and duration of pregnancy
        (1) Microinvasive disease follows same guidelines as for nonpregnant intraepithelial disease; continuation of pregnancy and vaginal delivery with postpartum therapy
        (2) Invasive cancer is treated immediately in first half of pregnancy; if detected in latter half, can wait for fetal viability and maturation
- Heart disease
  1. Incidence—rheumatic heart disease almost nonexistent in United States because of better management and resources; congenital heart disease accounts for half of pregnancy heart problems
  2. Heart disease accounts for 5–15% of maternal deaths
  3. Etiology—cardiac output increases in pregnancy by 30–50%, half of which occurs by the 8th week; reaches maximum level by midpregnancy
  4. Symptoms
     a. Progressive dyspnea
     b. Nocturnal cough
     c. Hemoptysis
     d. Syncope
     e. Chest pain
  5. Clinical findings
     a. Cyanosis
     b. Clubbing of fingers
     c. Neck vein distension
     d. Systolic murmur grade 3/6 or greater
     e. Diastolic murmur
     f. Cardiomegaly
     g. Persistent arrhythmia
     h. Persistent split-second sound
  6. Diagnosis—normal changes of pregnancy make diagnosis difficult
     a. EKG
     b. Echocardiography
     c. Chest radiograph
  7. Functional classification of cardiac disease—based on past and present disability, uninfluenced by physical signs
     a. Class I—uncompromised; no limit on activity; no symptoms of cardiac insufficiency, no anginal pain
     b. Class II—slightly compromised; ordinary activity results in excessive fatigue, palpitation, dyspnea, or anginal pain

c. Class III—markedly compromised; marked limitation of activity; less than normal activity causes symptoms manifested in Class II

d. Class IV—severely compromised; symptoms manifested in Class II and Class III develop at rest and become more intense with activity

8. Antepartum management of the patient with Class I and Class II cardiac disease with regard to the following:

a. Preventative measures—avoid upper respiratory infection (URI) contact; provide pneumococcal and flu vaccines

b. No smoking

c. No illicit drugs, especially cocaine and amphetamines

d. Instruct client regarding signs and symptoms of developing congestive heart failure:

   (1) Nocturnal cough

   (2) Basilar rales

Questions

Select the best answer.

1. M. S. comes to the office indicating her period is 1 month overdue. Her level of pregnancy diagnosis is?
   a. Positive
   b. Presumptive
   c. Possible
   d. Probable

2. R. L. states that she is trying to get pregnant and had unprotected intercourse on day 14 of her usual 28-day menstrual cycle. However, the pregnancy test was negative 3 days later. Appropriate management would be to:
   a. Order an ultrasound
   b. Prescribe progesterone
   c. Repeat the test in a week
   d. Order a serum pregnancy test

3. Pregnancy tests detect:
   a. Estrogen
   b. Human chorionic gonadotropin
   c. Human placental lactogen
   d. Progesterone

4. During the first few weeks of pregnancy, progesterone is secreted by the:
   a. Placenta
   b. Corpus luteum
   c. Endometrium
   d. Trophoblasts

5. Blood in the chorionic villi pertains to whose circulation?
   a. Mother
   b. Mother and fetus
   c. Placenta
   d. Fetus

6. The vessels of the umbilical cord are:
   a. One vein with oxygenated blood and two arteries with deoxygenated blood
   b. One vein with deoxygenated blood and two arteries with oxygenated blood
   c. Two veins with oxygenated blood and one artery with deoxygenated blood
   d. Two veins with deoxygenated blood and one artery with oxygenated blood

7. The uterus is palpable at the symphysis pubis at:
   a. 6 weeks
   b. 8 weeks
   c. 12 weeks
   d. 16 weeks

8. Implantation occurs _____ after fertilization.
   a. 24–48 hours
   b. 3–4 days
   c. 6–7 days
   d. 9–10 days

9. Placental transport of oxygen and glucose occurs by:
   a. Simple perfusion
   b. Facilitated diffusion
   c. Active osmosis
   d. Active perfusion

10. The human zygote consists of:
    a. 46 chromosomes from each parent
    b. 2 pairs of sex chromosomes
    c. 23 chromosomes
    d. 23 pairs of chromosomes

11. The trophoblast will ultimately become the:
    a. Placenta
    b. Embryo
    c. Blastocyst
    d. Umbilical cord

12. At her initial visit, M. R. was a healthy primigravida, but you heard a Grade I systolic murmur. Your management would be:
    a. A cardiology consult
    b. Chest radiograph
    c. Immediate referral
    d. No intervention

13. The drop in diastolic blood pressure during normal pregnancy is partly the result of:
    a. Plasma volume expansion
    b. Progesterone's effect on vessel walls
    c. Increased cardiac output
    d. Pooling of plasma in tissues

14. Changes in the respiratory system due to pregnancy may cause:
    a. Tachypnea
    b. Cough
    c. Increased chest diameter
    d. Pale nasal mucosa

15. C. D., a primigravida, came in for a visit at 34 weeks stating that she has "a lot of vaginal discharge" but no other symptoms or problems. On exam you see a white, odorless discharge of moderate quantity. Your next step would be:
    a. Treat for candida
    b. Check for trichomoniasis
    c. Reassure that this is normal
    d. Send a vaginal culture

16. R. P. comes for a 24-week visit and mentions that her interest in sex has increased greatly. You respond to her concern because you know that increased libido is:
    a. A normal variation of response in pregnancy
    b. An abnormal response of changing image
    c. Reflective of repressed desire to disrupt the pregnancy
    d. The early sign of a parenting disorder

17. R. Q., at her 36-week visit, tells you that she is having night-mares that include labor as well as fears of having an abnormal baby. Your best response is:
    a. Tell her there is nothing to worry about because most babies are fine
    b. Encourage her to tell you more about the nightmares and her fears
    c. Make her an appointment with a mental health nurse practitioner
    d. Reassure her that there are dangers about which we all have to worry

18. Initial management of constipation in pregnancy should include suggestions for:
    a. Increased protein intake
    b. Limitation of calcium-rich foods
    c. Use of a laxative
    d. Increased intake of fiber and fluids

19. P. J. has had three spontaneous abortions and is now pregnant for the fourth time. The term that defines her status is:
    a. Multipara
    b. Nullipara
    c. Primigravida
    d. Primipara

20. The calculation of estimated date of birth (EDB) by Naegele's rule is based on:
    a. A 28-day menstrual cycle
    b. Average length of pregnancy of 290 days
    c. A 32-day cycle
    d. Length of pregnancy of 270 days

21. A. B. is pregnant for the third time. Her obstetric history indicates she has had two miscarriages at 16 and 18 weeks and one twin birth at 36 weeks. One twin died, but the other is alive and well. The four-digit descriptor of this history is:
    a. 0121
    b. 0221
    c. 2021
    d. 2201

22. D. M. comes for her first antepartal visit. When asked the date of her last menstrual period, she indicates she has not had one since she has been nursing her 6-month-old daughter. You diagnose that she is pregnant. How would you determine estimated date of birth (EDB)?
    a. Determine when she expected to get her period and calculate from there
    b. Document quickening and extrapolate from there
    c. Send her to fetal assessment unit for an ultrasound
    d. Get good sexual history and use last coitus as the basis for calculation

23. R. P., G1 P0, comes for her 20-week visit. Her abdominal exam shows the uterine fundus to be half way between the symphysis and the umbilicus. This finding leads you to consider:
    a. Intrauterine growth restriction (IUGR)
    b. Nothing, since it is normal
    c. Oligohydramnios
    d. She is not eating and gaining enough weight

24. In an abdominal exam using Leopold's maneuvers, the first step is to determine fetal:
    a. Attitude
    b. Position
    c. Engagement
    d. Lie

25. D. P. presents for her first antepartal visit. She is 10 weeks pregnant and requests that you listen for the FHT. Your response would be:
    a. "No, there is no reason to because it cannot be heard yet anyway."
    b. "Sure, I will listen, but we may not hear it yet."
    c. "Sure we can listen because it will be there now."
    d. "We do not usually do that at this visit."

26. Normal findings on speculum and pelvic examination of a pregnant woman include:
    a. Bluish color of the cervix
    b. Pale vaginal mucosa
    c. Open cervical os
    d. Firm, slightly enlarged cervix

27. Clinical pelvimetry of a woman with an adequate pelvis would provide which of the following findings?
    a. Ischial tuberosities of 10 cm and a flat sacrum
    b. Convergent sidewalls
    c. Pubic arch of 90 degrees with diagonal conjugate of longer than 11.5 cm
    d. Protuberant ischial spines

28. The value of clinical pelvimetry rests in its ability to:
    a. Predict successful vaginal birth
    b. Identify the characteristics of the woman's pelvis
    c. Determine whether the woman will have a breech presentation
    d. Predict an occiput posterior position

29. F. R., a primigravida at 16 weeks, states that she is concerned because she has not felt the baby move yet. Your response should be:
    a. "Most women with a first pregnancy do not feel movement until around 20 weeks."
    b. "You are worrying too much, just relax."
    c. "I will order an ultrasound just to be sure everything is fine."
    d. "I would like you to return in a week so we can recheck it."

30. Maternal serum alphafetoprotein screening is performed in what time frame?
    a. 8–12 weeks
    b. 12–15 weeks
    c. 15–19 weeks
    d. 20–24 weeks

31. CDC recommends screening for group B streptococcus (GBS) at what point?
    a. At the first visit
    b. When labor starts
    c. At 20 weeks
    d. At 35–37 weeks

32. The triple screen tests for:
    a. AFP, progesterone, hCG
    b. AFP, estriol, hCG
    c. Estriol, progesterone, hPL
    d. Estradiol, progesterone, AFP

33. A nonstress test containing two fetal heart accelerations lasting 15 seconds that are 15 beats per minute above the baseline is:
    a. Negative
    b. Positive
    c. Nonreactive
    d. Reactive

34. The recommended folic acid supplement for a woman with a past history of a baby with a neural tube defect is:
    a. 4 mg per day starting before conception
    b. 0.4 mg per day starting with a missed period
    c. 2 mg per day prior to conception
    d. 0.4 mg per day throughout pregnancy

35. B. D. comes for her first antepartal visit. She is 5 ft 4 in and weighs 190 lb (BMI 33). Weight goal for the pregnancy should be:
    a. Maintain current weight
    b. Gain 11–20 lb
    c. Gain 25–35 lb
    d. Lose 10–15 lb

36. Exercise guidelines for healthy pregnant women include suggestions to:
    a. Discontinue exercise at 20 weeks
    b. Begin intense program of exercise, especially if prepregnant weight was high
    c. Modify the existing program if symptoms occur
    d. Limit fluids before exercising

37. Anticipatory guidance concerning sexual activity during pregnancy includes:
    a. Sexual intercourse may continue until early third trimester in an uncomplicated pregnancy
    b. Sexual intercourse is contraindicated throughout pregnancy if there is a past history of preterm labor
    c. The pregnant woman's sexual desire may change throughout pregnancy
    d. Most pregnant women do not desire sex after the first trimester

38. Breastfeeding should be encouraged for:
    a. All women whose families strongly support the idea
    b. All pregnant women who are not HIV positive
    c. Women with adequate breast tissue
    d. Women who desire to do so

39. M. D. comes for her first antepartal visit at 8 weeks and tells you she has nausea every morning but is able to eat and drink in the afternoon. Your management at this point would include:
    a. Prescription for antinausea medicine
    b. Vitamin B_6 50 mg bid

c. Advising her to eat small, frequent meals
d. Advising her to drink a carbonated beverage on rising

40. The fatigue of early pregnancy is best managed by:
    a. Ruling out a thyroid problem
    b. Encouraging increased exercise
    c. Encouraging increased amounts of caffeinated drinks
    d. Reassurance and rest

41. Leg cramps may be relieved by:
    a. Pointing the toes
    b. Hot compresses
    c. Flexion of the foot
    d. Hot tub baths

42. R. T. comes for her 36-week visit, during which she mentions that her hands and feet are somewhat swollen. She has gained 2 lb since her visit 2 weeks ago; her BP is 128/76 mm Hg and she has no protein in her urine. What is your plan?
    a. Refer to perinatologist for impending preeclampsia
    b. Explain the edema at this stage is normal and see her in a week
    c. Order bed rest with return visit in a week
    d. Restrict salt and fluid intake

43. T. G. asks about the value of childbirth preparation classes during a second-trimester visit. You tell her that the evidence indicates that they are associated with:
    a. Reduced use of analgesics/anesthesia during labor
    b. Improved parenting skills
    c. Decreased Cesarean rates
    d. Less use of IVs in labor

44. Diabetes screening recommendations during pregnancy for the woman who is obese include:
    a. Fasting blood glucose each trimester
    b. Testing hemoglobin A_{1c} in the first trimester
    c. Routine screening early in pregnancy and at 24–28 weeks
    d. The same as for the normal weight woman

45. G. H. comes for her 34-week visit, at which time the fundus measures 39 cm. Abdominal palpation reveals a large uterus and difficulty feeling fetal parts. The most likely diagnosis is:
    a. Multiple gestation
    b. Macrosomic fetus
    c. Uterine fibroid
    d. Polyhydramnios

46. W. T., during her initial prenatal visit, mentions that she had a rubella immunization 3 weeks before conceiving this baby. Your plan is to:
    a. Advise her to consider termination of the pregnancy
    b. Continue regular care
    c. Consult with an infectious disease specialist
    d. Refer to a perinatologist

47. On physical examination at an initial prenatal visit of a 25-year-old woman who is at 14 weeks' gestation, you feel a 1-cm mobile, well-defined, nontender mass in the upper, outer quadrant of her right breast. Your plan is to:
    a. Explain this is normal with the hormonal changes of pregnancy
    b. Advise her you will watch at each visit to assess for any change
    c. Schedule a mammogram to be done in the third trimester
    d. Refer for further evaluation with biopsy

48. A pregnant woman who is 5 ft 3 in tall has a prepregnancy weight of 115 lb. Which of the following represents the most appropriate weight for her by the end of her pregnancy?
    a. 120 lb
    b. 125 lb
    c. 145 lb
    d. 165 lb

49. The biophysical profile (BPP) assesses fetal well-being with:
    a. A combination of nonstress test and ultrasound evaluation to assess five variables
    b. Both a contraction stress test and ultrasound evaluation of amniotic fluid volume
    c. Serial ultrasounds to evaluate amniotic fluid volume as well as fetal breathing and body movement and tone
    d. Evaluation of fetal movement with kick counts after administration of oxytocin or nipple stimulation

50. An appropriate plan of care for a woman at 40 weeks' gestation with a BPP score of 8 that includes a 2 score for amniotic fluid volume includes:
    a. Order a contraction stress test
    b. Repeat the BPP in 48 hours
    c. Schedule a return visit after 1 week
    d. Admit for induction of labor and delivery

51. Evaluation of fetal lung maturity is a required procedure for a:
    a. Scheduled delivery after 39 weeks' gestational age
    b. Scheduled delivery before 38 weeks' gestational age
    c. Laboring woman at 37 weeks' gestational age
    d. Laboring woman at 35 weeks' gestational age

52. W. M., who is 11 weeks pregnant, calls you from the ER to say she sustained a laceration and they want to give her a tetanus booster. You would tell her:
    a. All vaccinations are contraindicated in pregnancy
    b. It is not a problem because she does not need the tetanus booster
    c. The tetanus booster can be given in pregnancy if needed
    d. She should wait until the third trimester

53. Drugs from which one of the following categories may be given to a pregnant woman when the potential benefit justifies the potential fetal risk?
    a. Category A
    b. Category B
    c. Category C
    d. Category X

54. A woman who is pregnant for the second time and whose first pregnancy ended with a spontaneous abortion at 10 weeks is a:
    a. Multigravida
    b. Multipara
    c. Primigravida
    d. Primipara

55. A pregnant woman presents for her 24-week visit, at which time she relates that she does not feel very interested in sex anymore. Your response is to:
    a. Tell her this is common and she should not be concerned
    b. Assure her the interest will return in the third trimester
    c. Tell her to get more rest and her interest will increase
    d. Get her to talk about what she is feeling and thinking about sex

56. The screening test for group B streptococcus requires that the specimen be obtained from the:
    a. Ectocervix and vaginal sidewalls
    b. Ectocervix and endocervical os
    c. Endocervical os and rectum
    d. Vaginal introitus and rectum

57. Pregnancy loss and the woman's need for appropriate grieving occur across the reproductive spectrum. Maladaptive grief reactions are best addressed by:
    a. Telling the woman to put the baby's things away
    b. Listening to whatever the woman has to say
    c. Encouraging the woman to be strong so she will get past it
    d. Making the woman an appointment with a therapist

58. Recommended routine screening tests at an initial antenatal visit during the first trimester include:
    a. Group B streptococcus culture
    b. Syphilis serology
    c. Triple marker screen
    d. Ultrasound

59. Which of the following statements concerning influenza vaccination for pregnant women is correct?
    a. Vaccination is recommended for all women who will be pregnant during the influenza season
    b. Pregnant women with HIV infection should not receive this vaccination
    c. The pregnant woman should be offered the option of either the injection or nasal administration of the vaccine
    d. Vaccination should be given only in the second or third trimester

60. RDA of calories and protein during pregnancy is:
    a. 3000 kcal and 50 g/day
    b. 3500 kcal and 60 g/day
    c. 3800 kcal and 60 g/day
    d. 2500 kcal and 60 g/day

61. R. H. presents for her 36-week visit. Abdominal exam reveals a likelihood of polyhydramnios. In response to her question of where does the fluid come from, you answer:
    a. From the mother's blood volume
    b. From a combination of maternal serum and fetal urination
    c. From amniotic epithelium and fetal functions
    d. From fluid ingested by the mother

62. D. B., a 24-year-old primigravida, during her initial visit asks how the fetus has genes from both her husband and herself. Your response is based on which fact?
    a. Mitosis occurs, producing half the number of chromosomes
    b. Meiosis occurs, producing half the number of chromosomes
    c. The egg is a somatic cell
    d. Sperm is a somatic cell

63. Which of the following are parts of the placenta?
    a. Trophoblasts, chorion, amnion
    b. Trophoblasts, chorion, endometrium
    c. Chorion, amnion, umbilical cord
    d. Intervillous spaces, endometrium, trophoblasts

64. The term *conceptus* means:
    a. The embryo and placenta
    b. The embryo and membranes

c. The embryo, membranes, and placenta

d. The embryo, membranes, placenta, and endometrium

65. Which structure in human reproduction produces the most diverse and greatest quantity of steroid and protein hormones?

a. Trophoblast

b. Blastocyst

c. Chorion laeve

d. Deciduas basalis

66. At her 32-week visit, B. R. asks you to tell her what you are looking for or feeling when doing her abdominal exam with Leopold's maneuvers. You respond that you are:

a. Determining the placement of the placenta

b. Finding which direction the fetus is lying

c. Evaluating the size of the uterus

d. Evaluating adequacy of fetal growth

67. T. D. comes for an 18-week visit. Appropriate routine screening tests at this visit include:

a. Gestational diabetes testing

b. Chlamydia and gonorrhea tests

c. CBC or hematocrit

d. Multiple marker screen

68. R. D. at 37 weeks calls to say she feels like the fetus is moving less. After further inquiry you decide to send her for an NST. She asks what this is. You explain that it is an assessment of fetal well-being based on:

a. Evaluation of body movements

b. Breathing movements

c. Fetal heart rate response to fetal movement

d. Fetal body tone

69. P. R. comes for a first visit at 11 weeks' gestation. Her history reveals her concern about sore gums that sometimes bleed. Your thinking is:

a. She most likely needs to see a periodontist

b. Gingivitis is common in pregnancy with increased vascularity of connective tissue

c. She should be started on antibiotics to prevent systemic infection

d. She should be placed on a soft diet until the problem is resolved

70. A woman presents at 32 weeks' gestation with vaginal bleeding for the past 6 hours, back pain, and irregular abdominal cramping pain. Exam reveals diffuse abdominal tenderness and increased uterine tone. You suspect:

a. Marginal placenta previa

b. Placental abruption

c. Preterm labor

d. Pyelonephritis

71. A postterm pregnancy is best diagnosed by:

a. Certain LMP

b. Third-trimester ultrasound

c. Fundal growth

d. Quickening

72. Serial beta hCG levels are done after uterine evacuation for hydatidiform mole to:

a. Ensure that the woman is not pregnant in the first year after treatment

b. Monitor for persistent trophoblastic proliferation

c. Identify a pregnancy early so appropriate care can be provided

d. Assess for a possible undetected ectopic pregnancy

73. P. R. indicates she is afraid of Pitocin because her sister had a uterine rupture when she was induced. Your response would be:

a. Reassurance because she will not need induction anyway

b. Discussing how Pitocin is given with assurance that nothing will go wrong

c. Discussing alternate methods to promote uterine readiness and contractions

d. Saying that Pitocin is the best way to get through labor and not a problem

74. L. M. is a G2 P1001 whose initial visit reveals a healthy pregnant woman. Her urinalysis and culture and sensitivity (C&S) report indicates a colony count of greater than 100,000 organisms/mL. You would:

a. Refer her to a urologist to evaluate for underlying renal disease

b. Encourage fluids and repeat C&S in 2 weeks

c. Initiate treatment with antibiotics

d. Advise her to contact you if she has any UTI symptoms

75. Antepartal care for the woman who is HIV positive should focus mainly on:

a. Ensuring fetal well-being at all cost

b. Frequent drug testing to ensure she is not using IV street drugs

c. Testing her partner and treating him if necessary

d. Maintaining her health and preventing neonatal transmission

76. On reviewing the record of a currently pregnant woman, you see that she is P1112. What obstetric history can you derive from this information?

a. Two previous pregnancies of which one infant was term and one was a premature stillbirth

b. You are unable to determine an obstetric history from this information

c. Three pregnancies with one term birth and premature twins

d. Three pregnancies of which one was term, one premature, and one an abortion

77. Polyhydramnios is defined as:

a. AFI greater than 10 cm

b. Single pocket greater than 5 cm

c. AFI greater than 15 cm

d. Single pocket greater than 8 cm

78. Etiology of polyhydramnios is associated with:

a. Maternal overhydration

b. Fetal anomalies of GI tract

c. Fetal anomalies of cardiovascular system

d. Maternal preeclampsia with edema

79. The fetal system most associated with oligohydramnios is the:

a. GI system

b. Central nervous system

c. Renal system

d. Cardiovascular system

80. When speaking with a primigravida about the way a baby develops, you would describe the embryonic stage as the:
    a. Period between the second and eighth weeks
    b. Time from implantation to 12 weeks into pregnancy
    c. Period when drugs are least likely to affect development
    d. Period from fertilization to 4 weeks

81. During the embryonic stage, all major organ systems are formed *except*:
    a. Heart
    b. Reproductive organs
    c. Liver
    d. Lungs

82. Determining an accurate estimated date of birth (EDB) is critical because:
    a. It is the basis for making decisions toward the end of the pregnancy
    b. Mothers want to know the exact date the baby will be born
    c. It is all that is needed to plan a 37-week elective C-section
    d. Families want to make plans around the baby's birth

83. Which of the following would *not* be a normal physical examination finding during pregnancy?
    a. Blue color of vaginal mucosa and cervix
    b. Hypertrophy of nasal mucosa and gums
    c. Mildly enlarged, nodular thyroid
    d. Thickening of vaginal mucosa

84. During the last 8 weeks of pregnancy, the fetus:
    a. Finishes the final formation of the renal system
    b. Completes the development of reproductive organs
    c. Experiences the closure of the foramen ovale
    d. Increases weight through fat accumulation

85. The determination of an accurate EDB is best accomplished by using:
    a. The first day of the last menstrual period
    b. A complete menstrual history
    c. The use of Naegele's rule
    d. The date when symptoms of pregnancy began

86. Dating of pregnancy by USG is most accurate in the first trimester using:
    a. Crown rump length (CRL)
    b. Head circumference
    c. Abdominal circumference
    d. Femur length

87. Which of the following statements most accurately reflects the growth of the pregnant uterus?
    a. At 14 weeks it begins to rise out of the pelvis, and at 24 weeks is at the umbilicus
    b. At 14 weeks it is halfway to the umbilicus, and at 20 weeks is at the umbilicus
    c. At 12 weeks it begins to rise out of pelvis, and at 20 weeks is at the umbilicus
    d. At 10 weeks it begins to rise out of the pelvis, and at 16 weeks is at the umbilicus

88. Which of the following is a presumptive sign of pregnancy seen in the vagina?
    a. Hegar's
    b. Piskacek's
    c. Goodell's
    d. Chadwick's

89. The pregnancy is maintained through hormones produced by:
    a. Egg sac and placenta
    b. Corpus luteum and chorion
    c. Corpus luteum and placenta
    d. Ovary and placenta

90. Of the four pelvic types, which is more likely to lead to a posterior position with higher possibility of dystocia?
    a. Android
    b. Platypelloid
    c. Anthropoid
    d. Gynecoid

91. The characteristic gait of pregnancy results from:
    a. Shift in the center of gravity as uterus enlarges
    b. Effects of relaxin and estrogen
    c. Effects of relaxin and progesterone
    d. Effects of increasing amounts of estrogen and progesterone

92. The effect of pregnancy on the cardiovascular system is most clearly seen in:
    a. Lower diastolic blood pressure in third trimester
    b. 10% cardiac volume increase that peaks in midpregnancy
    c. Resting pulse increase of 10–15 beats in first trimester
    d. Slight decrease in cardiac output in second trimester

93. The usual 1-g drop in hemoglobin during pregnancy is due to:
    a. Blood volume increase of 30–50%
    b. Decrease in iron absorption
    c. Decrease in production of RBCs
    d. Increasing iron needs of the fetus

94. Which of the following is considered a risk factor for psychological well-being in pregnancy?
    a. Limited support network
    b. Introversion at any point
    c. Ambivalence any time
    d. Concern about the danger signs

95. The maternal mortality ratio is defined as the number of maternal deaths that result from the reproductive process per:
    a. 1000 live births
    b. 100,000 live births
    c. 100,000 pregnant women
    d. 100,000 reproductive-age women

96. G. R. comes for her first pregnancy visit. Her obstetric history includes one spontaneous abortion, one termination of pregnancy, one infant born at 36 weeks, and one born at 41 weeks. Both infants are living. Her parity is:
    a. 2022
    b. 2122
    c. 1212
    d. 1122

97. The pelvic planes of obstetric significance are the:
    a. Inlet, midplane, and outlet
    b. Inlet, posterior outlet, and anterior outlet
    c. Inlet, posterior midplane, and anterior midplane
    d. Linea terminalis, posterior outlet, and anterior outlet

98. Which of the elements of clinical pelvimetry defines the midplane?
    a. Diagonal conjugate
    b. Intertuberous diameter
    c. Ischial spines distance and sacrum
    d. Pubic arch

99. Amniocentesis is used in early pregnancy to:
    a. Screen for fetal anomalies
    b. Diagnose fetal genetic well-being
    c. Evaluate maternal genetic problems
    d. Determine AFI and muscle tone

100. Chorionic villous sampling (CVS) has an advantage over amniocentesis because:
    a. It can be done 3–4 weeks earlier
    b. There is less risk for infection
    c. There is less risk for limb deformities
    d. There is greater specificity in test results

101. When considering the use of fetal movement counting for a particular woman, it is important to know that:
    a. Fetuses move constantly, so the counting can be done at any time
    b. Fetal movement is strongest at 29–38 weeks
    c. Most women do not feel the fetus move before 24 weeks
    d. There is only one way to perform fetal movement counts

102. The basis for the nonstress test (NST) to assess fetal well-being is that:
    a. Fetal movement will increase the mother's heart rate
    b. The fetus responds to an increase in heart rate by accelerating movement
    c. Fetal movement should cause no significant change in FHR
    d. Fetal heart rate accelerates in association with fetal movement

103. Contraindications to the contractions stress test (CST) include:
    a. Gestational age greater than 37 weeks
    b. History of ectopic pregnancy
    c. Nonreactive nonstress test (NST)
    d. Placenta previa

104. Cordocentesis may be used:
    a. As an adjunct to chorionic villus sampling (CVS)
    b. To obtain blood samples for fetal fibronectin test
    c. To provide fetal blood transfusion
    d. To relieve pressure on a prolapsed cord

105. Substances classified as addictive:
    a. Are only illegal drugs
    b. Include only those inhaled or injected
    c. Include both legal and illegal drugs
    d. Do not include alcohol

106. Which of the following is most common during pregnancy?
    a. Binge drinking
    b. Cigarette smoking
    c. Marijuana smoking
    d. Occasional alcohol use

107. When faced with a woman who manifests clear evidence of being a victim of violence, your first goal is to:
    a. Evaluate her safety
    b. Get her to a shelter
    c. Tell her to press charges
    d. Get photos of all injuries

108. Correct information concerning pregnancies with first-trimester bleeding includes:
    a. Approximately 10% of women have some bleeding in the first trimester
    b. Bleeding that occurs between 10 and 12 weeks is often caused by implantation

    c. Cervical incompetence is a common cause of first-trimester bleeding
    d. Ninety percent of pregnancies in which FHT are heard will continue to term after early bleeding

109. A patient presents with an LMP of 8 weeks ago and a positive urine pregnancy test. She is having a small amount of bleeding for the past 12 hours, along with some mild abdominal cramping. A pelvic exam reveals a closed cervix and a slightly enlarged uterus. Differential diagnosis for this woman includes:
    a. Complete abortion and threatened abortion
    b. Ectopic pregnancy and inevitable abortion
    c. Ectopic pregnancy and threatened abortion
    d. Incomplete abortion and inevitable abortion

110. An example of an autosomal recessive disease is:
    a. *BRCA2* breast cancer
    b. Cystic fibrosis
    c. Hemophilia
    d. Trisomy 21

111. A 34-week-pregnant woman presents stating she noticed a small amount of blood on her underwear this morning about an hour after having sexual intercourse. She is not having any pain or contractions. Your initial differential diagnosis for this woman would include:
    a. Cervicitis
    b. Incompetent cervix
    c. Placental abruption
    d. Premature rupture of membranes

112. Risks to the fetus in a postterm pregnancy are related to all of the following *except*:
    a. Fetal macrosomia
    b. Meconium aspiration
    c. Polyhydramnios
    d. Uteroplacental insufficiency

113. Symmetric growth restriction is more likely than asymmetric growth restriction to:
    a. Be related to multiple gestation
    b. First become apparent in late pregnancy
    c. Occur as a result of maternal medical illness
    d. Result from maternal cigarette smoking

114. Loss of a fetus in the second trimester is most frequently related to:
    a. Hydatidiform mole
    b. Inevitable abortion
    c. Ectopic pregnancy
    d. Incompetent cervix

115. As a result of an early USG, a low-lying placenta is verified for B. T. What do you tell her regarding this?
    a. Approximately 30% of women with low-lying placenta in early pregnancy will have placenta previa in the third trimester
    b. Approximately 30% of women have a low-lying placenta in the first trimester
    c. Regular vaginal examinations will be done in the third trimester to monitor any obstruction of the cervix
    d. Vaginal delivery is contraindicated if there is a marginal placenta previa

116. A pregnant woman has the following history: vaginal delivery at 38 weeks; spontaneous abortion at 8 weeks; elective abortion at 13 weeks; vaginal delivery at 34 weeks; 2 living children; is now 28 weeks pregnant. Her gravity and parity are:
    a. G5 P1122
    b. G5 P0222
    c. G3 P2002
    d. G3 P2112

117. Which of the following tests is diagnostic rather than screening?
    a. MSAFP
    b. Nuchal translucency US
    c. Amniocentesis
    d. USG at 10 weeks

118. An elevated maternal AFP result is associated with which of the following?
    a. Down syndrome
    b. Neural tube defect
    c. Autosomal recessive gene
    d. X-linked recessive inheritance

119. Which of the following factors would predispose a pregnant woman to having a baby with GBS disease?
    a. History of previous GBS-positive infant
    b. Bacterial vaginosis in current pregnancy
    c. Frequent urinary tract infections prior to pregnancy
    d. Streptococcal pharyngitis in the third trimester

120. V. R. comes for her 38-week visit, during which she reports that her friend gave birth last week and had a placental abruption. She is now concerned that she might have the same. What information would you share with her about this?
    a. In the event of bleeding near term, 50% of cases are related to placental abruption
    b. In the third trimester, she has a 30% chance of having a placental abruption
    c. The likelihood of her having a placental abruption occur is basically zero at this time
    d. A placental abruption is associated with risk factors such as hypertension, smoking, and trauma

121. *Genotype* refers to:
    a. The expression of genes present in an individual
    b. The dominant genes that will be inherited by a fetus
    c. The pair of genes for each characteristic inherent in an individual
    d. The recessive genes that will be passed on to a fetus

122. Which of the following women should receive RhoGAM postpartum?
    a. Nonsensitized Rh negative mother with an Rh negative baby
    b. Nonsensitized Rh negative mother with an Rh positive baby
    c. Sensitized Rh negative mother with an Rh negative baby
    d. Sensitized Rh negative mother with an RH positive baby

123. Aneuploidy describes which of the following situations?
    a. Down syndrome
    b. *BRCA1* and *BRCA2* inheritance
    c. Cystic fibrosis genes
    d. Sickle cell anemia

124. B. T., G2 P0010, comes for her first antepartal visit. Her history indicates she had a pregnancy loss at 18 weeks. She is gravely concerned that it will happen again in this pregnancy. You discuss cervical cerclage, mentioning the following facts:
    a. Will be done after 12–14 weeks and is 80–90% successful
    b. Will be done after 16–20 weeks and is 80–90% successful
    c. Will be done after 16–20 weeks and is 50–60% successful
    d. Will be done after 12–14 weeks and is 50–60% successful

125. CDC's recommended treatment for primary syphilis in a 10-week-pregnant woman is:
    a. Benzathine penicillin G 2.4 units IM × 1 dose after the first trimester
    b. Benzathine penicillin G 2.4 units IM × 1 dose at the time of diagnosis
    c. Benzathine penicillin G 2.4 units IM weekly × 3 doses
    d. Benzathine penicillin G 2.4 units IM at the time of diagnosis and repeat in 4 weeks if no decline in RPR titer

126. At an initial prenatal visit, a woman is diagnosed with bacterial vaginosis. She is not having any symptoms of vaginal infection. You will advise her that:
    a. All pregnant women should be treated if they have asymptomatic bacterial vaginosis
    b. Pregnant women who are at risk for preterm delivery should be treated if they have asymptomatic bacterial vaginosis
    c. Only pregnant women at risk for preterm delivery should be treated for symptomatic bacterial vaginosis
    d. Pregnant women who are at risk for preterm delivery should be tested for asymptomatic bacterial vaginosis in early third trimester

127. CDC's recommended treatment for trichomoniasis during pregnancy is:
    a. Metronidazole 2 g orally
    b. Clindamycin 300 mg orally bid × 7 days
    c. Azithromycin 1 g orally
    d. Ceftriaxone 125 mg IM

128. Symmetric intrauterine growth restriction:
    a. Generally becomes evident in midpregnancy
    b. Is usually associated with placental abnormalities
    c. Is caused by conditions that result in a reduction in cell size
    d. Is a neonatal diagnosis made when the infant falls below the 10th percentile

129. M. K. is a 34-year-old G5 P4004. Her 1-hour 50-g glucose challenge test at 28 weeks was 154 mg/dL. Follow-up 100-g glucose tolerance test produced the following results: 100, 192, 185, and 160 mg/dL. Your plan for M. K. includes:
    a. Obtaining fasting glucose tests at 32 and 36 weeks to ensure that levels stay at or below 100 mg/dL
    b. Referring her to a nutritionist to help her limit further weight gain to no more than 10 lb
    c. Referring her to a perinatologist for periumbilical blood sampling to determine fetal blood glucose levels
    d. Screening for diabetes at 6–12 weeks postpartum

130. At 20 weeks' gestation a pregnant woman was seen and fundal height was 1 cm below the umbilicus. At today's 24-week visit, fundal height is at the umbilicus. She is feeling regular fetal movement and fetal heart rate is 140 bpm. The most appropriate management for this patient is:
    a. Ordering a biophysical profile
    b. Ordering an ultrasound

c. Performing a nonstress test at this visit

d. Scheduling her next visit for 4 weeks from today

131. Ectopic pregnancy is consistent with no intrauterine sac on transvaginal ultrasound and an hCG titer of less than:

    a. 100 IU/L

    b. 1500 IU/L

    c. 6500 IU/L

    d. 10,000 IU/L

132. L. H. is an 18-year-old female who is 16 weeks pregnant. She has a positive chlamydia test. Appropriate management includes:

    a. Erythromycin base 500 mg orally qid for 7 days and ceftriaxone 125 mg IM

    b. Azithromycin 1 g orally in a single dose and perform test of cure in 3–4 weeks

    c. Ofloxacin 300 mg orally bid for 7 days and rescreen in the third trimester

    d. Spectinomycin 2 g IM now and repeat in 1 week

133. M. I. is a 29-year-old G4 P2012 at 41 weeks today. She complains of occasional cramping, denies leaking/bleeding, but states she passed her "mucus plug" yesterday. She asks how she will know if she is in labor because both her previous births were induced. You respond that:

    a. True labor occurs when contractions are 7–8 minutes apart and last for 45 seconds

    b. Real labor is when contractions are 2–3 minutes apart and are very painful

    c. Labor contractions usually become more regular and more intense over time

    d. Contractions begin slowly; once they are 4–5 minutes apart, it is real labor

134. Hyperthyroidism in pregnancy is diagnosed by:

    a. Elevated free thyroxine (FT_4) levels

    b. Low free T_3 levels

    c. Elevated TSH

    d. Elevated total thyroxine (TT_4) levels

135. ABO incompatibility occurs in which percentage of pregnancies?

    a. 15%

    b. 20–25%

    c. 25–40%

    d. 5–8%

136. T. W., a 32-year-old G2 P1001, is Rh negative. Her first pregnancy was uneventful, and she received RhoGAM after the birth. She read on the Internet that problems were much more likely with the second pregnancy. You respond that:

    a. Because she reports she has had no transfusions since the previous birth, there is no problem

    b. The RhoGAM she received in the last pregnancy will prevent any problems in this pregnancy

    c. She was not sensitized in the first pregnancy, and you will provide monitoring and treatment to prevent it in this pregnancy

    d. It is likely that her fetus is Rh–, so there is no real concern that she will have any problems related to this

137. At 28 weeks' gestation, a patient's Hgb is 12.4. g/dL. At her initial first-trimester visit, her Hgb was 12.8 g/dL. Management will include:

    a. Obtaining a CBC and ferritin level

    b. Asking if she is having difficulty tolerating her iron supplement and changing to a different type if needed

    c. Rechecking her history to see if she may be at risk for an inherited anemia

    d. Encouraging her to continue getting dietary iron and taking her iron supplement

138. Folic acid deficiency anemia is characterized by:

    a. Hemoglobin at 9 g/dL or less

    b. Low ferritin levels

    c. Elevated serum iron-binding capacity

    d. Macrocytic erythrocytes

139. Which of the following statements is true concerning sickle cell hemoglobinopathies:

    a. Trait indicates that one parent has sickle cell disease

    b. Disease is present when the person inherits a sickle cell gene from each parent

    c. G-6-PD deficiency is a potential complication of sickle cell disease

    d. 1 in 100 African Americans has sickle cell trait

140. Normal changes of pregnancy may confound a diagnosis of appendicitis. With this in mind, you should note the following as critical signs or symptoms pointing to possible appendicitis in pregnancy:

    a. Persistent abdominal pain and tenderness

    b. Intermittent lower abdominal cramping

    c. Elevated WBC level

    d. Nausea and vomiting

141. M. D., a 32-year-old P1, during a discussion of infant care and breastfeeding says, "My first baby did not like the breast, then I did not have enough milk, so I stopped breastfeeding after two weeks." What is your response to her statement?

    a. Tell her she probably misinterpreted what was going on and should not have stopped nursing

    b. Delve further into what occurred and how she came to the conclusions that led her to stop breastfeeding

    c. Let her know she probably was not drinking enough fluids, so did not have enough milk to feed the baby

    d. Reassure her that she was listening to her body and had done the right thing for herself and her infant

142. M. B., G1 P0, comes for her 36-week visit with a piece of paper in her hand. "I am really confused about this birth plan business. What am I supposed to do about my birth? Don't I just show up when I am in labor?" How will you counsel her today?

    a. "It really does not matter what you write because the hospital has its own plan"

    b. "You will need to be very detailed about each element of the birth experience so you get what you want"

    c. "The plan provides the opportunity for you to make choices about events associated with the birth"

    d. "The healthcare provider who is there when you are in labor will tell you what is best for you and how to do it"

143. Y. L., G2 P1001, comes for her first visit. She is concerned about the possibility of a UTI since her sister was recently hospitalized for pyelonephritis. What facts would you give her to enhance her understanding?
    a. UTIs do occur in about 10% of pregnancies
    b. 25% of women with UTI in pregnancy will develop pyelonephritis
    c. If she has a history of UTIs before pregnancy, she will be screened with a urine culture each trimester
    d. Pregnant women are typically screened for asymptomatic bacteriuria in early pregnancy

144. Who is at greatest risk for developing a UTI in pregnancy?
    a. Adolescents
    b. Woman pregnant with twins
    c. Women older than 35 years
    d. Woman with diabetes

145. L. T. returns for the reading of the PPD that was placed during her first prenatal visit. You read the result as 10 mm of induration. L. T. is American-born, healthy, and has no known history of contact with the disease. How do you interpret this result for her?
    a. It is positive and she needs referral to an infectious disease specialist
    b. It is unclear and she should have a chest radiograph to be certain
    c. It is positive and you should give her a prescription for INH
    d. It is negative because she has no high-risk characteristics for the disease

146. Which of the following statements concerning HIV in women is correct?
    a. The main route of acquiring the infection in women is IV drug use
    b. Viral load is the strongest predictor for transmission of infection to the infant during the birth process
    c. C-section is the recommended route of delivery for all HIV-infected women to reduce the risk of transmission of infection to the infant
    d. Breastfeeding should be recommended only if the mother's viral load is less than 200 copies/mL

147. S. R. has reached her 39th week of pregnancy. On abdominal exam you measure a fundal height of 42 cm. Leopold's maneuvers provide you with an EFW of 4200 g. What factors would help to ease your mind about the fetal size?
    a. She has wide hips and will have no problem with a big baby
    b. She is 5 ft 10 in with an anthropoid pelvis and her husband is 6 ft 4 in
    c. She is totally unconcerned and knows this baby will fit
    d. The fetus is not yet engaged, so the height is greater than expected

148. A patient who is 32 weeks pregnant has had symptoms of preterm labor and has a history of preterm delivery at 34 weeks. A fetal fibronectin test is negative. You advise her that:
    a. She has a 60% chance of going into labor within the next week
    b. It is really too early in her pregnancy for this test to be of much value
    c. The result offers some reassurance that she will not go into labor in the next 2 weeks
    d. It is really too late in her pregnancy for this test to be of much value

149. A decision is made to start tocolytic therapy for a 30 weeks' gestation woman in preterm labor. Betamethasone IM has also been ordered. This is done because the administration of corticosteroids:
    a. Decreases the respiratory side effects of tocolytic drugs
    b. Decreases the incidence of premature rupture of membranes
    c. Enhances the effects of tocolytic drugs
    d. Reduces the incidence of newborn respiratory distress syndrome

150. G. F. comes for her 32-week visit, and you determine she has a breech presentation. Your plan for her is to:
    a. Send her to Maternal Fetal Medicine for external cephalic version
    b. Refer her to a perinatologist for a care decision and treatment
    c. Send her for ultrasound to confirm breech presentation
    d. Wait until 36 weeks to see if spontaneous version has occurred

151. A pregnant woman presents for her 32-week visit with no complaints. All findings from previous visits have been normal. Today she has blood pressure of 145/95 mm Hg. Expected additional findings if she has mild preeclampsia include:
    a. Lower extremity edema
    b. Serum creatinine > 1.1 mg/dL
    c. Right upper epigastric pain
    d. Elevated liver function tests

Answers with Rationales

1. b. Presumptive
    Amenorrhea is a presumptive sign of pregnancy. *Presumptive signs of pregnancy* refers to signs and symptoms that may be caused by something else. Amenorrhea may be caused by sickness or stress.

2. c. Repeat the test in a week
    R. L. performed the test too early, so she needs to repeat the test in 1 week. Sensitive urine pregnancy tests can detect pregnancy approximately 1 week after conception.

3. b. Human chorionic gonadotropin
    Human chorionic gonadotropin (hCG) hormone is secreted by the placenta to help maintain corpus luteum function and production of progesterone; levels found in serum and urine assays of pregnant women are detected in pregnancy tests.

4. b. Corpus luteum
    Progesterone is secreted by the corpus luteum. Progesterone is essential in preparing the uterus for implantation of the fertilized ovum and maintaining the pregnancy.

5. d. Fetus
The chorionic villi develop from the outer wall of the blastocyst, which establishes an intimate connection with the endometrium and gives rise to the placenta.

6. a. One vein with oxygenated blood and two arteries with deoxygenated blood
The vessels of the umbilical cord are two arteries that carry fetal deoxygenated blood to the placenta and that are smaller in diameter than the vein, and one vein that carries oxygenated blood from the placenta to the fetus and that is characterized by twisting or spiraling to minimize snarling.

7. c. 12 weeks
The uterus is palpable at the symphysis pubis at 12 weeks. This is also the time that the fetus begins to make spontaneous movements in utero.

8. c. 6–7 days
Implantation occurs 6–7 days after fertilization and usually in the upper, posterior wall of the uterus.

9. b. Facilitated diffusion
Both oxygen and glucose are transported across the placenta via facilitated diffusion.

10. d. 23 pairs of chromosomes
The human zygote consists of the haploid number of chromosomes: 23 pairs. It possesses half the diploid or normal number of pairs of chromosomes, 46 pairs, found in somatic, or body, cells.

11. a. Placenta
The trophoblast is an essential component of the placenta.

12. d. No intervention
Ninety percent of pregnant women develop a physiologic systolic heart murmur and may have exaggerated splitting of S1, audible third sound, or soft transient diastolic murmur.

13. b. Progesterone's effect on vessel walls
Diastolic blood pressure is lower in the first two trimesters because of the development of new vascular beds and the relaxation of peripheral tone by progesterone, which result in decreased flow resistance.

14. c. Increased chest diameter
Thoracic circumference increases by 5–6 cm and residual volume decreases.

15. c. Reassure that this is normal
Absent any other symptoms besides increased vaginal discharge in a 34-week pregnant woman, and without odor or other presenting abnormal findings, reassurance may be given to the mother that an increase in vaginal discharge is normal in pregnancy. If further concern, rule out pathology.

16. a. A normal variation of response in pregnancy
Increase libido is a normal variation of response in pregnancy.

17. b. Encourage her to tell you more about the nightmares and her fears
It is the healthcare provider's role to listen and facilitate a patient's expression of feelings and to provide a nonjudgmental environment.

18. d. Increased intake of fiber and fluids
The first line of treatment for constipation is to increase fluids and fiber. Other strategies are to recommend prune juice or a warm beverage in the morning and to encourage exercise and stool softeners.

19. b. Nullipara
Nullipara is the term for a woman who has not carried a baby to 500 g or 20 weeks.

20. a. A 28-day menstrual cycle
The calculation of estimated date of birth (EDB) by Naegele's rule is based on a 28-day menstrual cycle, accounting for the average length of pregnancy to be 280 days or 10 lunar months.

21. a. 0121
A. B. has not had any term pregnancies, which accounts for the first number, 0. She had a preterm delivery at 36 weeks of twins, which accounts for the second number, and even though these were twins, they still count as one number, thus, a 1. She had two miscarriages under 20 weeks, which accounts for the third number, a 2. The fourth number is the total number of living children. One of A. B.'s twins died; therefore, she has only one living child

22. c. Send her to fetal assessment unit for an ultrasound
If uncertain of last menstrual period (LMP), ultrasound may be used to calculate estimated gestational age.

23. a. Intrauterine growth restriction (IUGR)
The fundus is typically found at the umbilicus at 20 weeks.

24. d. Lie
The first maneuver for Leopold's is to palpate the fetal lie, followed by the presentation, position, and attitude.

25. b. "Sure, I will listen, but we may not hear it yet."
Fetal heart tones can be auscultated by Doppler as early as 10 weeks, but this is done more commonly at 12 weeks.

26. a. Bluish color of the cervix
A normal finding in pregnancy is the Chadwick's sign—the changing of the color of the cervix to a bluish hue.

27. c. Pubic arch of 90 degrees with diagonal conjugate of longer than 11.5 cm
The pubic arch is formed by the descending rami of pubic bones and the inferior margin of the symphysis pubis; the angle should be at least 90 degrees.

28. b. Identify the characteristics of the woman's pelvis
Identifying the characteristics of the woman's pelvis is clinically significant because the pelvis is the bony canal through which the fetus passes.

29. a. "Most women with a first pregnancy do not feel movement until around 20 weeks."
Quickening is the maternal perception of fetal movement, which usually occurs between 18 and 20 weeks for primiparas; it occurs earlier for multigravidas at about 14–18 weeks.

30. c. 15–19 weeks
Second-trimester screening (also known as "multiple marker screening") is performed between 15 and 20 weeks to detect neural tube defects and trisomy 18 and 21. Serologic testing measuring maternal serum alphafetoprotein (MSAFP), estriol, and hCG is called a "triple screen"; with the addition of inhibin A, this becomes a "quad screen."

31. d. At 35–37 weeks
Group B streptococcus (GBS) screening is performed at 35–37 weeks by swabbing the vaginal introitus and rectal specimens.

32. b. AFP, estriol, hCG

Second-trimester screening (also known as "multiple marker screening") is performed between 15 and 20 weeks to detect neural tube defects and trisomy 18 and 21. Serologic testing measuring maternal serum alphafetoprotein (AFP), estriol, and human chorionic gonadotropin (hCG) is called a "triple screen," and with the addition of inhibin A, this becomes a "quad screen."

33. d. Reactive

Reactive constitutes two or more accelerations in fetal heart rate of 15 or more beats per minute lasting for 15 seconds or more within a 15- to 20-minute period.

34. a. 4 mg per day starting before conception

A 0.4-mg daily supplement of folic acid is recommended for childbearing-aged women, and 4-mg daily supplement prior to and during pregnancy is recommended for women with history of previous infant with neural tube defect.

35. b. Gain 11–20 lb

For obese women who have a prepregnancy BMI > 30 the recommended weight gain is 0.4–0.6 lb per week in the second and third trimesters for total of 11–20 lb gain.

36. c. Modify the existing program if symptoms occur

In the absence of either medical or obstetric complications, 30 minutes or more of moderate exercise a day on most, if not all, days of the week is recommended for pregnant women.

37. c. The pregnant woman's sexual desire may change throughout pregnancy

Changes in sexual desire throughout pregnancy are influenced by hormones, energy level, relationship, body image, fears of hurting the baby, and cultural beliefs and practices.

38. b. All pregnant women who are not HIV positive

Breastfeeding is recommended for all women except for women who are HIV positive, are untreated, have active tuberculosis (TB), use illicit drugs, or take prescribed cancer chemotherapy agents.

39. c. Advising her to eat small, frequent meals

Nausea and vomiting of pregnancy are most common in the first trimester. It is recommended that patients eat small, frequent meals, with no restriction on the kind of food or how often. Education includes to discontinue prenatal vitamins with iron until nausea and vomiting have resolved but to continue folic acid. Other recommendations may include consuming raspberry tea, peppermint tea, carbonated beverages, or hard candy; using acupressure, including sea bands for wrists; taking ginger 1 g per day in divided doses, pyridoxine (vitamin B_6) 25 mg bid or tid orally, doxylamine 12.5 mg bid or qid with pyridoxine orally, metoclopramide 5 to 10 mg g q6–8h orally, or promethazine 25 mg q4h per rectal suppository.

40. d. Reassurance and rest

Provide patients with reassurance that fatigue is a normal first-trimester problem and will pass. Other recommendations include getting mild exercise and good nutrition, decreasing activities and planning rest periods, decreasing fluid intake in the evening to decrease nocturia.

41. c. Flexion of the foot

Leg cramps may be relieved by flexing the ankle to stretch the calf, decreasing phosphate in the diet, drinking no more than two glasses of milk per day, massaging the affected leg, keeping the legs warm, walking, exercising, and taking calcium tablets and magnesium tablets.

42. b. Explain the edema at this stage is normal and see her in a week

R.T. is gaining appropriate weight and is normotensive, without protein in her urine, and without any severe features of preeclampsia. She can be reassured that edema at this stage in the pregnancy is normal and that if she exhibits any other symptoms, she would need to be evaluated by a healthcare provider.

43. a. Reduced use of analgesics/anesthesia during labor

Preparation for childbearing ultimately aids in reducing need for analgesics and anesthetics during labor.

44. c. Routine screening early in pregnancy and at 24–28 weeks

High-risk women need to be screened for diabetes as soon as possible using standard diagnostic testing.

45. d. Polyhydramnios

Polyhydramnios is indicated by uterine size larger than expected for gestational age (GA), difficulty auscultating fetal heart rate (FHR) and palpating fetal parts, and mechanical pressure exerted by the large uterus.

46. There are no documented cases of congenital rubella syndrome from vaccine, but recommend giving at least 4 weeks before attempting a pregnancy or postpartum; the vaccine may be given while breastfeeding.

47. b. Advise her you will watch at each visit to assess for any change

This well-defined, nontender mass has benign characteristics and would be okay to watch. Malignant breast mass is usually nontender, firm, irregularly shaped, and fixed to underlying tissue.

48. c. 145 lb

Weight gain recommendations in pregnancy: for underweight women (BMI less than 18.5), 1.0–1.3 lb per week in second and third trimesters for total of 28–40 lb; for normal weight women (BMI 18.5–24.9), 0.8–1.0 lb per week during second and third trimesters for total of 25–35 lb; for overweight women (BMI 25.0–29.9), 0.5–0.7 lb per week in second and third trimesters for total of 15–25 lb; for obese women (BMI 30.0 or higher), 0.4–0.6 lb per week in second and third trimesters for total of 11–20 lb.

49. a. A combination of nonstress test and ultrasound evaluation to assess five variables

A biophysical profile consists of five parameters: nonstress test, breathing, movement, tone, amniotic fluid volume.

50. c. Schedule a return visit after 1 week

A BPP score of 8/10 is a reassuring, normal score. BPP scoring interpretation criteria are as follows: 8–10 is normal; 6 is equivocal, repeat testing; 4 or less is considered abnormal and needs further evaluation.

51. b. Scheduled delivery before 38 weeks' gestational age

To help prevent iatrogenic prematurity and respiratory distress syndrome, there should be an evaluation of fetal lung maturity if labor induction or Cesarean delivery is electively scheduled for prior to 39 weeks' gestation.

52. c. The tetanus booster can be given in pregnancy if needed

Tetanus vaccination during pregnancy can protect at-risk newborns against neonatal tetanus; in maternal trauma, it may be indicated.

53. c. Category C

For drugs in Category C, animal studies have shown an adverse effect or no animal studies have been conducted, and there are no adequate and well-controlled studies in pregnant women.

54. a. Multigravida

Multigravida is a woman pregnant two or more times, regardless of the result of the pregnancies.

55. d. Get her to talk about what she is feeling and thinking about sex

It is the healthcare provider's role to listen and facilitate the patient's expression of feelings and to provide a nonjudgmental environment.

56. d. Vaginal introitus and rectum

Group B streptococcus (GBS) screening is performed at 35–37 weeks by swabbing the vaginal introitus and rectal specimens.

57. b. Listening to whatever the woman has to say

It is the healthcare provider's role to listen and facilitate the patient's expression of feelings and to provide a nonjudgmental environment.

58. b. Syphilis serology

Obtaining syphilis serology is a recommended routine screening for the first initial antenatal visit during the first trimester.

59. a. Vaccination is recommended for all women who will be pregnant during the influenza season

The trivalent inactivated influenza vaccine (TIV) is recommended for all pregnant women during influenza season; live attenuated nasal influenza vaccine is contraindicated during pregnancy.

60. d. 2500 kcal and 60 g/day

Recommended Dietary Allowance for pregnancy is 2500 kcal/day and 60 g/day of protein.

61. c. From amniotic epithelium and fetal functions

Amniotic fluid is produced by amniotic epithelium. Water transfers across the amnion and through fetal skin. In the second trimester, the fetus starts to swallow, urinate, and inspire amniotic fluid.

62. b. Meiosis occurs, producing half the number of chromosomes

Meiosis is the process of two successive cell divisions, producing cells, egg, or sperm, that contain half the number of chromosomes found in somatic cells.

63. a. Trophoblasts, chorion, amnion

Parts of the placenta are trophoblasts, chorion, amnion and chorionic villi, intervillous spaces, and decidual plate.

64. c. The embryo, membranes, and placenta

A conceptus comprises all tissue products of conception: embryo (fetus), fetal membranes, and placenta.

65. a. Trophoblast

Human trophoblasts produce more diverse steroid and protein hormones and in greater amounts than does any endocrine tissue in all of mammalian physiology.

66. b. Finding which direction the fetus is lying

Leopold's maneuvers consist of four abdominal palpation maneuvers used to determine the following fetal characteristics: lie, presentation, position, attitude.

67. d. Multiple marker screen

Second-trimester screening (also known as "multiple marker screening") is performed between 15 and 20 weeks to detect neural tube defects and trisomy 18 and 21.

68. c. Fetal heart rate response to fetal movement

A nonstress test (NST) is a method to assess fetal well-being by observing the fetal heart rate response to fetal movement.

69. b. Gingivitis is common in pregnancy with increased vascularity of connective tissue

Gingivitis is common and may result in bleeding of gums.

70. b. Placental abruption

Placental abruption is premature separation of the placenta from the uterus that may be partial or complete. Signs of placental abruption include vaginal bleeding, uterine tenderness and rigidity, contractions or uterine irritability and/or tone, and fetal tachycardia or bradycardia.

71. a. Certain LMP

Dating a pregnancy is most accurate with a certain last menstrual period (LMP).

72. b. Monitor for persistent trophoblastic proliferation

Weekly serial beta hCG levels are recommended after surgical evacuation for hydatidiform mole to monitor for persistent trophoblastic proliferation and identify metastatic disease including choriocarcinoma.

73. c. Discussing alternate methods to promote uterine readiness and contractions

Pitocin (oxytocin injection) may be utilized to help initiate or facilitate labor by stimulating contraction of the uterine smooth muscle. There are other methods to promote uterine readiness and contractions such as nipple stimulation.

74. c. Initiate treatment with antibiotics

A diagnosis of a urinary tract infection can be made by finding 100,000 colonies of pathogenic bacteria in a urinary culture. Treatment with appropriate antibiotics is necessary. Untreated asymptomatic bacteriuria may lead to pyelonephritis, which may cause serious complications for both mother and baby.

75. d. Maintaining her health and preventing neonatal transmission

Maintaining health of the woman and preventing vertical transmission to the neonate are the priority when caring for women with HIV.

76. d. Three pregnancies of which one was term, one premature, and one an abortion

The numbers represent a woman's obstetric history, TPAL: one term delivery, one preterm delivery, one abortion (spontaneous or elective), and two living children.

77. d. Single pocket greater than 8 cm

Polyhydramnios is an excess of amniotic fluid diagnosed as Amniotic Fluid Index greater than or equal to 24 cm or a maximum deepest vertical pocket of equal to or greater than 8 cm.

78. b. Fetal anomalies of GI tract

Etiology of polyhydramnios may be due to central nervous system or gastrointestinal tract fetal anomalies.

79. c. Renal system
    Oligohydramnios is associated with genitourinary abnormalities in the fetus.

80. a. Period between the second and eighth weeks
    Embryonic development is the period of organogenesis, which begins in the third week after fertilization, and spans for 8 weeks; this is around the time a woman may miss her next menstrual period and when pregnancy tests would turn positive by detecting human chorionic gonadotropin (hCG).

81. d. Lungs
    All major organ systems are formed during the embryonic stage except for the lungs.

82. a. It is the basis for making decisions toward the end of the pregnancy
    Determining an accurate estimated date of birth (EDB) is critical because an accurate estimation of the date of birth is the basis for making decisions toward the end of the pregnancy.

83. c. Mildly enlarged, nodular thyroid
    Having a mildly enlarged, nodular thyroid is an abnormal physical exam finding. The other findings are normal findings in pregnancy.

84. d. Increases weight through fat accumulation
    During 32–36 weeks, the fetus continues to increase weight as more subcutaneous fat accumulates.

85. a. The first day of the last menstrual period
    A complete menstrual history, which includes determining the first day of the LMP and the length of menstrual cycles, allows for a more accurate EDB.

86. a. Crown rump length (CRL)
    In the first trimester, the most accurate parameter for dating is crown rump length (CRL) measurement.

87. c. At 12 weeks it begins to rise out of pelvis, and at 20 weeks is at the umbilicus
    At 12 weeks' gestation, the uterus becomes an abdominal organ and rises out of the pelvis. At 20 weeks, the uterus is typically found at the umbilicus.

88. d. Chadwick's
    Chadwick's sign is a presumptive sign of pregnancy. *Presumptive sign of pregnancy* refers to signs and symptoms that may be caused by pregnancy. Amenorrhea may be caused by sickness or stress.

89. c. Corpus luteum and placenta
    Corpus luteum is responsible for the secretion of progesterone to maintain the endometrium and pregnancy until the placenta takes over production.

90. a. Android
    An android pelvic type is commonly known as a "male" pelvis, and 32.5% of white women and 15.7% of nonwhite women have this type of heavy, heart-shaped pelvis that leads to increased posterior positions, dystocia, and operative births.

91. c. Effects of relaxin and progesterone
    Relaxin and progesterone affect cartilage and connective tissue, resulting in a loosening of the sacroiliac joint and symphysis pubis.

92. b. 10% cardiac volume increase that peaks in midpregnancy

Cardiac volume increases by about 10% and peaks at about 20 weeks, and resting pulse increases by 10–15 beats per minute with the peak at 28 weeks.

93. a. Blood volume increase of 30–50%
    Blood volume increases 30–50% from nonpregnant levels and plasma volume expands, which result in a physiologic anemia.

94. a. Limited support network
    Risk factors for psychological well-being include limited support network, high levels of stress, psych/mental health issues, and problem pregnancies.

95. b. 100,000 live births
    Maternal mortality ratio is the number of maternal deaths that result from the reproductive process/100,000 live births.

96. d. 1122
    TPAL represents a woman's obstetric history. G.R. has one term pregnancy, one preterm, two abortions, and two live children.

97. a. Inlet, midplane, and outlet
    Three planes are of obstetric significance—inlet, midplane, and outlet.

98. c. Ischial spines distance and sacrum
    The distance between the ischial spines normally measures 10 cm, is the smallest diameter of the pelvis, and defines the midplane.

99. a. Screen for fetal anomalies
    Amniocentesis is used in early pregnancy to obtain amniotic fluid to be sent for chromosomal studies.

100. a. It can be done 3–4 weeks earlier
     An advantage of chorionic villous sampling (CVS) over amniocentesis is that CVS can be performed between 10 and 13 weeks, 3–4 weeks earlier.

101. b. Fetal movement is strongest at 29–38 weeks
     Fetal movement is strongest between 29 and 38 weeks. Fetal movement counting is a safe, simple, no-cost, noninvasive fetal assessment technique. Research has demonstrated that fetal activity is a good predictor of well-being. Dramatic decrease or cessation of movement is cause for concern.

102. d. Fetal heart rate accelerates in association with fetal movement
     The nonstress test (NST) is a method to assess fetal well-being by observing the fetal heart rate response to fetal movement.

103. d. Placenta previa
     Contraindications for contractions stress test (CST) include previous classic C-section or myomectomy, placenta previa, at risk for preterm labor, gestational age less than 37 weeks, and multiple gestation.

104. c. To provide fetal blood transfusion
     Cordocentesis is the process in which a needle is introduced under real-time ultrasound through the maternal abdomen and then into the umbilical cord. Blood is then aspirated or blood and/or medications are introduced into the fetus.

105. c. Include both legal and illegal drugs
     Both legal and illegal substances have the potential to be addicting.

106. b. Cigarette smoking
     According to the Substance Abuse and Mental Health Services Administration National Survey on Drug Use and Health, 2010, 16.3% of pregnant women smoked cigarettes in the past month,

10.8% reported current alcohol use, 3.7% engaged in binge drinking, 4.4% were current illicit drug users.

107. a. Evaluate her safety

The healthcare provider's primary goal when caring for a woman who is abused is to evaluate her safety.

108. d. Ninety percent of pregnancies in which FHT are heard will continue to term after early bleeding

Ninety percent of pregnancies with bleeding will continue to term after fetal heart tones (FHT) are observed. Other information to discuss with your patient includes the following: 40% of women have some bleeding in the first trimester, and 80% of spontaneous abortions occur in the first 12 weeks.

109. c. Ectopic pregnancy and threatened abortion

Differential diagnosis for bleeding in the first trimester includes implantation bleeding, threatened abortion, ectopic pregnancy, cervicitis, cervical polyps, vaginitis, trauma/intercourse, disappearing twin, and autoantibody/autoimmune disorder.

110. b. Cystic fibrosis

Autosomal recessive trait is expressed only when both copies of the gene are the same, for example, cystic fibrosis and sickle cell anemia.

111. a. Cervicitis

Painless bleeding after sexual intercourse at 34 weeks may be due to irritation of the cervix from cervicitis. There is usually painful bleeding associated with placental abruption. Premature rupture of membranes is typically associated with loss of fluid.

112. c. Polyhydramnios

Postterm pregnancy is typically associated with decreased amniotic fluid and not excess.

113. d. Result from maternal cigarette smoking

Symmetric growth restriction is associated with maternal use of drugs such as tobacco, alcohol, Dilantin (phenytoin), cocaine, and heroin.

114. d. Incompetent cervix

Second-trimester fetal loss is most likely due to incompetent cervix. The other stated causes of fetal loss, hydatidiform mole, inevitable abortion, and ectopic pregnancy, are related to first-trimester loss.

115. b. Approximately 30% of women have a low-lying placenta in the first trimester

One-third of women have low-lying placenta in the first trimester. Most will resolve, and only 1% have previa in the third trimester.

116. a. G5 P1122

The woman has five total pregnancies, including her current pregnancy, one term delivery, one preterm delivery, two abortions, and two living children.

117. c. Amniocentesis

Amniocentesis is a diagnostic test for genetic evaluation or assessment of neural tube defects.

118. b. Neural tube defect

An elevated maternal serum alphafetoprotein (AFP) is associated with neural tube defects, multiple gestation, and placental abruption.

119. a. History of previous GBS-positive infant

Risk factors for group B streptococcus (GBS) disease include history of previous GBS-positive infant, delivering early (before 37 weeks' gestation), developing fever during labor, having a long period between water breaking and delivery, and having a previous infant with early-onset disease.

120. d. A placental abruption is associated with risk factors such as hypertension, smoking, and trauma

Placental abruption risk factors include hypertension—chronic or gestational, trauma, smoking, cocaine use, multiparity, and uterine anomalies or tumors.

121. c. The pair of genes for each characteristic inherent in an individual

Genotype refers to the total hereditary information present in an individual, the pair of genes for each characteristic.

122. b. Nonsensitized Rh negative mother with an Rh positive baby

A nonsensitized Rh negative mother with an Rh positive baby needs RhoGAM postpartum to prevent future sensitization. A sensitized Rh negative mother does not need RhoGAM because she is already sensitized. A nonsensitized Rh negative mother with an Rh negative baby also does not need RhoGAM.

123. a. Down syndrome

Aneuploidy is an abnormal number of chromosomes in a cell. An abnormal number of chromosomes, the presence of extra chromosome 21, can be found in Down syndrome.

124. a. Will be done after 12–14 weeks and is 80–90% successful

Cervical cerclage is done after 12–14 weeks with a success rate of 80–90%. There is a risk of ruptured membranes or infection. There is a need to monitor cervical length via transvaginal ultrasound.

125. b. Benzathine penicillin G 2.4 units IM × 1 dose at the time of diagnosis

The treatment for early syphilis in pregnant women is one dose of benzathine penicillin G 2.4 million units IM.

126. b. Pregnant women who are at risk for preterm delivery should be treated if they have asymptomatic bacterial vaginosis

Treatment recommended for all pregnant women with symptoms of bacterial vaginosis: metronidazole 500 mg PO BID × 7 days OR metronidazole 250 mg PO TID × 7 days OR clindamycin 300 mg PO BID × 7 days.

127. a. Metronidazole 2 g orally

The treatment for trichomoniasis in pregnancy is metronidazole 2 g PO × 1 at any stage of pregnancy.

128. a. Generally becomes evident in midpregnancy

Symmetric growth restriction appears around 18–20 weeks and is caused by congenital infections, chromosomal abnormalities, maternal drug use—tobacco, alcohol, Dilantin (phenytoin), cocaine, heroin, and increased risk of adverse long-term sequelae.

129. d. Screening for diabetes at 6–12 weeks postpartum

M. K.'s 1-hour oral glucose tolerance test results are abnormal, and a diagnosis for gestational diabetes can be made. Thus, a screening for pregestational diabetes at 6–12 weeks postpartum is necessary.

130. b. Ordering an ultrasound

Ordering an ultrasound is the most appropriate management of the patient to evaluate fetal size and gestation. The patient is too early in gestation for a biophysical profile and a nonstress test. Waiting 4 weeks for an evaluation is too long to wait—the patient needs to be evaluated much sooner.

131. c. 6500 IU/L
Ninety percent of ectopics have b-hCG less than 6500 IU/L.

132. b. Azithromycin 1 g orally in a single dose and perform test of cure in 3–4 weeks
Recommended treatment for chlamydia: azithromycin 1 g PO × 1 OR amoxicillin 500 mg orally TID × 7 days. Alternative regimens:
   • Erythromycin base 500 mg PO QID × 7 days
   • Erythromycin base 250 mg PO QID × 14 days
   • Erythromycin ethylsuccinate 800 mg PO QID × 7 days
   • Erythromycin ethylsuccinate 400 mg PO QID × 14 days

133. d. Contractions begin slowly; once they are 4–5 minutes apart, it is real labor
Labor usually begins with slow contractions that gradually become more regular and closer together. When contractions are 4–5 minutes apart, this is a sign of real labor.

134. a. Elevated free thyroxine (FT_4) levels
Elevated serum free thyroxine (FT_4) or free thyroxine index (FTI) levels indicate hyperthyroidism in pregnancy.

135. b. 20–25%
Twenty percent to 25% of pregnancies are ABO incompatible.

136. c. She was not sensitized in the first pregnancy, and you will provide monitoring and treatment to prevent it in this pregnancy
The patient is Rh negative and received RhoGAM postpartum with her first pregnancy. She was not sensitized in the first pregnancy. She can be monitored and provided RhoGAM to prevent sensitization in this pregnancy.

137. d. Encouraging her to continue getting dietary iron and taking her iron supplement
Average hemoglobin level in pregnancy is 12.5 g/dL. The patient's hemoglobin level is slightly below normal, and she can be encouraged to continue getting dietary iron and taking her iron supplement.

138. d. Macrocytic erythrocytes
Folic acid deficiency anemia is characterized by laboratory tests showing macrocytic erythrocytes, hypersegmentation of neutrophils, and bone marrow megaloblastic erythropoiesis.

139. b. Disease is present when the person inherits a sickle cell gene from each parent
Sickle cell anemia (SS disease) disease is present when the person inherits a sickle cell gene from each parent.

140. a. Persistent abdominal pain and tenderness
Persistent abdominal pain and tenderness are the most critical symptoms of appendicitis.

141. b. Delve further into what occurred and how she came to the conclusions that led her to stop breastfeeding
It is the healthcare provider's role to listen and facilitate the patient's expression of feelings and to provide a nonjudgmental environment.

142. c. "The plan provides the opportunity for you to make choices about events associated with the birth"
It is the healthcare provider's role to listen and facilitate the patient's expression of feelings and to provide a nonjudgmental environment.

143. d. Pregnant women are typically screened for asymptomatic bacteruria in early pregnancy

Urinary tract infection (UTI) occurs in 2–7% of all pregnancies. UTI may be asymptomatic (asymptomatic bacteriuria), and 25–30% will progress to pyelonephritis if left untreated.

144. d. Woman with diabetes
Women with diabetes are at greatest risk for urinary tract infection (UTI). Other risk factors include sickle cell trait and pregnancy.

145. d. It is negative because she has no high-risk characteristics for the disease PPD (purified protein derivative of tuberculin) test interpretation by risk factors:
   a. 5 mm is positive for very high risk—HIV positive, with abnormal chest radiograph, recent contact with active case
   b. 10 mm is positive for high risk, that is, foreign born, HIV-negative, IV drug user, low-income populations, associated medical problems
   c. 15 mm is positive for those with none of these risks

146. b. Viral load is the strongest predictor for transmission of infection to the infant during the birth process
Viral load is the strongest predictor for vertical transmission.

147. b. She is 5 ft 10 in with an anthropoid pelvis and her husband is 6 ft 4 in
S.R.'s anthropoid pelvis shape favors a posterior position of the fetus and is adequate for a vaginal birth of a large infant.

148. c. The result offers some reassurance that she will not go into labor in the next 2 weeks
A negative result on a fetal fibronectin test is useful in ruling out imminent (within 14 days) preterm birth before 37 weeks' gestation (predictive value up to 94%).

149. d. Reduces the incidence of newborn respiratory distress syndrome
Corticosteroids such as betamethasone and dexamethasone are commonly used in women at risk for preterm delivery to reduce the risk of respiratory distress and cerebral hemorrhage in the newborn.

150. d. Wait until 36 weeks to see if spontaneous version has occurred
The incidence of breech is 14% between 29 and 32 weeks and 3.5% at term. Anticipatory guidance regarding plan for version as well as plans for persistent breech should be reviewed with the patient.

151. b. Serum creatinine > 1.1 mg/dL
Preeclampsia is the development of blood pressure higher than or equal to 140/90 mm Hg on two occasions at least 4 hours apart after 20 weeks of gestation and proteinuria greater than or equal to 300 mg per 24-hour urine collection or protein/creatinine ratio greater than or equal to 0.3 or, if other quantitative methods are unavailable, a dipstick result of 1+. In the absence of proteinuria, diagnosis parameters for pre-eclampsia include new-onset hypertension with any of the following:
   • Thrombocytopenia: platelet count < 100,000/microliter
   • Renal insufficiency: serum creatinine > 1.1 mg/dL or doubling of serum creatinine concentration without renal disease
   • Impaired liver function: doubling of normal levels of liver transaminases
   • Pulmonary edema
   • Cerebral or visual symptoms

Bibliography

ACIP Adult Immunization Work Group, Bridges, C. B., Woods, L., & Coyne-Beasley, T. (2013). Advisory Committee on Immunization Practices (ACIP) recommended immunization schedule for adults aged 19 years and older—United States, 2013. Retrieved from http://www.cdc.gov/mmwr/preview/mmwrhtml/su6201a3.htm

Alford, C., & Nurudeen, S. (2013). Physiology of reproduction in women. In A. H. DeCherney, L. Nathan, N. Laufer, & A. S. Roman (Eds.), *CURRENT Diagnosis & Treatment: Obstetrics & Gynecology* (11th ed.). New York, NY: McGraw-Hill Medical. Retrieved from http://www.accessmedicine.com/content.aspx?aID=56963628

American College of Obstetricians and Gynecologists. (2004). Nausea and vomiting of pregnancy (ACOG Practice Bulletin No. 52). Washington, DC: Author.

American College of Obstetricians and Gynecologists. (2007). Management of herpes in pregnancy (ACOG Practice Bulletin No. 82). Washington, DC: Author.

American College of Obstetricians and Gynecologists. (2008, July). Anemia in pregnancy (ACOG Practice Bulletin No. 95). Washington, DC: Author.

American College of Obstetricians and Gynecologists. (2012). Prediction and prevention of preterm birth (ACOG Practice Bulletin No. 130). Washington, DC: Author.

American College of Obstetricians and Gynecologists. (2013a, November). Definition of term pregnancy. *Committee Opinion*, 579. Retrieved from https://www.acog.org/About_ACOG/ACOG_Departments/~/media/Committee%20Opinions/Committee%20on%20Obstetric%20Practice/co579.pdf

American College of Obstetricians and Gynecologists. (2013b). Fetal growth restriction (ACOG Practice Bulletin No. 134). Washington, DC: Author.

American College of Obstetricians and Gynecologists. (2013c). Gestational diabetes mellitus (ACOG Practice Bulletin No. 137). Washington, DC: Author.

American College of Obstetricians and Gynecologists. (2013d). *Hypertension in pregnancy*. Washington, DC: Author. Retrieved from http://www.acog.org/~/media/Task%20Force%20and%20Work%20Group%20Reports/HypertensioninPregnancy.pdf

American College of Obstetricians and Gynecologists. (2013e). Repeated miscarriage. *Frequently Asked Questions 100*. Retrieved from http://www.acog.org/~/media/For%20Patients/faq100.pdf?dmc=1&ts=20140505T1552299642

American Diabetes Association. (2012). Standards of medical care in diabetes—2012. *Diabetes Care, 35*(Suppl. 1), S11–S63.

Barrett, K. E., Barman, S. M., Boitano, S., & Brooks, H. L. (2012). Chapter 22. Reproductive development & function of the female reproductive system. In K. E. Barrett, S. M. Barman, S. Boitano, & H. L. Brooks (Eds.), *Ganong's review of medical physiology* (24th ed.). New York, NY: McGraw-Hill Medical. Retrieved from http://www.accessmedicine.com/content.aspx?aID=56263207

Bernstein, H. B., & VanBuren, G. (2013). Chapter 6. Normal pregnancy and prenatal care. In A. H. DeCherney, L. Nathan, N. Laufer, & A. S. Roman (Eds.), *CURRENT Diagnosis & Treatment: Obstetrics & Gynecology* (11th ed.). New York, NY: McGraw-Hill Medical. Retrieved from http://www.accessmedicine.com/content.aspx?aID=56964326

Blackburn, S. (2007). *Maternal, fetal, and neonatal physiology: A clinical perspective* (3rd ed.). St. Louis, MO: Saunders Elsevier.

Centers for Disease Control and Prevention. (n.d.) *Diabetes and pregnancy: Gestational diabetes*. Retrieved from http://www.cdc.gov/pregnancy/documents/Diabetes_and_Pregnancy508.pdf

Centers for Disease Control and Prevention. (2010). *Gestational Diabetes and Pregnancy*. Retrieved from http://www.cdc.gov/pregnancy/diabetes-gestational.html

Centers for Disease Control and Prevention. (2013). *Birth: Final Data for 2012*. Retrieved from http://www.cdc.gov/nchs/data/nvsr/nvsr62/nvsr62_09.pdfv

Centers for Disease Control and Prevention. (2009). Table 4. Chlamydia—women–reported cases and rates by state/area and region listed in alphabetical order: United States and outlying areas, 2004–2008. 2008 sexually transmitted diseases surveillance. Retrieved from http://www.cdc.gov/std/stats08/tables/4.htm

Centers for Disease Control and Prevention. (2010). *Sexually transmitted disease treatment guidelines, 2010*. Atlanta, GA: Author. Retrieved from http://www.cdc.gov/mmwr/pdf/rr/rr5912.pdf

Centers for Disease Control and Prevention. (2012). Sexually Transmitted Disease Surveillance. Retrieved from http://www.cdc.gov/std/stats12/gonorrhea.htm

Centers for Disease Control and Prevention. (2012). Update to CDC's *sexually transmitted diseases treatment guidelines, 2010*: Oral cephalosporins no longer a recommended treatment for gonococcal infections. Retrieved from http://www.cdc.gov/mmwr/preview/mmwrhtml/mm6131a3.htm?s_cid=mm6131a3_w

Centers for Disease Control and Prevention. (2013). TB and pregnancy. Retrieved from http://www.cdc.gov/TB/topic/populations/pregnancy/default.htm

Centers for Disease Control and Prevention. (2014a). Natality data summary. Retrieved from http://wonder.cdc.gov/wonder/help/natality.html#Fertility-Rates

Centers for Disease Control and Prevention. (2014b). Tuberculosis: Data and statistics. Retrieved from http://www.cdc.gov/tb/statistics/

Centers for Disease Control and Prevention, Division of STD Prevention. (2013). *Incidence, prevalence, and cost of sexually transmitted infections in the United States*. Retrieved from http://www.cdc.gov/std/stats/STI-Estimates-Fact-Sheet-Feb-2013.pdf

Centers for Disease Control and Prevention, National Center for HIV/AIDS, Viral Hepatitis, STD, and TB Prevention, Division of STD Prevention. (2014). Syphilis—CDC fact sheet. Retrieved from http://www.cdc.gov/std/syphilis/STDFact-Syphilis.htm

Centers for Disease Control and Prevention. (2014). Vaccines and Immunizations, Tdap for Pregnant Women: Information for Providers. Retrieved from http://www.cdc.gov/vaccines/vpd-vac/pertussis/tdap-pregnancy-hcp.htm

Cunningham, F. G., Leveno, K. J., Bloom, S. L., Hauth, J. C., Rouse, D. J., & Spong, C. Y. (2009a). Chapter 5. Maternal physiology. In *Williams obstetrics* (23rd ed.). New York, NY: McGraw-Hill. Retrieved from http://www.accessmedicine.com/content.aspx?aID=6043606

Cunningham, F., Leveno, K., Bloom, S., Hauth, I., Rouse, D., & Spong, C. (2009b). *Williams obstetrics* (23rd ed.). New York, NY: McGraw-Hill.

Demian, E., Rizk, M. (2011). Preconception Care. In South-Paul JE, Matheny SC, Lewis EL. South-Paul, J. E., Matheny, S. C., Lewis, E. L. (Eds). *CURRENT Diagnosis & Treatment in Family Medicine, 3e.* Retrieved from http://accessmedicine.mhmedical.com/content.aspx?bookid=377&Sectionid=40349408

Feinstein, G., Budd, R., Gabriel, S., McInnes, I., & O'Dell, J. (2012). *Firestein: Kelley's textbook of rheumatology* (9th ed.). Philadelphia, PA: Elsevier Saunders.

Gibbs, R., Karlan, B., Haney, A., & Nygaard, I. (2008). *Danforth's obstetrics and gynecology* (10th ed.). Philadelphia, PA: Lippincott Williams & Wilkins.

Institute of Medicine. (2009). *Weight gain during pregnancy: Reexamining the guidelines.* Washington, DC: Author.

Javorsky, B. R., Findling, J. W., & Tyrrell, J. B. (2011). Chapter 4. Hypothalamus and pituitary gland. In D. G. Gardner & D. Shoback (Eds.), *Greenspan's basic & clinical endocrinology* (9th ed.). New York, NY: McGraw-Hill Medical. Retrieved from http://www.accessmedicine.com/content.aspx?aID=8400541

King, T., Brucker, M., Kriebs, J., & Fahey, J. (2013). *Varney's midwifery* (5th ed.). Burlington, MA: Jones & Bartlett Learning.

Mason, R., Broaddus, C., Martin, T., King, T., Schraufnagel, D., Murray, J., … Nadel, J. (2010). *Mason: Murray and Nadel's textbook of respiratory medicine* (5th ed.). Maryland Heights, MO: Saunders Elsevier.

Rakel, R., & Rakel, D. (Eds.). (2011). *Textbook of family medicine* (8th ed.). Philadelphia, PA: Elsevier.

Rhoads, J., & Peterson, S. (2014). *Advanced health assessment and diagnostic reasoning.* Burlington, MA: Jones & Bartlett Learning.

Robertson, G. L. (2012). Chapter 340. Disorders of the neurohypophysis. In D. L. Longo, A. S. Fauci, D. L. Kasper, S. L. Hauser, J. L. Jameson, & J. Loscalzo (Eds.), *Harrison's principles of internal medicine* (18th ed.). New York, NY: McGraw-Hill Professional. Retrieved from http://www.accessmedicine.com/content.aspx?aID=9140410

Rogers, V. L., & Worley, K. C. (2013). Chapter 19. Obstetrics and obstetric disorders. In M. A. Papadakis, S. J. McPhee, M. W. Rabow, & T. G. Berger (Eds.), *CURRENT Medical Diagnosis & Treatment 2014.* New York, NY: McGraw-Hill Medical. Retrieved from http://www.accessmedicine.com/content.aspx?aID=9353

Samuels, M. A. (2009). Chapter 27. The hypothalamus and neuroendocrine disorders. In A. H. Ropper & M. A. Samuels (Ed.), *Adams and Victor's principles of neurology* (9th ed.). New York, NY: McGraw-Hill Professional. Retrieved from http://www.accessmedicine.com/content.aspx?aID=3634491

Satterwhite, C. L., Torrone, E., Meites, E., Dunne, E. F., Mahajan, R., Ocfemia, M. C., … Weinstock, H. (2013). Sexually transmitted infections among U.S. women and men: Prevalence and incidence estimates, 2008. *Sex Transmitted Disease, 40*(3), 187–193.

Substance Abuse and Mental Health Services Administration. (2009). Results from the 2008 national survey on drug use and health: National findings. (Office of Applied Studies, NSDUH Series H-36, HHS Publication No. SMA 09-4434). Rockville, MD: Author. Retrieved from http://www.samhsa.gov/data/nsduh/2k8nsduh/2k8Results.htm

Tharpe, N., & Farley, C. (2014). *Clinical practice guidelines for midwifery and women's health* (4th ed.). Burlington, MA: Jones & Bartlett Learning.

U.S. Agency for International Development MEASURE Evaluation Population and Reproductive Health. (n.d.). Perinatal mortality rate (PMR). Retrieved from http://www.cpc.unc.edu/measure/prh/rh_indicators/specific/nb/perinatal-mortality-rate-pmr

U.S. Department of Health and Human Services. (2013). National Diabetes Information Clearing House: What I need to know about diabetes. Retrieved from http://www.diabetes.niddk.nih.gov/dm/pubs/gestational/index.aspx#3

World Health Organization. (2013). WHO vaccine-preventable diseases: Monitoring system. 2013 global summary. Retrieved from http://apps.who.int/immunization_monitoring/globalsummary/incidences?c=US

7

Intrapartum and Postpartum

Kimberly K. Trout and Jamille Nagtalon-Ramos

© Kheng Guan Toh/ShutterStock, Inc.

Initial Assessment

- Reason for visit: ("chief complaint or concern")
- Sociodemographics
  1. Age—opposite ends of the age spectrum create risks
     a. Adolescents
        (1) Prone to late entry to care and poor compliance with prenatal care schedule
        (2) At risk for low birth weight and prematurity
        (3) Increased risk for
            (a) Pre-eclampsia
            (b) Premature labor
            (c) Preterm birth
            (d) Intrauterine growth restriction (IUGR)
            (e) Infant mortality
        (4) Risk probably multifactorial with associated socioeconomic factors
            (a) Parity
            (b) Race
            (c) Marital status
            (d) Educational level
     b. Advanced maternal age for pregnancy is older than age 35 years
        (1) Higher incidence of infertility and first-trimester spontaneous abortion and ectopic pregnancy
        (2) Proportional increase in rates of genetic abnormalities with advancing age
        (3) Increased rates of complications including:
            (a) Hypertensive disorders of pregnancy
            (b) Preterm delivery
            (c) Gestational diabetes
            (d) Dysfunctional labor leading to Cesarean section
            (e) Relationship to underlying disease processes
            (f) Placenta previa and abruption
  2. Race/ethnicity
     a. Increased rate of low-birth-weight babies born to African American women
     b. Certain genetic disorders are increased within specific ethnic groups
  3. Socioeconomic status
     a. Lower socioeconomic status directly proportional to poor obstetric outcome, including premature labor and delivery
     b. Can be related to limited access to prenatal care and necessary resources such as appropriate food sources
- Gravidity and parity
  1. Length of labor
     a. Nullipara average longer labors
     b. Multipara average shorter labors
     c. Grand multiparous women (parity > 5) can have prolonged dysfunctional labors
  2. Obstetric complications
     a. Increased parity associated with increased rates of
        (1) Abruptio placenta
        (2) Placenta previa
        (3) Multifetal pregnancy
        (4) Postpartum hemorrhage
     b. Grand multiparity can contribute to abnormal presentation, including transverse lie
- Estimated gestational age (EGA)—Based on determination of estimated date of delivery (EDD). Synonymous terms for EDD include: estimated date of birth (EDB) and estimated date of confinement (EDC) (this term traditionally used but less frequently because of negative connotations of the word "confinement")
  1. Menstrual dating (using Naegele's rule)—add 7 days to the first day of the last menstrual period and subtract 3 months
  2. Ultrasound dating—most accurate if performed in the first trimester
  3. Anatomic dating by fundal height measurement
- Review of the antepartum course—preferably using prenatal chart
  1. History of prenatal visits
     a. Timing of first visit
     b. Compliance with visit schedule
     c. Unscheduled visits/consults
  2. Weight gain
     a. Prepregnancy weight/body mass index (BMI)

b. Appropriateness of interval weight gain

c. Total weight gain

3. Blood pressure

a. Initial blood pressure

b. Changes in blood pressure values throughout pregnancy

4. Fundal height growth

5. Ultrasound results

6. Current medications

7. Obstetric complications/unscheduled visits

- Laboratory data

1. Blood type and Rh factor

2. Hemoglobin/hematocrit

3. Hepatitis B surface antigen status

4. Rubella status

5. Pap test result

6. Sexually transmitted infection (STI) screening results (including HIV, RPR)

7. Glucose screening

8. Group B streptococcus culture

9. Genetic testing results

a. Chorionic villus sampling

b. Amniocentesis

c. Multiple marker screening (quad or penta)

d. Nuchal translucency combined with human chorionic gonadotropin (hCG) and pregnancy-associated plasma protein (PAPP-A) levels

e. Cell-free fetal DNA

- Family history

1. Obstetric complications

2. Genetic diseases, including chromosomal abnormalities and ethnicity-based disorders

3. Congenital defects or syndromes

4. Medical disorders

a. Hypertension (HTN)

b. Diabetes

c. Cardiac disease

- Obstetric history

1. Gravidity—total number of pregnancies

2. Parity—outcome of previous pregnancies

a. Expressed as a four-digit number (TPAL)

b. First digit is number of full-term infants (T); second digit is number of preterm infants (P); third digit is number of abortions (spontaneous/elective) (A); fourth digit is number of living children (L)

3. Description of previous pregnancies

a. Duration of gestation

b. Birth weight

c. Duration of labor

d. Type of delivery

e. Analgesia/anesthesia

f. Complications of the antepartum, intrapartum, or postpartum period

g. Place of delivery

h. Provider

- Past medical history

1. Allergies

2. Medical conditions

3. Previous surgeries

4. Medication (over-the-counter and prescription) and herb/supplement use

- Review of systems

1. Genitourinary

2. Respiratory

3. Cardiovascular

4. Gastrointestinal

5. Neurologic

6. Musculoskeletal

- Labor status

1. Onset of contractions

2. Description of contractions

a. Frequency

b. Duration

c. Intensity

3. Status of membranes

a. Time of rupture

b. Amount

c. Color

4. Frequency of fetal movements

5. Presence or absence of bloody show

6. Other subjective symptoms

a. Nausea and vomiting

b. Rectal pressure

Physical Examination

- Vital signs

- Abdominal examination

1. Leopold's maneuvers for fetal presentation and position during labor

a. Determination of attitude is more difficult secondary to fetal descent

b. Location of fetal back provides best determination of fetal position without pelvic examination

2. Palpation of contraction intensity

3. Presence of fetal movement

4. Location of fetal heart tones

- Pelvic examination

1. External perineal inspection

a. Presence of bloody show

b. Presence of amniotic fluid

c. Presence of lesions

2. Internal examination

a. Sterile speculum examination—*before digital examination* if ruptured membranes are suspected, frank bleeding is present, or inspection for herpetic lesions is necessary

b. Digital examination

(1) Dilation

(2) Effacement

(3) Station—relationship of the leading edge of the fetal presenting part to the ischial spines (in centimeters)

(a) 0 station—the presenting part is at the level of the spines

(b) −3, −2, −1 station—number of centimeters of the presenting part above the level of the ischial spines

(c) +1, +2, +3 station—number of centimeters of the presenting part below the level of the ischial spines

(4) Presenting part—the anatomic part of the fetus that first descends into the pelvis

(5) Position—relationship between the denominator of the presenting part and the maternal pelvis

   (a) Cephalic presentation—the denominator is the occiput

   (b) Breech presentation—the denominator is the sacrum

   (c) Shoulder presentation—the denominator is the scapula

   (d) Face presentation—the denominator is the mentum

(6) Status of membranes

(7) Clinical pelvimetry—determination of adequacy of bony pelvis

   (a) The pelvis is composed of four bones

      i. Two innominate

      ii. Sacrum

      iii. Coccyx

   (b) Symphysis pubis joins the two innominate (pubic) bones anteriorly

   (c) True pelvis defines the birth canal

      i. Inlet boundaries are at the level of the sacral promontory (posteriorly), the linea terminalis (laterally), and the upper margins of the pubic bones (anteriorly)

      ii. Midplane of the pelvis is known as " the plane of least dimensions" and the boundaries are the sacrum at the junction of the 4th and 5th sacral vertebrae (posteriorly), the ischial spines (laterally), and the inferior border of the symphysis pubis (anteriorly)

      iii. Outlet boundaries are the saccrococcygeal joint (posteriorly), the inner surface of the ischial tuberosities (laterally), and the lower border of the symphysis pubis (anteriorly)

   (d) Classification of pelvic types

      i. Gynecoid

         a) Round shaped pelvis

         b) Transverse diameter only slightly longer than anteroposterior

         c) Incidence—50% of white women

         d) Excellent prognosis for vaginal birth

      ii. Android

         a) Heart-shaped or triangular shaped pelvis

         b) Posterior pelvis wider than anterior

         c) Poor prognosis for vaginal birth requiring operative delivery or C-section

      iii. Anthropoid

         a) Oval-shaped pelvis

         b) Anteroposterior diameter is longer than transverse diameter

         c) Incidence—40.5% of nonwhite

         d) Good prognosis of vaginal birth—higher incidence of occiput posterior position

      iv. Platypelloid

         a) Flattened gynecoid shape pelvis

         b) Wide transverse diameter with very short anteroposterior diameter

         c) Incidence—3%

         d) Poor prognosis for vaginal birth

- Fetal heart rate assessment
  1. Continuous—by external electronic fetal monitor
     a. Determination of the fetal heart rate
     b. Assessment of variability
     c. Determine presence or absence of periodic changes, including decelerations, tachycardia, or bradycardia
  2. Continuous—by internal monitoring via fetal scalp electrode
     a. Measures the actual R-to-R interval of the fetal QRS complex; more accurate surveillance
  3. Intermittent by Doppler
     a. Auscultation of fetal heart rate at prescribed intervals based upon stage of labor to assess fetal tolerance of labor
     b. Unable to determine variability or isolated decelerations
  4. Fetal heart rate tracings classification (National Institute of Child Health and Human Development, 2008)
     a. Category I: Normal, no action required
     b. Category II: Indeterminate, require continued evaluation and close monitoring
     c. Category III: Associated with abnormal fetal acid–base status, prompt action required
- Head-to-toe examination
  1. General affect and coping abilities
  2. Head, eyes, ears, nose, and throat
     a. Absence of facial edema
     b. Absence of upper respiratory infection (URI) signs
  3. Heart and lungs
     a. Heart sounds without murmurs, rubs, or gallops—may have split S1, I-II/VI systolic murmur, audible S3
     b. Lungs clear to auscultation
  4. Abdomen
     a. Fundal height and appropriateness to gestational age
     b. Leopold's maneuvers if not performed previously
     c. Presence of scars or lesions
     d. Intensity of contractions by palpation
     e. Location of fetal heart tones
  5. Pelvic examination—described in detail in this chapter
  6. Extremities
     a. Presence or absence of edema
     b. Presence or absence of varicosities
     c. Reflexes

Diagnostic Studies

- Type of studies—dependent upon policies of birthing facility
  1. Complete blood count (CBC)
  2. Blood type and Rh—may need to type and screen or cross-match depending on maternal risk status

3. Repeat testing for HIV, syphilis, or hepatitis if indicated by history, examination findings, or required by law (varies by state and local municipalities)

- Urine testing
  1. Protein
  2. Glucose
  3. Ketones
- Cervical/vaginal/perineal cultures performed during sterile speculum examination if indicated
  1. Cervical culture if suspect active infection or has prolonged rupture of membranes (PROM)
  2. Culture of any suspicious lesions
  3. Vaginal and rectal cultures for group B streptococcus (GBS) if rupture of membranes before 37 weeks and not yet laboring

Management and Teaching

- Based upon birth facility's policies, client desire, and risk status for discussion, consultation and management options
- Admission versus outpatient management
  1. Generally admit during active labor; client may desire outpatient management
  2. Factors to consider in decision making
     a. Stage of labor
     b. Nullipara versus multipara
     c. Functional versus prodromal labor
     d. Labor support at home
     e. Need for increased fetal surveillance
- Intravenous access
  1. If intravenous access is necessary via saline lock or IV catheter, most common IV fluids are:
     a. Lactated Ringer's solution
     b. 5% dextrose with lactated Ringer's solution (D5LR)
     c. 0.9% NaCl solution
  2. Factors to consider in decision making
     a. Hydration status, including presence of ketonuria
     b. Need for oxytocin induction or augmentation
     c. Need for antibiotics
     d. Predisposing factors for postpartum hemorrhage such as an overdistended uterus
     e. Abnormal placentation
     f. Grand multiparity
     g. Need for pain medication or regional anesthesia
- Limitations of activity level
  1. Clients can be encouraged to ambulate to help labor progress and coping abilities
  2. Factors to consider in decision making
     a. Unstable lie or malpresentation
     b. Need for increased fetal surveillance and monitoring
     c. Membrane status and station of the presenting part
     d. Hypertensive disorders of pregnancy
     e. Maternal exhaustion level
- Nutrition and fluid status
  1. Energy levels can be positively influenced by oral intake
  2. Factors to consider in decision making
     a. Gastrointestinal motility/absorption

b. Potential need for anesthesia during labor
c. Birthing facility policy
3. Can consider gastrointestinal protective agents such as magnesium/aluminum hydroxide, calcium carbonate/magnesium hydroxide, and sodium citrate/citric acid combinations

- Monitoring of vital signs
  1. Dependent upon stage of labor and risk status
  2. Patients with ruptured membranes require more frequent vital signs, especially temperature
- Pain management/coping during labor and delivery
  1. Nonpharmacologic methods
     a. Can allow the woman to feel more in control of the birth process
     b. Can be used without significant risk of side effects—especially helpful in latent labor
        (1) Ambulation and movement/use of birthing ball
        (2) Hydrotherapy
        (3) Breathing and relaxation/hypnotherapy
        (4) Music
        (5) Position changes
        (6) Acupuncture/acupressure
        (7) Sterile water injections
        (8) Touch and massage; warms compresses such as a heating pad or rice sock
        (9) Aromatherapy
  2. Analgesia
     a. Used to ameliorate the pain sensation; may change and alter consciousness; some medications have amnesiac effect
     b. Can be used in latent and active phase
     c. Avoid within 1 hour of birth because of the potential respiratory depressant effect on the fetus
        (1) Hypnotic
        (2) Sedatives
        (3) Opioids
  3. Anesthesia
     a. Provides complete neurologic block
     b. Can interfere with muscular action
     c. Possible effect on the labor progress; may cause an increase in need for obstetric intervention
     d. Can have systemic effects, including hypotension (most common) and fever
     e. Inadvertent dural puncture can cause spinal headache
        (1) Spinal/intrathecal
        (2) Epidural
  4. Local blocks—provide pain blockade at site of pain for brief periods of time
     a. Paracervical
     b. Pudendal
     c. Local infiltration
- Fetal well-being monitoring—method used dependent upon risk status of mother, policy of the birth facility, and provider preferences in combination with mother's desires
  1. Intermittent auscultation
     a. Facilitates increased mobility
     b. Increased patient comfort
     c. Equivalent to continuous fetal monitoring when performed at appropriate intervals

d. Requires one-to-one labor attendance

e. Associated with decreased rates of intervention

2. Continuous fetal monitoring

a. May be indicated for antepartum or intrapartum risk factors

b. Reactive fetal monitor tracing (Category I) is predictive of a well-oxygenated fetus

c. Interpretation of fetal well-being can be equivocal in the presence of Category II fetal heart rate tracings

- Support people and their roles

1. Labor support can improve a woman's perception of her labor

2. One-to-one labor support can assist the woman to cope better with labor

3. Especially when provided by a doula (someone who is there solely to support the woman and who has no medical responsibilities); dedicated labor support has been found to decrease use of obstetric interventions

- Management of membranes

1. Intact membranes provide a barrier to bacterial introduction to the uterus

2. Intact membranes can facilitate rotation of the head during pelvic descent

3. Early rupture of membranes with unengaged vertex can increase risk of cord prolapse

4. Artificial rupture of membranes (AROM) may assist in the augmentation of labor if dysfunctional or arrested

- Physician role

1. Clarify with the client the Certified Nurse–Midwife (CNM) role in relation to the consulting physician

2. Indications for physician involvement should be reviewed

- Birth preferences

1. Birth plan should be reviewed with client upon admission and discussed in relation to status at that time

2. Discussion with client regarding inability to control labor process

Mechanisms of Labor

- The 4 Ps of labor

1. Power of contractile efforts

a. Adequacy of strength

b. Assess need for augmentation of labor

2. Passenger

a. Lie

b. Presentation

c. Position

d. Size

e. Synclitism versus asynclitism

(1) The relationship of the sagittal suture line to the maternal sacrum and symphysis pubis

(2) Synclitism denotes the sagittal suture is midway between these two bones; biparietal diameter is parallel to the planes of the pelvis

(3) Asynclitism denotes that the sagittal suture is oriented toward the pubis or the sacrum

(a) Posterior asynclitism—the sagittal suture is closer to the symphysis pubis

(b) Anterior asynclitism—the sagittal suture is closer to the sacrum

(c) Can be the cause of labor dystocia

(d) Lax abdominal musculature contributes to asynclitism

3. Passageway

a. Clinical pelvimetry

b. Classification of the pelvic structure

4. Psyche

a. Woman's view of labor/birth and her ability to handle it

b. Appropriateness of emotional support

c. Education or preparation of labor

d. Meaning of the pregnancy

e. Ability to achieve birth plan

f. History of sexual abuse

- Labor assessment and progress

1. Stages of labor—Friedman's concepts presented, but more recent research conflicts with some of Friedman's findings (as indicated below)

a. First stage—from onset of regular contractions through full dilatation (10 cm)

(1) Latent labor—from onset of labor until 4–6 cm

(a) Contraction pattern

i. Every 10–20 minutes lasting 15–20 seconds to every 5–7 minutes lasting 30–40 seconds

ii. Mild to moderate intensity

(b) Length

i. Per Friedman curve, nullipara should be 20 hours or less

ii. Per Friedman curve, multipara should be 14 hours or less

(2) Active labor—from 4–6 to 10 cm, begins with the acceleration phase that may not occur until 6 cm dilatation in some women. Recent research findings also suggest that there is not a normally occurring deceleration phase (as previously described by Friedman) in active labor just prior to complete dilatation

(a) Contraction pattern

i. Become more frequent, regular, and intense

ii. In active labor, every 2 to 3 minutes lasting at least 60 seconds

iii. Moderate to strong by palpation

(b) Length

i. Nullipara

ii. Multipara

(c) Strength of contractions

i. Externally measured by palpation

ii. Internally

a) By intrauterine pressure catheter (IUPC)

b) Adequacy is considered 200 Montevideo (mVu) in a 10-minute period

(d) Descent

i. Nullipara

ii. Multipara

b. Second stage of labor—from full dilatation until the birth of the baby; pushing or expulsive phase

2. Abnormal labor progress—according to Friedman
   a. Abnormal latent phase
      (1) Nullipara, more than 20 hours
      (2) Multipara, more than 14 hours
   b. Abnormal active phase
      (1) Nullipara progress, less than 1.2 cm/hour
      (2) Multipara progress, less than 1.5 cm/hour
      (3) Less than 200 mVu in 10 minutes by IUPC
   c. Descent
      (1) Nullipara, less than 1 cm/hour
      (2) Multipara, less than 2.1 cm/hour
3. Zhang's findings—Zhang et al. (2010) used modern statistical interval measure techniques to analyze more than 54,000 births and demonstrated a hyperbolic, not a linear or sigmoidal, labor curve, with dilation occurring more rapidly with advanced labor and without a deceleration phase (as previously described by Friedman)
   a. Nullipara—median time to dilate from 4 to 10 cm: 3.7 hours, 95 percentile: 16.7 hours
   b. Multipara—median time to dilate from 4 to 10 cm: 2.4 hours for parity 1, 2.2 hours for parity 2+, 95 percentile: 14.2 hours

Management of the First Stage of Labor

- Assessment of maternal status
  1. Psychological status of client
     a. Perception of pain/coping
     b. Coping ability and coping strategies
     c. Presence and support of people
     d. Client's perception of need for admission to the birthing facility
  2. Physical status of the client
     a. Vital signs
        (1) Temperature
           (a) Slightly elevated (< 100°F) during labor, highest in the time preceding and immediately following the birth
           (b) Epidural anesthesia can artificially elevate temperature
        (2) Blood pressure
           (a) Systolic blood pressure increases 10–20 mm Hg during contractions
           (b) Diastolic blood pressure increases 5–10 mm Hg during contractions
           (c) Blood pressure returns to prelabor levels between contractions
           (d) Pain and fear can contribute to elevations in blood pressure
        (3) Pulse
           (a) Because of the increased metabolic rate during labor, pulse rate is slightly elevated
           (b) Inversely proportional to action of the contraction, increases during increment and decreases at acme

   (4) Respiration
      (a) Slightly increased rate during labor
      (b) Hyperventilation is common and related to pain response and can lead to alkalosis
- Assessment of labor progress
  1. Vaginal examinations
     a. Allows assessment of labor progress related to cervical dilatation and/or fetal descent
     b. Frequency of vaginal examinations dependent upon phase of labor, provider choice, client's wishes, and status of membranes
  2. Partographs—graph of labor curve
     a. Designed by Dr. Emmanuel Friedman to chart labor progress to ensure adequacy
     b. Expectation of standard progress of labor by Friedman's formula not universally accepted
     c. Research by Philpott and Castle (1972) suggests that aggressive management interventions (such as oxytocin augmentation) should not be initiated unless dilatation averages less than 0.56–0.64 cm/hour in active labor. Recent evidence on the normal progress of the first stage of labor (Zhang, 2010) supports the use of an individualized approach
- Pain management
  1. Basis of labor pain
     a. Physiologic
        (1) Intensity of contractions
        (2) Degree of cervical dilatation
        (3) Descent of fetus causing pressure on pelvic structures
        (4) Fetal size
        (5) Fetal position
        (6) Hypoxia of uterine muscle cells during action of contractions
     b. Psychological
        (1) Fear
        (2) Anxiety
        (3) Lack of knowledge regarding labor process
        (4) Lack of support
        (5) Cultural influences
  2. Negative physiologic responses related to labor pain
     a. Hyperventilation
     b. Stress responses—related psychological effect causes increased cortisol and decreased placental perfusion
     c. Increased cardiac output and blood pressure
  3. Factors influencing pain management decisions
     a. Patient choice or birth plan
     b. Stage of labor
     c. Fetal status
     d. Other factors contributing to pain response
     e. Possible routes of medication administration
     f. Availability of pain medication modalities
     g. Nursing staff availability
  4. Pain management methods
     a. Nonpharmacologic pain relief
        (1) Relaxation and breathing techniques
        (2) Hydrotherapy—tub, shower, Jacuzzi
        (3) Position changes; ambulation
        (4) Massage

(5) Environmental measures (i.e., quiet surroundings, aromatherapy, music)

(6) Acupuncture/acupressure

(7) Hypnosis

b. Pharmacologic pain relief

(1) Sedatives/hypnotics used for false labor or prolonged latent phase of labor, facilitate rest/relaxation

    (a) Diphenhydramine 25–50 mg by mouth

    (b) Prochlorperazine 25 mg per rectum or 5-10 mg by mouth

(2) Ataractics—do not affect contraction pattern, have a calming effect, may be used in conjunction with opioids

    (a) Promethazine 25–50 mg IM or 25 mg IV

    (b) Hydroxyzine 25–100 mg IM or by mouth (MUST NOT BE GIVEN IV)

(3) Opioid analgesics given in labor but should be avoided with active labor

    (a) Morphine sulfate for prodromal labor 10–15 mg IM OR

    (b) Fentanyl 50–100 micrograms IV or IM OR

    (c) Meperidine 50–75 mg IM or 25–50 mg IV

(4) Mixed agonist-antagonist opioid analgesics

    (a) Butorphanol 1–2 mg IV or 2 mg IM

    (b) Nalbuphine 10–20 mg IM or 5 mg IV

c. Anesthesia

(1) Spinal/intrathecal

(2) Epidural

(3) Pudendal

(4) Nitrous oxide: Combination of 50% nitrous oxide and 50% oxygen self-administered via inhalation mask

- Assessment and evaluation of fetal well-being

1. Physiology of fetal heart rate (FHR) regulation

a. Parasympathetic/sympathetic nervous system—responsible for the variability of the FHR

b. Baroreceptors

(1) Increased pressures can cause vagal response in the fetus

(2) Located in the carotid arteries

c. Chemoreceptors

(1) Located in the aortic arch and carotid sinus

(2) Sensitive to changes in the fetal pH, O_2 level, and CO_2 level and respond by increasing fetal blood pressure and heart rate

d. Sympathetic nervous system—controls the baseline fetal heart rate

2. Evaluation of the FHR in labor

a. Baseline

(1) Normal range for a fetus at term 110–160 beats per minute (bpm)

(2) FHR between 110 and 120 bpm can be normal at term with appropriate variability

(3) Judged over approximately 10 minutes, the mean FHR in the absence of periodic changes rounded to the nearest 5 beats should be documented

b. Bradycardia

(1) FHR at less than 110 bpm for 10 or more minutes

(2) Marked bradycardia is less than 100 bpm for 10 or more minutes

(a) Causes

    i. Cord compression

    ii. Rapid descent

    iii. Vagal stimulation

    iv. Medications

    v. Anesthesia or medications

    vi. Placental insufficiency

    vii. Fetal cardiac anomalies

    viii. Terminal condition of the fetus

c. Tachycardia

(1) FHR of more than 160 bpm for more than 10 minutes

(a) Causes

    i. Maternal fever

    ii. Infection

    iii. Medications, especially beta sympathomimetics

    iv. Chronic fetal hypoxia

    v. Can be compensatory after temporary fetal hypoxia event

    vi. Undiagnosed prematurity

    vii. Excessive fetal movement

d. Variability

(1) Combination of influences between the sympathetic and parasympathetic nervous systems

(2) Baseline variability—fluctuations in the baseline of the fetal heart rate

(a) Absent—undetectable amplitude

(b) Minimal—amplitude range ≤ 5 bpm

(c) Moderate—amplitude range 6–25 bpm

(d) Marked—amplitude ≥ 25 bpm

e. Accelerations—sign of fetal well-being, cannot be produced by acidotic fetus (indicates fetal pH of more than 7.20)

(1) Greater than 32 weeks—a peak of ≥ 15 bpm above the baseline lasting ≥ 15 seconds but less than 2 minutes from beginning to end of acceleration

(2) ≤ 32 weeks—a peak of ≥ 10 bpm above the baseline lasting ≥10 seconds but less than 2 minutes from beginning to end of acceleration

f. Periodic changes

(1) Variable decelerations

(a) Abrupt (onset to nadir < 30 seconds) periodic or nonperiodic decrease in the FHR that differs in shape from one deceleration to another. The decrease in FHR from the baseline is ≥ 15 bpm lasting ≥ 15 seconds but less than 2 minutes

(b) FHR deceleration does not reflect the shape of the contraction

(c) Can occur at any time in relation to the contractions

(d) Nonconsistent shape; can look like a U, V, or W

(e) Generally with an abrupt drop below the FHR baseline and a rapid return to baseline

(f) Generally caused by cord compression

(g) Implications

    i. With rapid recovery to baseline and good variability, generally considered an uncompromised fetus

ii. Suspect fetal compromise with slow recovery to baseline, increasing length or depth of deceleration, absent variability, or increasing frequency of deceleration

(h) Management

i. Position change

ii. IV fluid bolus

iii. O_2 at 10 liters per minute (LPM) via face mask

iv. Pelvic examination, to rule out cord prolapse and provide scalp stimulation

v. Contact consulting physician if warranted

vi. Consider amnioinfusion

(2) Early decelerations

(a) Uniformly shaped slowing of the FHR that mirrors the contractions

(b) Gradual descent to the nadir ($\geq$ 30 seconds) with gradual return

(c) FHR usually remains within the normal range and deceleration usually less than 90 seconds

(d) Deceleration begins, peaks, and ends with the contraction

(e) Generally caused by head compression, vagal stimulation

(f) Generally considered a benign pattern

(g) Management

i. Surveillance

(3) Late decelerations

(a) Uniformly shaped gradual ($\geq$ 30 seconds) slowing of the FHR that begins with the peak of the contraction and does not return to baseline until after the completion of the contraction

(b) FHR may or may not remain within the normal fetal heart range

(c) Can occur in an isolated fashion but more ominous when occurs repetitively

(d) Possible causes

i. Uteroplacental insufficiency

ii. Fetal hypoxia

iii. Uterine hyperstimulation

iv. Decreased placental blood flow

v. Maternal hypotension

vi. Abruptio placenta

vii. Medication effect

(e) Management

i. Left lateral position

ii. IV fluid bolus

iii. O_2 at 10 LPM

iv. Attempt to correct underlying cause

v. Consult with physician

3. Fetal monitoring techniques

a. All women require some method of fetal monitoring in labor

b. Modality is based upon maternal/fetal risk status, birth site, and client desire

c. For low-risk women, intermittent auscultation is equivalent to continuous fetal monitoring to detect fetal compromise

d. FHR monitoring techniques

(1) Intermittent FHR auscultation by fetoscope or Doppler

(a) Should be considered for low-risk pregnancies

(b) Frequency of auscultation—dependent also on facility protocol

i. Auscultate for 60 seconds after a contraction every 30 minutes in the first stage of labor if low risk, every 15 minutes if high risk

ii. Every 15 minutes during the second stage of labor if low risk, every 5 minutes if high risk

(2) Continuous fetal monitoring

(a) Recommended for high-risk pregnancies or when intermittent monitoring is not indicated

(b) Frequency of FHR tracing review

i. Every 15 minutes in the first stage

ii. Every 5 minutes in the second stage

(c) Modalities for continuous fetal monitoring

i. External FHR—ultrasound detection and tracing of the FHR through the abdominal wall

ii. Internal FHR

a) Via fetal scalp electrodes (FSE)

b) Directly measures fetal heartbeat by measuring the R-to-R interval during heartbeats

c) Indications include inability to externally monitor (such as inability to maintain an external tracing in the obese client)

d) Fetal heart rate tracing classifications

i. Category I—normal tracing, associated with normal acid–base balance

• Normal baseline

• Moderate FHR variability

• Absent late or variable decelerations

• Present or absent early decelerations

• Present or absent accelerations

ii. Category II—indeterminate tracing, not predictive of fetal acid–base status, require continued monitoring and evaluation

• Baseline rate of either bradycardia or tachycardia

• Minimal, absent with no recurrent decelerations, or marked variability

• No accelerations despite fetal stimulation

• Recurrent variable decelerations with minimal or moderate baseline variability

• Prolonged decelerations between 2 and 10 minutes

• Recurrent late decelerations with moderate baseline variability

• Variable decelerations that have "overshoots" or "shoulders"

iii. Category III—abnormal tracings, associated with abnormal fetal acid–base status. Prompt corrective action required. Characterized by absent FHR variability in conjunction with any of the following:
- Bradycardia
- Recurrent variable decelerations
- Recurrent late decelerations
- Sinusoidal pattern

e. Direct fetal testing

(1) Fetal scalp stimulation

(a) During vaginal examination, fetal head is stimulated

(b) Expected result should be FHR acceleration of more than 15 beats off baseline for more than 15 seconds

(c) Expected result correlates to fetal pH of more than 7.20

(d) Cannot be reliably performed during deceleration or bradycardia; must wait for FHR recovery

(e) Validity and reliability not well established

4. External uterine monitoring

a. Tocodynameter—senses the changes in pressures against the strain gauge resulting from the change in abdominal wall contour

(1) Records contraction interval and duration

(2) Cannot determine intensity of contractions

b. Palpation

5. IUPC—can accurately measure the intensity of contractions in mm Hg so that adequacy of contractions can be calculated in Montevideo units

- Fetal positions during birthing process

1. Mechanisms of labor and cardinal movements based on occiput anterior (OA) position

a. Left occiput anterior (LOA) is the most common position of birth

b. Position and appropriate cardinal movements are facilitated in the gynecoid pelvis

c. Cardinal movements of labor

(1) Descent—usually in the left occiput transverse (LOT) position if engagement occurs during labor with rotation to LOA

(2) Flexion—vertex begins partially flexed, is completely flexed when reaches pelvic floor, changing presenting diameter to suboccipitobregmatic of 9.5 cm

(3) Internal rotation—rotation of 45 degrees to OA allows the head to maximize the anterior-posterior (AP) diameter of the gynecoid pelvis

(4) Extension—fulcrum of the neck under the symphysis pubis allows birth of the head

(5) Restitution—vertex rotates 45 degrees as the shoulders begin entering the AP diameter

(6) External rotation—as head rotates another 45 degrees, shoulders complete the remainder of the rotation to allow delivery in direct AP diameter

2. Mechanisms of labor and cardinal movements with occiput posterior (OP) position

a. Incidence of OP presentation is 15–30%

b. Right occiput posterior (ROP) is five times more common than left occiput posterior

c. More common in android pelvis and anthropoid pelvis

d. 90% of OP presentations rotate to OA via long arc rotation of 135 degrees (ROP to ROT to ROA to OA)

e. Short arc rotation of 45 degrees results in direct OP (or deep transverse pelvic arrest if failure to completely rotate)

f. Cardinal movements for persistent OP position (short arc rotation)

(1) Descent—head enters pelvis at an oblique angle (more often ROP than LOP)

(2) Flexion presents smaller diameter through pelvis

(3) Internal rotation—head rotates 45 degrees to OP position

(4) Flexion/Extension—once rotation is complete, birth of the head occurs by movements of flexion until the sinciput impinges beneath the symphysis pubis and then the remainder of the head is born by extension

(5) Restitution—fetal head rotates 45 degrees to either ROP or LOP position

(6) External rotation—head rotates another 45 degrees as shoulders complete remainder of rotation to the anterior-posterior diameter of the outlet to facilitate birth

- Emotional support

1. Psychological

a. Calm environment

b. Perception of safety and support for mother and baby

c. Maintenance of privacy and modesty

d. Participation in the plan of care

2. Role of the labor support person

a. Reinforcement of and positive encouragement for the laboring woman

b. Participation in the birth process

(1) Providing oral fluids and/or ice chips

(2) Encouraging position changes

(3) Relaxation techniques

(4) Massage

(5) Coaching with breathing techniques

Management of the Second Stage of Labor

- Begins with complete dilatation and ends with the birth of the infant

- Maternal status

1. Vital signs

a. Blood pressure (BP)—every 5–15 minutes

(1) BP must be taken between contractions

(2) BP can be elevated 10 mm Hg in the second stage of labor because of pushing effort

b. Pulse and respiratory rate every 5–15 minutes

c. Temperature every 2 hours if membranes intact, every 1 hour if membranes ruptured

2. Hydration and fluid status
   a. IV or oral fluids should be encouraged because of
      (1) Increased metabolism
      (2) Increased respiratory efforts/hyperventilation of transition
      (3) Diaphoresis
      (4) Nausea and vomiting
   b. Bladder status
      (1) Bladder distention can compromise pelvic capacity
      (2) Inability to void may require catheterization
      (3) Prevent problem by having client void (or catheterize) when full dilatation approaches
3. Behaviors and coping ability
   a. Assessment of maternal fatigue
   b. Coping ability
   c. Response to pain and pressure
4. Pain control
   a. Evaluate level of sensation in epiduralized client to determine whether anesthetic level is hindering pushing efforts
   b. Pudendal anesthesia is occasionally used in client without epidural as fetal descent occurs, causing perineal distention and pain
5. Expulsive effort
   a. Client should be coached to achieve effective pushing effort
   b. Allow women with an epidural a resting period of passive descent or "laboring down" before active pushing
   c. Types of pushing
      (1) Open glottis physiologic pushing
      (2) Closed glottis "Valsalva" pushing—can decrease cardiac output and blood flow to the uterus, associated with more fetal heart rate decelerations and a higher incidence of perineal trauma
   d. Client should be instructed to pant at the time of crowning; "control the mother, not the head"
6. Integrity of the perineum
   a. Maternal preference is generally avoidance of episiotomy
   b. Indications for episiotomy
      (1) Need to expedite birth secondary to fetal bradycardia
      (2) Anticipation of shoulder dystocia
      (3) Operative birth
      (4) Short perineum
- Fetal status
  1. Vaginal examination
     a. Evaluation of descent with pushing effort
     b. Normalcy of fetal position and adaptation to the maternal pelvis
        (1) Molding/caput succedaneum
        (2) Synclitism versus asynclitism
        (3) Appropriate rotation to facilitate delivery
  2. FHR monitoring
     a. Need for increased frequency of FHR evaluation
        (1) Evaluation at least every 15 minutes
        (2) More commonly every 5 minutes or after each contraction
     b. Periodic changes (early and variable decelerations) in FHR common
        (1) Decelerations secondary to head compressions

- Pain relief
  1. Breathing techniques
     a. Controlled breathing as contraction begins and ends assists in focusing efforts
     b. Promote relaxation between pushing efforts
  2. Opioid analgesia
     a. Should *not* be given within 1 hour of birth
     b. Can cause respiratory depression in the neonate
  3. Regional anesthesia
     a. Effectively lessens the pain and pressure sensations of the second stage
     b. Can lengthen second stage secondary to pelvic musculature relaxation and decreased pressure sensations
     c. Pudendal—lidocaine 1% up to 10 cc on each side
        (1) Provides dense nerve block to the perineum
        (2) Does not inhibit pushing efforts
        (3) Needs to be timed well for best anesthetic effect
           (a) Primiparas when vertex is at +2
           (b) Multiparas shortly before complete dilation
  4. Local anesthesia
     d. Perineal infiltration—lidocaine 1–2% usually 10 cc in divided dosing (up to 30 cc maximum of 1% solution)
        (1) Used prior to cutting of an episiotomy
        (2) For repair of episiotomy or laceration(s)
- Emotional support
  1. Encouragement
  2. Participation of labor support persons
  3. Adherence to birth plan
- Cardinal movements of labor
  1. Eight basic movements that take place to allow birth in vertex presentation
     a. Engagement—biparietal diameter of fetal head passes through pelvic inlet
     b. Descent—occurs secondary to forces of uterine contractions, change in the tone of pelvic musculature and maternal pushing
     c. Flexion—occurs when the fetal head meets the resistance of the pelvic floor during descent and forces the smaller suboccipitobregmatic diameter to enter the pelvis first
     d. Internal rotation—causes the fetal head to rotate to the anteroposterior diameter of the maternal pelvis, most commonly causing the occiput to rotate to the anterior portion of the pelvis
     e. Extension—mechanism by which the birth of the fetal head occurs; the fetal head follows the curve of Carus; the suboccipital region of the fetal head pivots under the maternal pubic symphysis
     f. Restitution—rotation of the head 45 degrees and realignment to the shoulders
     g. External rotation—occurs as the shoulders rotate 45 degrees, bringing the shoulders into the anteroposterior diameter of the pelvis; the head also rotates another 45 degrees
     h. Birth of the body occurs by lateral flexion of the shoulders via the curve of Carus

Delivery Management

- Maintenance of pelvic integrity
  1. Anatomy
     a. Pelvic floor musculature
        (1) Function to support pelvic organs
        (2) Aids in the anterior rotation of the fetus during pelvic descent and birth
        (3) Consists of two muscle groups
            (a) The levator ani, made up of:
                i. Pubococcygeus, made up of:
                   a) Pubovaginalis
                   b) Puborectalis
                   c) Pubococcygeus proper
                ii. Illiococcygeus
            (b) Coccygeus
     b. Perineal musculature
        (1) Perineum is divided into two triangles and is more superficial than the pelvic floor musculature
            (a) Anteriorly as the urogenital triangle
                i. Superficial transverse perineal muscle
                ii. Ischiocavernosus muscle
                iii. Bulbocavernosus
                iv. Deep transverse perineal muscle
            (b) Posteriorly as the anal triangle
                i. Sphincter ani externus
                ii. Anococcygeal body
  2. Factors interfering with perineal integrity
     a. Size of fetus
     b. Distensibility of perineum
     c. Control of expulsive efforts
     d. Operative delivery modalities (i.e., forceps or vacuum extraction)
     e. Occiput posterior position
     f. Use of lubricants
     g. Maternal position for birth
     h. Episiotomy (median or mediolateral)
  3. Strategies to minimize perineal trauma
     a. Antepartum perineal massage
        (1) Begin at 36–37 weeks
        (2) Increases elasticity and maternal tolerance to perineal stretching
     b. External perineal massage from the time of perineal distension—of note, vigorous massage and stretching of the perineum in the second stage of labor has not been shown to be effective and may actually predispose the woman to an increased risk of lacerations
     c. Warm compresses during second stage
        (1) Increases circulation to perineum
        (2) Promotes elasticity
        (3) Assists in the relaxation of the musculature
     d. Lateral positioning for birth
     e. Counter pressure to maintain flexion of the fetal head during birth
     f. Education of the mother regarding the importance of controlled delivery of the head
     g. Support of the perineum at the time of birth (this is controversial, some providers adopt a "hands-off" approach to birth)
- Episiotomy—surgical incision performed to enlarge the vaginal opening to allow delivery of the fetal head
  1. Anatomy
     a. Muscles cut during median episiotomy
        (1) Bulbocavernosus (sphincter vaginalis)
        (2) Ischiocavernosus
        (3) Superficial and deep transverse perineal muscles
  2. Technique
     a. Median episiotomy
        (1) Place index and middle fingers, slightly separated and palm side down, in vagina
        (2) Insert scissors into the introitus in an up and down position with one blade placed externally and one blade placed internally
        (3) Depth of insertion should correspond to the length of intended episiotomy
        (4) Cut tissue in one motion deliberately and purposefully
        (5) Evaluate adequacy of incision; repeat if indicated
     b. Mediolateral episiotomy—generally used if patient has a short perineum to avoid a laceration into the anal sphincter
        (1) Used much less frequently in United States—less than 10%
        (2) Same procedure except that the direction of the scissors is a 45 degree angle from the base of the introitus directed either right or left
        (3) The angle of the incision should be aimed toward the corresponding ischial tuberosity
        (4) Much more difficult to repair
  3. Lacerations
     a. First degree—involves the vaginal mucosa, posterior fourchette, and perineal skin
     b. Second degree—involves same structures as above plus perineal muscles
     c. Third degree—involves same structures as a second degree plus tearing through the entire thickness of the rectal sphincter
     d. Fourth degree—involves all the structures as above plus tearing of the rectal mucosa
  4. Repair
     a. Fundamentals of repair
        (1) Use of aseptic technique
        (2) Adequate anesthesia
        (3) Visibility through good hemostasis
        (4) Appropriate suture material including needle size
        (5) Minimize local tissue trauma through gentle and limited blotting
        (6) Minimize the amount of suture used
        (7) Good approximation of tissues decreasing dead space
     b. Suture material
        (1) Vicryl is the most common suture material
        (2) Chromic catgut is alternately used for repair
        (3) Suture gauge
            (a) 3-0
                i. Vaginal mucosa

ii. Subcutaneous tissue
iii. Subcuticular tissue
(b) 4-0 for finer repairs
i. Periurethral
ii. Periclitoral
iii. Anterior wall of the rectum
(c) 2-0 for areas requiring more tensile strength
i. Vaginal wall lacerations
ii. Cervical lacerations
iii. Deep interrupted sutures for repair of pelvic musculature
(4) Needle selection
(a) Atraumatic general closure needles are preferable
(b) Small, fine GI needles should be used for fine stitching
(c) Cutting needles should not be used
c. Mechanisms of repair of median episiotomy or second-degree laceration
(1) Inspection of tissues to assess depth and extent of laceration
(2) Identify all appropriate anatomic structures
(3) Begin repair approximately 1 cm beyond the apex of the laceration to the vaginal mucosa
(4) Close the mucosa using continuous locked stitches to the level of the hymenal ring
(5) Pass needle under hymenal ring and continue using blanket stitches (nonlocked) to the level of the bulbocavernosus muscle
(6) Repair bulbocavernosus muscle with a crown stitch using a separate 2-0 suture if desired
(7) If laceration is deep, consider several deep interrupted stitches using 2-0 suture
(8) Using the 3-0 suture again, repair the subcutaneous layer with continuous stitching to the perineal apex
(9) Using mattress stitches, perform subcuticular closure
(10) At the level of the hymenal ring, bury the suture and tie off
• Management decisions for birth
1. Birth setting
a. Hospital
b. Birth Center
c. Home
Timing for the preparation of the birth related to location (i.e., setting up instrument table and donning personal protective equipment)
2. Delivery position for birth
a. Semi-sitting
b. Squatting
c. Lateral
d. Hands and knees
e. Supine or lithotomy (least appropriate, but commonly used)
3. Determine need for an episiotomy
4. Need for/type of additional anesthesia/analgesia
5. Use of perineal support during birth
6. Use of the Ritgen maneuver—assistance, if needed, in delivering fetal head by applying upward pressure to the fetal chin through the rectum during extension

7. Need for additional personnel (i.e., nurse, second midwife, consulting physician, pediatric provider)
8. Placement of newborn upon delivery
9. Timing of umbilical cord cutting
• Hand maneuvers for birth in the OA position
1. Apply counter pressure to the fetal head during crowning to maintain flexion and control extension using nondominant hand
2. If using perineal support, place thumb and index finger laterally on the distended perineum with palmar surface supporting perineal body
3. Control birth of head during extension
4. After birth of head, slide fingers of dominant hand around fetal head to posterior neck to feel for umbilical cord
5. If nuchal cord is present:
a. Gently slip over baby's head if loose
b. If not easily reduced over the head, slip cord over baby's shoulders as the baby is born
c. If tight:
(1) Somersault maneuver direct baby to maternal thigh OR
(2) Doubly clamp and cut and unwind cord before delivery of the shoulders
6. Wipe fluid from the baby's face, nose, and mouth with a soft cloth. Routine suctioning with a bulb syringe is not necessary
7. After restitution and external rotation, place the palmar surface of each hand laterally on the baby's head
8. With gentle downward traction, and maternal pushing effort, deliver anterior shoulder. Some recommend waiting for the next contraction
9. With upward traction, lift the baby's head toward ceiling to deliver the posterior shoulder while observing the perineum
10. Glide posterior hand along head and posterior shoulder to control the posterior arm as it delivers
11. As the baby delivers, maintain posterior hand under the baby's head with support by the wrist and forearm
12. The anterior hand follows the body of the baby during birth and grasps the lower leg of the baby
13. Rotate the baby into the football hold with the head in the palm and the legs between what was the posterior arm and attendant's body
14. Keep the baby's head below its hips, and slightly to the side, to facilitate drainage and suctioning
• Suctioning
1. Routine suctioning of nasal and oral passages is no longer recommended because it can cause physical injury to the nares or oropharynx
2. Most healthy babies can clear their airways with no additional help
3. Bulb syringe
a. Generally sufficient to clear oral and nasal passages of fluid and mucus after birth if suctioning is indicated
b. Minimizes pharyngeal stimulation and tissue trauma (as compared to suction catheters)

Management of the Third Stage of Labor

- Begins with delivery of the infant and ends with the delivery of the placenta
  1. Physiologic management versus
  2. Active management of the third stage of labor (AMTSL) shown to decrease risk of postpartum hemorrhage in general population. 3 components of AMTSL per International Confederation of Midwives (ICM) and International Federation of Gynecology and Obstetrics (FIGO)
     a. Controlled cord traction (once pulsation stops)- World Health Organization (WHO) recommends this step only with skilled birth attendant, citing evidence of possible harm
     b. Use of a uterotonic agent (such as oxytocin)
     c. Fundal massage after delivery of the placenta
- Delivery of the placenta
  1. Timing—generally 5–30 minutes after the birth
  2. Method of placental separation
     a. Placenta separates from the uterine wall because of change in uterine size
     b. Hematoma forms behind the placenta along the uterine wall
     c. Separation of the placenta completes
     d. Descent of the placenta to the lower uterine segment or vagina
     e. Expulsion
  3. Signs and symptoms of placental separation
     a. Sudden increase in vaginal bleeding
     b. Lengthening of the umbilical cord
     c. Uterine change in shape from discoid to globular
     d. Uterus rises in the abdomen
  4. Mechanisms of placental delivery
     a. Schultz
        (1) Presents at the introitus with fetal side showing
        (2) More common than Duncan
        (3) Separation is thought to occur centrally first
        (4) Majority of bleeding is contained
     b. Duncan
        (1) Presents at the introitus with maternal side showing
        (2) Less common
        (3) Separation occurs initially at placental margin
        (4) Bleeding is more visible
        (5) Higher incidence of hemorrhage due to incomplete separation of placenta
  5. Management of placenta delivery
     a. Obtain cord bloods after clamping of the cord
     b. Inspect cord for number of vessels
     c. Guard the uterus while waiting for placenta separation
        (1) No fundal massage before separation
        (2) No traction on umbilical cord until separation
     d. Use modified Brandt-Andrews to assess for separation
     e. When separation has occurred, use Brandt–Andrews maneuver to stabilize the uterus and controlled cord traction to deliver the placenta
     f. May have mother push to assist expulsion
     g. Deliver placenta via the curve of Carus
     h. If membranes are trailing behind the placenta, carefully deliver membranes by:
        (1) Using a Kelly clamp or sponge stick clamp onto membranes, gently apply lateral and outward traction
        (2) Holding the bulk of the placenta and twisting the placenta over and over until the membranes are delivered
        (3) Inspecting placenta and membranes for completeness
- Appropriate diagnostic tests
  1. Cord blood
     a. Fetal blood type and Rh
     b. Direct Coombs' testing
  2. Maternal blood
     a. Kleihauer–Betke test if mother is Rh negative
     b. CBC if hemorrhage suspected
- Use of oxytocics
  1. Oxytocin
     a. Used prophylactically against postpartum hemorrhage
     b. Causes intermittent uterine contractions to decrease uterine size and the placental bed exposure
     c. Administration
        (1) Intravenous
           (a) 20–40 units in 1000 cc of IV fluid (normal saline or lactated Ringer's) with first liter running rapidly, second liter at 150 cc/hour
           (b) Can use up to 40 units per liter
           (c) Never give undiluted as a bolus injection
        (2) Intramuscular—10 units intramuscularly if no IV access
  2. Methylergonovine
     a. Causes a sustained, tetanic uterine contraction
     b. Can be used emergently as one-time dosing or as a series of doses for sustained effect
     c. Contraindicated in hypertensive patients because it causes peripheral vasoconstriction
     d. Administration
        (1) Intramuscular—0.2 mg IM, can be repeated once in 5 minutes, thereafter, every 2–4 hours
        (2) Oral
           (a) Generally given as a series of six doses over the first 24 hours postpartum
           (b) 0.2 mg orally every 6 hours
  3. Misoprostol
     a. Administration: 800 micrograms per rectum is usual dose
     b. Side effects—shivering, fever, diarrhea, and abdominal pain possible
  4. 15-methyl-F2alpha-prostaglandin (Hemabate)
     a. Used only in severe hemorrhage situations
     b. Administration
        (1) 250 micrograms
        (2) Can be given IM or intramyometrially
        (3) Contraindicated in women with asthma, active cardiac, pulmonary, renal, or hepatic disease
- Placental abnormalities and variations
  1. Battledore placenta—peripheral cord insertion, at placental margin

2. Succenturiate lobe
   a. Most common abnormality—occurrence 3%
   b. Accessory placental lobe within the fetal sac that had continuous vascular connections with main placenta
   c. Can cause retained placenta or hemorrhage
3. Velamentous cord insertion
   a. Cord insertion into fetal sac, not directly into placental bed, generally 5–10 cm away from placenta
   b. Can cause shearing of blood vessels during labor or delivery of placenta, causing hemorrhage
   c. More common in multiple gestation
4. Circumvallate placenta
   a. Opaque ring of fibrous-appearing tissue on fetal side of the placenta, caused by a double layer of chorion and amnion
   b. Can be seen in IUGR pregnancies but usually of no clinical significance

Management of Immediate Newborn Transition

- Apgar scoring
  1. Devised in 1952 by Dr. Virginia Apgar to identify infants requiring assistance adapting to the extrauterine environment
  2. Comparable to the biophysical profile scoring in utero
  3. Significance of scoring
     a. One-minute Apgar scoring reflects initial stabilization
     b. Five-minute Apgar scoring has a relationship to neonatal morbidity and mortality
        (1) Apgars of less than 7 at 5 minutes indicate need for pediatric/neonatal involvement
        (2) Apgars of less than 4 at 5 minutes correlate with neonatal mortality
        (3) Low Apgar scores by themselves are not predictive of later neurologic dysfunction
     c. Not as valid an assessment for preterm infants
- Indications for pediatric/neonatal involvement
  4. Any condition or circumstance that may compromise the adaptation of the neonate to extrauterine life
     a. Obstetric conditions
        (1) Known IUGR
        (2) Birth prior to 37 weeks
        (3) Oligohydramnios
        (4) Maternal systemic disease
        (5) Congenital abnormalities
     b. Intrapartum conditions
        (1) Opioid analgesia at less than 1 hour prior to birth
        (2) Chorioamnionitis
        (3) Operative delivery including Cesarean section
        (4) Category III fetal heart rate tracings

Special Considerations and Deviations from Normal

- Premature labor

1. Definitions
   a. Premature labor—onset of regular uterine contractions between 20 and 37 weeks' gestation with spontaneous rupture of membranes or progressive cervical changes
   b. Premature birth—delivery prior to 37 weeks' gestation
      (1) Very preterm: <32 0/7 weeks of gestation
      (2) Moderately preterm: 32 0/7 weeks of gestation through 33 6/7 weeks of gestation
      (3) Late preterm: 34 0/7 weeks of gestation through 36 6/7 weeks of gestation
   c. Term birth—delivery between 37 and 42 weeks' gestation
      (1) Early term: 37 0/7 weeks of gestation through 38 6/7 weeks of gestation
      (2) Full term: 39 0/7 weeks of gestation through 40 6/7 weeks of gestation
      (3) Late term: 41 0/7 weeks of gestation through 41 6/7 weeks of gestation
      (4) Postterm: 42 0/7 weeks of gestation and beyond
   d. Small for gestational age (SGA)—birth weight at less than 10th percentile for gestational age; corresponds to IUGR
2. Incidence—approximately 10% of all births in the United States
3. Etiology
   a. Idiopathic and multifactorial; in most cases the cause of premature labor is unknown
   b. Maternal factors
      (1) Systemic diseases
         (a) Hypertensive disorders of pregnancy
         (b) Renal disease
         (c) Autoimmune disease
         (d) Infection
      (2) Structural uterine abnormalities
         (a) Müllerian defects
         (b) Fibroids
      (3) Overdistended uterus
         (a) Multiple gestation
         (b) Polyhydramnios
      (4) Cervical insufficiency
      (5) History of premature labor
      (6) Low socioeconomic factors
   c. Fetal factors
      (1) Premature rupture of membranes—implicated in 30% of all premature labor
      (2) Fetal anomalies
      (3) Placental insufficiency
4. Signs and symptoms
   a. Menstrual-like cramping with increasing frequency and intensity
   b. Pelvic pressure, especially suprapubic
   c. Backache, especially low backache
   d. Passage of amniotic fluid
   e. Change in the character of vaginal secretions
   f. Bloody show/spotting
   g. Progressive cervical dilatation
5. Physical findings
   a. Uterine contractions documented by electronic fetal monitoring (EFM) or palpation
   b. Cervical dilation on digital examination

c. Documented ruptured membranes

6. Differential diagnosis
   a. Urinary tract infection/pyelonephritis
   b. Round ligament pain
   c. Braxton Hicks contractions
   d. Renal colic
   e. Appendicitis

7. Diagnostic tests to consider
   a. Fern and/or nitrazine test if suspect rupture of membranes
   b. Urinalysis with culture and sensitivity
   c. Other tests for suspected infections—chlamydia, gonococcal infection (GC), wet prep
   d. Fetal fibronectin—collect before digital examination; recent sexual activity or blood may affect results
   e. Ultrasound—cervical length and funneling, placental location and status, biophysical profile, and amniotic fluid index
   f. Amniocentesis—fetal surfactant and lecithin/sphingomyelin (L/S) ratio
   g. CBC with differential

8. Management—consultation with physician regarding need for transfer of care versus co-management
   a. Nonpharmacologic
      (1) Hydration
      (2) Left-lateral bed rest
   b. Tocolysis—generally used to delay birth more than 48 hours in order to give steroids to hasten lung maturity
      (1) Contraindications to tocolysis—any conditions causing a hostile uterine environment
         (a) Placental abruption
         (b) Chorioamnionitis
         (c) Severe pre-eclampsia
         (d) Placenta previa
         (e) Category III FHR tracing
         (f) Lethal fetal anomalies
         (g) IUGR without interval growth
      (2) Most effective tocolytics—calcium channel blockers (nifedipine)
         (a) Drug action—nonspecific smooth muscle relaxant; prevents influx of extracellular calcium ions into myometrial cells; effect not specific to uterus
         (b) Side effects
            i. Maternal hypotension
            ii. Flushing
            iii. Nausea/vomiting
         (c) Drug interactions
            i. Beta-agonists
            ii. Magnesium sulfate
         (d) Contraindications
            i. Do not use in presence of intrauterine infection, maternal hypertension, or cardiac disease
            ii. Do not use in combination with beta-agonists or magnesium sulfate
         (e) Administration and dosing
            i. Route—PO
            ii. Initial dose of 10 mg
            iii. If contractions continue, repeat doses every 20 minutes for total of 30 mg in 1 hour

iv. Once contractions decrease, may give 10 mg every 6 hours or 30–60 mg sustained release dose per day
         (3) Magnesium sulfate ($MgSO_4$)
            (a) Drug action—acts on vascular smooth muscle causing vasodilatation
            (b) Side effects
               i. Flushing
               ii. Palpitations
               iii. Feeling of warmth
               iv. Lethargy
               v. Muscle weakness
               vi. Dizziness
               vii. Nausea/vomiting
               viii. Respiratory depression
               ix. Pulmonary edema
            (c) Drug interactions—calcium channel blockers
            (d) Contraindications
               i. Do not use concurrently with calcium channel blockers
               ii. Toxic effects at serum level of more than 7 mg/dL
               iii. Antidote is calcium gluconate
            (e) Administration and dosing
               i. Generally IV, can be given IM
               ii. Loading dose 4–6 g in 100 cc intravenous fluid (IVF) over 20–30 minutes
               iii. Initial maintenance dose 2 g/hour
               iv. If contractions continue, increase by 0.5 g/hour every 30 minutes to a max dose of 4 g/hour
               v. Maintain at effective level for 12 to 24 hours after contractions stop
               vi. No benefit for weaning when discontinued
   c. Other management decisions
      (1) Group B streptococcal prophylaxis
         (a) Penicillin 5 million units IV followed by 2.5 million units every 4 hours until delivery
         (b) Clindamycin or vancomycin as alternative therapy if allergic to penicillin
      (2) Corticosteroid administration
         (a) Stimulates fetal lung maturity and possibly protection from intraventricular hemorrhage
         (b) Betamethasone 12 mg IM in 2 doses 24 hours apart OR
         (c) Dexamethasone 6 mg IM every 12 hours for 4 doses
         (d) Should attempt to delay birth until 24 hours post administration

• Umbilical cord prolapse
1. Definition—umbilical cord lies below or beside the presenting part; danger is compression of the umbilical cord, thus compromising the blood supply to the fetus
2. Etiology/incidence
   a. Presenting part does not fill the pelvic inlet; can occur with the rupturing of membranes
   b. Incidence—1 in 400 pregnancies
3. Signs and symptoms/physical findings
   a. Umbilical cord visible at or outside introitus

b. Palpation of cord during vaginal examination

c. Presumptive diagnosis of occult prolapse if prolonged fetal heart rate deceleration occurs immediately following rupture of membranes

4. Management

a. Elevate presenting part off cord by continuous vaginal examination

b. Assist mother into knee–chest position or steep left-lateral Trendelenburg

c. Do not attempt to manipulate the cord as this may cause cord spasm; if protruding, wrap loosely with warm normal saline-soaked gauze

d. Do not rely on cord pulsations as indicator of fetal status—obtain ultrasound if unable to detect fetal heart tones

e. Immediately alert consulting physician and other staff of emergency

f. Discontinue oxytocin infusion if applicable

g. O_2 at 10 L/min

h. Intravenous fluid bolus

i. Monitor FHR

j. Consider terbutaline for tocolysis

k. Prepare for Cesarean section

- Placenta previa

1. Definition—placenta is located over or very near the internal os

a. Complete placenta previa—placenta completely covers the cervical os

b. Partial placenta previa—cervical os partially covered by placenta

c. Marginal placenta previa—edge of placenta within 1 cm of cervical os

2. Etiology/predisposing factors

a. Increased parity

b. Advanced maternal age

c. Previous Cesarean section

d. Multiple gestation

3. Signs and symptoms

a. *Painless* vaginal bleeding during the third trimester 70–80% of the time

b. Bleeding with contractions 10–20%

c. Can be diagnosed before hallmark bleed with ultrasound

4. Physical findings—no digital vaginal exam until placenta location is known; contraindicated with placenta previa

5. Differential diagnosis—placental abruption

6. Diagnostic testing—ultrasound confirmation

7. Management

a. Acute bleeding requires emergency Cesarean section

b. Otherwise dependent on severity of symptoms and gestational age

c. Bed rest and/or hospitalization usually indicated

d. RhoGAM for unsensitized Rh-negative mother

e. Delivered by C-section

- Placental abruption

1. Definition—premature separation of the placenta from the uterine wall prior to delivery of the fetus

2. Etiology

a. Maternal hypertension

b. Severe abdominal trauma

c. Sudden decrease in uterine volume such as rupture of membranes with polyhydramnios or multiple gestation

d. Cocaine use

e. Tobacco use

f. Previous abruption

3. Incidence

a. 1 in 80 deliveries

b. Can be marginal abruption and not catastrophic

4. Signs and symptoms/physical findings

a. With complete abruption, *painful* vaginal bleeding, uterine rigidity, shock

b. Less than complete abruptions have less severe presentations

c. Bleeding can be concealed

5. Differential diagnosis—placenta previa

6. Diagnostic testing—ultrasound confirmation if placenta previa, ultrasound not very sensitive for placental abruption

7. Management

a. Complete abruption

(1) Notify consulting physician

(2) Insert two large-bore IV catheters

(3) Prepare for STAT C-section

(4) Obtain blood type and cross-match for blood products, including clotting factors

(5) Trendelenberg position

(6) O_2 at 10 L/min

(7) Monitor fetal status

b. Partial abruption

(1) IV access

(2) Monitor fetal status

(3) Preparation in the event immediate surgical intervention is required

- Shoulder dystocia

1. Definition—difficulty in delivery of shoulders secondary to anterior shoulder becoming impacted on the pelvic rim

2. Etiology/risk factors

a. Gestational diabetes

b. History of macrosomic babies

c. Maternal obesity

d. Increased weight gain during pregnancy

e. Small/abnormal/contracted pelvis

f. Prior history of shoulder dystocia

g. Estimated weight of fetus 1 lb larger than previous infants in a multiparous woman

3. Incidence—less than 1% of all births

4. Morbidity and mortality

a. Maternal—extensive vaginal and perineal lacerations

b. Fetal

(1) Fractured clavicle

(2) Brachial plexus injury

(3) Hypoxia/anoxia

(4) Fetal death

5. Signs and symptoms

a. "Turtle sign"—the immediate retraction of the fetal head against the perineum after extension

b. Delayed restitution or need for facilitated restitution without descent

c. Inability to deliver anterior shoulder with usual traction effort

6. Management

a. Anticipation of shoulder dystocia should be an indication or signal of need for emergency preparedness

b. Immediately have any physician paged STAT

c. Notify other staff, including anesthesia and the pediatrics team

d. Perform McRobert's maneuver—place mother in exaggerated lithotomy position (knees to shoulders)

e. Have suprapubic pressure (*not* fundal pressure) applied while exerting downward traction on baby's head while mother is pushing

f. Cut or extend episiotomy—controversial (and if performed, intent is to increase space for hands to perform necessary maneuvers); catheterize woman to empty bladder

g. Attempt to rotate shoulders to oblique and repeat McRobert's maneuver and suprapubic pressure—insert a hand on either side of the fetal chest and attempt to rotate shoulders out of the anteroposterior diameter

h. Attempt Wood's screw maneuver

(1) Using the same techniques

(2) Rotate fetus 180 degrees (keeping the back anterior)

(3) If still impacted, continue rotation another 180 degrees

i. Have woman turn to knee–chest position (Gaskin maneuver)—may be difficult with epidural

j. Deliver posterior arm

(1) Insert hand behind posterior shoulder

(2) Splint arm and sweep across abdomen and chest until the hand can be grasped externally

k. Break the anterior clavicle—place thumbs along clavicle and force clavicle outward; controversial as have possibility of puncturing lung or injuring subclavian vessels

l. Zavanelli maneuver—rotate and flex head while replacing fetus into pelvic cavity followed by immediate C-section; controversial as associated with significant risk of infant morbidity and mortality

- Breech delivery—the elective vaginal delivery of infants in the breech presentation is no longer recommended by the American College of Obstetricians and Gynecologists. Vaginal delivery of breech presentation should be reserved only for breeches that present emergently and when birth is essentially inevitable

1. Definition—delivery of infant presenting with buttocks, feet, or knees

a. Complete breech—legs and thighs are flexed with buttocks presenting

b. Frank breech—legs extended on abdomen with flexed thighs and buttocks presenting; most common type of breech presentation

c. Footling breech—one or both feet presenting

d. Knee presentation—single or double knees are presenting (most rare)

e. Spontaneous vaginal breech delivery—birth without additional external assistance

f. Assisted vaginal delivery (partial breech extraction)—spontaneous delivery to the umbilicus, remainder of the body delivered with assistance

g. Total breech extraction—entire body extracted by birth attendant

2. Incidence

a. 3–4% at term

b. At 28 weeks, 25% of all fetuses are breech

c. Most convert to cephalic by 34 weeks' gestation

3. Etiology/risk factors

a. Presentation possibly related to the fetus accommodating to the shape of the uterus

(1) Preterm fetuses position the head in the upper portion of the uterus being the larger portion of the body

(2) At term, the largest part of the fetus is the head, thus causing it to descend into the pelvis

b. Maternal indications

(1) Gestational age

(2) Fibroids

(3) Uterine anomalies

(4) Abnormal placentation

(a) Placenta previa

(b) Cornual fundal implantation

(5) Oligohydramnios/polyhydramnios

c. Fetal factors

(1) Congenital anomalies—threefold increase in anomalies with breech presentation

(2) Short umbilical cord

4. Morbidity/mortality

a. Cord prolapse (1.5% of frank breech and 10% in other breech presentations)

b. Traumatic vaginal delivery

(1) Largest part of the fetus is delivered last

(2) Head entrapment causing injury to organs, brain, and skull

c. Increased perinatal morbidity and mortality

5. Management and treatment

a. Vaginal breech birth is a co-management situation

b. Criteria for candidates of vaginal breech birth

(1) Frank breech presentation

(2) EFW 2500–3800 g

(3) Flexion of the fetal head

c. Management decisions

(1) Continuous fetal monitoring

(2) IV access

(3) Use of oxytocin for protraction disorders very controversial; generally Cesarean section is indicated

(4) Generous episiotomy

(5) Empty bladder before second stage

(6) Should deliver as a double setup in operating room

6. Delivery sequence for partial breech extraction

a. "Hands off the breech" until the body is born to the umbilicus

b. Second provider should be maintaining head flexion through the abdominal wall during entire descent

c. Pull down loop of cord

d. From this point on, the mother is instructed to push continuously
e. If the legs have not delivered spontaneously, they should be gently guided out of the vagina
f. Downward traction then applied with the hands to baby's hips with thumbs in the sacroiliac region to encourage delivery of the anterior scapula
g. Attendant delivers anterior arm by moving hand up the infant's back and over the top of the anterior shoulder sweeping the arm down across the chest and under the pubis with attendant's finger
h. The infant is raised so the posterior arm can be delivered in the same manner
i. The back should spontaneously rotate anteriorly; it is important to NOT let the head rotate to the occiput posterior (OP) position
j. Employ the Mauriceau-Smellie-Veit maneuver to maintain flexion of the head if needed
   (1) With dominant hand palmar side up, place extended index finger in baby's mouth with chest and body resting on palm and legs straddling forearm
   (2) The other hand is placed on top of the baby with the index finger on one side and middle finger on the other side of the neck extending over the shoulder for traction
k. Again apply downward traction until the suboccipital region (the hairline is seen coming under the pubic symphysis)
l. Now apply upward traction while elevating body to deliver the head via the curve of Carus

- Face presentation
  1. Definition—cephalic presentation with attitude of head in complete extension with occiput proximal to the spine; usually begins labor as a brow presentation
  2. Incidence 1 in 250 births, higher in multiparas
  3. Etiology
     a. Can be an indicator of CPD
     b. Multiple loops of nuchal cord
     c. Tumors of the neck
     d. Anencephalic fetus
  4. Risk factors
     a. If mentum is not anterior, fetus is unable to pass under the pubic symphysis
  5. Diagnosis
     a. During Leopold's maneuver, occipital bone is easily palpated and prominent; head feels larger than expected, cephalic prominence located on same side as fetal back
     b. During vaginal examination, facial landmarks can be palpated
  6. Management
     a. Review clinical pelvimetry to ensure pelvic adequacy
     b. Confirm position is mentum anterior because mentum posterior is contraindicated for vaginal birth
     c. Collaborate with consulting physician if protraction disorder occurs
     d. Pediatric attendance at the birth
- Twin gestation—intrapartum twins are always a collaborative management situation
  1. Definitions—multiple gestation with two fetuses in the uterus

a. Monozygotic twins—zygotic division between 4 and 8 days
   (1) Identical twins
   (2) One placenta
   (3) Generally one chorion, two amnions
b. Dizygotic twins
   (1) Fraternal twins
   (2) Two placentas
   (3) Two chorions, two amnions
2. Incidence
   a. Monozygotic twinning rate stable at 1 per 250 births
   b. Dizygotic twinning rates increasing as a result of assisted reproductive technologies
3. Predisposing factors
   a. Family history
   b. Ovulation induction/in vitro fertilization
   c. Sub-Saharan African descent
4. Diagnosis
   a. Size larger than dates
   b. Auscultation of more than one fetal heartbeat
   c. Abnormal Leopold's maneuver findings
   d. Ultimate diagnosis by ultrasound
5. Morbidity
   a. Premature labor and birth
   b. Premature rupture of membranes
   c. Malpresentation of second twin
   d. Cord prolapse
   e. Operative delivery for second twin
   f. SGA and IUGR babies
   g. Twin-to-twin transfusion
6. Management decisions
   a. Physician should be collaborating for all intrapartum decisions and present for the birth
   b. Ultrasound confirmation of presentation
   c. Intravenous catheter insertion
   d. Type and screen blood upon admission; some facilities require type and cross-match
   e. Continuous fetal monitoring
   f. Anesthesia presence for birth
   g. Pediatric attendance for birth
   h. Ultrasound machine in delivery room
   i. Bladder should be emptied prior to pushing
7. Management
   a. Birth of the first twin in usual fashion—if nuchal cord is present, *do not* cut cord, attempt birth with cord intact
   b. Upon delivery, clamp cord and transfer baby to pediatric team
   c. Assistant can guide second twin into the pelvis depending upon presentation
   d. Confirm presentation of second twin based on ultrasound
   e. Timing of delivery is dependent upon fetal status
   f. Oxytocin augmentation can be used if contractions do not resume
   g. Birth of second twin
   h. Observe for postpartum hemorrhage
- Retained placenta
  1. Definition—placenta that has not separated from uterine wall after 60 minutes

2. Predisposing factors
   a. Premature delivery
   b. Chorioamnionitis
   c. Prior Cesarean section
   d. Placenta previa
   e. Grand multiparity
3. Etiology
   a. Structurally abnormal uterus
   b. Abnormal placentation—incidence has increased with increasing Cesarean rates
      (1) Placenta accreta—adherence to myometrium due to partial or total absence of decidua
      (2) Placenta increta—further extension into the myometrium with penetration into the uterine wall
      (3) Placenta percreta—further extension through the uterine wall to the serosa layer
4. Management
   a. Facilitate usual methods of placental separation
      (1) Allow baby to nurse/nipple stimulation
      (2) Assist mother into squatting position
      (3) Empty maternal bladder
   b. If third stage is more than 30 minutes, consider that placenta is retained; notify consulting physician
   c. Management in preparation for consulting physician
      (1) Monitor for bleeding or shock
      (2) Insert IV if none in place
      (3) Prepare mother for manual placenta removal
      (4) Notify anesthesia

- Postpartum hemorrhage
  1. Definition—blood loss of more than 500 cc for vaginal birth
     a. Immediate—within first 24 hours
     b. Delayed—after the first 24 hours but within the first 6 weeks
  2. Etiology
     a. Predisposing factors
        (1) History of postpartum hemorrhage
        (2) Grand multiparity
        (3) Overdistended uterus
           (a) Multiple gestation
           (b) Polyhydramnios
           (c) Macrosomia
     b. Intrapartum factors
        (1) Induced or augmented labor
        (2) Prolonged labor
        (3) Precipitous labor
        (4) Uterine atony
  3. Management
     a. Notify consulting physician
     b. Uterine massage, if related to atony
     c. Medications
        (1) Oxytocin
        (2) Methylergonovine
        (3) Misoprostol
     d. IV fluid bolus
     e. Bimanual compression if other measures unsuccessful
     f. Consider manual removal of placenta if not delivered
     g. Consider vaginal, sulcus, cervical lacerations as cause of bleeding

The Normal Postpartum

- Database
  1. Pregnancy highlights
     a. Gravidity/parity
     b. Obstetric history
     c. Pertinent medical history
     d. Pertinent pregnancy diagnostic tests
        (1) Blood type and Rh
        (2) Rubella titer status
        (3) Hepatitis B status
        (4) HIV status
  2. Birth information
     a. Type of birth
        (1) Type of delivery
        (2) Type of episiotomy/laceration
        (3) Type of operative birth
        (4) Reason for interventions
     b. Type of anesthesia/analgesia
     c. Sex of baby
     d. Weight of baby
     e. Apgar scores
     f. Method of feeding
- Physiologic and anatomic changes
  1. Uterus
     a. Immediately contracts to 2/3 to ¾ of the way between the umbilicus and symphysis pubis, but by 12 hours postdelivery is at the level of the umbilicus
     b. By 2 weeks, no longer palpated abdominally
     c. By 6 weeks, returns to slightly larger than prepregnant size
     d. Involution—process of the uterus returning to the prepregnant state
        (1) Involves three steps
           (a) Contraction of the uterus
           (b) Autolysis of myometrial cells
           (c) Regeneration of the epithelium
        (2) Results from cell size reduction not cell number reduction
  2. Lochia
     a. Consists of the breakdown of myometrial placental bed, eschar and decidual cells
     b. Three stages of discharge
        (1) Rubra—first 24–72 hours, superficial layer of decidua sloughs with debris and necrotic remains of the placenta
        (2) Serosa—from day 3 to day 10, serous to serosanguinous secretion
        (3) Alba—until cessation of flow, yellowish or white discharge
     c. Flow increases with additional activity initially but decreases progressively over the puerperium
     d. Total amount 150 to 400 cc
  3. Cervix, vagina, and perineum
     a. Cervix
        (1) Initially appears edematous, dilated 3–4 cm and bruised

(2) At 7 days, 1 cm dilated and by day 10–12, fingertip dilated

(3) Nonpregnant appearance and texture 1 month postdelivery

(4) Multiparous—at completion of involution, external os does not return to its prepregnant appearance; remains somewhat wider with a transverse opening resembling a "fish-mouth"

b. Vagina

(1) Initially edematous, relaxed, sometimes bruised with decreased tone

(2) Rugae return by 3 weeks postpartum

c. Perineum

(1) Edematous with decreased tone immediately after birth

(2) Laceration and episiotomy repair should be well approximated

(3) Skin should appear healed at 7 days with only linear scarring at 6 weeks

4. Breasts

a. Colostrum is produced upon birth of baby

b. Engorgement occurs approximately 72 hours after birth

(1) Human milk production begins in the upper-outer milk glands

(2) Filling then occurs medially and inferiorly

(3) Distention and stasis of vascular and lymphatic circulation causes engorgement as the ducts, lobules, and alveoli fill with milk

c. Milk ejection reflex develops within the first 1 to 2 weeks

5. Hematologic

a. Within the first hours post delivery, cardiac output increases 60–80%

b. Over first 48 hours, as diuresis occurs plasma volume decreases and cardiac output normalizes by 2 weeks

c. Transient bradycardia occurs in first 1–2 days postpartum

d. Can have transient leukocytosis in initial 48 hours

6. Renal system changes

a. Diuresis occurs within first 5 days as a result of extravascular fluid shifts

b. Bladder can be hypotonic and edematous immediately after the birth; resolves within 24 hours

7. Weight loss

a. Weight loss of up to 15 pounds initially, may return to prepregnant weight by 6 weeks postpartum

b. Weight loss facilitated by breastfeeding secondary to increased caloric requirements (350–500 calories more per day)

8. Gastrointestinal changes

a. Peristalsis decreased in first 24 hours; increases risk of ileus after Cesarean section

b. Liver enzymes including AST and ALT return to prepregnant values within 2 weeks

9. Abdominal changes

a. Diastasis recti found in 75–80% of postpartum women—if diastasis after the postpartum period, future pregnancies will lack sufficient abdominal support leading to back pain

b. Striae common in most postpartum women

10. Endocrine

a. Breastfeeding women

(1) Lactation is stimulated and prolactin secreted

(2) By negative feedback mechanism, ovulation and menstruation are inhibited by increased prolactin and resulting estrogen suppression

(3) Resumption of menses is variable with supplementation or food introduction

(a) Generally ovulation occurs 14–30 days after weaning

(b) First menses 14 days later

(c) Mean time to ovulation is 190 days

b. Nonbreastfeeding women

(1) Prolactin levels fall after initial engorgement

(2) Hormonal shifts to stimulate ovulation begin approximately 3–4 weeks postpartum

(3) First menses at 6–8 weeks postpartum, 70% by 12 weeks

11. Vital signs

a. Temperature

(1) Stabilizes during the first 24 hours postpartum

(2) Should not be over 100.4°F

b. Pulse

(1) Should remain within normal limits

(2) More than 100 bpm could be significant for infection or posthemorrhage anemia

c. Respiratory rate—remains normal

d. Blood pressure

(1) Remains normal

(2) Blood pressure of greater than 140/90 mm Hg, evaluate for postpartum preeclampsia

(3) Blood pressure of less than 90/60 mm Hg, evaluate causes of hypotension

(a) Blood loss

(b) Medication reaction

Assessment of Maternal Response to Baby

- Early attachment and bonding
1. First hour after birth—maternal sensitive period, benefits of immediate, continuous skin-to-skin contact during first hour of life

a. Initial bonding occurs during this time

b. Mother and baby should *NOT* be separated

c. Signs of attachment

(1) Initial touching with fingertips progressing to entire hand with stroking and massaging baby

(2) "En face" posturing between mother and baby

(3) Using high-pitched speaking voice

(4) Bonding is facilitated during the first hour of life, the quiet alert phase for the baby

2. Attachment
   a. Privacy should be arranged for parents as soon as possible after the birth
   b. Attachment is a progressive process during the initial postpartum period
- Psychological response to childbearing
  1. Positive reactions
     a. Sense of achievement in giving birth
     b. Sense of empowerment and strength
     c. Thrill of new baby
  2. Negative reactions
     a. Sense of loss if birth was not as anticipated
     b. Feeling of mistrust of body if unable to complete the birth process or if birth was premature
- Postpartum blues and depression
  1. Postpartum blues
     a. 80% of all women
     b. Begins within 3–5 days of birth, concurrent with profound hormonal shifts
     c. Very labile emotions (giddiness through sadness and crying), usually defy explanation
     d. Generally time limited over 1–2 weeks
     e. Supportive, sensitive care is usually all that is required
  2. Postpartum depression/psychosis
     a. Approximately 10% incidence of depression, true postpartum psychosis in less than 1% of women
     b. Onset of symptoms around 4–6 weeks, generally worsen over time
     c. Symptoms are the same as for major depression in nonpostpartum woman
     d. Symptoms can incapacitate women
        (1) Unable to perform activities of daily living
        (2) Can have suicidal or homicidal ideation
        (3) Apathy toward themselves and their babies
     e. Symptoms do not improve over time; more likely they worsen
     f. Diagnosis—screen all postpartum women for depression with scale such as Edinburgh Postnatal Depression Scale; rule out postpartum thyroiditis, anemia, infection, sleep deprivation
     g. Require psychiatric evaluation and treatment usually including medication
     h. Women previously treated for clinical depression have increased risk of postpartum depression
     i. Psychosis—disorganized thinking, behavior, speech; auditory or visual perceptual disturbances; delusions—medical emergency!
- Grief
  1. Can be related to losing a pregnancy, having a viable baby but not meeting expectations (i.e., congenital anomalies or organic cause, such as postpartum depression)
  2. Stages of grief
     a. Shock
     b. Suffering
     c. Resolution

Management Plan for the Postpartum Period

- Evaluation of maternal well-being
- Chart review
- History
  1. Family history
  2. Past medical, surgical, and obstetric history
  3. Review of prenatal care
  4. Review of intrapartum period
  5. Infant data
- Physical examination
  1. Vital signs
  2. General appearance and affect
  3. Breasts
     a. Condition of breasts and nipples
     b. Status of milk production
  4. Abdominal examination
     a. Uterine fundal examination
     b. Abdominal musculature
     c. Bladder status
  5. Perineum
     a. REEDA (redness, ecchymosis, erythema, drainage, and approximation)
     b. Lochia
     c. Status of lacerations/episiotomy
     d. Hemorrhoids
  6. Extremities
     a. Calf tenderness and warmth
     b. Edema
     c. Varicosities
  7. Pain assessment
  8. Emotional status
- Diet—after normal birth, regular diet immediately postpartum
- Activity
  1. Out of bed as desired
  2. Should be escorted out of bed for the first time, secondary to risk of syncope
- Hygiene
  1. Should receive instructions in perineal care
  2. Topical anesthetics if indicated
- Contraception
  1. Nonbreastfeeding women may ovulate prior to the 6-week visit; therefore, birth control should be offered prior to discharge
  2. Hormonal methods (combination hormonal methods—pills, patch, vaginal ring; progestin-only methods—progestin-only pills, depot medroxyprogesterone acetate [DMPA], subdermal implant, levonorgestrel intrauterine contraception)
     a. Combination hormonal methods not indicated for breastfeeding women initially postpartum and because postpartum woman is still in a hypercoagulable state until about 6 weeks after delivery
     b. DMPA, progestin-only pills, subdermal implant, and intrauterine contraception (IUC) types are good choices for breastfeeding women

3. Barrier methods
   a. Cervical cap/diaphragm—cannot be fit until involution is complete
   b. Male and female condoms—can be used immediately
4. Spermicides
   a. Foam, cream, vaginal contraceptive film, sponge
   b. Should delay use until lochia ceases
5. Intrauterine contraception (IUC)—levonorgestrel or copper-containing
   a. Can be placed immediately post delivery but has a 30% expulsion rate
   b. If not placed within 48 hours postpartum, need to wait until 4 to 6 weeks postpartum
6. Lactational amenorrhea method
   a. Full or nearly full breastfeeding
      (1) Feeding an average of every 4 hours during the day
      (2) Feeding an average of every 6 hours at night
      (3) Has not substituted solid foods for breastfeeding for any meals
   b. Infant less than 6 months old
   c. No menses
   d. Choose alternative method if woman and infant do not fit all three criteria
7. Tubal ligation
   a. Permanent method of contraception
   b. Most easily accomplished during hospital stay
   c. Generally need to obtain consent prior to birth
- Diagnostic tests
  1. Complete blood count
     a. Commonly performed first morning after birth
     b. Only profound anemia will change management
  2. Cord blood testing for blood type, Rh, and Coombs
  3. Kleihauer–Betke screen if Rh negative
- Immunizations
  1. Rubella vaccine may be given prior to discharge if not immune to rubella
  2. RhoGAM within 72 hours of birth if indicated

Postpartal Discomforts

- Involutional pain
  1. Uncommon in primigravidas, increases in intensity with each subsequent birth
  2. Increases with nursing
  3. Nonpharmacologic relief
     a. Maintain empty bladder and bowels
     b. Prone position may relieve pain
  4. Pharmacologic relief
     a. Acetaminophen, ibuprofen
     b. Opioids such as codeine—use with caution because some women are ultrametabolizers, thus putting infants at risk for respiratory depression due to rapid maternal conversion of codeine to morphine
- Diuresis—maintain fluids to prevent dehydration
- Breast engorgement
  1. Initiate breastfeeding early and often
  2. Supportive brassiere
  3. Warm compresses
  4. If bottle feeding, tight brassiere, ice packs, analgesics, reassurance about time limitation, iced cabbage leaves for comfort
- Perineal pain
  1. Evaluate by REEDA
  2. Topical medications/treatments
     a. Witch hazel pads
     b. Dibucaine, benzocaine
     c. Sitz baths
- Constipation
  1. Increase fluids and fiber; stool softener
  2. Encourage ambulation
  3. Laxatives
- Hemorrhoids
  1. Ice packs
  2. Topical anesthetics
  3. Referral if thrombosed

Questions

Select the best answer.

1. At 38 weeks' gestation, Ms. Jones presents to your birth center complaining of a small amount of watery, clear-to-whitish vaginal discharge for the past 8 hours. She has been having Braxton Hicks contractions for a couple of days; the baby is moving on a regular basis, but now she just "does not feel right." What would you do in your initial assessment related to her presenting symptoms?
   a. Obtain 20-minute fetal monitor strip to ensure reactivity
   • b. Perform sterile speculum exam to R/O rupture of membranes versus vaginal infection
   c. Contact consulting physician regarding premature rupture of membranes protocol
   d. Send Ms. Jones home with reassurance and instructions to rest until better labor pattern is established
2. Mrs. Hogan, a 37-year-old G4 P0 at 35 weeks, presents saying she is having bright red bleeding and clots for 2 hours since intercourse with her husband. She has saturated 2 pads in 2 hours. She is *not* having any pain. The most probable diagnosis is:
   • a. Placenta previa
   b. Cervical irritation from intercourse
   c. Placental abruption
   d. Normal bloody show
3. Tocolysis of premature labor contractions is most effectively achieved by:
   a. NSAIDs
   • b. Calcium channel blockers such as nifedipine

c. Intravenous fluids

d. Oxytocics

4. Which client is most at risk for placental abruption?

   a. 19-year-old G2 P0010 in preterm labor at 35 weeks

   b. 28-year-old G1 smoker pregnant with twins with spontaneous rupture of membranes at 37 weeks

   c. 28-year-old G3 P2002 with induced labor at 41 weeks

   d. 41-year-old G1 pregnant who had low-lying placenta in first trimester

5. What is the major risk of multifetal gestation?

   a. Eclampsia

   b. Gestational diabetes

   c. Cephalopelvic disproportion

   d. Preterm birth

6. The cardinal movements of labor and birth for occiput anterior position are which of the following?

   a. Flexion, descent, internal rotation, extension, restitution, external rotation

   b. Descent, flexion, extension, internal rotation, external rotation, restitution

   c. Descent, flexion, internal rotation, extension, restitution, external rotation

   d. Descent, flexion, internal rotation, extension, external rotation, restitution

7. The cardinal movement responsible for the birth of the fetal head in the cephalic presentation is:

   a. Flexion

   b. Restitution

   c. Extension

   d. External rotation

8. The definition of postpartum hemorrhage is:

   a. Blood loss in excess of 500 cc or more after the third stage of labor

   b. Blood loss in excess of 750 cc during the entire labor

   c. Blood loss of more than 500 cc before a C-section

   d. Blood loss of 750 cc or more after the third stage of labor

9. Which of the following statements concerning Apgar scores is correct?

   a. Scoring is especially useful in assessment of the preterm infant

   b. Scoring is less useful when the infant is postterm

   c. A score of less than 7 at 1 minute correlates with increased neonatal morbidity

   d. Five-minute scoring has a relationship to neonatal morbidity and mortality

10. Infants born to mothers with gestational diabetes are at increased risk for:

   a. Hyperbilirubinema

   b. IUGR

   c. Hyperglycemia

   d. Shoulder dystocia

11. A client who is a G3 P2002 at 38 weeks presents with regular uterine contractions every 4–6 minutes for 60 seconds for the past 8 hours. Her vaginal exam is 2 cm/30%/−2, vertex with intact membranes. She is very uncomfortable with the contractions and declines discharge to home at this time. At this time, the patient is in:

   a. Transitional labor

   b. Latent labor

   c. Active labor

   d. Not in labor

12. For the client described in the previous question, your management plan at this time is:

   a. Discharge home with instructions

   b. Ambulate for 2 hours and then reassess

   c. Contact consulting physician for augmentation of labor

   d. Need additional information prior to formulating a plan

13. Three hours later, you reassess this client. Contractions are now every 4 minutes for 60 seconds. Her exam is 3 cm/50%/−2, vertex with intact membranes. The fetal heart rate is 150 bpm with audible accelerations by Doppler. At this time your client is in:

   a. Prolonged latent phase

   b. Latent phase of labor

   c. Active phase of labor

   d. Cannot make a determination based on this information

14. Nine hours later the client has the same contraction pattern every 4 minutes for 60 seconds. Her exam is now 3 cm/100%/0, vertex with intact membranes. The fetal heart rate remains in the 140s to 150s with audible accelerations. The client is exhausted and is no longer coping well with the contractions and "just wants it over." Your diagnosis at this time is:

   a. Latent phase of labor

   b. Prolonged latent phase of labor

   c. Arrested labor

   d. Protracted active phase of labor

15. Your management plan at this time is:

   a. Discharge home with encouragement and instructions to return when the contractions become closer

   b. Contact consulting physician regarding your plan for oxytocin augmentation

   c. Encourage her to continue with her original plan for an unmedicated childbirth

   d. Offer medication of morphine 10 mg IM so she can get some sleep and potentially correct this dysfunctional labor pattern

16. C.S. presents to your office stating she is pregnant, and she wants to know her due date. The first day of her last period was February 4. Her due date by menstrual dating (Naegele's rule) would be:

   a. November 11

   b. October 28

   c. May 11

   d. November 4

17. The denominator of breech presentation is the:

   a. Symphysis pubis

   b. Sacrum

   c. Feet

   d. Shoulders

18. Your client is in active labor and is making appropriate progress thus far. Currently, her exam is 6 cm/100%/−2, vertex with intact membranes. During your exam, you notice the position of the vertex is LOT and sagittal suture of the fetus is closer to the maternal sacrum. Your diagnosis at this time is:

   a. Deep transverse pelvic arrest

   b. Anterior asynclitism

  c. Failure to descend

  d. Posterior asynclitism

19. Your management plan for this patient would be:

  a. Artificial rupture of membranes

  b. Epidural anesthesia

  c. Pitocin augmentation

  d. Encourage movement and position change

20. On the monitor strip of the same client, you notice the fetal heart rate has intermittently been 100–110 bpm for 20–30 seconds at a time for the past 10–15 minutes with good return to the baseline of 140 bpm. You would document this as:

  a. Variable decelerations

  b. Late decelerations

  c. Fetal bradycardia

  d. Cannot determine from this information

21. The most favorable diameter of the fetal head to present in labor is the:

  a. Verticomental

  b. Submentobregmatic

  c. Occipitofrontal

  d. Suboccipitobregmatic

22. Intermittent auscultation of the fetal heart rate during labor is:

  a. Inferior to continuous electronic fetal monitoring

  b. Acceptable only for out-of-hospital birth

  c. Acceptable for the fetal monitoring of certain patients

  d. Correlated to lower Apgar scores than for babies born after continuous fetal monitoring

23. Your patient states that she does *not* want an episiotomy no matter what happens. Your management of this situation would be:

  a. Discuss the indications for episiotomy and reinforce that you would obtain consent prior to performing the procedure if necessary

  b. Teach her perineal massage antenatally and hope that she will not need an episiotomy

  c. Explain to her that skilled midwives never perform episiotomies

  d. Explain that because this is her first baby she will probably need an episiotomy to prevent serious laceration

24. A client presents while you are covering Labor and Delivery. She is a 33-year-old G3 P2002 at term in labor with ruptured membranes. Your exam reveals 5 cm/90% effaced/0 station, but you are unable to palpate fontanels or sutures. You suspect that you feel the orbital ridge in the anteroposterior diameter and the chin at 3 o'clock. If this is the case, what is the presentation?

  a. ROT

  b. LMT

  c. RMT

  d. ROA

25. Three hours later, the same client is completely dilated/100% effaced/0 station with an urge to push. Your exam now reveals that the presentation is MA. What would your next step be?

  a. Prepare client for urgent C-section

  b. Manually attempt to flex the fetal head

  c. Encourage patient to push as effectively as possible

  d. Allow patient to push only in the hands and knees position to allow the fetal head to rotate

26. During an assisted breech birth, if a nuchal arm is encountered, what should you do?

  a. Exert steady downward traction on the entire fetus

  b. Slowly rotate the infant 180 degrees to attempt to dislodge the arm

  c. Raise the baby in a warm towel above the plane of the vagina

  d. Sweep the arm down by hooking the elbow and pulling the arm down

27. The most common cause of postpartum hemorrhage is:

  a. Sulcus tears

  b. Episiotomy extensions to third- and fourth-degree lacerations

  c. Uterine atony

  d. Cervical lacerations

28. The process of involution takes place over which of the following time frames?

  a. The first 6 weeks postpartum

  b. The first 24 hours postpartum

  c. The first 2 weeks postpartum

  d. The first year postpartum

29. The following is the clinical picture of your client. She is a G1 P0 at 39 weeks with an uncomplicated pregnancy. Her labor started at 4:00 a.m. with regular contractions. She was admitted at 8:00 a.m. when her exam was 2–3 cm/100%/–2 station, vertex, membranes intact.

  At 12:00 p.m., her exam was 3–4 cm/100%/–2, intact.

  At 4:00 p.m., her exam was 4 cm/100%/–2, intact.

  At 7:30 p.m., her exam was 5–6 cm/100%/–1, intact.

  At 8:15 p.m., she ruptured membranes for light meconium-stained fluid.

  At 10:00 p.m., her exam was 8 cm/100%/0 station.

  Based on the information provided, at 12:00 p.m. what was the most appropriate diagnosis related to your client's labor progress?

  a. Latent phase

  b. Protracted latent phase

  c. Unable to make determination with this information

  d. Active labor

30. For this patient, at 7:30 p.m. what was the most appropriate diagnosis?

  a. Unable to make determination based on the information provided

  b. Active phase of labor

  c. Latent phase of labor

  d. Arrest of labor in the active phase

31. At 10:00 p.m., she requests something for pain because she states the pain is intolerable now and she is feeling increased pelvic pressure. What would *not* be indicated for pain relief at this time?

  a. Epidural anesthesia

  b. Intravenous opioids

  c. Pudendal anesthesia

  d. Paracervical block

32. At 10:50 p.m., you notice on the fetal monitor strip early decelerations that occur with every contraction. The baseline heart rate is in the 140s with average variability. What do you suspect the cause of these decelerations is?

a. Maternal hypotension

b. Head compression

c. Uteroplacental insufficiency

d. Fetal distress related to the meconium fluid

33. The benefit of placing an internal scalp electrode on a fetus in labor is:

a. The ability to have a continuous tracing when external monitoring is insufficient

b. The ability to detect decelerations

c. It keeps the client in bed

d. The ability to assess variability

34. If you are performing scalp stimulation, what is the fetal response that indicates fetal well-being?

a. A FHR deceleration to 100 bpm for 2 minutes

b. An acceleration of 5 bpm over baseline for 5 seconds

c. A variable deceleration

d. A fetal heart rate acceleration of 15 bpm for 15 seconds

35. What is the most common position for birth?

a. ROA

b. LOA

c. ROP

d. LOP

36. The long arc rotation is most commonly performed by babies beginning labor in which presentation?

a. LOP

b. LSA

c. ROA

d. LOA

37. In the second stage of labor, how frequently should the BP of low-risk women be checked?

a. Every 30 minutes

b. Every 2 minutes

c. Every 60 minutes

d. Every 15 minutes

38. When is the most appropriate time to administer pudendal anesthesia for perineal pain relief in the multiparous client?

a. For the repair of any laceration or episiotomy

b. When the head distends the perineum and client complains of the "ring of fire"

c. When the vertex is at +2

d. At approximately 8–9 cm dilated

39. What is the largest group of muscles in the pelvic musculature?

a. Levator ani

b. Pubococcygeus

c. Bulbocavernosus

d. Sphincter ani

40. In a second-degree laceration, which structure is *not* involved?

a. Vaginal mucosa

b. Deep transverse perineal muscles

c. Rectal sphincter

d. Hymenal ring

41. The Ritgen maneuver is used to:

a. Slow down the descent of the fetal head during birth

b. Control expulsion of the fetal head at the time of birth

c. Avoid lacerations or the need for an episiotomy

d. Assist in the delivery of the fetal head during extension

42. What complication may be encountered if a placenta is delivered by the Duncan mechanism?

a. Increased perineal lacerations

b. Increased bleeding

c. Increased hemorrhoids due to extra maternal pushing effort

d. Uterine inversion

43. Which of the following would *not* be included in the differential diagnosis of premature labor?

a. Urinary tract infection

b. Appendicitis

c. Renal colic

d. Heartburn

44. The fetal heart rate variability is predominantly controlled by:

a. The parasympathetic/sympathetic nervous system

b. The baroreceptors

c. The chemoreceptors

d. The central nervous system

45. During uterine contractions, intervillous blood flow to the placenta

a. Increases

b. Decreases

c. Remains unchanged

d. Has not been studied in humans

46. Moderate variability of the fetal heart rate is a change of how many beats per minute from the baseline?

a. Fewer than 2

b. 2–6

c. 6–25

d. > 25

47. Which of the following would *not* cause an alteration in the variability of the fetal heart rate?

a. Medications

b. Congenital cardiac anomalies of the fetus

c. Placenta previa

d. Fetal activity patterns

48. Your client, who you are co-managing with your consulting physician, is 33 weeks and 4 days pregnant admitted with premature labor with a cervical exam of 2–3 cm/80%/−1, vertex, intact. She is currently on $MgSO_4$ at 3.0 g/hour with occasional contractions. During rounds, she complains of feeling flushed and hot, lethargic, and sort of short of breath, which usually gets better when she changes position. Which response would be best to address her complaints?

a. "The $MgSO_4$ commonly makes you feel like this, but hopefully they will start weaning the medication today"

b. "Well, because you are almost 34 weeks, I could ask the doctor if we can discontinue the medication now"

c. "I do not think that you should be having shortness of breath like you are; I am going to have the physician see you and order a chest radiograph"

d. "Being a little uncomfortable is so much better than giving birth to a 33-week-old infant"

49. Which of the following conditions would *not* necessitate continuous fetal monitoring?

a. Labor at 41 weeks and 1 day

b. Thick meconium-stained fluid

c. Nonreactive NST who is now in labor

d. IV narcotics

50. Mothers in premature labor are given glucocorticosteroids to:

a. Help stop the uterine contractions

b. Prevent infections, especially chorioamnionitis

c. Speed the maturation of the fetal respiratory system, including the production of surfactant

d. Prevent muscle wasting commonly seen in bed rest patients

51. Kelly Jones, a G3 P2002 at 37 weeks and 1 day, presents to Labor and Delivery with regular contractions every 2–3 minutes for 5 hours. Your vaginal exam reveals 6 cm/100%/–2, LSA with ruptured membranes positive for light meconium. What is your next step?

a. Admit for expectant management

b. Discuss with Kelly her birth plan

c. Await a reactive tracing before making a management plan

d. Notify your consulting physician and prepare for a C-section

52. A complete breech presentation is described as:

a. One or two feet are the presenting part

b. Legs and thighs are flexed with buttocks presenting

c. The baby is flexed at the hips

d. The knees are the presenting part

53. Your client, who is 41 weeks and 5 days pregnant, presents for postdates testing, including a nonstress test. When you assess the tracing after 20 minutes, the FHR is 140–145 bpm, there are no decelerations, the variability is moderate, but the tracing does not meet criteria for reactivity. What would you do?

a. Admit the client and induce labor

b. Begin a contraction stress test

c. Use the vibroacoustic stimulator

d. Continue nonstress test for another 20 minutes

54. The same client is now in labor, at 4 cm/100%/+1, vertex, and she is having contractions every 3–5 minutes for 50–70 seconds, which are moderate to palpation. The FHR baseline is still in the 140s, but she is having variable decelerations to the 110s with good return to baseline and average variability. What action would be contraindicated at this time?

a. Allowing the patient to get into the Jacuzzi

b. Beginning oxytocin augmentation

c. Inserting an intravenous catheter

d. Expectant management

55. The definition of engagement is:

a. The fetal head reaches the pelvic floor

b. The widest diameter of the presenting part descends to at or below the pelvic inlet

c. The biparietal diameter is just above the pelvic inlet

d. The head is on the perineum

56. When an IUPC is used for the assessment of uterine contractions, the adequacy is quantified in:

a. Millimeters of mercury

b. Mild, moderate, and strong

c. Montevideo units

d. Centimeters

57. By internal monitoring of uterine contractions, which of the following must be achieved in the course of 10 minutes in order to be considered adequate contractile strength to dilate the cervix?

a. 80–100 Montevideo units

b. 80–100 mm Hg

c. 180–200 Montevideo units

d. 180–200 mm Hg

58. Which of the following would represent a contraindication for the use of an IUPC?

a. Maternal birth plan

b. Breech presentation

c. HIV

d. Lack of labor progress

59. For low-risk laboring women, in the first stage of labor the interval for intermittent fetal heart rate auscultation is:

a. 15 minutes

b. 20 minutes

c. 30 minutes

d. 60 minutes

60. All of the following are risk factors for preterm labor *except*:

a. Age

b. Smoking

c. Race

d. Sex of fetus

61. Shelley Blank is seen in Labor and Delivery at 33 weeks and 1 day complaining of menstrual-type cramping for the past 3 hours. She denies bleeding or ruptured membranes. The fetus is active. The EFM reveals occasional uterine contractions approximately every 8–12 minutes. The FHR is 135–140 bpm. Which of the following tests would be most important in formulating your management plan?

a. Complete blood count

b. Cervical culture

c. Urine culture

d. Ultrasound

62. What would be the next step in your management plan?

a. Expectant management until the lab results are back

b. Tocolysis

c. Pain management

d. Additional information is necessary to formulate the management plan

63. Which of the following represents a risk factor for shoulder dystocia?

a. Advanced maternal age

b. Epidural anesthesia

c. Polyhydramnios

d. Maternal obesity

64. Which of the following elective vaginal births is no longer recommended?

a. Brow presentation

b. Face presentation

c. Breech presentation

d. Vertex presentation

65. During the birth of twins, which represents a maneuver that should *not* be performed?
    a. Artificial rupture of membranes
    b. Clamping and cutting of a nuchal cord
    c. McRobert's maneuver
    d. Breech delivery of the second twin

66. Which of the following represents a risk factor for retained placenta?
    a. Preterm delivery
    b. Multiple gestation
    c. Multiparity
    d. Postterm pregnancy

67. While repairing a first-degree laceration, you notice a continual "trickle" of bright red blood from the vagina. As you continue your repair, the bleeding becomes more brisk. What would be the next step after fundal massage in your management plan?
    a. Bimanual compression
    b. Adding 20 additional units of oxytocin in the IV
    c. Discussion with the consulting physician regarding management plan
    d. Methylergonovine IM if BP is normotensive

68. Thirty-six hours after birth, you find Megan, a 16-year-old, crying quietly with the baby in her room as you perform a.m. rounds. What would be the most helpful response?
    a. Prescribe an SSRI because adolescents are prone to postpartum depression
    b. Encourage her to focus on her baby's needs as her first priority now
    c. Explain that it is normal to have a combination of sadness and euphoria so close to the time of the birth
    d. Conduct a screening test for possible postpartum depression

69. During postpartum rounds, your multiparous client is very pleased with her birth and is clearly bonding with her new baby girl. She is successfully nursing her baby every 3 hours for 5 minutes. She is asking about early discharge and wants to go home as soon as possible. Her only complaint is that her left leg is sore because of her need to deliver in stirrups. What would be the most important piece of your assessment?
    a. Availability of assistance at home with her two other children to ensure her of rest
    b. Breast exam and assessment to check for milk production to ensure adequacy of feeding prior to discharge
    c. Dietary recall to ensure adequate kcal and fluids to produce adequate human milk
    d. Examination of the lower legs to be sure that the muscle strain that she is complaining about is simply related to positioning

70. The same client would like to resume birth control prior to discharge. Which method would be most appropriate for this client?
    a. DMPA
    b. IUD
    c. Combination birth control pills
    d. Diaphragm with spermicidal cream

71. For the high-risk client, during the second stage of labor, the fetal heart rate should be monitored:
    a. Every 5 minutes
    b. Every 15 minutes
    c. Every 30 minutes
    d. Continuously

72. A sudden bradycardia seen in the second stage of labor after an uneventful labor course and previously normal fetal heart tracing is commonly caused by:
    a. A vagal response in the fetus related to descent
    b. Fetal hypoxia related to length of labor
    c. Cord prolapse
    d. Uteroplacental insufficiency

73. Which of the following FHR tracings are indicative of a Category III FHR tracing?
    a. A prolonged deceleration with recovery to baseline with moderate variability
    b. Variable decelerations that become more pronounced during the second stage but with normal FHR between pushing efforts
    c. Late decelerations and an absence of variability
    d. Late decelerations with return to baseline and moderate variability between decelerations

74. The risk factor that is most predictive of a preterm birth during a current pregnancy is:
    a. Uterine contractions
    b. Prior preterm labor
    c. Prior preterm birth
    d. Pre-eclampsia

75. The pain of the second stage of labor is caused by:
    a. Uterine muscle hypoxia with lactic acid buildup and distention of the musculature of the pelvic floor
    b. Cervical and lower uterine segment stretching and traction on the ovaries, fallopian tubes, and pelvic ligaments
    c. Pressure on the bony pelvis, urethra, bladder, and rectum
    d. Fundal uterine displacement and extension of the fetal lie

76. Hemodynamic changes during the initial postpartum period include:
    a. Elevated cardiac output for up to 48 hours after the birth
    b. Decreased WBC during the first 72 hours postpartum
    c. Elevated blood pressure for 48 hours after the birth
    d. Decreased urine output for the first 24 hours

77. In the initial newborn period, a 10-minute Apgar score is performed:
    a. Routinely
    b. If the 1-minute Apgar score was less than 7
    c. If the 5-minute Apgar score was less than 7
    d. If the combined Apgar score at 1 and 5 minutes is less than 16

78. The bluish discoloration of the baby's hands and feet within the first 24–48 hours after birth is:
    a. Acrocyanosis
    b. Circumoral cyanosis
    c. Central cyanosis
    d. Mongolian spots

Answers with Rationales

1. b. Perform sterile speculum exam to R/O rupture of membranes versus vaginal infection
   A sterile speculum examination should be performed if ruptured membranes are suspected.

2. a. Placenta previa
   With placenta previa, 70–80% of the time, painless vaginal bleeding occurs.

3. b. Calcium channel blockers such as nifedipine
   Recent research has determined that calcium channel blockers are most effective for tocolysis.

4. b. 28-year-old G1 smoker pregnant with twins with spontaneous rupture of membranes at 37 weeks
   Tobacco use is a significant risk factor for placental abruption.

5. d. Preterm birth
   Preterm labor and birth are major risks in multifetal gestations.

6. c.
   The cardinal movements of labor are: Descent, flexion, internal rotation, extension, restitution, external rotation

7. c. Extension
   The fetal head is born by the process of extension.

8. a. Blood loss in excess of 500 cc or more after the third stage of labor for a vaginal birth
   Definition of postpartum, hemorrhage

9. d. Five-minute scoring has a relationship to neonatal morbidity and mortality
   Five-minute scoring is more predictive of neonatal morbidity and/or mortality than 1-minute scoring is.

10. d. Shoulder dystocia
    Gestational diabetes is one of the risk factors for shoulder dystocia.

11. b. Latent labor
    Latent phase of labor is from onset of labor until 4–6 cm.

12. b. Ambulate for 2 hours and then reassess
    Ambulation for 2 hours will allow the clinician to evaluate for cervical change (definition of labor). The client's perception of need for admission to the birthing facility is important in clinical decision making as well.

13. b. Latent phase of labor
    Latent phase of labor is from onset of labor until 4–6 cm.

14. b. Prolonged latent phase of labor
    Client is exhausted with abnormal latent phase.

15. d. Offer medication of morphine 10 mg IM so she can get some sleep and potentially correct this dysfunctional labor pattern
    Morphine is quite effective for maternal exhaustion due to prodromal/prolonged latent phase of labor.

16. a. November 11
    Naegele's rule is to add 7 days to the first day of the last menstrual period and subtract 3 months

17. b. Sacrum
    The sacrum is the denominator for breech presentations.

18. b. Anterior asynclitism
    Anterior asynclitism is noted when the sagittal suture is closer to the sacrum.

19. d. Encourage movement and position change
    Movement and position change can encourage the fetus to descend into a favorable position for birth.

20. a. Variable decelerations
    Variable decelerations are abrupt in nature with a decrease in FHR from baseline of ≥ 15 bpm lasting ≥ 15 seconds but less than 2 minutes.

21. d. Suboccipitobregmatic
    When the fetal head meets the resistance of the pelvic floor, flexion is encouraged so that the most favorable diameter (suboccipitobregmatic) presents.

22. c. Acceptable for the fetal monitoring of certain patients
    Intermittent auscultation is an acceptable method of assessing fetal well-being in low-risk clients.

23. a. Discuss the indications for episiotomy and reinforce that you would obtain consent prior to performing the procedure if necessary
    Although episiotomy is no longer a routine procedure, there are specific indications for its use and these should be discussed with the client.

24. b. LMT
    Face presentation—the denominator is the mentum.

25. c. Encourage patient to push as effectively as possible
    More than 90% of anterior face presentations deliver vaginally without complications (Posner, Dy, Black, & Jones, 2013, p. 250).

26. d. Sweep the arm down by hooking the elbow and pulling the arm down
    It is important to remain calm and guide the arm in a physiologic range of motion.

27. c. Uterine atony
    Uterine atony is the most common cause of postpartum hemorrhage.

28. a. The first 6 weeks postpartum
    Normal postpartum involution takes a full 6 weeks to be complete.

29. a. Latent phase
    Latent phase of labor is from onset of labor until 4–6 cm.

30. b. Active phase of labor
    Active phase of labor is from 4–6 cm until complete dilatation.

31. b. Intravenous opioids
    Intravenous opioids should not be used when birth is anticipated within an hour because of the risk for respiratory depression in the newborn.

32. b. Head compression
    Early decelerations are due to a vagal response from head compression and are considered benign.

33. a. The ability to have a continuous tracing when external monitoring is insufficient
    An internal scalp electrode allows for accurate, continuous fetal monitoring when an external monitor is not producing a reliable continuous tracing.

34. d. A fetal heart rate acceleration of 15 bpm for 15 seconds
    A fetal heart rate acceleration indicates a fetal pH of ≥ 7.20.

35. b. LOA

    Left occiput anterior (LOA) is the most common position for birth.

36. a. LOP

    Most babies who are in posterior position will undergo the long-arc rotation to anterior before birth.

37. d. Every 15 minutes

    Blood pressure should be evaluated every 15 minutes in the second stage of labor for low-risk women.

38. d. At approximately 8–9 cm dilated

    The correct timing for administration of pudendal anesthesia is just prior to complete dilatation in a multiparous client.

39. a. Levator ani

    The largest group of muscles in the pelvic musculature is the levator ani.

40. c. Rectal sphincter

    A second-degree laceration involves the vaginal mucosa, posterior fourchette, the perineal muscles, and perineal skin.

41. d. Assist in the delivery of the fetal head during extension

    The Ritgen maneuver can be used to expedite the delivery of the fetal head when necessary.

42. b. Increased bleeding

    Bleeding is more visible and likely to be increased because of incomplete separation of the placenta.

43. d. Heartburn

    The other conditions, urinary tract infection, appendicitis, and renal colic, may mimic the signs/symptoms of preterm labor, whereas heartburn does not.

44. a. The parasympathetic/sympathetic nervous system

    Fetal heart rate variability is predominantly controlled by the autonomic nervous system (parasympathetic/sympathetic).

45. b. Decreases

    During a uterine contraction, the intramyometrial pressure exceeds that of the spiral arteries, resulting in decreased intervillous blood flow.

46. c. 6–25

    Moderate variability is defined by an amplitude range of 6–25 bpm.

47. c. Placenta previa

    The other choices, medications, congenital cardiac anomalies, and fetal activity, are known factors that influence fetal heart rate variability.

48. c. "I do not think that you should be having shortness of breath like you are; I am going to have the physician see you and order a chest radiograph"

    Shortness of breath is not a typical side effect of magnesium sulfate and should be investigated.

49. a. Labor at 41 weeks and 1 day

    Forty-one weeks and 1 day is normal gestation (i.e., not preterm or postdates). The other choices—thick meconium-stained fluid, nonreactive nonstress test, and IV narcotics—entail risk factors that would necessitate continuous fetal monitoring.

50. c. Speed the maturation of the fetal respiratory system, including the production of surfactant

    Corticosteroid administration accelerates fetal lung maturity.

51. d. Notify your consulting physician and prepare for a C-section

    LSA indicates that the fetus is in breech presentation. At 6 cm, delivery is not imminent, thus a Cesarean birth is indicated.

52. b. Legs and thighs are flexed with buttocks presenting

    A complete breech has both legs and thighs flexed and is the most common type of breech presentation.

53. d. Continue nonstress test for another 20 minutes

    The fetus has sleep/wake cycles, so nonreactivity may be due to fetal sleep. Extending the time of the test is common practice to account for this.

54. a. Allowing the patient to get into the Jacuzzi

    Variable decelerations are an indication for continuous monitoring (which cannot be accomplished in the Jacuzzi tub).

55. b. The widest diameter of the presenting part descends to at or below the pelvic inlet

    The widest diameter of the fetal head is the biparietal diameter. The definition of engagement is when the biparietal diameter has cleared the pelvic inlet. Functionally, once the head is engaged, the leading edge of the fetal head is at the level of the ischial spines (0 station).

56. c. Montevideo units

    While the IUPC quantifies the strength of the contractions in millimeters of mercury, adequacy is determined by the average Montevideo units over a 10-minute period.

57. c. 180–200 Montevideo units

    Adequate contraction strength is indicated by 180–200 Montevideo units over a 10-minute period.

58. c. HIV

    Attempts should be made to minimize possible transmission of maternal blood to the fetus, as could occur with placement of an IUPC.

59. c. 30 minutes

    This is the low-risk protocol for auscultation of the FHR.

60. d. Sex of fetus

    The other risk factors—age, smoking, and race—are evidence-based risk factors for preterm labor. Research does not support sex of the fetus as a risk factor for preterm labor.

61. c. Urine culture

    A urinary tract infection can mimic (and is a risk factor for) preterm labor.

62. d. Additional information is necessary to formulate the management plan

    The information listed is incomplete to formulate a management plan.

63. d. Maternal obesity

    Maternal obesity is a risk factor for a macrosomic infant. Macrosomic infants are at greater risk for shoulder dystocia.

64. c. Breech presentation

    Vaginal delivery of breech presentations should be reserved only for breeches that present emergently and when birth is essentially inevitable.

65. b. Clamping and cutting of a nuchal cord

    If nuchal cord is present, it should not be cut, and birth should be attempted with the cord intact.

66. a. Preterm delivery

    Preterm birth is a predisposing factor for retained placenta.

67. d. Methylergonovine IM if BP is normotensive
    Methylergonovine causes sustained, tetanic uterine contractions but is contraindicated in hypertensive patients.

68. c. Explain that it is normal to have a combination of sadness and euphoria so close to the time of the birth
    Provide the patient with an explanation of normal psychological response to childbirth.

69. d. Examination of the lower legs to be sure that the muscle strain that she is complaining about is simply related to positioning
    It would be important to examine her lower extremities to assess for possible deep vein thrombosis (DVT).

70. a. DMPA
    DMPA is an acceptable contraceptive method that can be administered prior to discharge.

71. b. Every 5 minutes
    This is the frequency for auscultation in the second stage as per ACOG for the high-risk client.

72. a. A vagal response in the fetus related to descent
    With rapid descent a vagal response can occur.

73. c. Late decelerations and an absence of variability
    A Category III tracing shows an absence of FHR variability.

74. c. Prior preterm birth
    Prior preterm birth is a very strong risk factor for subsequent preterm birth.

75. c. Pressure on the bony pelvis, urethra, bladder, and rectum
    The descent of the fetus causes pressure on pelvic structures.

76. a. Elevated cardiac output for up to 48 hours after the birth
    Within the first hours post delivery, cardiac output increases 60–80%.

77. c. If the 5-minute Apgar score was less than 7
    Apgar scores are performed routinely at 1 and 5 minutes, with a 10-minute Apgar usually performed only if the 5-minute Apgar is less than 7.

78. a. Acrocyanosis
    The bluish discoloration of the baby's hands and feet is normal in the first 24–48 hours after birth and is known as acrocyanosis.

Bibliography

Blackburn, S. T. (2013). *Maternal, fetal, and neonatal physiology: A clinical perspective* (4th ed.). Maryland Heights, MO: Elsevier Saunders.

Butarro, T. M., Trybulski, J., Bailey, P. P., & Sandberg-Cook, J. (2013). *Primary care: A collaborative practice* (4th ed.). St. Louis, MO: Mosby Elsevier.

Coad, J., & Dunstall, M. (2012). *Anatomy and physiology for midwives* (3rd ed.). Edinburgh, Scotland: Elsevier.

Creasy, R., & Resnik, R. (2009). *Maternal fetal medicine: Principles and practice* (6th ed.). Philadelphia, PA: W. B. Saunders.

Cunningham, F. G., Leveno, K., Bloom, S., Hauth, I., Rouse, D., & Spong, C. (Eds.). (2010). *Williams obstetrics* (23rd ed.). New York, NY: McGraw-Hill.

Davidson, M. R., London, M. L., & Ladewig, P. A. W. (2012). *Olds' maternal-newborn nursing and women's health across the lifespan* (9th ed.). Upper Saddle River, NJ: Pearson Education.

Enkin, M., Keirse, M. J. N. C., Neilson, J., Crowther, C., Duley, L, Hodnett, E., & Hofmeyr, J. (2000). *A guide to effective care in pregnancy and childbirth* (3rd ed.). Oxford, England: Oxford University Press.

Gabbe, S. G., Niebyl, J. R., Simpson, J. L., Landon, M. B., Galen, H.L., Jauniaux, E. R. M., Driscoll, D. A. (2012). *Obstetrics: Normal and problem pregnancies* (6th ed.). Philadelphia, PA: Mosby Elsevier.

Gibbs, R., Karlan, B., Haney, A., & Nygaard, I. (2008). *Danforth's obstetrics and gynecology* (10th ed.). Philadelphia, PA: Lippincott Williams & Wilkins.

Hatcher, R. A., Trussell, J., Nelson, A., Cates, W., Kowal, D., Pollicar, M. (2011). *Contraceptive technology* (20th ed.). New York, NY: Ardent Media.

Jordan, R. G., Engstrom, J. L., Marfell, J. A., & Farley, C. L. (2014). *Prenatal and postnatal care: A woman-centered approach.* Ames, IA: Wiley.

King, T. L., Brucker, M. C., Kriebs, J. M., Fahey, J. O., Gegor, C. L., & Varney, H. (2015). *Varney's midwifery* (5th ed.). Burlington, MA: Jones & Bartlett Learning.

Lowdermilk, D., & Perry, S. (2012). *Maternity and women's health* (10th ed.). Philadelphia, PA: Mosby Elsevier.

Nagtalon-Ramos, J. (2014). *Maternal-newborn nursing care.* Philadelphia, PA: F. A. Davis.

Philpott, R. H., & Castle, W. M. (1972). Cervicographs in the management of labour in primigravidae. I. The action line and treatment of abnormal labour. *Journal of Obstetrics and Gynaecology of the British Commonwealth, 79,* 599–602.

Posner, G. D., Dy, J, Black, A. Y., & Jones, G. D. (2013). *Oxorn-Foote human labor and birth* (6th ed.). New York, NY: McGraw-Hill.

Riordan, J., & Auerbach, K. (2010). *Breastfeeding and human lactation* (4th ed.). Burlington, MA: Jones & Bartlett Learning.

Seidel, H. M., Rosenstein, B. J., Pathak, A., & McKay, W. (2006). *Primary care of the newborn* (4th ed.). St. Louis, MO: Mosby.

Tharpe, N., Farley, C., & Jordan, R. G. (2012). *Clinical practice guidelines for midwifery and women's health* (4th ed.). Burlington, MA: Jones & Bartlett Learning.

Zhang, J., Troendle, J., Mikolajczyk, R., Sundarum, R., Beaver, J., & Fraser W. (2010). The natural history of the normal first stage of labor. *Obstetrics & Gynecology, 1154,* 705–710.

8

Midwifery Care of the Newborn

Kimberly K. Trout

Physiologic Transition to Extrauterine Life

- Immediate extrauterine transition—immediate transition from intrauterine to extrauterine life depends on changes in four major areas: respiration, circulation, thermoregulation, and glucose regulation
- Respiratory changes
  1. Must immediately begin respiration upon delivery
  2. Factors in initiation of respiration
     a. Biochemical—relative hypoxia at the end of labor
     b. Physical stimuli—cold, gravity, pain, light, noise
     c. Recoil from pressure on thorax while passing through vagina
  3. Sustained respiration depends on coordinated response of the following:
     a. Central nervous system (CNS) respiratory center
     b. Aortic and carotid chemoreceptors
     c. Thoracic mechanoreceptors
     d. Diaphragm and respiratory muscles
  4. Initial breathing serves the following purposes:
     a. Assist in conversion from fetal to extrauterine circulation
     b. Clear lungs of fluid
     c. Establish lung volume and expand alveoli
  5. Characteristics of normal newborn respiration
     a. Respiratory rate 30 to 60 breaths per minute
     b. Irregular/fluctuating pattern
     c. Diaphragmatic and abdominal breathing
     d. Obligate nose breathing
     e. Absence of nasal flaring, grunting, and retractions
- Circulatory changes
  1. Transition from fetal to adult circulation begins with clamping of the umbilical cord and continues throughout the first weeks of life
  2. Characteristics of fetal circulation

  a. Low-pressure system, including placenta (low-resistance circuit)
  b. Minimal circulation to lungs; bypassed via foramen ovale and ductus arteriosus
  c. Foramen ovale favors circulation of most oxygen-rich blood to the brain
  3. Transition from fetal to neonatal circulation
     a. Increased systemic resistance due to loss of placental circuit
     b. Increased pressure in left atrium causes functional closure of foramen ovale
     c. Initial respiration opens pulmonary vasculature, favoring circulation to lungs
     d. Increased oxygenation of circulating blood causes constriction and functional closure of ductus arteriosus
     e. Absence of placental circulation closes ductus venosus
- Thermoregulation
  1. Mechanisms of neonatal heat loss
     a. Convection
     b. Conduction
     c. Radiation
     d. Evaporation
  2. Neonate creates heat in three ways:
     a. Shivering (inefficient)
     b. Muscle activity (limited benefit)
     c. Thermogenesis by metabolism of brown adipose tissue (BAT)
        (1) BAT stores are decreased in preterm and growth-restricted fetuses
        (2) Hypoglycemia decreases efficiency of BAT metabolism
  3. Consequences of cold stress
     a. Increased oxygen consumption, leading to relative hypoxia and acidosis
     b. Metabolism of BAT and release of fatty acids decreases pH
     c. Increased use of glucose, depletion of glycogen stores, and hypoglycemia
     d. Worsening hypoglycemia and acidosis may result in respiratory distress

4. Management
   a. Skin-to-skin on mother's chest or abdomen with blanket over both
   b. Prewarm blankets and resuscitation area
   c. Dry the newborn immediately and replace wet blankets
   d. Regulate room temperature and minimize exposure to air convection
   e. Postpone newborn bath at least 2 hours
   f. Keep newborn warm and wrapped
- Glucose regulation
  1. Glycogen stores
     a. Predominantly in liver
     b. Accumulated in third trimester
  2. Risk factors for neonatal hypoglycemia
     a. Infants of diabetic mothers
     b. Intrauterine growth restriction
     c. Preterm or postterm
     d. Intrapartum—perinatal acidemia, beta-agonist tocolysis, IV glucose administration
     e. Maternal substance abuse
  3. Glucose regulation in the healthy neonate
     a. Normal physiologic decrease in blood glucose
        (1) Lowest at 1–1.5 to 5 hours after birth
        (2) Stabilizes at 3 to 4 hours after birth
        (3) Should not drop below 40 mg/dL
     b. Mean glucose levels from 4 to 72 hours are 60 to 70 mg/dL
     c. Sources and mechanisms of glucose maintenance
        (1) Intake of human milk or formula
        (2) Glycogenolysis (use of glycogen stores)
        (3) Gluconeogenesis (production of glucose from amino acids)
  4. Signs and symptoms of hypoglycemia
     a. Weak cry
     b. Jitteriness
     c. Cyanosis
     d. Apnea
     e. Lethargy
     f. Poor feeding
  5. Management
     a. Encourage feeding as soon as possible
     b. Observe for signs/symptoms of hypoglycemia
     c. Assess glucose levels if signs/symptoms or risk factors are present
        (1) Profound severity at less than 20–24 mg/dL
        (2) Moderate severity at 25–34 mg/dL
        (3) Minimal severity at 35–45 mg/dL
     d. Indications for treatment with intravenous dextrose
        (1) Symptomatic infants, or those with initial serum glucose less than 25 mg/dL
        (2) Asymptomatic infants with persistent serum glucose less than 40 mg/dL

Ongoing Extrauterine Transition

- Changes in the blood
  1. Red blood cells (RBCs)

a. Hemoglobin F
   (1) Predominates in fetal circulation
   (2) High affinity for oxygen
   (3) Gradually eliminated in first month of life
b. Short RBC life span leads to increased bilirubin and physiologic jaundice
c. Cord clamping
   (1) Evidence of benefit for infant with delayed cord clamping (till pulsation stops, mean of approximately 2 minutes) versus immediate cord clamping
   (2) Neutral position on maternal abdomen is preferable
   (3) Below introitus—may cause placental transfusion and polycythemia
d. Normal values
   (1) Hemoglobin
       (a) Newborn 13.7–20.0 g/dL
       (b) Slight rise in first few days of life due to decreased plasma volume
       (c) Mean value at 2 months of age 12.0 g/dL
   (2) Hematocrit 43–63%
   (3) RBC count 4.2–5.8 million/mm³
   (4) Reticulocytes 3–7%
2. White blood cells (WBCs) normal value—10–30,000/mm³
3. Platelets
   a. Normal value—150–350,000/mm³
   b. Relatively low levels of vitamin-K-dependent clotting factors
4. Obtaining blood samples
   a. Venous stasis in extremities may lead to false values from heel-stick samples
   b. Maximize blood flow by using heel warmer before obtaining sample
   c. Confirm abnormal results with venipuncture sample
- Changes in the gastrointestinal (GI) system
  1. Relatively mature aspects of the neonatal GI system
     a. Suckling/swallowing
     b. Gag and cough reflexes
  2. Relatively immature aspects of the neonatal GI system
     a. Limited ability to digest fats and proteins
     b. Better absorption of monosaccharides than polysaccharides
     c. Frequent regurgitation due to
        (1) Incomplete development of cardiac sphincter
        (2) Limited stomach capacity (less than 30 cc)
     d. "Gut closure"
        (1) Maturation process of intestinal lining and its enzymes and antibodies
        (2) Vulnerability to bacteria, viruses, and allergens until process is complete
        (3) Promoted by breastfeeding
     e. Large intestine
        (1) Less efficient water conservation than adult
        (2) Predisposes infant to dehydration
- Changes in the immune system
  1. Natural immunity
     a. Physical and chemical barriers (skin, mucosa, gastric acid)
     b. Phagocytes (neutrophils, monocytes, macrophages)
        (1) Immature phagocytic response
        (2) Relative inability to localize infection

2. Acquired immunity
   a. Maternal IgG crosses placenta, conferring passive immunity to viruses the mother has encountered
   b. Breast milk provides maternal antibodies
   c. Active production of IgG develops slowly throughout childhood as passive immunity diminishes
3. Immaturity of natural and acquired immune systems predisposes the newborn to infection and sepsis

- Changes in the renal system
  1. Limited renal circulation
  2. Decreased glomerular filtration rate
  3. Immature tubular function
     a. Relative inability to concentrate urine
     b. Predisposition to fluid and electrolyte imbalances

Immediate Care and Assessment of the Healthy Newborn

- Assessment prior to birth of pertinent maternal history
  1. Genetic history
     a. Family history of structural or metabolic defects
     b. History of genetic syndromes
  2. Maternal elements
     a. Demographic factors
        (1) Maternal age of younger than 16 years or older than 35 years
        (2) Overweight or underweight prior to pregnancy
        (3) Maternal education less than 11 years
        (4) Family history of inherited disorders
     b. Medical factors
        (1) Cardiac disease
        (2) Pulmonary disease
        (3) Renal disease
        (4) Gastrointestinal disease
        (5) Endocrine disorders, particularly diabetes or thyroid disease
        (6) Chronic hypertension
        (7) Hemoglobinopathies
        (8) Seizure or other neurologic disorders
     c. History of present pregnancy
        (1) Late or no prenatal care
        (2) Rh sensitization
        (3) Fetus large or small for gestational age
        (4) Premature labor or delivery
        (5) Hypertensive disorders of pregnancy
        (6) Multiple gestation
        (7) Polyhydramnios
        (8) Premature or prolonged rupture of membranes
        (9) Antepartum bleeding
        (10) Abnormal presentation
        (11) Postmaturity
        (12) Abnormal results in fetal testing
        (13) Anemia
     d. Psychosocial history
        (1) Inadequate financial, housing, or social resources
        (2) Minority status
        (3) Malnutrition
        (4) Parental occupation
        (5) Significant relationships, marriage status
        (6) Violence or abuse
        (7) Smoking during pregnancy
        (8) Alcohol use during pregnancy
        (9) Drug use/abuse

- Assessment at birth
  1. During and immediately following birth
     a. Assess tone and skin color
     b. Gross inspection of anatomy
     c. Place infant on maternal abdomen or radiant warmer
     d. Can palpate cord to assess heart rate
  2. Apgar scoring
     a. Scale—0 to 10
        (1) Heart rate—0 = absent, 1 = < 100, 2 = > 100
        (2) Respiratory effort—0 = absent, 1 = slow/irregular, 2 = strong cry
        (3) Tone—0 = flaccid, 1 = flexion of extremities, 2 = active motion
        (4) Reflex irritability—0 = no response, 1 = grimace, 2 = strong cry
        (5) Color—0 = general cyanosis, 1 = acrocyanosis, 2 = completely pink
     b. Assigned at 1 and 5 minutes; may be assigned at additional 5-minute intervals when prolonged resuscitation efforts are required
     c. Primary purpose of Apgar score—objective method of quantifying the newborn's condition and response to resuscitation
     d. Poor predictor of long-term outcome
     e. Poor predictor of acidemia
     f. Apgar score is not used to determine the need for resuscitation, which resuscitation steps are necessary, or when to use them

- Review of neonatal resuscitation (American Academy of Pediatrics [AAP], 2010)
  1. Midwives and nurse practitioners who care for women in the intrapartum setting should be trained and certified in neonatal resuscitation; the information presented here is a review, not a substitute for training and certification
  2. Approximately 10% of newborns require some assistance to begin breathing at birth; about 1% require extensive resuscitation
  3. Evaluation is based upon three signs
     a. Respirations
     b. Heart rate
     c. Color
  4. ABCs of resuscitation
     a. Establish an open *Airway*
        (1) Position the infant on back or side with the neck slightly extended
        (2) Suction mouth and nose, and trachea as indicated
        (3) Insert endotracheal (ET) tube to ensure open airway if necessary
     b. Initiate *Breathing*
        (1) Use tactile stimulation to initiate respirations
        (2) Use positive-pressure ventilation (PPV) with 100% oxygen when necessary

    c. Maintain *Circulation*—stimulate and maintain circulation with chest compressions and/or medications when necessary

5. Overview of resuscitation in the delivery room
    a. Initial steps
      (1) Place infant under radiant warmer
      (2) Suction trachea if meconium present and infant is not vigorous
      (3) Dry infant; remove wet linen
      (4) Suction mouth and nose
      (5) Provide tactile stimulation
    b. Evaluate respirations, heart rate, and color
      (1) If no respirations, or heart rate less than 100 beats per minute (bpm), provide positive-pressure ventilation (PPV) with oxygen
        (a) If heart rate is below 60 bpm after 30 seconds of effective PPV, continue PPV and initiate chest compressions
        (b) If heart rate is above 60 bpm, continue PPV without chest compressions
    c. Medications
      (1) Medications are initiated when the heart rate remains below 60 bpm after 30 seconds of coordinated chest compressions and PPV
      (2) Dosage based on infant weight
      (3) Medications include
        (a) Epinephrine—increases strength and rate of cardiac contractions and causes peripheral vasoconstriction
        (b) Volume expanders—recommended solution is normal saline
        (c) Sodium bicarbonate—may be beneficial in correcting acidosis during prolonged resuscitation
        (d) Naloxone—narcotic antagonist used when there is severe respiratory depression and a history of maternal opioid administration within the last 4 hours

6. Newborns with meconium-stained amniotic fluid
    a. If the baby has a normal respiratory effort, normal tone, and heart rate greater than 100 bpm, use bulb syringe or suction catheter to clear secretions and meconium from mouth and nose—endotracheal suctioning is not indicated
    b. If the baby is not vigorous, as evidenced by depressed respirations, depressed tone, or heart rate less than 100 bpm, endotracheal suctioning of meconium is indicated

Care During the First Hours After Birth

- Transitional period
1. Time when the infant stabilizes and adjusts to extrauterine life
2. Three stages
    a. First period of reactivity
    b. Period of unresponsive sleep
    c. Second period of reactivity
3. May be altered when the infant is significantly stressed in labor and delivery

4. Preferred management for first hour of life; some say during hospital stay
    a. Maintain contact with the mother
    b. Limit or defer examinations and procedures, or perform them unobtrusively

- First period of reactivity
1. Begins immediately after birth
2. Lasts approximately 1–2 hours
3. Assessment findings
    a. Rapid heart rate and respirations—near upper limits of normal
    b. Respiratory rales present, disappearing by 20 minutes of age
    c. Behavior—alert, eyes open, may exhibit startle, cry, and/or rooting
    d. Bowel sounds usually present by 30 minutes after birth; may pass stool
4. Encourage breastfeeding during first period of reactivity
    a. Facilitated by infant's alert, active state
    b. Ameliorates physiologic drop in blood glucose at 1 to 1.5 hours after birth

- Period of unresponsive sleep
1. Lasts from 1 to 4 hours after birth
2. Assessment findings
    a. Heart rate decreases—usually to less than 140 bpm
    b. Murmur may be present because of incomplete closure of ductus arteriosus
    c. Slower, more regular respirations
    d. Bowel sounds present but diminished

- Second period of reactivity
1. Lasts from 2 to 8 hours after birth
2. Assessment findings
    a. Labile heart rate
    b. Rapid changes in color
    c. Respiration—rate less than 60 breaths/minute without rales or rhonchi
3. Early feeding
    a. Infant may be interested in feeding during the second period of reactivity
    b. Prevention of hypoglycemia
    c. Stimulation of stool passage
    d. Prevention of jaundice

- Bonding and parent–newborn attachment
1. Definitions vary; generally referring to the process occurring in the time after birth whereby the mother (and/or other family members) form a unique, lasting relationship with the newborn
2. Factors that may influence attachment
    a. Parental background
      (1) Care that parents received from their parents
      (2) Social/cultural factors
      (3) Couple and family relationships
      (4) Experiences in previous pregnancies
    b. Care practices
      (1) Interventions and assessments before and after birth
      (2) Behavior of healthcare providers
      (3) Care and support received in Labor and Delivery
      (4) Institutional rules and policies

c. Facilitating factors
(1) Skin-to-skin contact
(2) Breastfeeding
(3) Visual contact
(4) Holding, touching, "getting acquainted"
3. Limitations of bonding and attachment theories
a. Formation of relationships probably evolves out of many experiences rather than a single critical event
b. Little evidence that early separation has permanent effects on mother–infant or parent–child relationships
c. May lead to judgmental responses among healthcare providers, or guilt among parents, when bonding expectations are not met

Plan of Care for the First Few Days of Life

- Feeding
  1. Demand feeding
     a. Indicated for both breast- and bottle-fed infants
     b. Most infants will stop sucking and may fall asleep when full and satisfied
  2. Breastfeeding
     a. Breastfed infants average 8 to 12 feedings per day
     b. Intake is adequate if the infant seems satisfied and wets 4 to 6 diapers per day
     c. Frequent assessment, reassurance, and anticipatory guidance are essential for breastfeeding mothers and infants in the first few days of life
     d. Discourage supplementary bottle feedings to promote development of maternal and infant breastfeeding skills and to ensure adequate milk supply
  3. Formula feeding
     a. Formula-fed infants average 6 to 8 feedings per day
     b. Limited stomach capacity
        (1) Infant may take only 20 to 30 mL of formula at initial feedings
        (2) Most infants should take 60 to 120 mL formula per feeding by the third day of life
     c. Demonstrate positioning and burping techniques
- Voiding/stooling
  1. Record time and characteristics of first passage of urine and stool
  2. Stool will progress from meconium to yellow-green
  3. Absence of voiding for 24 hours is an indication for pediatric evaluation
- Skin
  1. Full baths and use of antibacterial soap are discouraged
  2. "Dry care"—skin is dried and skin folds are wiped clean with gauze
  3. Warm sponge bath late in first day of life to clear blood and meconium
  4. Discourage use of skin lotions, powders, creams, oils
- Medications
  1. Gonorrhea/chlamydia prophylaxis
     a. 0.5% erythromycin ointment

b. Should be deferred until after the first period of reactivity
2. Vitamin K
   a. Prevention of hemorrhagic disease
   b. May be administered intramuscularly or orally
3. Hepatitis B vaccination
   a. First dose prior to discharge
   b. Second dose at 1 to 2 months of age
   c. Third dose no earlier than 24 weeks of age
- Health promotion and safety
  1. All caregivers should wash hands thoroughly before handling infant
  2. Follow policies/procedures for infant identification
  3. Follow policies/procedures for infant security
  4. Teaching—safety and signs of illness (see following section on discharge teaching)

Discharge Planning

- Discharge teaching
  1. Formula feeding
     a. Use iron-fortified formula
     b. Clean nipples and bottles thoroughly prior to use
     c. 1.5–4 oz every 3 to 4 hours, increasing gradually based on infant cues of hunger/satiety
     d. Supplementary water or juice not recommended
  2. Breastfeeding
     a. On demand, at least every 2 to 5 hours
     b. Average 8 to 12 feeds every 24 hours
     c. Allow infant to remain on breast until signs of satiety demonstrated
     d. Adequate maternal rest and fluid intake
     e. Sore nipples usually indicate incorrect positioning or latch-on
  3. Voiding/stooling
     a. Bottle-fed infant stools—yellow-green, firm to pasty, straining is normal and not necessarily indicative of constipation
     b. Breast-fed infant stools—yellow-gold, loose or liquid, frequency varies, stooling with each feed or every other day
     c. 4 to 6 wet diapers per day is usually indicative of adequate intake
  4. Physiologic jaundice
     a. Occurs in more than 50% of newborns
     b. Temporary condition, rarely indicative of disease
     c. Usually peaks at 3 to 4 days of life
     d. Yellowing of sclera should be evaluated by pediatric provider
  5. Skin
     a. Sponge bath every day or every other day
     b. Tub baths after cord stump falls off
     c. Mild, unscented soap
     d. Lotions, oils, and powders are unnecessary
     e. Dry/peeling skin is normal and resolves spontaneously
     f. Diaper rash may be treated with petroleum jelly and air exposure, but notify pediatric provider if persistent
  6. Cord care
     a. In developed countries, antiseptic solutions no longer typically applied to cord. Keep the area dry
     b. Diaper should be fastened below cord

    c. Avoid immersion of cord stump in water

    d. Cord will usually drop off at approximately 2 weeks

    e. Redness around the cord base, foul odor, or drainage from cord should be reported to pediatric provider

7. Safety

    a. Infant car seats for every car ride

    b. Hand-held carrier versus body carrier—pros and cons

    c. Bottle propping is dangerous because of choking risk

    d. Avoid handling hot liquids while handling newborn

    e. Avoid exposure to direct sunshine; sunscreens are not necessarily safe for newborns

    f. Install smoke and carbon monoxide detectors

    g. Avoid exposure to cigarette smoke

    h. Infant should sleep in supine position

8. Expected infant behavior

    a. Hiccups are common and do not require treatment

    b. Sneezing is normal and does not necessarily indicate illness

9. Signs of illness

    a. Poor feeding, irritability, lethargy, skin rash, cord problems, vomiting, diarrhea, decreased urine output, rectal temperature greater than 100°F, or change in infant's behavior

    b. Emphasize that neonatal infection is not always accompanied by fever

- Psychosocial barriers/considerations to discharge

1. Current maternal substance abuse

2. Present or historical maternal psychiatric illness

3. Severe illness or physical disability of the mother

4. History of abuse or neglect of a previous child

5. Inappropriate maternal behavior

6. Homelessness or inadequate living arrangements

- Physical barriers to discharge

1. Feedings—newborn must demonstrate adequate intake of human milk or formula prior to discharge

2. Prematurity

    a. Any newborn less than 37 weeks' gestation or less than 2500 g should be observed for minimum of 3 days or in accord with pediatric/neonatal department policy

    b. Premature infants must demonstrate ability to maintain normal body temperature outside incubator for 24 hours prior to discharge

3. Neonatal drug withdrawal

    a. Newborn should be held for observation

    b. Social work evaluation and referral to drug treatment, if indicated

    c. Referral to child protective services is indicated if withdrawal symptoms occur or if newborn's urine toxicology is positive

    d. If medication is required to treat withdrawal, newborn must be held until medication is no longer necessary

    e. Newborn should be asymptomatic for 48 to 72 hours

4. Congenital abnormalities

    a. Heart murmurs suspected to be pathologic should be evaluated prior to discharge

    b. Dislocated hips should be evaluated by orthopaedic specialist and treatment begun prior to discharge

    c. Abnormal renal findings on prenatal ultrasound should be evaluated prior to discharge

5. Infections

    a. Sepsis—infant at risk for sepsis should be treated with antibiotics until blood cultures negative for 72 hours

    b. Syphilis—infants with congenital syphilis or infants of mothers with untreated syphilis should receive spinal tap and be treated within 10 days with intramuscular or intravenous penicillin

    c. Pneumonia—infants with pneumonia should be held in hospital for 7 to 14 days for antibiotic treatment

6. Hyperbilirubinemia

    a. Physiologic jaundice

      (1) Not visible in first 24 hours

      (2) Rises slowly and peaks at day 3 or 4 of life

      (3) Total bilirubin peaks at less than 13 mg/dL

      (4) Lab tests reveal predominance of unconjugated (indirect) bilirubin

      (5) Not visible after 10 days

    b. Possible pathologic jaundice

      (1) Visible during first 24 hours

      (2) May rise quickly to greater than 5 mg/dL/24 hours

      (3) Total bilirubin is greater than 13 mg/dL

      (4) Greater amounts of conjugated (direct) bilirubin

      (5) Visible jaundice persists after 1 week

    c. Labs—serum total bilirubin (STB), blood type, Rh, Coombs

    d. Phototherapy, if indicated, may be arranged through home healthcare agency

    e. Infants with elevated bilirubin but without hemolytic disease may be discharged if outpatient pediatric follow-up can be arranged

- Criteria for early discharge

1. General criteria

    a. Following uncomplicated birth, most infants may be discharged at 12–24 hours after birth depending on hospital/birth center policy

    b. Joint decision by midwife, pediatric provider, and family

    c. Uncomplicated antepartum, intrapartum, and postpartum course

    d. Early discharge increases importance of patient and family education to assess newborn

    e. Adequate support for mother at home, including home healthcare referral

2. Neonatal criteria

    a. Uncomplicated vaginal delivery

    b. Full-term infant with adequate growth (2500 to 4500 g)

    c. Normal findings on neonatal examination

    d. May be minimum 6-hour hospitalization but at least sufficient time under provider care to demonstrate:

      (1) Thermal homeostasis

      (2) Ability to feed

    e. Normal laboratory results confirmed

3. Maternal criteria

    a. Demonstrated ability with chosen feeding method

    b. Demonstrated ability with cord care

    c. Demonstrated ability to assess newborn's temperature with thermometer

    d. Verbalizes understanding of signs of newborn well-being and illness

- Discharge evaluation
  1. Complete physical examination with emphasis on the following:
     a. Frequency and duration of breast feedings or frequency and amount of bottle feedings
     b. Number of voids/stools
     c. Present weight and birth weight
  2. Discharge evaluation should be performed in the presence of parents for teaching, answering questions, and providing anticipatory guidance
- Follow-up care
  1. Pediatric follow-up should be arranged prior to discharge
  2. Factors influencing time of first pediatric visit
     a. Medical condition of newborn
     b. Length of hospital stay
     c. Experience of mother and family in caring for newborns
     d. Size of newborn
     e. Mother/family psychosocial factors
     f. Adequacy of newborn feeding

Newborn Assessment

- History—see the section titled "Immediate Care and Assessment of the Healthy Newborn" earlier in this chapter
- Physical examination
  1. General
     a. Whole
        (1) Proportions
        (2) Symmetry
        (3) Facies
        (4) Gestational age (approximate)
     b. Skin
        (1) Color
        (2) Subcutaneous tissue
        (3) Imperfections (bands and birthmarks)
        (4) Vernix and lanugo
        (5) Cysts and masses
     c. Neuromuscular
        (1) Movements
        (2) Responses
        (3) Tone (flexor)
  2. Head and neck
     a. Head
        (1) Shape
        (2) Circumference
        (3) Molding
        (4) Swellings
        (5) Depressions
     b. Fontanelles, sutures
        (1) Size
        (2) Tension
     c. Eyes
        (1) Size
        (2) Separation
        (3) Cataracts
     d. Ears
        (1) Placement
        (2) Complexity
        (3) Preauricular tags
     e. Mouth
        (1) Symmetry
        (2) Size
        (3) Clefts
     f. Neck
        (1) Swellings
        (2) Fistulas
  3. Chest
     a. Inspect for deformities (nipples, clavicles, sternum)
     b. Observe respiratory function with abdomen
     c. Palpate—breast bud size; clavicle for crepitus and/or swelling
  4. Lungs and respiration
     a. Retractions
     b. Grunting
     c. Quality of breath sounds
  5. Heart and circulation
     a. Rate
     b. Rhythm
     c. Murmurs—may be present for 1–2 days after birth until ductus arteriosus closes
     d. Sounds
  6. Abdomen
     a. Musculature
     b. Bowel sounds
     c. Cord vessels—number and type
     d. Distension
     e. Scaphoid shape
     f. Masses
     g. Liver edge may be palpable at 2–3 cm below right costal margin
     h. Normal spleen and kidneys are not easily felt
     i. Femoral pulses are felt when the infant is quiet
  7. Genitalia and anus
     a. Placement
     b. Identify ambiguous genitalia
     c. Scrotum—size, skin is wrinkled; determine whether testes are descended
     d. Phallus—size, placement of urethra
     e. Labia—palpate for masses; identify all structures and determine patency of vaginal orifice
     f. Anus—determine patency and relative position to other genital structures
  8. Musculoskeletal
     a. Posture
     b. Hands—digits; polydactyly, syndactyly, webbing, overlapping, shape and texture; "fisting"
     c. Feet—degree of flexion, shape, position
     d. Neck—rotation
     e. Joints—normal range of motion
     f. Long bone fractures—distortion, swelling, crepitus

9. Spine
   a. Symmetry
   b. Scoliosis
   c. Sinuses
- Gestational age assessment
  1. Dubowitz (detailed assessment of gestational age) and New Ballard (abbreviated version of Dubowitz) scales
     a. Estimation of gestational age and maturity based on observation and examination—score for 40-week infant total equals 40
     b. Elements include posture and tone, and characteristics of skin, lanugo, plantar surface, breast tissue, eyes/ears, and genitals
  2. Posture and tone—premature infant generally demonstrates extended posture, less tone, and less resistance to flexion of extremities
  3. Skin—premature infant has redder/pinker, translucent skin; postmature infant has cracked, wrinkled skin
  4. Lanugo is sparse to absent in the postmature or very premature infant and is most abundant in midterm infant (28 to 30 weeks)
  5. Plantar surface
     a. Assessed by length of foot from heel to tip of great toe in the premature infant
     b. Creases appear by 28 to 30 weeks of gestation and cover the entire surface at term
  6. Breast tissue and areola—progressive development throughout gestation
     a. Preterm—flat areola with no palpable breast bud
     b. Term infant—raised areola with 3- to 4-mm palpable breast bud
  7. Eye/ear
     a. Eyelids are fused in very premature neonate
     b. More mature infants will exhibit more cartilaginous ear tissue that exhibits greater firmness and recoil when flexed
  8. Male genitalia—increasing rugation of scrotum and descent of testes with advancing gestational age
  9. Female genitalia—increasing development of labia majora and decreasing prominence of clitoris and labia minora with advancing gestational age
  10. Anterior vascular capsule of ocular lens—more prominent vasculature at early gestational ages
- Measurements
  1. Weight
     a. Normal weight for a term newborn is 2501 to 4000 g
     b. Less-than-normal birth weight—definitions
        (1) Extremely low birth weight—less than 1000 g
        (2) Very low birth weight—1000–1500 g
        (3) Low birth weight—1501–2500 g
     c. Usual growth patterns
        (1) Infants typically lose 10% to 15% of birth weight in first 3 days of life
        (2) Should regain birth weight by 10 to 14 days of age
        (3) Double birth weight by 4 to 6 months of age
        (4) Triple birth weight by 12 months of age
  2. Length
     a. Most accurately measured by placing head against a firm surface, extending legs, then marking the surface
     b. Normal length for a term newborn is 48 to 53 cm

3. Head circumference
   a. Measured from the occiput around head and above eyebrows
   b. Normal head circumference for a term newborn is 33 to 35 cm
4. Chest circumference
   a. Measured under armpits across nipple line
   b. Normal chest circumference is 30 to 33 cm and 2 to 3 cm less than head circumference
5. Be aware of genetic pool of parents (i.e., one or both of small stature)
- Assessment for birth defects
  1. Minor malformations are relatively common, but three or more minor malformations on physical examination is suggestive of a major underlying condition
  2. Minor malformations
     a. Large fontanelles
     b. Epicanthic eye fold
     c. Hair whorls
     d. Widow's peak
     e. Low posterior hair line
     f. Preauricular skin tags or pits
     g. Minor ear anomalies—low-set, rotated, protruding
     h. Darwinian tubercule—small nodule on upper helix of ear
     i. Digital anomalies—curved, webbed, or bent fingers
     j. Transverse palmar crease
     k. Shawl scrotum
     l. Redundant umbilicus
     m. Widespread or supernumerary nipples
- Neurologic examination
  1. Level of alertness
     a. Most sensitive of all neurologic functions
     b. Varies depending on gestational age, time of last feeding, sleep patterns, recent stimuli, and recent experiences
     c. Findings associated with level of alertness
        (1) Response to arousal attempts (e.g., gentle shaking, sound, light)
        (2) Level and character of motility
  2. Neuromotor findings
     a. Tone and posture
     b. Motility and power
     c. Tendon reflexes—brachioradialis, patellar, Achilles
     d. Plantar response—flexion or extension of toes
     e. Eyes—red reflex, pupillary reflex, doll's eye reflex, blink reflex
  3. Assess for normal, absent, diminished, or exaggerated reflexes—abnormal reflexes suggest nervous system depression, spinal lesion, or central nervous system disorder or lesion
  4. Primary neonatal reflexes (Volpe, 2008)
     a. Palmar grasp
        (1) Newborn grasps object or finger placed on his/her palm
        (2) Typically disappears by 2 months of age
     b. Tonic neck response
        (1) Elicited by rotation of the head to one side
        (2) Newborn extends arm on the side to which the head is rotated and flexes the contralateral arm ("fencing posture")
        (3) Typically disappears by 7 months of age

c. Moro reflex
  (1) "Startle" response, evidenced by abduction and extension of arms with hands open and thumb and index finger semiflexed to form a C
  (2) Elicited by jarring examination table, allowing the infant to fall backward onto the examiner's hand, or making a loud noise
  (3) Typically disappears by 6 months of age

d. Placing and stepping ("walking")
  (1) Elicited by holding the infant upright and placing soles of feet in contact with flat surface or table edge
  (2) Typically disappears by 4 weeks of age

- Metabolic screening
  1. No federal guidelines; requirements vary state to state
  2. Metabolic screening tests mandated in most states, e.g.:
     a. Phenylketonuria
     b. Biotinidase deficiency
     c. Congenital adrenal hyperplasia
     d. Congenital hypothyroidism
     e. Cystic fibrosis
     f. Galactosemia
     g. Homocystinuria
     h. Branched-chain ketoaciduria
     i. Sickle cell disease
     j. Tyrosinemia
  3. Timing of metabolic screening
     a. Generally, after 24 hours of age—allowing time for feeding to be established and accumulation of toxic metabolites if disease is present
     b. Preferably 48 to 72 hours of age
     c. Recommended repeat screening at 2- to 4-week pediatric visit
     d. Law may mandate screening before discharge—for early discharge, repeat screening must be done

Primary Care of the Newborn for the First 6 Weeks

- Well-child surveillance
  1. All newborns should have at least two physical examinations before discharge
  2. Well-child visit
     a. Within 3 to 5 days for early discharged newborns
     b. Within 10 to 14 days for newborns held 48 hours
     c. Purpose—reexamine newborn, review teaching, perform metabolic screening
     d. Assessment includes
        (1) Review of maternal, perinatal, and newborn history
        (2) Observation of parents and assessment of family adjustment
        (3) Newborn interval history, including feeding, behavior, voiding/stooling
        (4) Physical examination
     e. Schedule follow-up visits

- Newborn behavior
  1. Sleep–wake states as classified by Brazelton
     a. Quiet sleep
     b. Active sleep
     c. Drowsy
     d. Quiet alert
     e. Active alert
     f. Crying
  2. Alert state
     a. Determine infant's ability to feed and interact with environment
     b. Comprises approximately 15% of daytime hours
  3. Crying
     a. May express need for feeding, holding, stimulation, or sleep
     b. May be indicative of pain
     c. Parental responsiveness to crying does not promote "spoiling" of infant—responsiveness is essential to newborn's development
  4. Sleeping
     a. Infant may exhibit varying respiratory patterns while sleeping, e.g., decreased depth and rate or periodic breathing (intermittent cessation of breathing for up to 10 seconds)
     b. Normal infants sleep up to 60% of the time

- Sensory capabilities
  1. Sensory threshold—level of tolerance for stimuli within which the infant can respond appropriately
     a. Infant may become fatigued or stressed when overstimulated; signs of stress and fatigue include:
        (1) Color changes
        (2) Irregular respiration
        (3) Irritability or lethargy
        (4) Vomiting
     b. Varies significantly among individuals; markedly low in premature or neurologically impaired newborns
  2. Visual capabilities
     a. Normal term infant can visually fix and track objects
     b. Sharp focus limited to distance of 10 to 12 inches
     c. Preference for striped patterns and strong contrasts
     d. Limited color perception
     e. Ability to recognize mother visually and respond to facial expressions within the first few weeks of life
  3. Newborns can detect and discriminate odors
  4. Taste capabilities
     a. Newborns react strongly to variations in taste
     b. Preference for sweets and flavors from maternal diet (prenatal and postnatal flavor learning)
  5. Hearing is acute, with ability to localize sounds and preference for mother's voice
  6. Touch—sensitive to light touch, as demonstrated by reflex responses

- Regulation of behavior
  1. Ability to respond appropriately to stimuli and maintain behavioral states
  2. Full-term infants should demonstrate smooth transition between states from sleep to active alertness; consistently abrupt or unpredictable changes are a cause for concern

3. Ability to maintain active alert state varies among individuals—some have difficulty becoming or remaining alert, whereas irritable infants progress rapidly from alertness to crying

4. Overstimulated infants may require "time-out"; relative isolation from stimuli and time to recover

5. Organization—ability to integrate physiologic and behavioral systems in response to the environment without disruption in state or physiologic functions

   a. Maintenance of stable vital signs
   b. Smooth state transitions
   c. Coordination of movements and responses in interacting with environment
   d. Consolable with ability for self-consolation (frequently characterized by hand-to-mouth movements)
   e. Habituation—ability to block out noxious stimuli

- Developmental milestones in first 6 weeks as measured by Denver II

  1. Personal/social skills—spontaneous and responsive smiling, attentiveness to a face
  2. Visual tracking—follows dangling object from midline through 45 degrees
  3. Spontaneous vocalization
  4. Response to sound of bell
  5. Gross motor—lifting head momentarily and symmetrical body movements

- Psychological tasks of early infancy as defined by Erikson

  1. Development of basic trust
     a. Birth through 12 to 18 months
     b. Definition—belief that world is a place where people and things can be relied upon and needs and wishes will be met
     c. Essential for formation of human attachments throughout life
  2. Development of differentiation—ability to discriminate between self and other
  3. Ability to elicit caregiving is essential to early development
  4. Secure attachment depends on caregivers':
     a. Emotional availability
     b. Sensitivity and stimulation
     c. Appropriate response to infant cues
     d. Consistency
  5. In the first year of life, securely attached infants will venture out and return to mother
  6. Results of insecure attachment
     a. Anxious or unable to cope with changes or distance from mother
     b. More negative infant behavior
     c. Avoidance/detachment
     d. Research suggests long-term impairment, including school problems and delinquency
  7. Counseling or parenting classes may be helpful when mothers/caregivers are experiencing problems in forming secure attachment

- Circumcision

  1. Increased prevalence in United States during 1950s
  2. Significant role of cultural, religious, and family traditions

3. Medical complications are rare but serious; include bleeding, infection, and inappropriate operative result

4. Controversial impact on sexual and psychological functioning; no clear evidence

5. The American Academy of Pediatrics (2012) has concluded that there is some benefit of reduced sexually transmitted infections (STIs), urinary tract infections (UTIs), and cancer of the penis in men who are circumcised. Therefore, although they conclude that the evidence for health benefits is not strong enough to recommend routine circumcision for all newborns, the benefits are sufficient enough to ensure access to this procedure for those families who have chosen to have circumcision performed. Opponents maintain that modern sanitary conditions and hygienic practices are more important factors underlying those medical conditions that have shown reductions with circumcision. It is important to fully inform the family of all of the known risks and benefits so that they may make an informed, conscious decision

6. Provide pain control if family chooses circumcision

7. Care of circumcised infant
   a. Apply petroleum jelly gauze strip to prevent adhesion of tissue to diaper
   b. Continue to use petroleum jelly on affected tissue until healed
   c. Notify care provider if bleeding, exudate, swelling, or inability to void occur

8. Uncircumcised infant
   a. Foreskin should separate and become freely mobile by 4 to 7 years of age
   b. Never forcefully retract the foreskin
   c. Infant hygiene—"only clean what can be seen"
   d. As the child matures, he should be taught to retract the foreskin and clean

- Nonnutritive sucking

  1. Thumb sucking and use of pacifiers subject to mother/family preferences and attitudes
  2. Common behavior in utero
  3. Infant may use nonnutritive sucking to regulate behavior state or self-console
  4. Avoid:
     a. Use of empty bottle for nonnutritive sucking (promotes ingestion of air, dental caries, and may contribute to otitis)
     b. Placing pacifier on string around baby's neck
     c. Prolonged use of and serious dependence on pacifiers

Common Variations from Normal Newborn Findings

- Jaundice

  1. Incidence—up to 50% of newborns
  2. Physiologic versus pathologic jaundice
     a. Physiologic jaundice does not occur within first 24 hours of life
     b. Total serum bilirubin concentrations increasing by more than 5 mg/dL per day indicate pathologic jaundice

c. Physiologic jaundice rarely results in total serum bilirubin concentrations greater than 15 mg/dL

d. Direct serum bilirubin levels greater than 1.5 mg/dL indicate pathologic jaundice

3. More common and slower to resolve in breastfed infants

4. Can be detected by blanching skin of nose, palms, or soles of feet—if jaundiced, skin will blanch yellow

5. Treatment

   a. Supplementation of breastfed infants with oral glucose water is not helpful and may be harmful

   b. Frequent feeding to stimulate GI elimination

   c. Management algorithm (values reflect total serum bilirubin concentrations)

      (1) Consider phototherapy for values of 12 to 17 mg/dL

      (2) Phototherapy indicated for values of 15 to 20 mg/dL

      (3) Exchange transfusion indicated for values of 20 to 25 mg/dL

      (4) Treatment thresholds are lower at earlier ages (24 to 48 hours after birth)

   d. Phototherapy may be indicated; some sources recommend exposing newborn to indirect sunlight for short periods several times per day

- Obstructed lacrimal ducts

  1. Incidence—50% of newborns will exhibit excessive tearing and mucoid discharge from eyes

  2. Treatment

     a. Massage—apply gentle, firm pressure in a circular motion on the lateral aspect of the nose adjacent to inner canthus of eye

     b. Clear drainage with cotton ball moistened with warm water, proceeding from inner to outer canthus

     c. Repeat treatment 3 to 4 times per day

- Dacryocystitis

  1. Definition—acute infection of lacrimal ducts

  2. Presentation—purulent discharge, swelling, tenderness adjacent to inner canthus of eye

  3. Treatment

     a. Same hygiene routine as described for obstructed lacrimal ducts

     b. Aseptic technique to prevent cross-contamination

     c. Topical or systemic antibiotics are indicated

- Skin problems

  1. Cradle cap

     a. Definition—dermatitis resulting from accumulation of sebum on scalp

     b. Presentation—characteristic yellow, crusting patches on anterior scalp, often in area of anterior fontanelle

     c. Treatment

        (1) Vigorous cleansing with mild shampoo and washcloth

        (2) Apply baby oil to area 30 minutes prior to shampooing

        (3) Rub affected area with dry washcloth gently but firmly to remove crusting

        (4) If severe, antiseborrheic shampoo may be indicated

  2. Diaper dermatitis

     a. Definition—general term for a variety of skin conditions that can occur in the diaper area

     b. Primary—caused by exposure to moisture and friction

     c. Secondary

        (1) Caused by colonization of affected area by pathogen; most commonly *Candida albicans*

        (2) Presentation—"fire-engine red" erythema, circumscribed pustulovesicular lesions, often with satellite lesions

     d. Treatment

        (1) Change diapers frequently

        (2) Avoid use of baby wipes

        (3) Rinse area with tepid water after every voiding; use tepid water and mild soap after stooling

        (4) Clean and dry skin thoroughly

        (5) Allow exposure of skin to air, especially before reapplying diaper

        (6) Some infants are sensitive to irritants in disposable diapers; change brands or use cloth diapers

        (7) For infants with diarrhea, apply zinc oxide ointment to clean, dry skin to provide a barrier

        (8) Severe irritation may be treated with 1% topical hydrocortisone

        (9) Nystatin topical cream, applied at each diaper change, for *Candida albicans* dermatitis

- Thrush

  1. Definition—oral fungal infection usually caused by *Candida albicans*

  2. Peak incidence around second week of life

  3. Often occurs after antibiotic therapy

  4. Presentation—characteristic white patches on the buccal mucosa, gums, tongue, and/or palate; lesions may be friable

  5. May cause feeding difficulty if extensive

  6. Treatment

     a. Nystatin suspension orally 4 times a day for 1 week

     b. Instill one dropper-full into each buccal pocket

     c. "Paint" lesions with cotton-tipped applicator

     d. Bottle-fed infants—boil nipples after use

     e. Breastfed infants—treat mother's nipples simultaneously with topical antifungal agents (nystatin, miconazole, clotrimazole) or with oral fluconazole, if topical treatment fails

- Regurgitation

  1. Definition—effortless "spitting up" of small amount of formula or breast milk

  2. Exacerbated by excessive swallowing of air, resulting from underfeeding or delayed feeding and prolonged crying, improper positioning, sucking on empty formula bottle

  3. Treatment

     a. Normal self-limiting condition, no treatment necessary

     b. May be reduced if infant is positioned sitting upright at 50 to 60 degree angle for 30 to 60 minutes after feeding

- Colic

  1. Definition—sudden, loud, and/or continuous unexplained crying often accompanied by flushed facies, mild abdominal distension, adduction of legs, or clenched fists

  2. Affects 10% of infants

  3. No proven organic basis; suggested but unproved causative factors may include:

     a. Overfeeding, especially in bottle-fed infants

b. Allergy to constituents of formula or breastfeeding mother's diet (milk products often suggested)

c. Anxiety in primary caregiver or tension in household; possibly symptomatic rather than etiologic

d. Immaturity of digestive system

4. Treatment

a. Attempt to identify factors associated with colic episodes for the individual infant

b. Correct overfeeding

c. Trial elimination of milk products from breastfeeding mother's diet

  (1) Efficacy is unknown; anecdotally effective in many cases

  (2) If bovine allergens are implicated, a trial longer than 1 week is necessary to clear mother's system

  (3) Maternal calcium supplementation is suggested with this approach

d. Some infants respond to warmth, wrapping in a blanket, limitation of stimuli, rhythmic soothing motion, gentle repetitive massage, or soft monotonous music

e. Probably most important factor is supportive care for parents, including reassurance and respite opportunities

f. As a last resort for exhausted parents, infant may be positioned safely and left to cry for limited periods of time

Deviations from Normal

- Danger signs of neonatal morbidity
1. Central nervous system signs
   a. Lethargy
   b. High-pitched cry
   c. Jitteriness
   d. Abnormal eye movement
   e. Seizure activity
   f. Abnormal fontanelle size or bulging fontanelles
2. Respiratory signs
   a. Intermittent cessation of breathing for more than 15 seconds, usually accompanied by bradycardia or cyanosis
   b. Tachypnea
   c. Nasal flaring, expiratory grunting, and/or chest retractions
   d. Persistent rales and/or rhonchi
   e. Asynchronous breathing movements
3. Cardiovascular signs
   a. Abnormal rate and rhythm
   b. Murmurs
   c. Changes in blood pressure
   d. Marked differential between upper and lower extremity blood pressure
   e. Alterations and/or differentials in pulses
   f. Changes in perfusion and skin color
4. Gastrointestinal signs
   a. Refusal to feed
   b. Absent or uncoordinated feeding reflexes
   c. Vomiting
   d. Abdominal distension
   e. Changes in stool patterns

5. Genitourinary signs
   a. Hematuria
   b. Absence of urine or failure to pass urine
6. Metabolic alterations
   a. Hypoglycemia
   b. Hypocalcemia
   c. Hyperbilirubinemia and jaundice, especially jaundice occurring within the first 24 hours of life
7. Fluid balance alterations
   a. Decreased urine output
   b. 5–15% weight loss in one day
   c. Dry mucous membranes
   d. Sunken fontanelles
   e. Poor skin turgor
   f. Increased hematocrit
8. Temperature instability
- Preterm infants
1. Definition—infants born before 37 completed weeks of gestation
2. Associated complications
   a. Respiratory complications
   b. Necrotizing enterocolitis
   c. Intraventricular hemorrhage
   d. Hypothermia
   e. Hypoglycemia
   f. Infection
   g. Hyperbilirubinemia
3. Maternal factors associated with prematurity
   a. Obstetric—uterine malformation, multiple gestation, cervical insufficiency, premature rupture of membranes, hypertensive disorders of pregnancy, placenta previa, history of previous preterm birth, isoimmunization
   b. Medical—diabetes, hypertension, urinary tract infection, other acute illness
   c. Psychosocial—poor prenatal care, low socioeconomic status, malnutrition, adolescent pregnancy, substance abuse
- Small for gestational age infants
1. Definition—birth weight below 10th percentile
2. Symmetric growth restriction
   a. Results from early and prolonged insult(s)
   b. Associated with decreased brain size and intellectual disability
   c. Growth restriction continues after birth
3. Asymmetric growth restriction
   a. Results from insult(s) late in pregnancy
   b. Head circumference is near normal for gestational age
   c. Rapid postnatal growth and development with normal cognitive development
4. Maternal factors associated with growth restriction
   a. Obstetric—history of infertility, history of abortions, grand multiparity, hypertensive disorders of pregnancy
   b. Medical—heart disease, renal disease, hypertension, sickle cell disease, phenylketonuria, diabetes
   c. Psychosocial—malnutrition, low socioeconomic status, extremes of maternal age, poor prenatal care, substance abuse

- Postterm infants
  1. Definition—born after 42 completed weeks' gestation
  2. Associated complications
     a. Meconium aspiration
        (1) Physical barrier to gas exchange
        (2) Causes chemical irritation and thickening of the alveolar walls
        (3) Vasoconstriction/vasospasm may cause pulmonary hypertension and persistent fetal circulation
     b. Hypoglycemia
     c. Polycythemia
     d. Hypothermia
  3. Associated maternal and fetal factors
     a. Maternal—primigravid, grand multiparity, previous postterm delivery
     b. Fetal—anencephaly, trisomies
- Large for gestational age infants
  1. Definition—birth weight above 90th percentile; sometimes defined as birth weight above 4000 or 4500 g
  2. Associated complications
     a. Birth injuries, including fractures and intracranial hemorrhage
     b. Hypoglycemia
     c. Polycythemia
     d. Perinatal asphyxia
  3. Maternal factors associated with excessive fetal growth
     a. Gestational diabetes
     b. Genetic predisposition
     c. Excessive maternal weight gain during pregnancy
  4. Infants of diabetic mothers (IDM)
     a. Gestational diabetes and hyperglycemia more likely to result in excessive fetal growth (macrosomia)
     b. Chronic or severe maternal diabetes with vascular changes more likely to result in growth restriction
     c. Pregestational diabetes associated with congenital anomalies, including central nervous system anomalies, congenital heart defects, and tracheo-esophageal fistula
- Neonatal infection
  1. Signs of infection in the newborn
     a. Often subtle and nonspecific
     b. Early signs—lethargy, refusal to feed, vomiting, temperature instability
     c. May show subtle changes in color—cyanosis, pallor, mottling
     d. May be related to involved organ system(s)
        (1) CNS infections—jitteriness, seizures
        (2) Pulmonary infections—respiratory distress, apnea
        (3) Intestinal infections—diarrhea
  2. Signs of chronic intrauterine infection
     a. Growth restriction
     b. Microcephaly
     c. Hepatosplenomegaly
  3. Sepsis
     a. Increased susceptibility because of immature immune function
     b. Evaluation includes blood and cerebrospinal fluid (CSF) cultures, complete blood count (CBC) with differential, IgM titer, chest radiograph; toxoplasmosis, rubella, cytomegalovirus, and herpes screening

  4. Bacterial infections
     a. Group B b-hemolytic streptococcus (GBS)
        (1) Most common pathogen in neonatal infections
        (2) Etiology—maternal colonization, transmitted to neonate during labor and delivery
        (3) Preterm newborns at highest risk
        (4) Early-onset GBS disease—develops within first 24 hours of life, characterized by respiratory involvement, may be fatal
        (5) Late-onset GBS disease—onset usually after second week of life, characterized by CNS involvement, rarely fatal, but may result in permanent neurologic damage
     b. Listeria
        (1) Presentation—diffuse papular rash on trunk and pharynx, respiratory distress, cyanosis, sepsis
        (2) Etiology—maternal colonization, transmitted to neonate during labor and delivery
     c. *Escherichia coli*
        (1) Major cause of neonatal meningitis and sepsis
        (2) Etiology—maternal colonization, transmitted to neonate during labor and delivery
     d. *Neissieria gonorrhoeae*
        (1) Pathogenic for ophthalmia neonatorium
        (2) May cause blindness if untreated
        (3) Prophylaxis—administration of silver nitrate or erythromycin ointment to eyes after birth
        (4) Rarely, may invade joint capsules causing septic arthritis
     e. Tuberculosis
        (1) Congenital disease is rare unless mother has untreated, advanced disease
        (2) Primarily affects newborn liver when acquired before birth
        (3) Separation of newborn from mother is unnecessary if mother has negative chest radiograph, negative sputum culture, and is receiving treatment
  5. Viral and protozoal infections
     a. Toxoplasmosis
        (1) Associated with raw meat and infected feces, especially cat
        (2) Mother is often asymptomatic
        (3) Signs of infection in the newborn include microcephaly, cerebral calcifications, chorioretinitis, hepatosplenomegaly, and jaundice
        (4) Treatment limits further disease but does not correct damage to the central nervous system
     b. Syphilis
        (1) Signs of infection in the newborn include intrauterine growth restriction (IUGR), ascites, rhinitis, jaundice, anemia
        (2) Spontaneous abortion, stillbirth, or newborn demise occurs in 40% of cases when mother is untreated; another 40% will result in congenital syphilis
        (3) Congenital syphilis may result in multisystem organ damage and/or death

c. Rubella
   (1) Infection in utero may result in IUGR, cardiac anomalies, deafness, blindness, and/or intellectual disability
   (2) Effects depend on gestational age at transmission and duration of infection
d. Cytomegalovirus (CMV)
   (1) No effective means of treatment or prevention
   (2) Effects of congenital CMV infection—30% incidence of death in infancy, 90% of survivors will have CNS, visual, and/or auditory damage
e. Herpes
   (1) Transmission typically occurs during intrapartum period; prenatal infection is rare
   (2) Newborns are susceptible to systemic disease, which may involve hepatitis, pneumonia, encephalitis, and/or disseminated intravascular coagulopathy
   (3) Primary maternal infection is associated with 50% newborn mortality rate and high rates of permanent neurologic damage
   (4) Recurrent maternal infection rarely results in severe systemic disease
f. Hepatitis B
   (1) Often results in prematurity and low birth weight
   (2) Onset of disease occurs 4 to 6 weeks after birth and is marked by poor feeding, jaundice, and hepatomegaly
   (3) Most infants infected perinatally demonstrate carrier state without acute disease
g. Chlamydia
   (1) Most common cause of blindness worldwide
   (2) Intrapartum transmission may result in conjunctivitis, pneumonia, and/or otitis media
   (3) Chlamydial conjunctivitis is not prevented by ocular administration of silver nitrate; erythromycin ophthalmic ointment is preferred
h. Human immunodeficiency virus (HIV) and acquired immune deficiency syndrome (AIDS)
   (1) Maternal antiretroviral therapy during pregnancy dramatically reduces vertical transmission; Cesarean section prior to the start of labor is recommended for all women with a viral load ≥ 1000 copies/mL to further reduce risk of vertical transmission
   (2) Can be transmitted via breast milk
   (3) May result in prematurity, growth restriction, and/or microcephaly
   (4) Opportunistic infection usually manifests within the first months of life

- Plexus injuries—prognosis is good; 88–92% of affected infants recover fully within first year of life
  1. Thought to result from lateral traction on shoulder or head during delivery; some evidence of intrauterine effect also exists
  2. Erb's palsy
     a. Accounts for 90% of all plexus injuries
     b. Involves upper part of the plexus (C5 through C7 and occasionally C4)
     c. Shoulder and upper arm are affected
     d. Decreased biceps reflex is present
     e. When C4 is involved, diaphragmatic dysfunction is present

3. Total palsy
   a. Accounts for 8–9% of all plexus injuries
   b. Diffuse plexus involvement (C5 to T1)
   c. Upper arm, lower arm, and hand are affected
   d. Biceps and triceps reflexes are decreased
4. Klumpke paralysis
   a. Accounts for less than 2% of all plexus injuries
   b. Involves C8 to T1
   c. Lower arm and hand are affected
5. Associated injuries—clavicle fracture, humerus fracture, shoulder dislocation, facial nerve injury
6. Management usually consists initially of limiting movement of the affected extremity, and then gradual introduction of gentle range-of-motion exercises

- Neonatal fractures
  1. Fracture of the clavicle—not a significant newborn fracture
     a. Most common neonatal fracture
     b. Signs—hematoma, crepitus, asymmetric tone/movement of upper extremities
     c. Sometimes associated with plexus injuries
  2. Fracture of humerus or femur—significant fractures, may be nosocomial
     a. Rare; usually associated with breech deliveries
     b. Ecchymosis, hematoma, or hemorrhage may occur at fracture site
  3. Skull fracture
     a. Rare; may be associated with forceps delivery
     b. Linear fracture—usually benign, resolves without treatment
     c. Depressed fracture—may be associated with seizures and/or permanent neurologic injury
     d. Signs—cephalohematoma, palpable depression in bone

- Infants with hemolytic disease
  1. Definition—destruction of red blood cells resulting in hyperbilirubinemia and jaundice
  2. Causes—maternal antibodies, enzymatic disorders, infections
  3. Rh incompatibility
     a. Occurs when mother is Rh negative and fetus is Rh positive
     b. Positive result on direct Coombs' test indicates presence of maternal antibodies
     c. May necessitate exchange transfusion
  4. ABO incompatibility
     a. Occurs when mother is serologic type O and fetus is type A or B; infrequently when mother is type A and fetus is type B
     b. Very rare incidence of hydrops or stillbirth
     c. May result in neonatal jaundice; rarely causes severe hemolysis or anemia

- Hyperbilirubinemia and severe jaundice
  1. Associated with many neonatal complications, including hemolytic disease, prematurity, impaired hepatic function, sepsis, metabolic disorders, hematomas, impaired intestinal function, and others
  2. Kernicterus
     a. Encephalopathy caused by deposition of bilirubin in brain cells
     b. Classic signs—lethargy, diminished reflexes, hypotonia, and seizures

    c. Contributing factors—prematurity, hypothermia, asphyxia, acidosis, sepsis

    d. Complications include hearing impairment, cerebral palsy, and intellectual disability

  3. Phototherapy

    a. Oxidizes unconjugated bilirubin in the skin, rendering it water soluble and facilitating elimination

    b. Precautions

      (1) Protect infant's eyes from high-intensity light

      (2) Monitor fluid status and temperature

- Infants affected by maternal substance abuse

  1. Fetal alcohol spectrum disorders (FASD)

    a. Fetal/neonatal effects—microcephaly, facial abnormalities, cardiac defects, malformation of joints, failure to thrive, intellectual disability

    b. May result in withdrawal syndrome in the neonate characterized by irritability, tremors, tachypnea, tachycardia, poor feeding

  2. Cocaine abuse

    a. Fetal/neonatal effects—prematurity, low birth weight, IUGR, genitourinary abnormalities, seizures, congenital heart disease, irritability, frantic or poor feeding

    b. May result in long-term behavioral impairment

  3. Opiate abuse

    a. Minimal long-term effects compared to cocaine and alcohol; primarily affects immediate neonatal period

    b. Abstinence syndrome (opiate withdrawal)

      (1) Onset shortly after birth

      (2) CNS signs—irritability, tremors, high-pitched cry, hyperstimulability, possible seizure activity

      (3) Other signs—tachypnea, tachycardia, poor or disorganized feeding, hyperthermia, vasomotor instability

      (4) Care is primarily supportive, although methadone or buprenorphine may be necessary with severe symptoms

  4. Marijuana abuse

    a. Little or no evidence for teratogenic effects

    b. Possible newborn behavioral effects—fine tremor, prolonged startle response, irritability, poor habituation to visual stimuli

    c. No behavioral effects demonstrated to persist beyond infancy

  5. Prescription drugs of abuse potential

    a. Amphetamines

      (1) Fetal/neonatal effects—genitourinary, cardiac, and/or central nervous system abnormalities, behavioral state disorganization

      (2) May result in long-term learning disabilities

    b. Benzodiazepines—fetal/neonatal effects include hypotonia, hypothermia, low Apgar scores, respiratory depression, poor feeding, possible association with midline cleft defects

- Congenital anomalies

  1. Central nervous system anomalies

    a. Spina bifida occulta

      (1) Absent or incomplete closure of one or more vertebral arches

      (2) Dimple or hair tuft may be present over site

      (3) Often asymptomatic without requiring treatment

    b. Meningocele/myelomeningocele

      (1) Meningocele—extrusion of meninges and cerebrospinal fluid (CSF) through defect in vertebral column

      (2) Myelomeningocele—meningocele with extrusion of spinal cord

      (3) Surgical repair is necessary to prevent rupture and infection

      (4) Myelomeningocele results in loss of sensory and motor function below the level of the defect

    c. Anencephaly

      (1) Congenital absence of cranial vault and underlying brain tissue

      (2) Newborn may manifest heart rate and respiration but will die within a few hours after birth

    d. Hydrocephalus

      (1) Abnormal accumulation of cerebrospinal fluid in ventricles of the brain

      (2) Signs—increased head circumference, separation of cranial sutures, bulging tense fontanelles, high-pitched cry, and downward deviation of eyes ("setting sun sign")

      (3) Surgical treatment involves placement of a shunt to drain excess fluid

  2. Respiratory anomalies

    a. Choanal atresia

      (1) Definition—congenital blockage of posterior nasal passages

      (2) Respiratory distress will be evident at birth if both nares are blocked

      (3) Treatment includes respiratory support and surgical repair

    b. Diaphragmatic hernia

      (1) Definition—defect of diaphragm, allowing herniation of abdominal contents into thoracic cavity and displacement of heart and lung tissue

      (2) Presentation—respiratory distress and scaphoid abdomen apparent at birth

      (3) Treatment is surgical repair

    c. Pulmonary hypoplasia/agenesis

      (1) Definition—underdevelopment or absence of one or both lungs

      (2) Strong association with other anomalies

      (3) Rare condition with high mortality rate

      (4) Presentation—acute respiratory distress with thoracic asymmetry

  3. Cardiovascular anomalies

    a. Anomalies resulting in increased pulmonary blood flow

      (1) Atrial septal defect, ventricular septal defect, patent ductus arteriosus, and atrioventricular canal defect

      (2) Surgical repair required

      (3) Prognosis is usually good

    b. Anomalies resulting in decreased pulmonary blood flow

      (1) Tetralogy of Fallot—pulmonary stenosis, ventricular septal defect, overriding aorta, and right ventricular hypertrophy

      (2) Aortic stenosis—narrowing or stricture of the aortic valve, causing resistance to blood flow in the left ventricle, with decreased cardiac output

(3) Tricuspid atresia—results in no direct communication between right atrium and right ventricle; further resulting in hypoplastic right ventricle and enlarged left ventricle

(4) Coarctation of the aorta—narrowing near the insertion of the ductus arteriosus, resulting in increased pressure proximal to the defect and decreased pressure distal to the obstruction

(5) Pulmonic stenosis—narrowing at the entrance of the pulmonary artery; results in decreased pulmonary blood flow and right ventricular hypertrophy resulting from resistance to blood flow

(6) Surgery is generally more complicated

c. Anomalies resulting in mixed blood flow (saturated and desaturated blood mix within the heart or great arteries)

(1) Transposition of the great vessels—aorta arises from right ventricle and pulmonary artery arises from left ventricle, resulting in circulatory bypass of lungs and circulation of unoxygenated blood to the body

(2) Truncus arteriosus—failure of embryonic structure to divide into aorta and pulmonary artery

4. Gastrointestinal anomalies

a. Cleft lip and palate

(1) Definition—incomplete fusion of lip and palate during prenatal development

(2) May interfere with feeding and weight gain

(3) Surgical repair usually results in good cosmetic and functional results

b. Esophageal atresia and tracheoesophageal fistula

(1) Definition—abnormal development of trachea and esophagus, resulting in "blind pouch" esophagus and/or communication between the two structures

(2) Presentation—copious drooling, poor feeding with reflux, acute respiratory distress and cyanosis with feeding

(3) Repaired surgically, with good prognosis

c. Pyloric stenosis

(1) Definition—obstruction of pylorus (distal opening of stomach)

(2) Affects males three to four times more often than females

(3) Presentation—vomiting, visible gastric peristalsis, constipation

(4) Repaired surgically, with good prognosis

d. Omphalocele

(1) Definition—defect of abdominal wall with herniation of abdominal viscera through umbilical ring

(2) Protruding abdominal viscera usually covered by membrane

(3) Frequently associated with other anomalies

(4) Repaired surgically; prognosis depends on extent of lesion and nature and extent of associated anomalies

e. Gastroschisis

(1) Definition—defect of abdominal wall and evisceration of abdominal organs

(2) Rarely associated with other anomalies

(3) Management at birth—cover eviscerated organs with sterile gauze moistened with sterile saline solution

(4) No oral intake until after repair; IV therapy for fluid and electrolyte maintenance

(5) Repair may require several surgeries; prognosis depends on extent of lesion

5. Genitourinary anomalies

a. Hypospadias

(1) Definition—in males, urethral opening is located on ventral aspect of penis

(2) Circumcision contraindicated—foreskin tissue is often used in surgical repair

(3) Rare in females, with urethral opening located in the vagina

b. Epispadias

(1) Definition—congenital opening of urethra on dorsum of penis

(2) Often associated with other genitourinary anomalies

(3) Repaired surgically

c. Ambiguous genitalia

(1) Definition—anomalies of the external genitalia precluding identification of the newborn's sex

(2) May be associated with anomalies of the internal genitalia

(3) Chromosome studies can determine genotypic sex

(4) Gender identity problems are frequent; reconstructive surgery is controversial

d. Exstrophy of the bladder

(1) Definition—exposure of bladder outside the abdominal wall

(2) Repaired surgically; often complicated by associated genitourinary anomalies

e. Patent urachus

(1) Definition—persistence of fetal opening between bladder and umbilical cord

(2) Repaired surgically

6. Musculoskeletal anomalies

a. Congenital hip dysplasia

(1) Definition—abnormal development of the acetabulum, resulting in dislocation of femoral head

(2) Presentation—asymmetry of gluteal folds, positive Ortolani sign

(3) Treatment—reduction and stabilization of femoral head into acetabulum to allow development of stable hip capsule

(4) Stabilization is accomplished by use of Frejka pillow or Pavlik harness

b. Talipes equinovarus

(1) Definition—congenital deformity of ankle and foot

(2) Orthopaedic treatment involves application of splints or successive plaster casts to correct position of foot and allow normal development

(3) Success of treatment depends on early treatment; with early treatment, prognosis is good

7. Chromosomal abnormalities

a. Down syndrome

(1) Results from extra chromosome at pair 21

(2) Signs include close-set, slanting eyes; narrow palpebral fissures; flattened nose; large, protuberant tongue; short, thick fingers with incurving of fifth digit; simian palmar crease; nuchal thickening

(3) Involves varying degrees of intellectual impairment

(4) Associated with multiple congenital anomalies, including cardiac and GI tract defects

  b. Trisomies 13 and 18

(1) Clinically similar to but more severe than Down syndrome

(2) High mortality rates; poor life expectancy

8. Inborn errors of metabolism

  a. Phenylketonuria

(1) Definition—deficiency of phenylalanine hydroxylase, resulting in inability to metabolize phenylalanine

(2) Results in toxic accumulation of abnormal metabolites of phenylalanine, eventually leading to CNS damage

(3) Treatment—dietary restriction of foods high in phenylalanine

(4) Should be identified and treated before 3 weeks of age

  b. Galactosemia

(1) Definition—inability to convert galactose to glucose

(2) Results in toxic accumulation of galactose in the bloodstream

(3) Treatment—dietary restriction of foods containing galactose

- Sudden infant death syndrome (SIDS)
  1. Definition—sudden unexplained death of infant between birth and 1 year of age
  2. Prevalence—2 out of 1000 infants

  a. Most prevalent between 2 and 4 months of age

  b. Rarely occurs before 3 weeks or after 9 months

3. Unknown cause

  a. Theory of delayed development of "arousal" and cardiorespiratory control

  b. Earlier research had suggested apnea as cause, but subsequent research has not shown a strong association between apnea and SIDS

  c. No evidence that home cardiorespiratory monitoring saves lives

4. Risk factors

  a. Gender—SIDS occurs more often in male than female infants

  b. Premature birth

  c. IUGR

  d. Low socioeconomic status

  e. Young maternal age

  f. Short interpregnancy interval

  g. Maternal smoking or use of cocaine or opiates

  h. More common in cold weather months

  i. More common after midnight and before 8:00 a.m.

  j. Higher incidence in African American or Native American infants

5. Recommendations

  a. "Back to sleep"—infants should be positioned in supine position to sleep

  b. Avoidance or reduction of modifiable risk factors

  c. Infants should sleep on a firm surface

  d. Avoid loose bedclothing

Questions

Select the best answer.

1. Which of the following infants is *least* at risk for neonatal hypoglycemia?
   a. The infant of a mother with diabetes mellitus
   b. The infant of a mother with gestational diabetes
   c. An infant who had intrapartum fetal monitoring findings suggestive of perinatal acidemia
   d. The infant of an opioid-abusing mother

2. Which of the following best describes the appearance and behavior of an overstimulated infant?
   a. Tremors, tachycardia, nonnutritive sucking, nasal flaring, and grunting
   b. Color changes, irregular respiration, irritability or lethargy, and vomiting
   c. Lethargy, flaccid tone, pallor, and inability to maintain alert active state
   d. Habituation to noxious stimuli and attempts to self-console

3. The midwife performs a physical examination on a newborn 2 hours after birth. Which of the following findings indicate a need for pediatric consultation?
   a. Respiratory rate of 50 breaths per minute
   b. Intermittent episodes of apnea, lasting less than 10 seconds each

  c. Yellow blanching of skin when pressure is applied to the infant's nose

  d. Preauricular skin tag

4. Ms. G. has just given birth, and the midwife's initial impression is that resuscitation may be necessary. According to American Academy of Pediatrics (AAP) and American Heart Association (AHA) guidelines, the midwife's initial steps are, in sequential order:

  a. Place the infant under a radiant heater, dry the infant and remove wet linen, suction the mouth and nose, and provide tactile stimulation while assessing for the presence or absence of spontaneous respirations

  b. Place the infant under a radiant heater, suction the mouth and nose, and evaluate heart rate by palpating the base of the umbilical cord or femoral pulse

  c. Place the infant under a radiant heater, evaluate heart rate by palpating the base of the umbilical cord or femoral pulse, dry the infant and remove wet linen, suction the mouth and nose, and continue to provide tactile stimulation

  d. Place the infant under a radiant heater, suction the mouth and nose, evaluate for the presence or absence of spontaneous respirations, and dry the infant and remove wet linen

5. Following the steps listed in question 4, the midwife notes that spontaneous respiration and tone are normal, the infant is crying vigorously, and the heart rate is 120 beats per minute. Continuing to follow AAP/AHA guidelines, the midwife then:
   a. Initiates positive-pressure ventilation with 100% oxygen
   b. Returns the infant to the mother to facilitate bonding and initiate breastfeeding
   c. Evaluates the infant's color and provides oxygen if acrocyanosis or general cyanosis are present
   d. Evaluates the infant's color and provides oxygen only if general cyanosis is present

6. With respect to question 5, how would the midwife proceed differently if meconium staining of the amniotic fluid had been noted on rupture of membranes?
   a. Suction the trachea after drying the infant and removing wet linen
   b. Suction the trachea on the perineum before delivery of the thorax
   c. Suction the mouth, nose, and pharynx only—endotracheal suctioning is not indicated
   d. Suction the trachea after drying the infant and providing tactile stimulation

7. Which of the following statements about the newborn transitional period is *not* true?
   a. Rapid changes in the infant's color during the period from 2 to 6 hours after birth are an ominous sign and require further evaluation
   b. The three stages, in order, are: (1) the first period of reactivity, (2) the period of unresponsive sleep, and (3) the second period of reactivity
   c. Respiratory rales are normally present during the first 20 minutes of life
   d. A period of unresponsive sleep typically begins within 1 hour after birth and continues until about 4 hours after birth

8. Ms. F., a primipara, is discussing infant feeding with her midwife. Which statement would indicate to the midwife that further teaching is necessary to correct a misunderstanding?
   a. "As long as my baby is suckling well and wetting diapers, I don't have to worry about whether he's getting enough milk."
   b. "Because I'm bottle feeding, I'm going to stick to a regular 2-hour feeding schedule."
   c. "My baby is 5 days old, but according to the scale on the side of the bottle, she's only taking about 20 or 30 mL of formula at each feeding. I'm worried: shouldn't she be eating more than that by now?"
   d. "I'm letting my baby feed until he seems satisfied at every feeding."

9. Which of the following statements about prophylaxis for newborn eye infections is *untrue*?
   a. Because of the rapid onset of ophthalmia neonatorum, administration of silver nitrate or erythromycin should take priority over family bonding and initiation of breastfeeding
   b. Erythromycin is preferred over silver nitrate because it provides coverage against the two most common pathogens
   c. Chlamydial conjunctivitis is the most common cause of blindness worldwide
   d. The two major pathogens for newborn eye infections are *Neisseria gonorrhoeae* and *Chlamydia trachomatis*

10. Ms. H., who has a 1-month-old infant, contacts the midwife on call. Ms. H. sounds distraught and tells the midwife that her baby "just cries and cries, all the time, and cries so hard that he gets red in the face. He's starting to drive me crazy!" The midwife asks questions about the baby's temperature, feeding habits, and voiding and stooling, all of which appear to be normal despite the baby's behavior. The midwife correctly tells Ms. H. that:
    a. She should take the baby to the emergency room immediately
    b. The baby's behavior is normal and getting used to the demands of an infant is a normal part of adjusting to motherhood
    c. Some babies are prone to this behavior, and one of the biggest problems is the effect on the baby's parents—when it gets to be too much, position the baby safely in his crib and go outside for a "sanity break"
    d. The baby's problem results from lack of stimulation—put on some upbeat music, turn on all the lights, make sure he can move freely, and engage him in active play

11. At her 6-month well-child checkup, Ms. J.'s baby weighs 12 lb, compared to a birth weight of 6 lb. Ms. J. says that she seems to breastfeed well but frequently spits up afterward. The midwife:
    a. Obtains a consultation with the pediatrician
    b. Recommends supplementation of formula in addition to continuing breastfeeding
    c. Orders metabolic screening, including screening for phenylketonuria
    d. Reassures Ms. J. that the baby's weight gain is normal and reinforces her breastfeeding technique

12. Which of the following is *not* characteristic of normal newborn behavior states?
    a. Abrupt, unpredictable changes between Brazelton's sleep–wake states
    b. Difficulty becoming and remaining alert
    c. Irritability and rapid progression from alertness to crying
    d. Overstimulation, requiring "time-out" with limitation of stimuli

13. The midwife wishes to estimate a newborn's gestational age. Which standard instrument is appropriate?
    a. Denver II
    b. New Ballard
    c. Erikson
    d. Erb-Duchene

14. Which of the following statements about the major psychological tasks of early infancy is *untrue*?
    a. Secure attachment is facilitated by caregivers who demonstrate predictable responses and emotional availability
    b. The development of basic trust is essential for formation of relationships later in life
    c. Research has not been able to demonstrate any long-term effects of insecure attachment in early infancy
    d. A major issue is the infant's ability to elicit caregiving responses from his or her mother

15. The midwife's discussion about circumcision with the infant's parents should acknowledge that:
    a. There are no medical benefits to circumcision
    b. The risks of circumcision, while rare, are potentially serious
    c. Research has proven that circumcision has a negative impact on long-term psychological and sexual functioning

d. Although there may be some modest benefit in reducing potential urinary tract and sexually transmitted infections, decisions about circumcision are largely based on personal, cultural, and religious considerations

16. Which of the following statements about hemolytic disease is true?
   a. ABO incompatibility is most common when the maternal blood type is A and the fetus's blood type is B
   b. Rh incompatibility may result in neonatal jaundice but rarely causes severe hemolysis or anemia
   c. A positive result on the direct Coombs' test indicates the presence of fetal blood cells in maternal circulation
   d. Hemolytic disease in the infant can be caused by maternal antibodies, enzymatic disorders, and some infections

17. The midwife suspects maternal opiate abuse as a result of which of the following clusters of newborn signs and conditions?
   a. Prematurity, low birth weight, genitourinary abnormalities, congenital heart disease, irritability, and frantic ineffective sucking
   b. Irritability, tremors, high-pitched cry, hyperstimulability, tachypnea, tachycardia, disorganized feeding, hyperthermia, and vasomotor instability
   c. Microcephaly, facial abnormalities, cardiac defects, and malformation of joints
   d. Lethargy, diminished reflexes, and hypotonia

18. Which of the following assessment findings are most consistent with prematurity?
   a. Translucent skin, sparse lanugo, flat areolae, prominent clitoris and labia minora, and highly flexible, nonrecoiling ear tissue
   b. Scant rugation of scrotum, undescended testes, and wrinkled, cracked, peeling skin
   c. Extended posture, flaccid tone, little resistance to flexion of extremities, and increased recoil of ear tissue
   d. Abundant lanugo, flexed posture, skin creases covering entire plantar surface, and relatively low-set position of ears

19. Prominent vasculature of the anterior lens capsule is most suggestive of which condition?
   a. Herpes virus exposure in the intrapartum period
   b. Relatively immature gestational age
   c. Gonococcal or chlamydial conjunctivitis
   d. Elevated total serum bilirubin concentration

20. Compared to fetal circulation, which of the following is *not* characteristic of circulation after birth?
   a. Increased pressure in the left atrium that facilitates closure of the foramen ovale
   b. Relatively low pulmonary vascular resistance that results in increased circulation to the lungs
   c. Decreased systemic vascular resistance due to loss of high-resistance placental circuit
   d. Increased oxygenation of circulating blood that causes constriction of the ductus arteriosus

21. Mr. N. is concerned about Ms. N.'s positive tuberculosis screening result. While awaiting results from Ms. N.'s chest radiograph and sputum culture, the midwife tells Mr. N. that:

a. Even if the chest radiograph is negative, Ms. N.'s exposure will necessitate a period of isolation from the newborn that may interfere with the initiation of breastfeeding
   b. Congenital tuberculosis is unlikely to be a problem for the newborn since Ms. N. shows no signs of active disease
   c. If the newborn acquires tuberculosis in utero, the most serious risk is for respiratory problems in the neonatal period
   d. Subclinical maternal tuberculosis infection is associated with a number of congenital malformations

22. Which of the following newborn assessment findings is/are *least* likely to be related to maternal gestational diabetes?
   a. High-pitched cry, plethora, tachypnea, and inconsolability
   b. Weak cry, jitteriness, cyanosis, apnea, poor feeding, and lethargy
   c. Serum glucose level below 40 mg/dL
   d. Absent Moro reflex on right side, and palpable crepitus between the right shoulder and neck

23. A defect in the vertebral column that results in extrusion of meninges and cerebrospinal fluid is best described as:
   a. Spina bifida occulta
   b. Hydrocephaly
   c. Myelomeningocele
   d. Meningocele

24. Which of the following conditions is most likely to result in loss of sensory and motor function below the level of the defect?
   a. Spina bifida occulta
   b. Hydrocephaly
   c. Myelomeningocele
   d. Meningocele

25. Within the first day of life, the midwife notices that Ms. O.'s baby drools copiously, feeds poorly with excessive reflux, and turns bluish-gray while feeding. Which condition does the midwife suspect?
   a. Tracheoesophageal malformation
   b. Pyloric stenosis
   c. Gastroschisis
   d. Oomphalocele

26. Increased oxygen consumption, hypoglycemia, hypoxia, acidosis, and respiratory distress can be caused in the immediate newborn period by:
   a. Congenital bacterial infections
   b. Maternal opioid abuse
   c. Patent ductus arteriosus
   d. Cold stress in the birthing room

27. Relatively mature capabilities of the newborn's gastrointestinal system include:
   a. Suckling, swallowing, and gag reflex
   b. Ability to digest fats and proteins
   c. Absorption of complex sugars
   d. Cardiac sphincter tone

28. At 1 minute of age, Baby P exhibits a strong cry, some flexion of the arms and legs, heart rate of 136 beats per minute, and acrocyanosis. Baby P's 1-minute Apgar score is:
   a. 6
   b. 7
   c. 8
   d. 9

29. At 5 minutes of age, Baby Q exhibits slow irregular respirations, some flexion of extremities, heart rate of 96 beats per minute, grimace in response to suction, and generalized cyanosis. Baby Q's 5-minute Apgar score is:
    a. 4
    b. 5
    c. 6
    d. 7

30. Which of the following statements about Apgar scores is true?
    a. The infant's Apgar score indicates whether or not resuscitation is needed and which steps of resuscitation procedure should be initiated
    b. The 1-minute Apgar score is more predictive of cord pH and long-term outcome than is the 5-minute Apgar score
    c. The 5-minute Apgar score is more predictive of cord pH, whereas the 1-minute Apgar score is more predictive of long-term outcome
    d. The Apgar score is only useful as a systematic way to assess the newborn's immediate adaptation to extrauterine life

31. In the initial examination of a male infant, the midwife notes drainage of urine from the stump of the umbilical cord. The newborn's condition is most likely:
    a. Patent urachus
    b. Epispadias
    c. Hypospadias
    d. Exstrophy of the bladder

32. Which of the following is *not* a true statement about the newborn's first breaths?
    a. The first inhalation requires less ventilatory pressure than later breaths
    b. The first breaths trigger the conversion from fetal to extra-uterine circulation
    c. Initial breathing serves to clear the lungs of fluid
    d. The first breaths establish lung volume and expand the alveoli

33. Which of the following is a true statement about thermoregulation in the transitional period?
    a. Shivering and muscular activity are the newborn's most effective means of thermogenesis
    b. Convection, conduction, radiation, and evaporation are important thermoregulatory mechanisms in the newborn period
    c. Metabolism of BAT is limited as a means of thermoregulation
    d. Alkalosis is a potentially serious consequence of ineffective thermoregulation in the newborn

34. Patient education about newborn skin care includes:
    a. "Cradle cap," a crusty yellowish-white accumulation on the anterior scalp, is caused by *Candida albicans* and must be treated with a topical antifungal agent
    b. Dry or peeling skin can be treated with baby oil, but if the condition does not resolve quickly, the healthcare provider should be notified
    c. Primary diaper dermatitis, characterized by circumscribed areas of bright red erythema and smaller outlying lesions, can be treated with thorough cleaning, baby powder, and air exposure

d. Tub baths should be avoided for the first 2 weeks of life or so until the cord stump has fallen off

35. Which of the following newborns is *not* a candidate for early discharge?
    a. Metabolic screening tests have not been completed; the baby has an appointment with the pediatric provider in 2 days
    b. Congenital hip dislocation is suspected; the baby has an orthopaedic appointment in 2 weeks for evaluation and treatment
    c. The infant's birth weight was 2625 g; gestational age assessment indicates term infant
    d. The infant requires phototherapy; a home health agency referral has been made

36. The midwife is examining Baby S prior to discharge. She notes that the head circumference is 34 cm, while the chest circumference is 31 cm. The midwife should:
    a. Assess for further signs of hydrocephalus, including separation of cranial sutures, bulging fontanelles, high-pitched cry, and downward deviation of the eyes
    b. Repeat the measurements—these findings are extremely unlikely
    c. Suspect diaphragmatic hernia—measurement of abdominal circumference and location of heart, lung, and bowel sounds may give some indication
    d. Proceed to the next component of the examination without further investigation of these findings

37. Evaluation of the newborn begins:
    a. Before the infant is born
    b. When the presenting part is crowning
    c. At the moment of birth
    d. After initial stabilization and resuscitation, if necessary

38. Which of the following statements is true of small for gestational age infants?
    a. Symmetric growth restriction results from chronic conditions and is typically associated with "catch-up growth" and good long-term outcome
    b. An infant is considered small for gestational age if he/she weighs less than 1500 g at birth
    c. An infant with head circumference above the 45th percentile and birth weight below the 10th percentile for gestational age would be described as asymmetrically growth restricted
    d. Asymmetric growth restriction is associated with acute insults in late pregnancy and is associated with poor long-term outcome

39. Baby U has the most abundant lanugo the midwife has ever seen. Baby U's gestational age is probably:
    a. 24 to 26 weeks
    b. 26 to 28 weeks
    c. 32 to 34 weeks
    d. 36 to 38 weeks

40. Which of the following is *not* associated with microcephaly?
    a. Prenatally acquired toxoplasmosis
    b. Prenatally acquired hepatitis B
    c. Fetal alcohol spectrum disorders
    d. Prenatally acquired HIV

41. At her 6-week postpartum visit, Ms. V. asks her midwife about sudden infant death syndrome (SIDS). In discussing SIDS with Ms. V., the midwife states that:
    a. SIDS almost never occurs after 6 weeks of age, so her baby is "in the clear"
    b. SIDS is extremely rare, affecting less than 2 in 100,000 infants
    c. The exact cause of SIDS is unknown
    d. Infants should be put to sleep in a prone or side-lying position

42. The normal newborn's sensory capacities are most limited in:
    a. Color perception
    b. Hearing
    c. Taste sensation
    d. Near vision focus

43. The organized infant is able to:
    a. Form significant relationships with others throughout life
    b. Hear high-pitched sounds
    c. Self-console and return to a stable behavioral state
    d. Sleep for 20–25% of daytime hours

44. Which of the following is a true statement about newborn metabolic disorders?
    a. Federal law mandates testing for phenylketonuria, galactosemia, and cystic fibrosis
    b. For early-discharge neonates, screening at 8 hours of life is acceptably reliable
    c. Most are characterized by enzyme deficiency, resulting in toxic accumulation of metabolites

    d. Breastfeeding is strongly recommended for infants with galactosemia

45. Which of the following is *not* an associated combination of intrapartum factor and neonatal finding?
    a. Forceps delivery—cephalohematoma
    b. Vertex presentation—asymmetry of gluteal folds
    c. Shoulder dystocia—asymmetric Moro reflex
    d. Breech presentation—positive Ortolani sign

46. Visible gastric peristalsis on observation of the abdomen is most suggestive of:
    a. Pyloric stenosis
    b. Esophageal fistula
    c. Colic
    d. Normal finding

47. Normal newborn respiratory findings include:
    a. Nasal flaring, expiratory grunting, and retractions
    b. Diaphragmatic and abdominal breathing
    c. Respiratory rate 40 to 80 breaths per minute
    d. Ventilation primarily through the mouth

48. Nonnutritive sucking
    a. Is *not* known to occur before birth
    b. Should be discouraged to prevent dental and facial malformations
    c. Is an example of behavioral self-regulation
    d. Can be promoted by placing a pacifier on a string around the baby's neck

Answers with Rationales

1. d. The infant of an opioid-abusing mother
   The other choices indicate risk factors for neonatal hypoglycemia. Opioid abuse is not a risk factor for hypoglycemia.

2. b. Color changes, irregular respiration, irritability or lethargy, and vomiting
   Infants may become fatigued or stressed when overstimulated. Color changes, irregular respiration, irritability or lethargy, and vomiting can be signs of such stress.

3. c. Yellow blanching of skin when pressure is applied to the infant's nose
   Jaundice in the first 24 hours of life is a pathologic finding that requires further evaluation and treatment.

4. a. Place the infant under a radiant heater, dry the infant and remove wet linen, suction the mouth and nose, and provide tactile stimulation while assessing for the presence or absence of spontaneous respirations
   This is the correct sequence of initial steps in neonatal resuscitation, as per Neonatal Resuscitation Program (NRP) guidelines.

5. d. Evaluates the infant's color and provides oxygen only if general cyanosis is present
   If the infant is crying vigorously, he or she does not require positive-pressure ventilation.
   The infant should not be returned to the mother until the color is assessed; oxygen is not necessary for acrocyanosis—this is a normal finding.

6. c. Suction the mouth, nose, and pharynx only—endotracheal suctioning is not indicated
   The infant is vigorous and therefore does not require endotracheal intubation. Stimulation is to be avoided until necessary suctioning is performed.

7. a. Rapid changes in the infant's color during the period from 2 to 6 hours after birth are an ominous sign and require further evaluation
   The other choices are true; rapid change in the infant's color in the transitional period is not necessarily an ominous sign (e.g., Harlequin's sign is normal).

8. b. "Because I'm bottle feeding, I'm going to stick to a regular 2-hour feeding schedule."
   Whether breastfed or bottle-fed, infants thrive best when fed on demand in response to cues of hunger.

9. a. Because of the rapid onset of ophthalmia neonatorum, administration of silver nitrate or erythromycin should take priority over family bonding and initiation of breastfeeding
   There is no increased risk for ophthalmia neonatorum if eye prophylaxis is delayed until after first period of reactivity. Eye contact during this period is considered important in the maternal-infant attachment process.

10. c. Some babies are prone to this behavior, and one of the biggest problems is the effect on the baby's parents—when it gets to be too much, position the baby safely in his crib and go outside for a "sanity break"

Colic affects approximately 10% of infants and can be quite frustrating for parents. Sometimes a short break of stepping out on the porch and breathing fresh air (when assured that the baby is safely in his/her crib) can be restorative and calming for the parent.

11. d. Reassures Ms. J. that the baby's weight gain is normal and reinforces her breastfeeding technique

Regurgitation is common in infants. The infant is thriving well and gaining weight appropriately.

12. a. Abrupt, unpredictable changes between Brazelton's sleep–wake states

Abrupt, unpredictable changes between Brazelton's sleep–wake states are not characteristic of normal newborn behavior.

13. b. New Ballard

The New Ballard instrument is the only one of the choices that estimates a newborn's gestational age.

14. c. Research has not been able to demonstrate any long-term effects of insecure attachment in early infancy

Research suggests long-term impairment, including school problems and delinquency, can result from insecure attachment in early infancy.

15. d. Although there may be some modest benefit in reducing potential urinary tract and sexually transmitted infections, decisions about circumcision are largely based on personal, cultural, and religious considerations

It appears that there is some benefit of reduced STIs, UTIs, and cancer of the penis in men who are circumcised, but opponents maintain that modern sanitary conditions and hygienic practices are more important factors in reducing the incidence of these diseases in comparison to the benefits from circumcision.

16. d. Hemolytic disease in the infant can be caused by maternal antibodies, enzymatic disorders, and some infections

Hemolytic disease can be caused by maternal antibodies, enzymatic disorders, or infections.

17. b. Irritability, tremors, high-pitched cry, hyperstimulability, tachypnea, tachycardia, disorganized feeding, hyperthermia, and vasomotor instability

Irritability, tremors, high-pitched cry, hyperstimulability, tachypnea, tachycardia, disorganized feeding, hyperthermia, and vasomotor instability are all signs of abstinence syndrome (opiate withdrawal) in the neonate.

18. a. Translucent skin, sparse lanugo, flat areolae, prominent clitoris and labia minora, and highly flexible, nonrecoiling ear tissue

Choices B, C, and D offer conflicting findings regarding gestational age assessment. Only option A lists all of the features that are consistent with prematurity.

19. b. Relatively immature gestational age

The vasculature of the anterior capsule of ocular lens is more prominent with early gestational ages.

20. c. Decreased systemic vascular resistance due to loss of high-resistance placental circuit

The placental circuit is low resistance, and the opposite is true after birth, when there is increased systemic vascular resistance with the loss of the placental circuit.

21. b. Congenital tuberculosis is unlikely to be a problem for the newborn since Ms. N. shows no signs of active disease

Congenital disease is rare unless the mother has untreated, advanced disease.

22. a. High-pitched cry, plethora, tachypnea, and inconsolability

Choices B, C, and D list findings that are more typically present in infants of diabetic mothers.

23. d. Meningocele

A meningocele is the extrusion of meninges and cerebrospinal fluid (CSF) through the vertebral column.

24. c. Myelomeningocele

Sensory and motor function loss below the level of the defect is noted with myelomeningocele.

25. a. Tracheoesophageal malformation

Copious drooling, poor feeding with reflux, and acute respiratory distress with feeding is characteristic of esophageal atresia and tracheoesophageal fistula.

26. d. Cold stress in the birthing room

Cold stress can result in all of the consequences listed, thus emphasizing the importance of thermoregulation of the neonate.

27. a. Suckling, swallowing, and gag reflex

Sucking, swallowing, and gag reflexes are all relatively mature in the term neonate.

28. c. 8

Perfect score for Apgar is 10. This infant receives only 1 point (out of 2) for color, 1 point (out of 2) for partial flexion of the extremities, 2 points for heart rate (> 100), and 2 points each for respiratory effort and reflex irritability (strong cry).

29. a. 4

Baby Q receives 0 points for color and only 1 point for each of the other four parameters, for a total of 4.

30. d. The Apgar score is only useful as a systematic way to assess the newborn's immediate adaptation to extrauterine life

The Apgar score is useful as a systematic way to assess the newborn's immediate adaptation to extrauterine life. The other statements are inaccurate.

31. a. Patent urachus

A patent urachus is the persistence of fetal opening between the bladder and the umbilical cord.

32. a. The first inhalation requires less ventilatory pressure than later breaths

The first inhalation requires more ventilatory pressure than later breaths.

33. c. Metabolism of BAT is limited as a means of thermoregulation

There is a limited supply of brown adipose tissue (BAT), thus limiting its metabolism as a means of thermoregulation.

34. d. Tub baths should be avoided for the first 2 weeks of life or so until the cord stump has fallen off

The infant should receive only sponge baths until the cord stump has fallen off because it is important to keep the area dry.

35. b. Congenital hip dislocation is suspected; the baby has an orthopaedic appointment in 2 weeks for evaluation and treatment

An infant with a suspected congenital hip dislocation would not be a good candidate for early discharge as compared with the other choices listed, who can be commonly followed on an outpatient basis.

36. d. Proceed to the next component of the examination without further investigation of these findings

The head circumference and chest circumference are normal; thus, the midwife should proceed with the next component of the exam.

37. a. Before the infant is born

    The infant's evaluation is begun even before birth via maternal history, risk factors, fetal testing results, and intrapartum factors.

38. c. An infant with head circumference above the 45th percentile and birth weight below the 10th percentile for gestational age would be described as asymmetrically growth restricted

    With asymmetric growth restriction, the head circumference is near normal for gestational age.

39. b. 26 to 28 weeks

    Lanugo is sparse to absent in the postmature or very premature infant and is most abundant in midterm infants (28–30 weeks).

40. b. Prenatally acquired hepatitis B

    Hepatitis B often results in prematurity and low birth weight, but not microcephaly.

41. c. The exact cause of SIDS is unknown

    There are theories surrounding the cause of SIDS, but the exact cause is unknown. An infant should always be put to sleep on his/her back.

42. a. Color perception

The normal newborn's sensory capacity is most limited in color perception.

43. c. Self-console and return to a stable behavioral state

    The organized infant is able to integrate physiologic and behavioral systems in response to the environment.

44. c. Most are characterized by enzyme deficiency, resulting in toxic accumulation of metabolites

    The organized infant is able to integrate physiologic and behavioral systems in response to the environment.

45. b. Vertex presentation—asymmetry of gluteal folds

    Asymmetry of gluteal folds is usually indicative of congenital hip dislocation. There is nothing inherent in a vertex presentation that would contribute to a hip dislocation.

46. a. Pyloric stenosis

    Visible gastric peristalsis, vomiting, and constipation are common features that present with pyloric stenosis.

47. b. Diaphragmatic and abdominal breathing

    Diaphragmatic and abdominal breathing are normal respiratory findings, whereas the other choices are incorrect.

48. c. Is an example of behavioral self-regulation

    Nonnutritive sucking is an example of a self-regulating behavior for self-consolation.

Bibliography

American Academy of Pediatrics. (2010). *Textbook of neonatal resuscitation* (6th ed.). Elk Grove, IL: Author.

American Academy of Pediatrics. (2012). Circumcision policy statement. *Pediatrics, 130*(3), 585–586.

Blackburn, S. T. (2013). *Maternal, fetal and neonatal physiology* (4th ed.). Maryland Heights, MO: Elsevier Saunders.

Centers for Disease Control and Prevention. (2014). *Birth–18 years and "catch-up" immunization schedule—United States, 2014*. Atlanta, GA: Author. Retrieved from http://www.cdc.gov/vaccines /schedules/hcp/child-adolescent.html

Hockenberry, M. J., & Wilson, D. (2011). *Wong's nursing care of infants and children* (9th ed.). St. Louis, MO: Elsevier-Mosby.

King, T. L., Brucker, M. C., Kriebs, J. M., Fahey, J. O., Gegor, C. L., & Varney, H. (2015). *Varney's midwifery* (5th ed.). Burlington, MA: Jones & Bartlett Learning.

Kliegman, R. M., Stanton, B. F., St. Geme, J. W., Schor, N. F., & Behrman, R. E. (2011). *Nelson textbook of pediatrics* (19th ed.). Maryland Heights, MO: Elsevier Saunders.

Kumar, V., Abbas., A. K., Fausto, N., & Aster, J. C. (2009). *Robbins and Cotran pathologic basis of disease, professional edition* (8th ed.). Maryland Heights, MO: Elsevier Saunders.

Lowdermilk, D., Perry, S., Cashion, M. C., & Alden, K. (2012). *Maternity and women's health* (10th ed.). St. Louis, MO: Elsevier Mosby.

Nagtalon-Ramos, J. (2014). *Maternal-newborn nursing care.* Philadelphia, PA: F. A. Davis.

Papalia, D. E., Olds, S. W., & Feldman, R. (2009). *Human development* (11th ed.). New York, NY: McGraw-Hill.

Riordan, J., & Auerbach, K. G. (2010). *Breastfeeding and human lactation* (4th ed.). Sudbury, MA: Jones and Bartlett.

Seidel, H. M., Rosenstein, B. J., & Pathak, A. (2006). *Primary care of the newborn* (4th ed.). St. Louis, MO: Mosby.

Tappero, E. P., & Honeyfield, M. E. (2009). *Physical assessment of the newborn* (4th ed.). Petaluma, CA: NICU Ink.

Volpe, J. J. (2008). *Neurology of the newborn* (5th ed.). Philadelphia, PA: W. B. Saunders.

9

Common Health Problems in Primary Care

Beth M. Kelsey and Jamille Nagtalon-Ramos

Cardiovascular Disorders

Hypertension

- Definition
  1. Systolic blood pressure (SBP) of 140 mm Hg or greater, or diastolic blood pressure (DBP) of 90 mm Hg or greater, based on the average of two or more properly measured, seated blood pressure (BP) readings on each of two or more office visits or taking antihypertensive medication (American Heart Association Statistics Committee and Stroke Subcommittee, 2014)
  2. Classification of blood pressure (7th Joint National Committee [JNC 7], 2003)

Classification	SBP	DBP
Normal	< 120	and < 80
Prehypertension	120–139	or 80–90
Stage 1 hypertension	140–159	or 90–99
Stage 2 hypertension	≥ 160	or ≥ 1003

  3. Evaluation of patients with documented hypertension has three objectives:
     a. To identify secondary causes
     b. To assess for target organ damage (TOD)—eye, brain, blood vessels, heart, and kidney
     c. To identify other cardiovascular risk factors or concomitant disorders that may define prognosis and guide therapy. Major cardiovascular risk factors include:
        (1) Smoking
        (2) Obesity (body mass index [BMI] ≥ 30)
        (3) Physical inactivity
        (4) Dyslipidemia
        (5) Diabetes mellitus
        (6) Microalbuminuria or estimated glomerular filtration rate (GFR) of less than 60 mL/min
        (7) Age older than 55 years in men and older than 65 years in women
        (8) Family history of premature cardiovascular disease (men age < 55 and women age < 65)
- Etiology/incidence
  1. Etiology
     a. Primary or essential
        (1) No discernible cause; a complex polygenic and multifactorial disorder
        (2) Comprises 90–95% of diagnosed cases
     b. Secondary
        (1) Underlying disease or condition identified; requires separate treatment
        (2) Comprises 5–10% of adult cases
  2. Incidence/prevalence (American Heart Association Statistics Committee and Stroke Subcommittee, 2014)
     a. One in three adults has high blood pressure (HBP)
     b. Approximately 6% of adults have undiagnosed HBP
     c. Men and women have similar percentages of HBP ages 45–64 years
     d. 57% of older women (ages 65+ years) have HBP compared with 54% of older men
     e. The prevalence of HBP is highest in non-Hispanic blacks (40.4%) compared with non-Hispanic whites (27.4%) and Hispanics (26.1%)
- Signs and symptoms
  1. Symptoms usually not present
  2. In cases of secondary hypertension, may be symptoms associated with secondary condition
     a. Weakness in primary aldosteronism
     b. Truncal obesity and purple striae in Cushing's syndrome
     c. Palpitations, tremor, and sweating in pheochromocytoma
  3. In chronic hypertension, may be symptoms associated with TOD
     a. Symptoms associated with peripheral vascular disease, coronary artery disease, and heart failure
     b. Symptoms associated with stroke or transient ischemic attack

- Physical findings
  1. Elevated blood pressure as noted in definition
  2. Findings associated with secondary causes or TOD
     a. Retinopathy
     b. S_4 gallop, S_3 gallop, precordial heave, and displaced point of maximal impulse
     c. Renal artery bruit in renal artery stenosis
     d. Delayed or absent femoral pulses and decreased blood pressure in lower extremities in coarctation of the aorta
     e. Diminished or absent peripheral pulses, edema
     f. Neurologic findings
- Differential diagnosis/secondary causes
  1. Sleep apnea
  2. Chronic kidney disease
  3. Primary aldosteronism
  4. Renovascular disease
  5. Chronic steroid therapy and Cushing's syndrome
  6. Pheochromocytoma
  7. Coarctation of the aorta
  8. Thyroid or parathyroid disease
  9. Drug-induced or drug-related
     a. Drug abuse—cocaine, amphetamines, alcohol
     b. Combination hormonal contraception
     c. Sympathomimetics—over-the-counter cold remedies
- Diagnostic tests/findings
  1. Recommended before initiating therapy to rule out secondary causes, determine the presence of risk factors, and assess for TOD
  2. Recommended initial laboratory tests
     a. Urinalysis
     b. Complete blood count (CBC)
     c. Blood glucose, serum potassium, creatinine or estimated GFR, calcium, lipid profile
        (1) Hypokalemia in primary aldosteronism
        (2) Elevated creatinine in renal disease
     d. Electrocardiogram (ECG) to assess evidence of ischemic heart disease or left ventricular hypertrophy (LVH)
  3. Optional studies
     a. Measurement of urinary albumin excretion or albumin/creatinine ratio
     b. Thyroid-stimulating hormone (TSH)
     c. Intravenous pyelogram (IVP) to rule out renovascular disease
     d. 24-hour urine for metanephrines and catecholamines to rule out pheochromocytoma
     e. Chest radiograph to rule out cardiomegaly and coarctation of the aorta
     f. Echocardiogram is more sensitive study to detect LVH
- Management/treatment—JNC 8 (James, et al., 2014)
  1. Goals of therapy
     a. Prevent/minimize TOD
     b. Focus on achievement of systolic BP goal; most patients will achieve diastolic goal once systolic BP is at goal (< 140/90 mm Hg)
     c. BP goal in patients with coronary heart disease (CHD), diabetes, abdominal aortic aneurysm, peripheral arterial disease, carotid artery disease, 10-year Framingham risk score

of 10% or greater, or renal disease is less than 130/80 mm Hg
  2. Nonpharmacologic—lifestyle modifications recommended for all patients (both prehypertension and hypertension)
     a. Weight reduction—maintain ideal body weight
     b. Adopt Dietary Approaches to Stop Hypertension (DASH) eating plan—diet rich in fruits, vegetables, and low-fat dairy products with a reduced content of saturated and total fat
     c. Dietary sodium reduction—6 g NaCl/day
     d. Physical activity—engage in aerobic physical activity at least 30 minutes per day most days of the week
     e. Moderation of alcohol consumption—no more than one drink/day for women
     f. Stop smoking
  3. Pharmacologic
     a. General principles of drug therapy for hypertension–JNC 8 (James, et al., 2014)
        (1) Set BP goal and initial BP-lowering medication based on age, diabetes, and chronic kidney disease (CKD)
        (2) BP goals
           (a) General population (no diabetes or CKD) age 60 years or older—BP goal is SBP less than 150 mm Hg and DBP less than 90 mm Hg
           (b) General population (no diabetes or CKD) age younger than 60 years—BP goal is SBP less than 140 mm Hg and DBP less than 90 mm Hg
           (c) All ages with diabetes and/or CKD present—BP goal is SBP less than 140 mm Hg and DBP less than 90 mm Hg
        (3) Initial BP-lowering medication
           (a) All ages, African American (no diabetes or CKD or diabetes without CKD)—thiazide-type diuretic or calcium channel blocker (CCB), alone or in combination
           (b) All ages, Caucasian (no diabetes or CKD or diabetes without CKD)—thiazide-type diuretic or angiotensin-converting enzyme inhibitor (ACEI) or angiotensin receptor blocker (ARB) or CCB, alone or in combination
           (c) All ages, all races with CKD present with or without diabetes—ACEI or ARB, alone or in combination with other drug classes
        (4) Select a drug treatment titration strategy
           (a) Strategy 1—maximize first medication before adding second medication OR
           (b) Strategy 2—add second medication before reaching maximum dose of first medication OR
           (c) Strategy 3—start with two medication classes separately or as a fixed-dose combination
        (5) If BP goal not met with titration strategies
           (a) Reinforce medication and lifestyle adherence
           (b) Strategy 1 or 2—add and titrate thiazide-type diuretic or ACEI or ARB or CCB (use medication class not previously selected; avoid combining ACEI and ARB)
           (c) Strategy 3—titrate does of initial medications to maximum

(d) If BP goal still not met, add and titrate thiazide-type diuretic or ACEI or ARB or CCB (use medication class not previously selected; avoid combining ACEI and ARB)

(e) If BP goal still not met, refer to physician with expertise in hypertension management

b. Classification of drugs for hypertension by drug action (see **Table 9-1**)

4. Patient education
   a. Lifelong nature of hypertensive condition
   b. Asymptomatic nature of hypertension
   c. Adherence to treatment regimens reduces complications and deaths
   d. Critical to comply with recommended follow-up and monitoring schedule

- Referral
  1. Evaluation and management of secondary causes
  2. Resistance to drug therapy; failure to respond to three-drug regimen that includes a diuretic

Heart Murmurs

- Definition
  1. Prolonged extra heart sounds heard during either systole or diastole; commonly associated with dynamics of regurgitation or stenosis
  2. Classification
     a. Innocent or functional murmurs
        (1) Transient; pose no direct threat to health
        (2) Most frequently heard during systole
        (3) No structural or functional cardiac abnormality
        (4) Often noted in pregnancy because of increased cardiac output
     b. Pathologic murmurs are indicative of heart or valvular disease (e.g., aortic or pulmonary stenosis, atrial septal defect, rheumatic heart disease)
- Etiology/incidence
  1. Etiology
     a. Turbulent blood flow into, through, or out of the heart can result in audible murmur
     b. Characteristics of sound depend upon the following factors:
        (1) Size of valve opening
        (2) Integrity of valve
        (3) Vigor of contraction
        (4) Rate of flow
        (5) Thickness of chest wall
  2. Incidence
     a. Innocent systolic murmurs occur in 50–70% of children and up to 50% of adults at some time
     b. Pathologic murmurs are less common, but incidence increases with age
        (1) Congenital—Marfan's syndrome, valve malformation
        (2) Acquired—rheumatic heart disease, mitral valve prolapse (MVP)
- Signs and symptoms
  1. Innocent murmurs—not symptomatic
  2. Pathologic

a. Possible chest pain
b. Shortness of breath on exertion
c. Orthopnea
d. Cough or wheeze
e. Paroxysmal nocturnal dyspnea
f. Growth failure

- Physical findings
  1. Innocent
     a. Usually none except audible murmur
     b. Soft (grade 1 or 2 intensity), medium pitch, systolic murmur
     c. Heard best when patient is supine
     d. Disappears with standing or straining
     e. Increases with increased cardiac output (e.g., fever, exercise)
  2. Pathologic
     a. Diastolic or pansystolic murmur or any murmur above grade 3
     b. Intensifies with exercise or Valsalva maneuver
     c. Mid or late systolic click, associated with MVP
     d. Cyanosis
     e. Jugular vein distension
     f. Hepatomegaly
     g. Pedal edema
     h. Diminished femoral pulses or unequal blood pressure in left and right arms
- Differential diagnosis—focused on differentiating innocent versus pathologic murmur
- Diagnostic tests/findings—indicated only if pathologic murmur suspected
  1. Echocardiography—confirms severity, location of clinically detected lesions
  2. Chest radiograph—suspected cardiac enlargement
  3. CBC—rule out anemia
  4. Thyroid function tests—rule out hyper- or hypothyroidism
- Management/treatment
  1. Low-grade, asymptomatic systolic murmur with low-risk history can be assumed innocent and followed up at next visit
  2. Pharmacologic—bacterial endocarditis prophylaxis for susceptible patients
     a. Patients with valvular heart disease, prosthetic heart valves, or other structural cardiac abnormalities
     b. Indicated dental, upper respiratory, gastrointestinal, and genitourinary procedures
     c. Give oral amoxicillin 2 g 1 hour before procedure
  3. Patient education
     a. Self-knowledge and self-disclosure in future encounters
     b. Follow-up schedule if indicated
- Referral
  1. Diastolic murmurs
  2. Suspected pathologic systolic murmurs

Thromboembolic Disease

- Definitions
  1. Thrombosis—blood clot that forms abnormally within blood vessels
  2. Embolus—blood clot that breaks free from its site of formation

▪ **Table 9-1** Hypertension Pharmacology (representative list)

Drug Name	Action	Side-effects	Interactions	Contraindications / Precautions
Thiazide diuretics				
Hydrochlorothiazide Indapamide Chlorthalidone	Inhibits sodium reabsorption from distal renal tubules; reduced sodium results in decreased vascular tone	Hypokalemia and other electrolyte disorders, hyperglycemia, hyperuricemia, orthostatic hypotension, volume depletion, worsening kidney function, transient hyperlipidemia	Enhances other classes of antihypertensives; may decrease oral sulfonylurea and insulin drug efficacy; digitalis and lithium toxicity; NSAIDs may reduce effect of thiazide and increase risk of acute renal failure	Sulfonamide allergy; use caution in patients with impaired renal function, diabetes, history of gout, and elderly who may be at more risk for orthostatic hypotension Second line as treatment choice during pregnancy, theoretical potential for intravascular volume depletion (ACOG, 2013). Other risks to fetus include a decrease in glucose, platelets, sodium, potassium levels, and possible death resulting from complications with the mother. (Briggs & Freeman, 2015). Low concentrations in breast milk, may reduce quantity of milk production (ACOG, 2013)
Beta-adrenoreceptor antagonists—Beta blockers				
Propranolol Atenolol Labetalol	Inhibits sympathetic stimulation of the heart; reduces sympathetic outflow to peripheral vasculature; blocks renin release from kidney	Bronchospasm, bradycardia, hypotension, heart failure, may mask insulin-induced hypoglycemia, insomnia, fatigue, decreased exercise tolerance	Additive effect with other antihypertensive agents and alcohol; altered effectiveness of hypoglycemic drugs	Asthma, A-V block, heart failure; use caution with diabetes, older adults Labetalol may be considered if needed for initial treatment of pregnant women with chronic hypertension; low concentrations of labetalol and propranolol in breast milk, high concentrations of atenolol (ACOG, 2013), The American Academy of Pediatrics (AAP) considers labetalol compatible with breastfeeding. Atenolol has been associated with cyanosis and bradycardia in infants of mothers taking this medication (Briggs & Freeman, 2015 and AAP, 2001)
Calcium channel antagonists—Calcium channel blockers (CCB)				
Nifedipine Diltiazem Verapamil	Blocks influx of calcium through transmembrane calcium channels that trigger smooth muscle contraction; results in prolonged vascular smooth muscle relaxation	Dizziness, hypotension, headache, GI symptoms, peripheral edema, heart failure Side effects less common with sustained release forms	Additive effect with other antihypertensive agents and alcohol; risk of digoxin and lithium toxicity; Drugs that inhibit CYP3A4 and grapefruit juice may increase free drug levels	Heart failure, A-V block; significant peripheral edema Avoid with GERD as may make worse Nifedipine may be considered if needed for initial treatment of pregnant women with chronic hypertension, no adverse effects have been reported with breastfeeding (ACOG, 2013), AAP considers nifedipine compatible with breastfeeding (Briggs & Freeman, 2015 and AAP, 2001)

Angiotensin-converting enzyme inhibitors—ACE inhibitors

Drug	Action	Side effects	Interactions	Considerations
Captopril Enalapril	Inhibits angiotensin-converting enzyme; prevents conversion of angiotensin I to angiotensin II thus enhancing vasodilation	Cough;, hypotension, rash; angioedema,	Additive effect with other antihypertensive agents and alcohol; increased risk for renal toxicity with NSAIDS; increased risk for hyperkalemia with potassium-sparing diuretics	ACE inhibitor associated or other angioedema bilateral renal artery stenosis, hyperkalemia Associated with fetal anomalies, not recommended for pregnant women, low concentrations in breast milk (ACOG, 2013) Enalapril is compatible with breast milk, as per the American Academy of Pediatrics (Briggs & Freeman, 2015 and AAP, 2001)

Angiotensin II receptor blockers—ARB

Drug	Action	Side effects	Interactions	Considerations
Losartian, Valsartan	Block binding of angiotensin II to receptor thus enhancing vasodilation	Similar to ACE inhibitors, but not likely to cause cough and less likely to cause angioedema	Same as with ACE inhibitors	Same as with ACE inhibitors with exception of angioedema Associated with fetal anomalies, not recommended for pregnant women (ACOG, 2013) Effects of valsartan on breastfeeding have been identified Valsartan is compatible with breastfeeding as per the American Academy of Pediatrics (Briggs & Freeman, 2015 and AAP, 2001)

3. Deep vein thrombosis (DVT)—formation of blood clots in deep veins of legs; may break off and lead to pulmonary embolism
4. Thromboembolism—DVT plus systemic embolism
5. Thrombophilia—refers to individuals who have tendency to develop thrombosis from either acquired or inherited causes, or both
6. Superficial phlebitis—inflammation of superficial veins as result of local trauma, venous stasis, or infection

- Etiology/incidence/risk factors
  1. Etiology
     a. Origin of most venous thrombi lie in Virchow's triad—endothelial damage, stasis, hypercoagulability
        (1) Endothelial damage secondary to trauma
        (2) Stasis secondary to immobility
        (3) Hypercoagulability secondary to protein deficiency states such as protein C or S, antithrombin III; nephrotic syndrome, chronic liver disease, and certain malignancies
     b. DVT occurs as blood clots form within the deep venous plexus of the calf or within the popliteal, femoral, iliac veins
     c. Approximately 40% of DVTs embolize to pulmonary circulation when thigh veins involved; risk minimal when only calf veins involved
     d. Prevention of pulmonary embolus (PE) necessitates prompt diagnosis and treatment of DVT
     e. Superficial thromboses usually occur in varicose veins
  2. Incidence—DVT/PE—500,000 cases annually
  3. Risk factors (acquired)
     a. Recent surgery—gynecologic or orthopedic procedures of the hip, knee
     b. Immobilization or venous stasis
     c. Trauma or fractures
     d. Malignancies
     e. Pregnancy and early postpartum
     f. Combination hormonal contraceptives
     g. Congestive heart failure or recent myocardial infarction (MI)
     h. Prior history of thromboembolic disease
     i. Obesity
     j. Inflammatory diseases
     k. Antiphospholipid syndrome
     l. Smoking
  4. Risk factors (inherited)
     a. Factor V Leiden
     b. Homocysteine abnormalities
     c. Prothrombin gene mutation
     d. Protein C or S deficiency
- Signs and symptoms
  1. Superficial phlebitis—localized area of edema, erythema, and tenderness over superficial vein
  2. DVT
     a. Acute onset of unilateral leg pain (calf)
     b. Leg edema
     c. Up to 50% have no symptoms
  3. PE
     a. Unilateral chest pain
     b. Anxiety, restlessness
     c. Dyspnea

- Physical findings
  1. Superficial phlebitis
     a. Localized area of edema, erythema, and tenderness over a superficial vein
     b. Increased temperature in surrounding skin
  2. DVT—often no findings
     a. Calf tenderness to compression; pain elicited with dorsiflexion of foot (Homan's sign); nonspecific finding
     b. Palpable venous cord
     c. Unilateral leg edema; skin may be warm and erythematous
  3. PE
     a. Cyanosis
     b. Diminished breath sounds over involved area
     c. Tachypnea
     d. Cough with hemoptysis
     e. Tachycardia
     f. Fever
- Differential diagnosis
  1. DVT
     a. Muscle strain or contusion
     b. Cellulitis—more diffuse redness
     c. Popliteal (Baker's) cyst
     d. Superficial phlebitis
  2. PE
     a. Myocardial infarction
     b. Pneumothorax
     c. Pneumonia
- Diagnostic tests/findings
  1. Superficial phlebitis—usually none indicated
  2. DVT
     a. Duplex ultrasound—use as initial test when probability of DVT is intermediate to high; good sensitivity and specificity in symptomatic patients; negative test if intermediate to high probability of DVT requires further testing
     b. Plasma D-dimer enzyme-linked immunosorbant assay (ELISA)
        (1) Measures active breakdown of thrombi
        (2) Elevated in 95–98% of DVT; useful in ruling out DVT if negative
        (3) Positive results are not diagnostic because several other conditions cause positive result (e.g., atrial fibrillation, impaired renal function, pregnancy, ongoing blood loss)
        (4) Best used as initial test if probability of DVT is low
     c. Contrast venography—best used for suspected calf vein thrombus or when clinical findings conflict with ultrasound
     d. Other lab tests for inherited or acquired anticoagulation deficiencies
        (1) Protein C, Protein S
        (2) Antithrombin III
        (3) Antiphospholipid antibodies
        (4) Factor V Leiden
  3. PE
     a. Ventilation-perfusion (V/Q) lung scan
     b. Arterial blood gases
     c. ECG and chest radiograph
     d. Plasma D-dimer ELISA
     e. Pulmonary angiogram

- Management/treatment
  1. Refer suspected DVT or PE for immediate medical management
  2. Superficial phlebitis
     a. Nonpharmacologic—elevation of leg and compression with an ace wrap
     b. Pharmacologic—nonsteroidal anti-inflammatory drugs
  3. Patient education—for high-risk patients
     a. During prolonged, confined travel—support hose, adequate fluids, passive intermittent contraction of calf muscles, rest breaks to stretch and exercise the legs
     b. May consider low-dose aspirin (81–365 mg) for individuals with risk for DVT who travel long distances
     c. Do not smoke
     d. Do not use estrogen-containing contraceptives

Dyslipidemia

- Definition
  1. Increased levels of total blood cholesterol and low-density lipoproteins (LDL) or triglycerides (TG); suppressed high-density lipoproteins (HDL), or any combination; risk factor for the development of coronary heart disease in adults
  2. Classifications using National Cholesterol Education Program (NCEP) Adult Treatment Panel III (ATP III) Guidelines (National Heart, Lung, and Blood Institute [NHLBI], 2001)
     a. Elevated LDL-C greater than 130 mg/dL
     b. Hypertriglyceridemia greater than 200 mg/dL
     c. Low HDL-C less than 40 mg/dL
     d. Metabolic syndrome—any three risk factors
        (1) Abdominal obesity/waist circumference
            (a) Men, greater than 40 inches
            (b) Women, greater than 35 inches
        (2) Triglycerides 150 mg/dL or greater
        (3) HDL-C
            (a) Men, less than 40 mg/dL
            (b) Women, less than 50 mg/dL
        (4) Blood pressure 130/85 mm Hg or greater
        (5) Fasting glucose 110 mg/dL or greater
- Etiology/incidence/prevalence
  1. Etiology
     a. Genetic predisposition
     b. Secondary causes
        (1) Obesity
        (2) Disease processes (e.g., endocrine and metabolic disorders, obstructive liver disease, renal disorders)
        (3) Drugs (e.g., corticosteroids, thiazide diuretics, beta blockers)
  2. Incidence/prevalence—estimated 65 million Americans have high cholesterol
- Signs and symptoms—none except those associated with CHD
- Physical findings
  1. Xanthomas
  2. Arcus senilis
  3. Central obesity
- Differential diagnosis—focused on ruling out secondary causes
- Diagnostic tests/findings

1. Screening schedule
   a. A fasting lipoprotein profile (total cholesterol, LDL-C, HDL-C, TG) should be obtained every 5 years in patients 20 years or older (NHLBI, 2001)
   b. If fasting opportunity not available at initial screen, obtain total cholesterol and HDL-C; if total cholesterol is greater than 200 mg/dL or HDL-C is less than 40 mg/dL, have patient return for fasting profile
2. Cholesterol and triglycerides classification—ATP III
   a. Total cholesterol
      (1) Less than 200 mg/dL—desirable
      (2) 200–239 mg/dL—borderline high
      (3) 240 mg/dL or greater —high
   b. LDL cholesterol
      (1) Less than 100 mg/dL—optimal
      (2) 100–129 mg/dL—near or above optimal
      (3) 130–159 mg/dL—borderline high
      (4) 160–189 mg/dL —high
      (5) 190 mg/dL or greater—very high
   c. HDL cholesterol
      (1) Less than 40 md/dL—low
      (2) 60 or greater mg/dL —high (protective against CHD)
   d. Triglycerides
      (1) Less than 150 mg/dL—normal
      (2) 150–199 mg/dL—borderline high
      (3) 200–499 mg/dL—high
      (4) 500 mg/dL or greater—very high
- Management/treatment
  1. Treatment of dyslipidemia is based on risk of CHD events
     a. Determine if patient has clinically manifested CHD or CHD risk equivalents—peripheral vascular disease, abdominal aortic aneurysm, symptomatic carotid artery disease, diabetes
     b. Determine if presence of major risk factors (other than high LDL):
        (1) Cigarette smoking
        (2) Hypertension (BP ≥ 140/90 mm Hg or on antihypertensive medication)
        (3) Low HDL cholesterol (< 40 mg/dl); HDL > 60 counts as negative risk factor—remove one risk factor from the total count
        (4) Family history of premature CHD (CHD in male first-degree relative < 55 years; CHD in female first-degree relative < 65 years)
        (5) Age (men ≥ 45 years; women ≥ 55 years)
     c. If patient has two or more risk factors, without CHD or CHD risk equivalent, determine the 10-year risk of a CHD event with the Framingham risk tool
        (1) Three risk categories
            (a) CHD or CHD risk equivalents = 10-year risk > 20%
            (b) 2+ risk factors without CHD or CHD risk equivalents = 10-year risk ≤ 20%
            (c) 0–1 risk factors = 10-year risk < 10%
     d. Assign a treatment goal for LDL-C based on risk category
        (1) CHD or CHD risk equivalents—LDL-C goal of less than 100 mg/dL

(2) 2+ risk factors without CHD or CHD risk equivalents—LDL-C goal of less than 130 mg/dL

(3) 0–1 risk factors without CHD or CHD risk equivalents—LDL-C goal of less than 160 mg/dL

2. Nonpharmacologic/therapeutic lifestyle changes

  a. Dietary modification

    (1) Cholesterol reduction from diet modification and dietary supplements can average 10–15%

    (2) Nutrition recommendations from NCEP

      (a) Total fat 25–35% of total calories/day; less than 7% from saturated fat, 20% or less from monounsaturated fat, 10% or less from polyunsaturated fat

      (b) Carbohydrate 50–60% of total calories/day

      (c) Protein approximately 15% of total calories/day

      (d) Cholesterol less than 200 mg/day

    (3) Foods/supplements to enhance LDL lowering

      (a) Fiber 20–30 g/day; 10–25 g/day soluble fiber

      (b) Plant stanols/sterols—2–3 g/day available in margarines and salad dressings

      (c) Nuts as a snack—walnuts, almonds

      (d) Substitute soy protein

      (e) Omega-3 fish oil capsules

  b. Encourage moderate-intensity exercise for 30 minutes/day for most days of the week—this can be walking

  c. Aggressive smoking cessation program

  d. Weight loss for overweight and obese patients (goal BMI < 25); initial weight loss goal of 5–10% of current weight

3. Pharmacologic

  a. For most patients at moderate risk, lifestyle changes should be prescribed and followed for 3 months before initiating drug therapy; early drug therapy indicated for patients with CHD and CHD equivalents

  b. Pattern of dyslipidemia directs drug choice

  c. Pharmacologic agents

    (1) HMG-CoA reductase inhibitors (statins)

      (a) Atorvastatin (Lipitor), fluvastatin (Lescol), lovastatin (Mevacor), pravastatin (Pravachol), rosuvastatin (Crestor), simvastatin (Zocor)

      (b) Drug action—inhibits HMG-CoA reductase, the enzyme that controls cholesterol biosynthesis in cells; effective decrease LDL-C, moderate increase HDL, moderate decrease triglycerides

      (c) Side effects—elevated liver enzymes and myopathy; monitor liver function

      (d) Drug interactions—combined with fibrates or niacin may increase risk of myopathy

      (e) Contraindications/precautions—severe liver disease; pregnancy Category X; not recommended while nursing

    (2) Nicotinic acid

      (a) Niacin/immediate release; Niaspan/extended release

      (b) Drug action—decreases synthesis of LDL-C by reducing hepatic synthesis of very low density lipoprotein (VLDL) cholesterol; increases HDL-C by decreasing its catabolism; decreases triglycerides

      (c) Side effects—flushing, pruritus/decreased if take acetylsalicylic acid (ASA, aspirin) 30 minutes before; dyspepsia, hyperglycemia, hyperuricemia, hepatotoxicity

      (d) Drug interactions—additive hypotensive effect with antihypertensives; monitor for myopathy if used with statins

      (e) Contraindications/precautions—liver disease, severe gout, peptic ulcer, diabetes; pregnancy Category C; not recommended in nursing mothers

    (3) Bile acid sequestrants

      (a) Cholestyramine (Questran), colestipol (Colestid), colesevelam (Welchol)

      (b) Drug action—binds cholesterol-containing bile acids in intestines, forming insoluble complex that is excreted; moderate decrease LDL-C; minimal increase HDL-C; no decrease, possible increase triglycerides

      (c) Side effects—gastrointestinal effects (e.g., constipation, bloating, nausea, cramping; no systemic toxicity)

      (d) Drug interactions—may interfere with absorption of other medications; administer other drugs 1 hour before or 3 hours after resin

      (e) Contraindications/precautions—patients with triglycerides greater than 400 mg/dL and patients with low HDL-C; pregnancy Category C; caution while nursing

    (4) Fibric acids

      (a) Gemfibrizil (Lopid), fenofibrate (Tricor)

      (b) Drug actions—acts primarily on triglyceride-rich lipoproteins, effective decrease triglycerides, minimal decrease in LDL-C, moderate increase in HDL-C

      (c) Side effects—dyspepsia, gallstones, myopathy

      (d) Drug interactions—may increase risk of myopathy when combined with statins; may potentiate effect of warfarin

      (e) Contraindications/precautions—severe renal or hepatic disease; pregnancy Category C; not recommended while nursing

    (5) Ezetimibe (Zetia)

      (a) Drug action—cholesterol absorption inhibiter, use alone or in combination with a statin

      (b) Side effects—back pain, arthralgia, diarrhea, abdominal pain; with statin, increase in serum transaminases

      (c) Drug interactions—not recommended for use with fibrates; separate dosing bile acid sequestrants

      (d) Contraindications/precautions—liver disease; pregnancy Category C; not recommended in nursing mothers

    (6) Combination medications

      (a) Statin plus aspirin

      (b) Statin plus calcium channel blocker

      (c) Statin plus cholesterol absorption inhibitor

      (d) Statin plus niacin

4. Patient education
   a. Therapeutic lifestyle changes
   b. Monitoring schedule
- Referral
  1. Nutritional consultation
  2. Lipid specialist with unusually severe, refractory, or complex disorders

Coronary Heart Disease (CHD)

- Definition—atherosclerotic changes to coronary vasculature; decreased blood flow through coronary arteries due to partial obstruction or vasospasm
- Etiology/incidence/risk factors
  1. Etiology
     a. Atherosclerosis develops with the formation of fatty streaks, fibrous plaques, and complicated lesions that narrow the lumen of the coronary arteries
     b. Angina pectoris—myocardial ischemia secondary to inability of the coronary arteries to supply oxygenated blood to meet myocardial oxygen demands
     c. Acute coronary syndromes—a plaque may rupture with thrombus formation that impedes/completely occludes the coronary lumen
        (1) Unstable angina
        (2) Acute myocardial infarction
  2. Incidence—CHD is the leading killer of women; CHD is the cause of one out of every three deaths in women each year
  3. Risk factors include:
     a. Cigarette smoking
     b. Hypertension
     c. Dyslipidemia
     d. Diabetes mellitus
     e. Genetic predisposition
     f. Obesity
     g. Sedentary lifestyle
     h. Sleep apnea
- Signs and symptoms
  1. May be asymptomatic
  2. Chronic stable angina pectoris
     a. Clinical syndrome characterized by discomfort in the chest, jaw, shoulder, back, or arm precipitated by exertion and relieved by rest or nitroglycerin
     b. Predictable frequency, severity, duration, and provocation
     c. Pattern remains the same unless there is acceleration of disease process
  3. Acute coronary syndromes—unstable angina and myocardial infarction
     a. May have a constellation of symptoms
     b. Chest pain—pressure, heaviness, squeezing, crushing, aching
     c. Pain generally involves sternum and/or epigastrum
     d. Pain may radiate to shoulder, arm, jaw, neck, back
     e. Associated nausea, vomiting, diaphoresis, dyspnea
- Physical findings
  1. May be no specific findings
  2. Elevated blood pressure
  3. Dyspnea, tachycardia, pallor, diaphoresis

4. Heart—changes in point of maximum impulse(s) and heart sounds may occur dependent on extent of heart damage or dysfunction
- Differential diagnosis
  1. Chronic stable angina
  2. Unstable angina
  3. Myocardial infarction
  4. Pulmonary disease—pulmonary embolism, pneumothorax, pneumonia
  5. GI disorders—gastroesophageal reflux, cholecystitis, peptic ulcer
  6. Musculoskeletal conditions—costochondritis, muscle strain
  7. Anxiety disorders
  8. Acute aortic dissection
  9. Herpes zoster
- Diagnostic tests/findings
  1. Electrocardiogram
     a. Acute episode of chronic stable angina—ST-segment depression, symmetric T-wave inversion in affected leads; reverts to normal during pain-free intervals
     b. Unstable angina, myocardial infarction—changes dependent on location of involved vessel, amount of myocardium involved, duration of ischemia
  2. Exercise or pharmacologic stress testing—ischemic changes or angina during test is clinically diagnostic
  3. Myocardial perfusion imaging—used to confirm and assess extent and location of coronary artery disease
  4. Coronary angiography—definitive test for coronary artery disease
  5. Laboratory tests—myocardial markers
     a. Troponin I and T—high sensitivity and specificity; become elevated within 3–4 hours of event and continue to be released for up to 7–14 days after cardiac event
     b. Myoglobin—released within 1–3 hours of myocardial cell injury; not as cardiac specific as troponins; normalizes in 24 hours
- Management/treatment
  1. Nonpharmacologic
     a. Primary prevention—smoking cessation; dietary management of hypertension, dyslipidemia, diabetes, obesity; regular aerobic exercise
     b. Secondary prevention—surgical revascularization
        (1) Percutaneous transluminal coronary angioplasty (PTCA)
        (2) Coronary artery bypass graft (CABG)
  2. Pharmacologic—the treatment of chronic stable angina has two major purposes: to prevent myocardial infarction and to reduce the symptoms of angina
     a. Primary prevention
        (1) Medications for treatment of hypertension, diabetes, hyperlipidemia, and smoking cessation
        (2) Aspirin 81–325 mg/day—inhibits platelet aggregation
     b. Secondary management of angina—may use a combination of medications for increased effectiveness
        (1) Sublingual nitroglycerine 0.4 mg as needed for symptomatic relief of anginal episodes (see "Long-acting nitrates" section later)

(2) Beta-adrenergic blockers—metoprolol, propranolol, atenolol; preferred initial therapy in absence of contraindications

    (a) Drug action—decrease myocardial demand by decreasing heart rate, systolic blood pressure, and contractility

    (b) Side effects—fatigue, dizziness, depression, bradycardia, hypotension, nausea, diarrhea, dyspnea, bronchospasm, rash

    (c) Drug interactions—may potentiate other antihypertensives, may antagonize effects of sympathomimetic drugs

    (d) Contraindications—sinus bradycardia, heart block greater than 1 degree, heart failure, cardiogenic shock; pregnancy Category C

(3) Calcium channel blockers—verapamil, amlodipine/long-acting formulations only

    (a) Drug action—promote peripheral arterial vasodilation, which decreases oxygen demand by decreasing afterload, also decrease coronary vasospasm

    (b) Side effects—hypotension, edema, bradycardia, constipation, dizziness, headache, fatigue, nausea, dyspnea, rash

    (c) Drug interactions—may potentiate beta blockers, other antihypertensives, digitalis; antagonized by rifampin, phenobarbital

    (d) Contraindications—severe left ventricular dysfunction, hypotension, heart block greater than 1 degree, cardiogenic shock; pregnancy Category C

(4) Long-acting nitrates—nitropaste, nitropatches, isosorbide dinitrate

    (a) Drug action—cause venous dilation, which decreases venous return to the heart and modest arterial vasodilation; results in decreased myocardial oxygen demand

    (b) Side effects—headache, dizziness, flushing, orthostatic hypotension, tachycardia, nausea, rash

    (c) Drug interactions—hypotension potentiated with alcohol, other vasodilators, calcium channel blockers

    (d) Contraindications—acute myocardial infarction; pregnancy Category C

3. Patient education

  a. Instructions on use and side effects of medications

  b. Education and support for lifestyle changes

- Referral

1. Patients with unstable angina

2. Patients with stable angina who cannot be controlled with medication

Eye, Ear, Nose, and Throat Disorders

Allergic Rhinitis

- Definition—inflammation of mucous membranes of nose in response to contact with specific allergens, triggering production of IgE antibodies, causing histamine release and subsequent edema, itching, discharge, and sneezing; the eyes, ears, sinuses, and throat can also be involved

- Etiology/incidence

1. Seasonal—occurs at specific times of year when pollens/allergens are present (hay fever)

  a. Trees—April to July

  b. Grasses—May to July

  c. Ragweed—August to October

2. Perennial—year-round symptoms usually related to dust mites, mold, cockroaches, and animal dander

3. Affects approximately 10–20% of adults; onset typically between ages 10–20 years

- Signs and symptoms

1. Nasal congestion, clear rhinorrhea, sneezing

2. Pruritus of nose, throat, eyes

3. Sore throat and cough from postnasal drip

- Physical findings

1. Pale, boggy nasal mucosa

2. Clear, thin rhinorrhea

3. Nasal crease—horizontal crease across lower bridge of nose caused by repeated upper rubbing of tip of nose with palm of hand

4. Injected conjunctiva, tearing

5. "Allergic shiners" or dark discoloration beneath both eyes

- Differential diagnosis

1. Vasomotor rhinitis—triggered by nasal irritants; smoke, perfume, certain medications, alcohol, spicy foods

2. Rhinitis medicamentosa—excessive topical use of topical vasoconstrictors; cocaine

3. Septal obstruction—nasal polyps, deviated septum, nasal neoplasms

- Diagnostic tests/findings

1. Usually none indicated for diagnosis

2. Skin tests to determine specific allergens; gold standard test

3. Serum allergy tests—RAST; measures amount of specific IgE to individual allergens, which correlates with the allergic sensitivity to that substance; can determine specific IgE to a number of different allergens at one time; expensive and not as sensitive as specific skin testing

- Management/treatment

1. Nonpharmacologic—allergen avoidance

  a. Bedroom must be the most allergen free

  b. Environmental control—vacuum, dust, remove carpeting, feather pillows, stuffed animals

  c. Eliminate or restrict exposure to pets; pets should not be in bedroom

  d. Air conditioning/air filters

2. Pharmacologic (see **Table 9-2**)

  a. Antihistamines

    (1) Generally considered first-line therapy

    (2) Highly effective in reducing itching, sneezing, rhinorrhea; minimal effect on nasal congestion

    (3) More effective if given before onset of symptoms

  b. Decongestants—use alone or in combination with antihistamines to treat nasal congestion

  c. Topical (nasal) corticosteroids

    (1) Given their effectiveness, increased use as first-line treatment

• Table 9-2 Antihistamines, Decongestants, and Anti-inflammatory Medications for Respiratory Disorders (representative list)

Drug	Action	Side-effects	Interactions	Contraindications/Precautions
Antihistamines				
1st generation Chlorpheniramine Diphenhydramine Meclizine	Block action of histamine; anticholinergic effects	Drowsiness, dry mucous membranes, blurred vision	Additive effects with alcohol, sedatives, anti-anxiety agents, MAO inhibitors, tricyclic antidepressants	No fetal malformations associated with use. Diphenhydramine is the antihistamine drug of choice in pregnancy (Briggs & Freeman, 2015). Secreted in breast milk and can cause neonatal sedation, may decrease milk supply due to anticholinergic effects. According to the product information for diphenhydramine, it is contraindicated in nursing women (Briggs & Freeman, 2015 and Parke-Davis, 1997)
2nd generation Loratidine Desloratidine Fexofenadine Cetirizine	Selective peripheral histamine receptor antagonist; no anticholinergic effects	Fewer sedating effects (with exception of cetirizine)	Additive CNS depressant effects with alcohol, barbiturates, tricyclic antidepressants, and loratidine and cetirizine	Caution in patients with renal or hepatic dysfunction Limited data, no known teratogenic associations, Loratadine is compatible with breastfeeding as per the American Academy of Pediatrics (AAP) (Briggs & Freeman, 2015 & AAP, 2001). Cetirizine has low molecular weight, and can be found in low concentration levels in breast milk, but probably compatible (Briggs & Freeman, 2015)
Azelastine HCL Intranasal	Inhibits histamine release from mast cells	Bitter taste, somnolence, headache	Potentiates other CNS depressants	No controlled human data on use in pregnancy or lactation (Briggs & Freeman, 2015)
Decongestants				
Pseudoephedrine Phenylephrine	Alpha-adrenergic agonists; vasoconstriction reduces engorgement of mucosa	Increases heart rate and BP CNS stimulation	Hypertensive crisis with MAO inhibitors	Contraindicated with severe hypertension, cardiovascular disease, MAO inhibitor use Some evidence of association between first-trimester use of pseudoephedrine and risk of infrequent specific birth defects Low concentration levels in breast milk, may reduce milk production No controlled human data on use of phenylephrine during pregnancy and lactation (Briggs & Freeman, 2015)
Nasal corticosteroids				
Budesonide Fulticasone	Anti-inflammatory effects; therapeutic benefit not immediate	Local irritation, epistaxis, headache; systemic absorption at recommended doses minimal	Cytochrome P450 effect	Not for relief of acute bronchospasm; avoid with Cushing's syndrome Very little of nasal corticosteroid is absorbed systemically, only minute concentrations in breast milk. Probably compatible (Briggs & Freeman, 2015)
Mast cell stabilizers				
Cromolyn	Prevents degranulation of mast cells and release of histamine; prophylactic drug	Local reactions: burning, stinging, sneezing	None known	Available data suggest no association with fetal toxicity or teratogenicity; No data on excretion in breast milk; harm to infant is not likely (Briggs & Freeman, 2015)

(2) Not helpful with ocular symptoms

(3) Slow onset of effect; may use prn; maximal effectiveness with daily use as maintenance therapy

d. Mast cell stabilizers/intranasal cromolyns—no direct anti-inflammatory or antihistamine effects; effective for prophylaxis

e. Montelukast (see **Table 9-3**)

3. Patient education

a. Identify and eliminate or avoid allergens (e.g., remove carpeting, pets, install air filters)

b. Appropriate use of medications, combinations, side effects, and overuse syndromes

- Referral—refer for skin tests to determine specific allergens

Conjunctivitis

- Definition—encompasses a broad group of conditions presenting as inflammation of the conjunctiva
- Etiology/incidence
  1. Viral conjunctivitis—adenovirus most common; herpes simplex and herpes zoster
  2. Bacterial conjunctivitis—staphylococci, streptococci, *C. trachomatis, Neisseria gonorrhea*
  3. Allergy—type I, IgE-mediated hypersensitivity reaction precipitated by small airborne allergens (e.g., pollen, animal dander, dust)
  4. Most common eye complaint in primary care
- Signs and symptoms
  1. Sensation of grit in eye, "scratchy"; mild discomfort
  2. Pain, photophobia, blurred vision that fails to clear with blink are not typical features of primary conjunctival process—may indicate corneal involvement
  3. Viral conjunctivitis
     a. Acute onset; may be unilateral or bilateral with a watery discharge
     b. Preauricular adenitis
     c. May be associated with upper respiratory infection
  4. Bacterial conjunctivitis
     a. Acute onset; symptoms begin in one eye and spread to other eye
     b. Mucopurulent discharge; patient reports eyelids are matted together on awakening
     c. Marked conjunctival injection of abrupt onset with copious purulent discharge associated with gonococcal infection; sight-threatening ocular infection
  5. Allergic conjunctivitis
     a. Major cause of chronic conjunctivitis
     b. Complaints of bilateral itching, tearing, redness, and mild eyelid swelling
     c. Discharge is clear and watery or stringy and mucoid
     d. Personal or family history of atopic disease
- Physical findings
  1. Characterized by dilation of superficial conjunctival blood vessels, resulting in hyperemia; hyperemia greatest at the periphery of the bulbar conjunctiva
  2. Discharge (see "Signs and symptoms" earlier)
  3. Cornea clear; pupils equal, round, reactive to light (PERRL)
  4. Visual acuity with no acute change

5. Preauricular adenopathy—most common with *N. gonorrhoeae* and viral ocular syndromes

- Differential diagnosis
  1. Foreign body
  2. Subconjunctival hemorrhage
  3. Blepharitis
  4. Episceritis/scleritis
  5. Keratitis
  6. Uveitis
  7. Acute angle closure glaucoma
- Diagnostic tests/findings
  1. Fluorescein stain—stain uptake suggests corneal involvement
  2. Conjunctival scrapings and cultures if suspect gonococcal or chlamydial infection; chronic or recurrent infection failure to respond to treatment
- Management/treatment
  1. Viral
     a. Self-limited with adenovirus infection
     b. Cold compresses and lubricants (liquid tears) for comfort
  2. Bacterial
     a. Broad-spectrum topical antibiotic—sodium sulfacetamide (Sulymid); polymixin B/trimethoprim (Polytrim); tobramycin (Tobrex)
     b. Systemic antibiotics for gonococcal and chlamydial infections—ceftriaxone, doxycycline, erythromycin
     c. Reserve fluoroquinolones for severe infections—emerging drug resistance
  3. Allergic
     a. Removal of offending allergen if possible
     b. Topical antihistamine—levocabastine (Livostin)
     c. Mast cell stabilizer—cromolyn (Crolom)
     d. Mast cell stabilizer/antihistamine—olopatadine HCL (Patanol)
     e. Topical nonsteroidal anti-inflammatory drugs (NSAIDs)—ketorolac (Acular)
  4. Prevention of transmission of viral or bacterial conjunctivitis
     a. Frequent, thorough hand washing for patient and close contacts
     b. Avoid close contact and sharing linens during acute phase when drainage occurs
     c. Discard opened eye makeup; replace contact lenses, cases, and opened solutions
- Referral
  1. Patients with pain, photophobia, blurred vision; circumcorneal erythema/ciliary flush
  2. Conjunctivitis caused by herpes simplex or herpes zoster
  3. No improvement after 48 hours of treatment

Acute Otitis Media

- Definition—infection of the middle ear that is often preceded by upper respiratory infection (URI) or allergies
- Etiology/incidence/risk factors
  1. Etiology
     a. Eustachian tube dysfunction secondary to URI (often viral) or allergies causes edema and congestion that impede flow of middle ear secretions; accumulation of secretions promotes growth of pathogens

■ **Table 9-3 Asthma Quick-Relief and Long-Term-Control Medications (representative list)**

Drug	Action	Side-effects	Interactions	Contraindications/ Precautions
Short-acting inhaled B$_2$-agonists				
Albuterol – metered dose inhaler (MDI), nebulizer solution	Relaxes bronchial smooth muscle by selective action on B$_2$-receptors Duration 2–6 hours	Tachycardia, nervousness, skeletal muscle tremor	May have increased cardiovascular effects with MAO inhibitors, tricyclic antidepressants, sympathomimetic agents; antagonized by beta-blockers	Caution with cardiovascular disease, diabetes, hyperthyroidism, seizure disorders No evidence of fetal harm with use; Albuterol is short-acting beta agonist of choice if needed during pregnancy; very low concentrations in breast milk, most likely compatible (Briggs & Freeman, 2015)
Inhaled corticosteroids				
Fluticasone MDI/dry powdered inhaler (DPI)* Budesonide DPI	Inhibits inflammatory response	Minimal systemic effects; oropharyngeal candidiasis, hoarseness	Cytochrome P450 effect; caution with CYP3A4 inhibitors (e.g., ketoconazole)	Not for treatment of acute attack Very little of nasal corticosteroid is absorbed systemically; budesonide is inhaled corticosteroid of choice if needed during pregnancy; only minute concentrations in breast milk; no data on effects of fluticasone exist, but due to low systemic effects, probably compatible with breastfeeding (Briggs & Freeman, 2015)
Oral corticosteroids				
Prednisone	Inhibits inflammatory response	Adrenal suppression; masks infection	Effects may be decreased by barbiturates, rifampin, other hepatic enzyme inducers; may be potentiated by ketoconazole, oral contraceptives, NSAIDs	Contraindicated with systemic mycoses; live vaccination Several studies show possible association with orofacial clefts to use of prednisolone in the first trimester (Briggs & Freeman, 2015). Low concentration levels in breast milk. Prednisone is compatible with breast feeding, as per the American Academy of Pediatrics (AAP) (Briggs & Freeman, 2015 and AAP, 2001)
Long-acting inhaled B$_2$-agonists				
Salmeterol DPI	Relaxes bronchial smooth muscle by selective action on B$_2$-receptors Duration 12 hours	Headache, pharyngitis, URI, tachycardia, tremor	May have increased cardiovascular effects with MAO inhibitors, tricyclic antidepressants, sympathomimetic agents; antagonized by beta-blockers	Allergy to milk proteins; should not be used for symptom relief or acute exacerbation; caution with cardiovascular disease, diabetes, hyperthyroidism, seizure disorder Preliminary data from human studies do not support an association with fetal harm; no human data on excretion in breast milk, probably compatible (Briggs & Freeman, 2015)

(continues)

■ **Table 9-3** Asthma Quick-Relief and Long-Term–Control Medications (representative list) *(continued)*

Drug	Action	Side-effects	Interactions	Contraindications/ Precautions
Leukotriene modifiers				
Montelukast	Suppresses leukotriene biosynthesis, leukotrienes cause the inflammation component of asthma	Headache, fatigue, fever, GI upset	Effects may be decreased with phenobarbital, erythromycin, thoephylline; effects may be increased by aspirin, rifampin	Not for treatment of acute attack No evidence of teratogenicity in animal studies; no controlled human data in pregnancy No human data on excretion in breast milk, compatibility with breast feeding is probable (Briggs & Freeman, 2015)
Mast cell stabilizers				
Cromolyn Nedocromil	Prevents mast cell release of histamine, leukotrienes Inhibits antigen-induced bronchospasm	Throat irritation, bad taste, cough	None identified	Not for treatment of acute attacks No evidence of teratogenicity in animal studies; no controlled human data in pregnancy; no data on excretion in breast milk; harm to infant is not likely (Briggs & Freeman, 2015)
Methylxanthines				
Theophylline	Relaxes bronchial smooth muscle	GI upset, headache, CNS stimulation, diuresis, arrhythmias, seizures	Cytochrome P450 effect; numerous drugs may effect serum concentration via induction or inhibition of P450 enzymes	Peptic ulcer disease, arrhythmias, seizure disorders Some teratogenicity in animal studies, no controlled human data during pregnancy; may occasionally cause stimulation and irritability in breastfed infant; compatible in pregnancy and lactation (Briggs & Freeman, 2015)

b. Common pathogens—*Streptococcus pneumoniae, Haemophilus influenzae, Moraxella catarrhalis,* rhinovirus, respiratory syncytial virus

2. Highest incidence in childhood, younger than age 10 years, seen infrequently in adults

3. Risk factors
   a. Recent/current URI
   b. Exposure to cigarette smoke, active or passive

- Signs and symptoms
  1. Rapid onset, short duration if uncomplicated
  2. Ear pain, decreased hearing, fever (adult less likely to have fever)
  3. Aural pressure
  4. Vertigo, nausea, and vomiting

- Physical findings
  1. Full or bulging tympanic membrane (TM) with absent or obscured landmarks
  2. Distorted light reflex
  3. Decreased/absent mobility of TM on pneumatic otoscopy
  4. Erythema of TM is an inconsistent finding
  5. Bullae on TM; often associated with *Mycoplasma pneumoniae*
  6. Preauricular or cervical lymphadenopathy

- Differential diagnosis
  1. Otitis externa
  2. Otitis media with effusion
  3. Temporomandibular joint (TMJ) syndrome
  4. Dental abscess
  5. Mastoiditis

- Diagnostic tests/findings
  1. Usually none indicated
  2. Tympanometry for recurrent infections; indicator fluid posterior to TM

- Management/treatment
  1. Most uncomplicated cases of acute otitis media resolve spontaneously without antibiotic treatment
  2. Requires follow-up with antibiotic treatment if symptoms worsen or do not improve within 48–72 hours of symptom onset
  3. Pharmacologic
     a. Antibiotics
        (1) Amoxicillin; for penicillin-allergic patients, trimethoprim/sulfamethoxazole or erythromycin; if inadequate response, change to amoxicillin-clavulanate
        (2) Side effects
            (a) Gastrointestinal (GI) upset, nausea, vomiting, diarrhea
            (b) Rashes, urticaria
        (3) Drug interactions—trimethoprim/sulfamethoxazole may potentiate oral anticoagulants, hypoglycemics
        (4) Contraindications/precautions
            (a) Hepatic impairment
            (b) Pregnancy Category B except sulfa drugs, which are Category C; sulfa not recommended while nursing
     b. No demonstrated benefit with use of decongestants
     c. Analgesics/antipyretics
        (1) Acetaminophen

        (a) Drug action—inhibits central nervous system (CNS) prostaglandin synthesis
        (b) Side effects—can cause serious or fatal hepatic injury
        (c) Drug interactions—increased risk of hepatotoxicity with chronic, heavy alcohol use
        (d) Contraindications/precautions—pregnancy Category B; use with caution while nursing
        (2) Nonsteroidal anti-inflammatory drugs (NSAIDs)
            (a) Ibuprofen, naproxen, ketoprofen
            (b) Drug action
                i. Inhibits cyclooxygenase, the enzyme that catalyzes the synthesis of prostaglandins and thromboxane from arachidonic acid
                ii. Analgesic, anti-inflammatory, and antipyretic effects
            (c) Side effects
                i. Hypersensitivity
                ii. Dyspepsia, GI bleeding
                iii. Tinnitus, drowsiness, headache
                iv. Nephrotoxiciy
                v. Hepatotoxicity
            (d) Interactions
                i. Decreased antihypertensive effect of ACE inhibitors, beta blockers, diuretics
                ii. Potentiates anticoagulants
            (e) Contraindications/precautions
                i. Aspirin allergy
                ii. Pregnancy Category C, but contraindicated in third trimester; not recommended while nursing

4. Patient education
   a. Appropriate ear canal hygiene
   b. Antibiotic use and side effects
   c. Need for additional care if no improvement in 2 to 3 days
   d. Cessation of smoking and avoidance of second-hand smoke exposure

- Referral
  1. For suspected extension of infection, mastoiditis, or perforation of tympanic membrane
  2. Persistent hearing loss after adequate treatment
  3. Adults with recurrent otitis media need ears, nose, and throat (ENT) referral to rule out underlying process (e.g., malignancy)

Sinusitis

- Definition—inflammation of the mucosal surface of the paranasal sinuses
- Etiology/incidence
  1. Etiology
     a. Acute sinusitis—caused by viral or bacterial infections and allergies; bacterial causes include *Streptococcus pneumoniae, Haemophilus influenzae, Moraxella catarrhalis*
     b. Infection usually involves maxillary and ethmoid sinuses
     c. Chronic sinusitis occurs with episodes of prolonged infection that resist treatment and/or repeated or inadequately treated acute infection; treatment failure secondary to failure of sinuses to drain, which may be associated with anatomic defect
  2. Incidence—accounts for 6% of primary care office visits

- Signs and symptoms
  1. Acute sinusitis
     a. Nasal congestion, facial pain, toothache, headache, fever, yellow/green nasal drainage
     b. Increased pain with bending over or sudden head movement
     c. Common cold and allergic/vasomotor rhinitis may precede infection
     d. "Double sickening"—URI symptoms with initial improvement followed by increasing nasal symptoms
  2. Chronic sinusitis
     a. Nasal congestion, discharge, and cough that last longer than 30 days
     b. Dull ache or pressure across forehead and/or midface
     c. Constant postnasal drip and chronic cough
- Physical findings
  1. Afebrile or low-grade fever
  2. Mucopurulent nasal discharge; postnasal discharge
  3. Nasal mucosa swollen, pale, dull red to gray
  4. Pain on firm palpation over sinus areas
- Differential diagnosis
  1. Uncomplicated URI
  2. Migraine headaches
  3. Allergic/vasomotor rhinitis
  4. Nasal polyps
  5. Dental abscess
  6. Trigeminal neuralgia
- Diagnostic tests/findings
  1. None for typical presentation
  2. CT scan—reserved for complicated disease and search for ethmoidal disease in patients with refractory symptoms
- Management/treatment
  1. Nonpharmacologic
     a. Saline nasal spray
     b. Steam inhalation
     c. Warm compresses
     d. Hydration
  2. Pharmacologic
     a. Antibiotics (see "Acute Otitis Media" section in this chapter)
        (1) If signs and symptoms are present 10 or more days after onset of upper respiratory symptoms
        (2) If signs and symptoms of acute sinusitis worsen within 10 days of initial improvement
     b. Oral/topical decongestants
        (1) Oral decongestants (see Table 9-2)
        (2) Topical decongestant/oxymetazoline spray 0.05%
           (a) Provides rapid relief
           (b) Should not be used for longer than 3–5 days to prevent rebound congestion
     c. Nasal steroids—to reduce mucosal inflammation (see Table 9-2)
     d. Antihistamines not recommended unless patient has allergies
     e. Pain management as needed with acetaminophen, NSAIDs, opioids if severe
  3. Patient education
     a. Avoidance of allergens, environmental irritants (e.g., cigarette smoke)
     b. Importance of maintaining adequate hydration

- Referral
  1. Severe facial pain, periorbital swelling
  2. Failure to respond to two courses of antibiotic
  3. Suspected anatomic abnormality
  4. Chronic sinusitis or more than three episodes of acute sinusitis per year

Common Cold

- Definition—an acute, mild, self-limited viral infection of the upper respiratory tract mucosa
- Etiology/incidence/risk factors
  1. Etiology
     a. Inflammation of the mucosal membranes from the nasal mucosa to the bronchi
     b. Rhinovirus, coronavirus, adenovirus
     c. Spread by airborne droplets and contact with infectious secretions on hands and environmental surfaces
     d. Incubation period 48–72 hours
  2. Incidence
     a. Peaks in winter months
     b. Children—6 to 8 infections per season
     c. Adults—2 to 4 per season
  3. Risks
     a. Repeated exposure to groups of children
     b. Close quarters, contact
- Signs and symptoms
  1. General malaise
  2. Nasal congestion and clear rhinorrhea
  3. Sneezing, coughing, sore throat, hoarseness
  4. Tearing, burning sensation of eyes
- Physical findings
  1. Low-grade fever
  2. Nasal mucosa swollen and erythematous
  3. Conjunctiva slightly red
  4. Throat erythematous with cervical lymphadenopathy
- Differential diagnosis
  1. Allergic rhinitis
  2. Streptococcal pharyngitis
  3. Influenza
  4. Otitis media
- Diagnostic tests/findings
  1. Generally none recommended
  2. Rapid strep screen/throat culture if streptococcal pharyngitis suspected
- Management/treatment
  1. Nonpharmacologic
     a. Inhalation of warm vapors
     b. Saline nasal drops or sprays
     c. Saline gargles/throat lozenges
     d. Increase fluids
  2. Pharmacologic
     a. Acetaminophen or NSAIDs (see "Acute Otitis Media" section in this chapter)
     b. Topical/oral decongestants (see Table 9-2)
     c. Cough suppressants—e.g., dextromethorphan
        (1) Drug action—depresses cough reflex by direct inhibition of cough center in the medulla

(2) Side effects—minimal CNS depressant action

(3) Drug interactions—hyperpyretic crisis with mono-amine oxidase inhibitors (MAOIs)

(4) Contraindications/precautions

(a) Persistent or chronic cough

(b) First trimester of pregnancy; caution while nursing

d. Expectorants—e.g., guaifenesin

(1) Drug action—may increase output of respiratory tract secretions, facilitating removal of mucus

(2) Side effects—GI upset, drowsiness, headache

(3) Drug interactions—may increase toxicity/effect of disulfiram, MAOIs, metronidazole, procarbazine

(4) Contraindications/precautions—pregnancy Category C; use with caution while nursing

3. Patient education

a. Infection control

b. Self-limited nature of infection

c. Symptoms of complications; secondary bacterial infection

Pharyngitis

- Definition—inflammation of the pharynx and tonsils
- Etiology/incidence
  1. Etiology
     a. Viral—most common cause is rhinovirus and adenovirus
     b. Bacterial
        (1) Group A beta-hemolytic streptococci (GABHS)
        (2) *Neisseria gonorrhoeae*
     c. Noninfectious causes—allergic rhinitis or postnasal drip
  2. Incidence
     a. One of the most frequent reasons for outpatient care in United States
     b. Accounts for 16 million office visits per year; 2.5% of visits to primary care providers
- Risks—crowded work or living conditions
- Signs and symptoms
  1. Viral pharyngitis
     a. Sore throat, fever, malaise, cough, headache, myalgia, and fatigue
     b. May also complain of rhinitis, congestion, conjunctivitis
  2. GABHS
     a. Sudden onset of sore throat, fever, chills, headache, nausea/vomiting
     b. Rhinitis, cough, conjunctivitis not typically present
- Physical findings
  1. Viral pharyngitis—mild erythema of the pharynx with little or no exudates
  2. Bacterial pharyngitis
     a. Marked erythema of the throat, exudates, tender anterior cervical lymphadenopathy
     b. Erythematous "sandpaper" rash/accentuation in groin and axillae with scarlet fever
- Differential diagnosis
  1. Peritonsillar abscess
  2. Infectious mononucleosis
  3. Pharyngeal candidiasis
  4. Diphtheria
  5. Epiglottitis

- Diagnostic tests/findings
  1. GABHS testing is not indicated in all adults with pharyngitis (5–15% of adult pharyngitis cases are caused by GABHS)
  2. Rapid streptococcal antigen test is recommended for adult with pharyngitis that meets two or more of the following criteria:
     a. Fever
     b. Lack of cough
     c. Tonsillar exudates
     d. Tender anterior cervical adenopathy
  3. Cultures are not recommended for routine evaluation of adult pharyngitis or for confirmation of negative rapid antigen tests
  4. Culture is useful if other pathogens (e.g., gonococcus) are being considered
- Management/treatment
  1. Nonpharmacologic
     a. Adequate hydration
     b. Saline gargles
     c. Topical anesthetics (e.g., lozenges, sprays)
  2. Pharmacologic
     a. GABHS
        (1) Penicillin V PO/benzathine penicillin IM
           (a) Drug action—bactericidal
           (b) Side effects—hypersensitivity reactions
           (c) Contraindications/precautions—penicillin allergy; pregnancy Category B
        (2) Erythromycin if penicillin allergy
     b. Gonococcal pharyngitis—ceftriaxone IM
        (1) Drug action—bactericidal
        (2) Side effects—injection site reaction, hypersensitivity reactions
        (3) Drug interactions—potentiated by probenecid
        (4) Contraindications/precautions—penicillin allergy; pregnancy Category B
        (5) Alternative agents—azithromycin, spectinomycin—obtain pharyngeal culture 3–5 days after treatment if use alternative regimen
- Referral
  1. Suspected peritonsillar abscess
  2. Epiglottitis

Infectious Mononucleosis (IM)

- Definition—an acute, self-limiting viral syndrome secondary to Epstein-Barr virus and some other viruses characterized by fever, malaise, pharyngitis, and lymphadenopathy
- Etiology/incidence
  1. Etiology
     a. Causal agent is most often Epstein-Barr virus (EBV)
     b. Mode of transmission is oropharyngeal route via saliva
  2. Incidence—rarely symptomatic in children younger than 5 years; most clinically apparent infections occur in individuals 10–30 years old; peak rate ages of 15–19 years
- Signs and symptoms
  1. Prodrome of headache, malaise, fatigue, anorexia
  2. Fever, sore throat, swollen lymph nodes (classic triad)
- Physical findings
  1. Tonsillar enlargement with exudate

2. Palatal petecchiae at junction of hard and soft palates (25% of cases)
3. Lymphadenopathy; particularly anterior and posterior cervical chain
4. Fever compatible with severity of infection
5. Hepatomegaly (25% cases)
6. Splenomegaly (40–100% cases)

- Differential diagnosis
  1. Streptococcal pharyngitis
  2. Other viral causes of pharyngitis
  3. Acute cytomegalovirus (CMV) infection
  4. Acute HIV infection
- Diagnostic tests/findings
  1. Monospot/heterophile antibody test
     a. Sensitivity 63–84%; specificity 84–100%
     b. Initially negative, usually positive by 1 to 2 weeks after onset of symptoms
  2. CBC—lymphocytic leukocytosis with 10% of cells atypical
  3. Liver function tests—may have elevated aminotransferases (AST, ALT), bilirubin
  4. Throat culture—frequent secondary infection with GABHS
- Management/treatment
  1. Nonpharmacologic—lozenges, gargles for relief of pharyngitis; treatment largely supportive
  2. Pharmacologic
     a. Acetaminophen, NSAIDs to reduce fever, aches (see "Acute Otitis Media" section in this chapter)
     b. Corticosteroids—prescribed for significant pharyngeal edema and obstructive tonsillar enlargement
  3. Patient education
     a. Rest during acute phase of illness; activity as tolerated
     b. Contact sports, heavy lifting, and strenuous activity should be avoided for at least 1 month if have splenomegaly
     c. Avoid alcohol for at least 1 month
     d. Seek immediate care with sudden onset of severe abdominal pain
- Referral
  1. Onset of abdominal pain—possible ruptured spleen
  2. Airway obstruction from pharyngeal edema

Lower Respiratory Disorders

Community-Acquired Pneumonia

- Definition—acute infection of the lower respiratory tract that is associated with at least two symptoms of active pneumonia infection in an individual who has not been hospitalized or resided in a long-term care facility for 14 days before the onset of symptoms
- Etiology/incidence/risk factors
  1. Etiology
     a. Bacterial—*Streptococcus pneumoniae, Haemophilus influenzae, Legionella pneumophila*
     b. Atypical, nonbacterial—*Mycoplasma pneumoniae, Chlamydia pneumoniae*
     c. Viral—influenza, adenovirus

2. Incidence—sixth leading cause of death; leading cause of death from infectious disease
3. Risk factors
   a. Preceding viral URI
   b. Cigarette smoking
   c. Age older than 65 years
   d. Chronic lung disease
   e. Corticosteroid use
   f. Immunosuppression

- Signs and symptoms
  1. May be masked or absent in very young, elderly, immunosuppressed, coexisting chronic disease
  2. Fever, chills, sweats
  3. Cough with/without sputum production
  4. Dyspnea, pleuritic chest pain
  5. Associated symptoms—lethargy, headache, anorexia, nausea, vomiting
- Physical findings
  1. Tachycardia
  2. Tachypnea, dyspnea
  3. Percussion
     a. Often normal in early disease
     b. Dullness over area of consolidation
  4. Auscultation
     a. Coarse rhonchi may clear or shift with cough
     b. Nonclearing rales
     c. Diminished breath sounds over consolidation
  5. Fever with chills, high spikes (102.2°F or above) especially if bacterial etiology
  6. Small areas of pneumonia cannot always be detected by physical examination
- Differential diagnosis
  1. Bronchitis
  2. Atelectasis
  3. Chronic obstructive pulmonary disease
  4. Congestive heart failure
  5. Malignancy
  6. Tuberculosis
  7. Pulmonary embolism
- Diagnostic tests/findings
  1. Chest radiograph
     a. Establishes diagnosis by revealing an infiltrate; helps distinguish pneumonia from acute bronchitis
     b. Demonstrates the presence of complications such as pleural effusion and multilobar disease
  2. Value of sputum collection for Gram's stain and culture is controversial—not recommended as routine for outpatients diagnosed with community-acquired pneumonia
  3. CBC with differential—white blood cell (WBC) elevation ($10,000/mm^3$ to $25,000/mm^3$) with a shift to left (e.g., bandemia, neutrophilia, especially if bacterial etiology)
- Management/treatment
  1. Nonpharmacologic
     a. Oral hydration and humidification
     b. Improve oxygenation (e.g., smoking cessation)
  2. Pharmacologic

a. Empiric antimicrobial therapy—American Thoracic Society (Mandell, et al., 2007)
  (1) Patients who are otherwise healthy with no risk factors for drug-resistant streptococcus pneumonia (DRSP)—advanced generation macrolide (azithromycin or clarithromycin)
    (a) Drug action—inhibits bacterial protein synthesis
    (b) Side effects—GI effects
    (c) Drug interactions—inhibits cytochrome P-450 enzymes; may inhibit metabolism of other drugs
    (d) Contraindications/precautions—hypersensitivity to macrolide antibiotics; pregnancy Category B; enters human milk/use caution
    (e) Alternative agent—doxycycline, use only if allergic to or unable to tolerate macrolides, contraindicated in pregnancy
  (2) Patients with comorbidity, risk factors for DRSP including age older than 65 years or nursing home residence, or use of antimicrobials within previous 3 months (use alternative from different class)—respiratory fluoroquinilone (levofloxacin, moxifloxacin, gemifloxacin)
    (a) Drug action—inhibits bacterial DNA synthesis
    (b) Side effects—GI upset, CNS toxicity
    (c) Drug interactions—avoid drugs that prolong QT interval; increased risk of tendon rupture with corticosteroids; inhibits cytochrome P-450 enzymes; may inhibit metabolism of other drugs
    (d) Contraindications/precautions—hypersensitivity or allergy, pregnancy Category C; not recommended for nursing mothers
    (e) Alternative agent—beta-lactam (penicillins, cephalosporins) plus a macrolide
b. Antipyretics—acetaminophen, NSAIDs (see "Acute Otitis Media" section in this chapter)
3. Patient education
  a. Infection containment principles
  b. Need for hydration
  c. Rest
  d. Avoid cough medicines if have a productive cough so can clear thick secretions
  e. Medication schedules and side effects
  f. Prevention—annual influenza vaccination; pneumonia vaccination for individuals age 65 years or older or at high risk for pneumonia; smoking cessation
- Referral/MD consult
1. Base decision to hospitalize on age, comorbid illness, physical examination, and laboratory findings
2. No improvement in 24 to 36 hours
3. Fever over 102°F, pallor or cyanosis, nasal flaring
4. Mental confusion

Asthma

- Definition
1. A chronic inflammatory disorder of the airways in which many cells and cellular elements play a role, in particular, mast cells, eosinophils, T lymphocytes, neutrophils, and epithelial cells; in susceptible individuals, this inflammation causes recurrent episodes of wheezing, breathlessness, chest tightness, and cough, particularly at night and the early morning; these episodes are associated with airflow obstruction that is often reversible; the inflammation also causes an associated increase in existing bronchial hyperresponsiveness to a variety of stimuli (NHLBI, 2007)
2. Classification correlates to treatment recommendations
  a. Intermittent—step 1
    (1) Symptoms 2 times/week or less; nocturnal symptoms 2 times/month or less
    (2) PEF/FEV_1 greater than 80% of predicted value; variability less than 20%; normal between exacerbations
  b. Mild persistent—step 2
    (1) Symptoms 3–6 times/week; nocturnal symptoms 3–4 times/month
    (2) PEF/FEV_1 greater than 80% of predicted value; variability 20–30%
  c. Moderate persistent—step 3
    (1) Daily symptoms; nocturnal symptoms more than 1 time/week but not nightly
    (2) PEF/FEV_1 greater than 60% but less than 80%; variability greater than 30%
  d. Severe persistent—step 4
    (1) Continual daily symptoms; frequent nocturnal symptoms
    (2) PEF/FEV_1 less than 60%; variability greater than 30%
- Etiology/incidence
1. Etiology
  a. Caused by single or multiple triggers
    (1) Allergic triggers
      (a) Airborne pollens, molds, dust mites, cockroaches, animal dander
      (b) Food additives or preservatives
      (c) Feather pillows
    (2) Nonallergic triggers
      (a) Smoke and other pollutants
      (b) Viral respiratory infections
      (c) Medications—ASA, NSAIDs, beta blockers
      (d) Exercise
      (e) Gastroesophageal reflux
      (f) Emotional factors
      (g) Menses, pregnancy
  b. In children there is generally a strong history of atopy; adult-onset asthma may be related to allergens, but nonallergic triggers likely to be a factor
2. Incidence
  a. Occurs in approximately 3% of the general population
    (1) Affects approximately 10% of children
    (2) Affects approximately 5% of adults
  b. Can occur at any age; increasing in prevalence in United States
- Signs and symptoms
1. Episodic wheeze, chest tightness, shortness of breath or cough; cough may be sole symptom
2. Symptoms worsen in presence of aeroallergens, irritants, and exercise

3. Symptoms occur or worsen at night; cause nighttime awakening
4. History of allergic rhinitis or atopic dermatitis; family history of asthma, allergic rhinitis, or atopic dermatitis
- Physical findings
  1. Hyperexpansion of thorax; hyperresonance with percussion
  2. Wheezing; prolonged expiratory phase
  3. Diminished breath sounds
  4. Tachypnea, dyspnea
  5. Atopic dermatitis/eczema or other skin manifestations of allergic skin disorders
  6. Increased nasal secretions, mucosal swelling, nasal polyps
- Differential diagnosis
  1. Acute infection—bronchitis, pneumonia
  2. Chronic obstructive pulmonary disease (COPD); may overlap with asthma
  3. Heart disease—heart failure
  4. Foreign body aspiration
  5. Pulmonary emboli
  6. Cough secondary to drugs such as ACE inhibitors
- Diagnostic tests/findings
  1. Pulmonary function tests/spirometry—to establish airway obstruction
     a. FEV_1 (forced expiratory volume in 1 second) less than 80% of predicted; FEV_1/FVC (forced vital capacity) less than 65% or below limit of normal
     b. Spirometry and peak flow rates improve with bronchodilator challenge; FEV_1 increases 12% and at least 200 mL after use of inhaled short-acting B_2-agonist
  2. If normal spirometry, assess diurnal variation in PEF (peak expiratory flow); 20% difference between two measures/PEF variability supports diagnosis of asthma
  3. Bronchoprovocation with methacholine, histamine, or exercise if diagnosis in question; negative test helps exclude diagnosis of asthma
  4. Chest radiograph if infection, large airway lesions, heart disease, or foreign body obstruction suspected
- Management/treatment
  1. Goals
     a. Minimize symptoms, normalize daily activity
     b. Maintain near-normal pulmonary function
     c. Minimal use of short-acting B_2-agonist
  2. Nonpharmacologic
     a. Peak flow monitoring
        (1) Establish patient's "personal best" and develop "Asthma Action Plan"
        (2) A drop in peak flow below 80% indicates an acute exacerbation and need to contact clinician for medication adjustment
        (3) A drop in peak flow below 50% indicates need for emergency treatment
     b. Avoidance of known allergens, triggers
     c. Adequate hydration and humidity
     d. Annual influenza vaccine; pneumococcal vaccine
  3. Pharmacologic—stepwise approach (see Table 9-3)
     a. Intermittent—step 1
        (1) No daily medications

(2) Short-acting inhaled B_2-agonist as needed for symptoms
(3) Course of systemic corticosteroids recommended for severe exacerbations
  b. Mild persistent—step 2
     (1) Low-dose inhaled corticosteroids
     (2) Alternative treatments—mast-cell stabilizer, leukotriene modifier, or theophylline
     (3) Short-acting inhaled B_2-agonist as needed for symptoms
  c. Moderate persistent—step 3
     (1) Low-medium dose inhaled corticosteroids and long-acting inhaled B_2-agonist
     (2) Alternative treatments: add leukotriene or theophylline; increase inhaled corticosteroid within medium dose range
     (3) Short-acting inhaled B_2-agonist as needed for symptoms
  d. Severe persistent—step 4
     (1) High-dose inhaled corticosteroids and long-acting inhaled B_2-agonist; oral corticosteroid if needed
     (2) Short-acting inhaled B_2-agonist as needed for symptoms
  e. Severe exacerbation (peak flow < 60%) can occur with any category of asthma; consider short course of oral steroids 40–60 mg/day for 5–10 days (NHLBI, 2007)
  f. Treatment of asthma in pregnancy (NHLBI, 2007)
     (1) Uncontrolled asthma increases the risk of perinatal mortality, preeclampsia, preterm birth, and low-birth-weight infants
     (2) It is safer for pregnant women to be treated for asthma than to have asthma symptoms and exacerbations
     (3) Albuterol is the preferred short-acting inhaled B_2-agonist and budesonide DPI is the preferred inhaled corticosteroid
  4. Patient education
     a. How to recognize signs of worsening asthma
     b. Use of peak flow meter
     c. Clear instructions on use of written "Asthma Action Plan"
     d. Proper use of inhaler for effective dosing
     e. Prophylactic medication (e.g., preexercise dosing)
     f. Control of environmental factors (e.g., allergens and irritants)
- Referral
  1. Failure to respond to emergency treatment; arrange for emergency room treatment if signs of severe obstruction present—peak flow reduced by 50%, pulsus paradoxus, use of accessory muscles of respiration
  2. Difficulty controlling asthma or if step 4 is required

Tuberculosis (TB)

- Definition—necrotizing bacterial infection caused by *Mycobacterium tuberculosis;* most commonly infects the lungs, but any organ can be affected
  1. Active TB disease/ATBD—signs, symptoms, and radiographic findings secondary to *M. tuberculosis;* disease may be pulmonary or extrapulmonary

2. TB infection/latent TB infection (LTBI)
    a. Positive tuberculin skin or blood test with no signs or symptoms of disease
    b. Chest radiograph negative or only granulomas/calcifications in lungs and/or regional lymph nodes
    c. Not infectious to others
- Etiology/incidence/risk factors
    1. Etiology—*Mycobacterium tuberculosis;* spread by small airborne particles
    2. Incidence/prevalence
        a. 10 to 15 million infected in United States; 90–95% of primary TB infections remain in a latent or dormant stage
        b. Incidence rising due to HIV infection
    3. Risk factors
        a. Individuals with weakened immune systems—HIV-infected, severe kidney disease, organ transplant, long-term corticosteroid therapy
        b. Individuals who are incarcerated, in long-term institutional living, or in crowded conditions
        c. Individuals who abuse drugs or alcohol
        d. Individuals who have immigrated from countries with high TB rates
        e. Individuals who work in institutions or facilities that serve high-risk individuals—hospitals, long-term care, correctional facilities, homeless shelters
        f. Household contacts of diagnosed cases
- Signs and symptoms
    1. TB infection/LTBI
        a. Asymptomatic state may last months to years
        b. 10% go on to develop active TB
    2. Active TB/ATBD
        a. Generalized symptoms
            (1) Night sweats, fever
            (2) Malaise, weakness
            (3) Anorexia
            (4) Weight loss
        b. Pulmonary symptoms
            (1) Productive cough, possible hemoptysis
            (2) Chest pain
            (3) Dyspnea
        c. Systemic symptoms (extrapulmonary sites)
            (1) Pelvic pain
            (2) Flank pain
- Physical findings
    1. Generally normal appearance in early disease, progressing to cachectic
    2. Unexplained fever
    3. Lung findings—increased tactile fremitus and dullness to percussion over consolidated areas; apical rales and whispered pectoriloquy
    4. Advanced disease—purulent green or yellow sputum
    5. Hemoptysis
- Differential diagnosis
    1. Pneumonia
    2. Malignancy
    3. Chronic obstructive pulmonary disease
    4. Silicosis
    5. Sarcoidosis
- Diagnostic tests/findings
    1. Purified protein derivative (PPD) skin test (antigen response) recommended for routine screening of individuals at risk of infection
        a. Positive test indicates exposure, not active disease
        b. Individual must return to office in 48–72 hours to interpret test results
        c. PPD interpretation
            (1) A reaction of 5-mm induration or greater is considered positive in patients with
                (a) HIV infection, immunocompromised/immunosuppressed individuals
                (b) Those with abnormal chest radiographs consistent with healed TB lesions
                (c) Recent close contact with infected person
            (2) A reaction of 10-mm induration or greater is considered positive among
                (a) Recent arrivals (< 5 years) from high-prevalence areas
                (b) Low socioeconomic status, homeless
                (c) Aged, nursing home resident, incarcerated individual
                (d) Individuals with chronic disease or predisposing conditions (e.g., gastrectomy, diabetes mellitus, or corticosteroid therapy)
            (3) A reaction of 15-mm induration or greater is considered positive among individuals without risk factors
        d. False negative
            (1) PPD administered after recent live virus vaccination
            (2) Immunosuppressed
            (3) Elderly
            (4) Incorrect administration—needs to be intradermal
        e. False positive
            (1) Previous BCG (Bacillus Calmette–Guérin) vaccination
            (2) Nontuberculosis mycobacterium
        f. "Positive converter"—previous negative PPD
    2. Interferon-gamma release assay (IRGA) blood test also used for routine screening, measures immune reaction to bacteria causing TB
        a. Requires only one visit; test results within 24 hours
        b. Not affected by prior BCG vaccination
        c. Reported as positive or negative
        d. More expensive
    3. Chest radiography, both anteroposterior and lateral views, indicated with positive skin or blood TB test result
        a. Identifies active pulmonary disease; negative chest radiograph rules out active TB
        b. Radiologic findings include apical scarring, hilar adenopathy with peripheral infiltrate and upper lobe cavitation
    4. Three sputum samples required for both smear and culture in patients suspected of pulmonary TB
        a. A presumptive diagnosis of TB can be made with detection of acid-fast bacilli in sputum smear
        b. A positive culture for *M. tuberculosis* is essential to confirm diagnosis

- Management/treatment
  1. LTBI
     a. Nonpharmacologic—not applicable
     b. Pharmacologic
        (1) Treatment goal—stop progression to active disease state
        (2) Recommended for individuals at high risk of exposure and those at high risk of progression from latent TB infection to active disease
            (a) Close contact of confirmed active TB
            (b) Foreign-born persons from endemic countries and in United States for 5 years or less
            (c) Residents and employees of congregate settings
            (d) Healthcare workers with high-risk patients
            (e) Persons with HIV or otherwise immunosuppressed
            (f) Others on a case-by-case basis assessment of risk for developing active disease
        (3) Screening procedures to identify appropriate individuals for preventive treatment
            (a) Exclude active disease with chest radiograph
            (b) Exclude individuals who have already been adequately treated
            (c) Identify contraindications to isoniazid
            (d) Identify individuals needing special consideration (e.g., pregnant, older than 35 years)
        (4) Treatment with isoniazid for 9 months
            (a) Drug action—inhibition of myocolic acid synthesis resulting in disruption of bacterial cell wall
            (b) Side effects—GI symptoms; hepatitis/monitor transaminase levels at baseline, 3, 6, and 9 months; peripheral neuropathy/dose with vitamin B_6 (pyridoxine)
            (c) Drug interactions—alcohol increases risk of hepatitis; pyridoxine deficiency increases risk of peripheral neuropathy
            (d) Drug contraindications/precautions—acute hepatic disease; pregnancy Category C
  2. Active disease treatment—consult/referral to specialist
     a. Nonpharmacologic
        (1) Well-balanced diet; additional caloric intake may be needed to maintain or gain weight
        (2) Outdoor exercise
     b. Pharmacologic
        (1) Typical regimen includes isoniazid, rifampin, pyrazinamide for 2 months; isoniazid and rifampin for 4 months; given resistance concerns include ethambutol in initial regimen until drug susceptibility tests are known
        (2) Directly observed therapy (DOT) is one method to ensure compliance; healthcare provider/designee observes patient ingest medications
  3. Patient education
     a. Importance of continuous treatment
        (1) Possibility of microbial resistance
        (2) Signs of developing side effects, drug interactions
     b. Infection control principles
        (1) Reducing respiratory droplet broadcast
        (2) Care with disposal of infected wastes, tissues
        (3) Avoiding crowded conditions, contact with susceptible individuals while infectious

     c. Follow-up requirements, liver function monitoring
     d. Necessity for contact evaluation and treatment
     e. Importance of general health maintenance
- Referral
  1. Patients with ATBD
  2. Report all cases to health department for monitoring, strain identification
  3. Health department follow-up for contact tracing, risk assessment

Gastrointestinal Disorders

Constipation

- Definition—infrequent or difficult evacuation of stool
  1. Constipation is a symptom rather than a disease
  2. May include incomplete evacuation of stool, straining during bowel movement, hard stools, less than three bowel movements in a week
- Etiology/incidence
  1. Etiology
     a. Functional causes—low-fiber diet, motility disorders (irritable bowel syndrome), sedentary lifestyle, dehydration
     b. Structural abnormalities—anal disorders (anal fissure), colon polyps or tumors, diverticulosis
     c. Hypothyroidism
     d. Neurologic, neuromuscular disorder—multiple sclerosis, spinal cord disorders
     e. Celiac disease
     f. Medications—laxative overuse, anticholinergics, narcotics, calcium channel blockers, iron supplements
     g. Pregnancy
  2. Prevalence—unknown because of frequent self-treatment; commonly reported by patients, especially elderly adults
  3. Risks—see "Etiology"; more common in elderly
- Signs and symptoms
  1. Typically fewer than three bowel movements per week
  2. Hard feces, difficult to pass
  3. Abdominal bloating or pain
  4. Hemorrhoids
  5. Sense of incomplete evacuation
  6. Having to use fingers to help stool passage
- Physical findings
  1. Firm-to-hard stool in rectum
  2. Fecal impaction
  3. Abdomen
     a. Normal bowel sounds
     b. Nontender with simple constipation
- Differential diagnosis—see "Etiology"; constipation is a symptom, not a disease
- Diagnostic tests/findings—indicated when "red flags" identified, constipation is persistent or fails to respond to treatment, or particular disorder suspected
  1. Red flags
     a. Abdominal pain, nausea/vomiting
     b. Weight loss

c. Melena, rectal bleeding

d. Rectal pain

e. Fever

f. New onset older than age 50 years

2. Diagnostic tests

  a. CBC, TSH

  b. Stools for hemoccult

  c. Flexible sigmoidoscopy/colonoscopy

- Management/treatment

1. Nonpharmacologic

  a. Increased fluid intake

  b. Increased physical activity

  c. High-fiber diet—bran, fruits, vegetables, whole grain cereals and bread

  d. Plan time for elimination, consistent time each day

2. Pharmacologic

  a. Bulk-forming agents—psyllium husk, methylcellulose, calcium polycarbophil

    (1) Drug action

      (a) Increased stool bulk, retention of stool water, reduces transit time

      (b) Used to prevent constipation, not useful treatment of acute constipation

    (2) Side effects

      (a) Must be taken with ample fluid to prevent esophageal/intestinal obstruction or fecal impaction

      (b) Abdominal distention and flatus

    (3) Drug interactions—decreased absorption of digitalis, salicylates, tetracyclines, nitrofurantoin, and others

    (4) Contraindications/precautions

      (a) Signs of fecal impaction

      (b) GI obstruction

      (c) Pregnancy Category B

  b. Stool softeners—docusate sodium

    (1) Drug action

      (a) Act as surfactants; lower surface tension, which facilitates penetration of water into stool

      (b) Useful for patients complaining of hard stools and those for whom straining at stool should be avoided

    (2) Side effects

      (a) Bitter taste, throat irritation

      (b) Mild abdominal cramping, diarrhea

    (3) Drug interactions—may increase absorption of mineral oil

    (4) Contraindications/precautions

      (a) Acute abdominal pain, intestinal obstruction

      (b) Pregnancy Category C

      (c) Because absorption minimal, should pose no risk to breastfeeding infant

  c. Osmotic laxatives—sorbitol, lactulose, polyethylene glycol

    (1) Drug action

      (a) Nonabsorbable disaccharide that acts as osmotic diuretic

      (b) Drug of choice after bulk-forming laxatives for chronic constipation

    (2) Side effects

      (a) Flatulence

      (b) Intestinal cramps, diarrhea

    (3) Drug interactions—antacids may inhibit osmotic laxative effect

    (4) Contraindications/precautions

      (a) Acute surgical abdomen, intestinal obstruction, fecal impaction

      (b) Galactose-restricted diets

      (c) Pregnancy Category B; caution in nursing mothers

  d. Saline laxatives—magnesium hydroxide/milk of magnesia

    (1) Drug action

      (a) Variety of poorly absorbed salts that draw water into intestinal lumen causing fecal mass to soften and swell; swelling stretches intestinal lumen and stimulates peristalsis

      (b) Treatment of acute constipation

    (2) Side effects

      (a) Diarrhea, abdominal cramps

      (b) Fluid and electrolyte disturbances

    (3) Drug interactions

      (a) Decreased absorption of quinolones and tetracyclines

      (b) Premature absorption of enteric-coated drugs

    (4) Contraindications/precautions

      (a) Renal failure

      (b) Acute surgical abdomen, intestinal obstruction, fecal impaction

      (c) Pregnancy Category B; no problems reported in nursing mothers

  e. Chloride channel activator—lubiprostone

    (1) Drug action

      (a) GI motility enhancer, increases fluid in the intestines

      (b) Treatment of chronic idiopathic constipation

    (2) Side effects

      (a) Nausea

      (b) Diarrhea, flatulence

      (c) Abdominal pain, distention

    (3) Drug interactions—none listed

    (4) Contraindications/precautions

      (a) Renal or hepatic impairment

      (b) Confirm absence of bowel obstruction before use

      (c) Pregnancy Category C, nursing mothers monitor infant for diarrhea

      (d) Take with food and water

      (e) Reevaluate periodically for need to continue—established as safe for up to 12 months

3. Patient education

  a. Plan time for defecation, do not ignore urge to defecate

  b. Avoid overuse of laxatives

  c. Drink adequate amounts of fluid to avoid dehydration

  d. Increase fiber in diet

- Referral—any suspected obstructive or serious systemic pathology

Diarrhea

- Definition—defecation of loose, watery stools 3 or more times a day
  1. Diarrhea is a symptom rather than a disease
  2. Acute—less than 1–2 weeks duration
  3. Chronic—more than 3 weeks duration, continuous or intermittent
- Etiology/incidence/risk factors
  1. Etiology
     a. Acute
        (1) Viral—Norwalk
        (2) Bacterial—*Salmonella, Shigella, E. coli* (traveler's diarrhea)
        (3) Protozoa—*Giardia lamblia, E. histolytica*
        (4) Bacterial toxins—*Staphylococcus, Clostridium*
        (5) Medications—antibiotics, laxatives, antacids
     b. Chronic or recurrent
        (1) Protozoa—*Giardia lamblia, E. histolytica*
        (2) Inflammatory—ulcerative colitis, Crohn's disease, ischemic colitis
        (3) Medications—antibiotics, laxatives, antacids
        (4) Functional—irritable bowel syndrome
        (5) Malabsorption—sprue, pancreatic insufficiency, lactase deficiency
        (6) Postsurgical—postgastrectomy dumping syndrome
        (7) Systemic diseases—diabetes, hyperthyroidism
  2. Incidence—estimated that the average adult in the United States experiences 1–2 acute diarrheal episodes per year
  3. Risk factors
     a. Travel to some countries in Africa, Asia, Latin America, Caribbean
     b. Close contact with infected persons (e.g., day care, institutionalization)
     c. Decreased immunity—more susceptible to organisms that generally do not cause symptoms in immunocompetent hosts
- Signs and symptoms
  1. Abrupt onset
  2. Increased frequency and volume of stools
  3. Crampy abdominal pain
  4. May be associated with nausea and vomiting
  5. Dehydration if severe
- Physical findings
  1. Acute
     a. Occasionally—low-grade fever; postural changes in pulse, blood pressure
     b. Abdominal examination—hyperactive bowel sounds; diffuse tenderness to palpation
  2. Chronic—signs associated with specific causes (e.g., thyromegaly, lymphadenopathy, cachexia, rectal mass, impaction)
- Differential diagnosis—see "Etiology"; diarrhea is a symptom, not a disease
- Diagnostic tests/findings
  1. Usually none indicated for symptoms lasting less than 72 hours unless associated with bloody diarrhea or patient appears ill

  2. If persistent or chronic
     a. Stool evaluation
        (1) For fecal leukocytes
        (2) For occult blood
        (3) For culture for bacterial pathogens
        (4) For ova and parasites
        (5) Giardia antigen assay
        (6) *Clostridium difficile* toxin assay
        (7) Qualitative fat (sudan stain)—fat content increased in presence of small bowel disease or pancreatic insufficiency
     b. HIV testing
     c. Hematologic evaluation for indications of underlying disease
        (1) CBC, electrolytes, and sedimentation rate for indications of infection, dehydration
        (2) TSH low in hyperthyroidism
        (3) Hyperglycemia in diabetes mellitus
- Management/treatment
  1. Nonpharmacologic
     a. Observation—acute diarrhea usually self-limited
     b. Hydration/electrolyte replacement
     c. Normal diet as soon as patient able to tolerate
     d. For lactase deficiency, limit milk products and consider exogenous lactase
  2. Pharmacologic
     a. Antimotility agents—loperamide, diphenoxalate/atropine
        (1) Drug action—slows intestinal transit, allowing more time for absorption
        (2) Side effects
           (a) Abdominal pain
           (b) Distention
           (c) Dizziness, fatigue
           (d) Rash
           (e) Anticholinergic effects
        (3) Drug interactions—diphenoxylate/atropine
           (a) Potentiates MAOIs
           (b) CNS depressant effects with alcohol use
        (4) Contraindications/precautions
           (a) Bloody diarrhea or severe illness
           (b) Acute dysentery
           (c) Pseudomembranous, ulcerative colitis
           (d) Pregnancy Category B/C; not recommended while nursing
     b. Antisecretory agents—bismuth subsalicylate
        (1) Drug action—may involve adsorption of bacterial toxins and/or local anti-inflammatory effect
        (2) Side effects—darkened tongue or stool
        (3) Drug interactions—potentiates oral anticoagulants and hypoglycemics; salicylism with aspirin
        (4) Contraindications/precautions—hypersensitivity to salicylates; influenza or varicella in teenagers; coagulation disorders, diabetes, pregnancy Category C/D (third trimester); not recommended in nursing mothers
     c. Antibiotics
        (1) Indicated only when pathogen identifiable

(2) May exacerbate simple episode

(3) Traveler's diarrhea—ciprofloxacin or trimethoprim-sulfamethoxazole for 3 days

3. Patient education

  a. Maintain adequate fluid intake

  b. Normal diet when tolerated

  c. Limit use of antidiarrheal agents

  d. Prevention of traveler's diarrhea

    (1) Don't drink tap water, use for brushing teeth, or as ice in drinks

    (2) Don't eat raw fruits and vegetables unless you have to peel them

    (3) Don't drink unpasteurized milk or milk products

    (4) Don't eat raw or rare cooked meats or fish

- Indications for referral

1. Blood in stools

2. Diarrhea accompanied by severe abdominal pain

3. Worsening symptoms

4. Definitive diagnosis and management of underlying disease

Hemorrhoids

- Definition

1. Varicosities of the hemorrhoidal plexus in the lower rectum or anus

2. Internal

  a. Originate above the anorectal line

  b. Covered by nonsensitive rectal mucosa

3. External

  a. Originate below the anorectal line

  b. Covered by well-innervated epithelium

- Etiology/incidence/risk factors

1. Etiology

  a. Thin-walled, dilated vessels; engorge with increased intra-abdominal pressure

  b. Prolapse may be secondary to passage of a large, hard stool; increase in venous pressure from pregnancy or heart failure; or straining due to lifting or defecation

2. One of the most commonly encountered anorectal conditions in general practice

3. Risk factors

  a. Constipation, straining at stool

  b. Pregnancy

  c. Low-fiber diet

  d. Pelvic congestion

  e. Poor pelvic musculature

  f. Loss of muscle tone with advanced age

- Signs and symptoms

1. Internal—painless, bright red bleeding with defecation

2. External—itching, pain, and bleeding with defecation

- Physical findings

1. Internal

  a. Usually not palpable unless thrombosed

  b. Usually not visible unless prolapsed

2. External

  a. Protrude with straining or standing

  b. Blue, shiny masses at the anus if thrombosed

  c. Painless, flaccid skin tags (resolved thrombotic hemorrhoids)

- Differential diagnosis

1. Condyloma accuminata

2. Rectal prolapse

3. Rule out other causes for bleeding

  a. Colorectal cancer

  b. Polyps

  c. Anal fissures

  d. Inflammatory bowel disease

  e. Colonic diverticulitis

- Diagnostic tests/findings

1. Anoscopic examination—with internal hemorrhoids bright red to purplish bulges

2. Additional testing if underlying pathology suspected

- Management/treatment—no treatment necessary if asymptomatic

1. Nonpharmacologic

  a. Increase bulk/fiber/fluids in diet

  b. Sitz baths

  c. Witch hazel pads or gel—may provide transient relief and help reduce inflammation

2. Pharmacologic

  a. Topical anesthetic/steroid suppositories and ointments

    (1) Drug action—anesthetic and anti-inflammatory action

    (2) Side effects

      (a) Local irritation, contact dermatitis, folliculitis

      (b) Dermal atrophy with topical steroid; possibility of systemic absorption

    (3) Drug interactions—none

    (4) Contraindication/precautions—some are pregnancy Category C; not recommended while nursing

  b. Bulk-forming agents (see "Constipation" section in this chapter)

  c. Stool softeners (see "Constipation" section in this chapter)

3. Patient education

  a. Regulation of bowel habits

  b. Dietary changes to maintain hydration, bulk

  c. Appropriate use of bulk laxatives, stool softeners, hemorrhoidal preparations

- Referral

1. Acute thrombosis of an external hemorrhoid

2. Failure to respond to conservative management

Irritable Bowel Syndrome (IBS)

- Definition

1. A chronic functional disorder characterized by altered bowel habits and abdominal pain

2. Rome III Criteria for Diagnosis of IBS (Longstreth et al., 2006)—recurrent abdominal pain or discomfort at least 3 days per month in the previous 3 months

  a. Associated with two or more of the following:

    (1) Improvement with defecation

    (2) Onset associated with change in stool frequency

    (3) Onset associated with change in stool form

b. One or more of the following symptoms on at least 25% of occasions for subgroup identification (constipation IBS, diarrhea IBS, mixed/alternating IBS)
  (1) Abnormal stool frequency—less than 3 times per week or more than 3 times per day
  (2) Abnormal stool form—lumpy/hard or loose/watery
  (3) Abnormal stool passage—straining, incomplete evacuation
  (4) Bloating, feeling of abdominal distention
  (5) Passage of mucus

- Etiology/prevalence/risk factors
  1. Etiology—proposed
     a. Altered bowel motility
     b. Visceral hypersensitivity
     c. Imbalance of neurotransmitters
  2. Prevalence—as high as 15% in general population; only 25% of persons with symptoms consistent with IBS seek care
  3. Risk factors—female to male ratio of 2:1; late teens, early adulthood

- Signs and symptoms
  1. Refer to Rome criteria
  2. Presence of the following symptoms suggest organic disease (alarm symptoms)
     a. Pain/diarrhea that interferes with sleep
     b. Recurrent nausea and vomiting
     c. Evidence of GI bleeding
     d. Unintentional weight loss (> 10% of ideal body weight)
     e. Persistent diarrhea or severe constipation

- Physical findings—mild left-lower quadrant tenderness on abdominal examination

- Differential diagnosis
  1. Food intolerance—lactose, fructose, sorbitol
  2. Colon cancer
  3. Infectious disease/parasitic infestation (*Giardia*)
  4. Inflammatory disease (ulcerative colitis, Crohn's disease)
  5. Laxative abuse

- Diagnostic tests/findings
  1. Not indicated for patients who are younger than age 50 years, meet Rome criteria, normal physical examination, lacking alarm symptoms
  2. Consider the following dependent on other history or physical examination findings
     a. CBC, chemistry panel, sedimentation rate
     b. Stool studies including fecal leukocytes, occult blood, ova, and parasites
     c. Flexible sigmoidoscopy
     d. 2-week trial of lactose-free, fructose-free, or sorbitol-free (one at a time) to rule out food intolerance if has bloating, gas, distention, and diarrhea
  3. Colonoscopy if patient older than 50 years, weight loss, anemia, evidence of GI bleeding, or risk factors for colon cancer or inflammatory bowel disease

- Management/treatment
  1. Nonpharmacologic
     a. Reassurance of benign nature of disease
     b. Diet
        (1) Decrease caffeine, alcohol, fatty foods, gas-forming foods, or products containing sorbitol; limit dairy products if lactose intolerance suspected
        (2) Increase fiber in diet or in the form of supplements if has constipation-IBS
     c. Stress management, relaxation techniques, identify "triggers"
     d. Regular physical activity
     e. Probiotics—theorized that may ameliorate IBS symptoms by stimulating immune response, reducing inflammation, altering composition of gut flora
  2. Pharmacologic—use patient's symptoms as a guide
     a. Pain predominant
        (1) Antispasmodic/anticholinergic—dicyclomine hydrochloride, *L*-hyoscyamine sulfate
           (a) Drug action—selectively inhibits gastrointestinal smooth muscle and may reduce pain and bloating
           (b) Side effects—drowsiness, anticholinergic effects
           (c) Drug interactions—alcohol, CNS depressants, additive anticholinergic effects with other anticholinergics
           (d) Contraindications/precautions
              i. Glaucoma
              ii. Unstable cardiovascular disease
              iii. GI or urinary tract obstruction
              iv. Pregnancy Category B/C; contraindicated in nursing mothers
        (2) Tricyclic antidepressants—amitryptyline, nortriptyline, desipramine
           (a) Drug action—analgesic and mood-enhancing properties; anticholinergic effects
           (b) Side effects—drowsiness, anticholinergic effects, constipation
           (c) Drug interactions—fluoxetine, MAO inhibitors, alcohol, CNS depressants
           (d) Contraindications/precautions
              i. During or within 14 days of MAO inhibitors; postacute MI
              ii. Pregnancy Category C; not recommended in nursing mothers
     b. Diarrhea predominant
        (1) Loperamide, diphenoxylate/atropine (see "Diarrhea" section in this chapter)
        (2) Alosetron
           (a) Drug action—a 5-HT$_3$ receptor antagonist, decreases intestinal secretion, motility, and afferent pain signals
           (b) Limited use for women with severe chronic diarrhea predominant IBS; unresponsive to conventional therapy and not caused by anatomic or metabolic abnormality
           (c) Side effects—possible severe adverse GI effects, including ischemic colitis and serious complications of constipation resulting in hospitalization, and rarely blood transfusion, surgery, and death

(d) Contraindications/precautions—only healthcare providers enrolled in Lotronex (alosetron) prescribing program should prescribe; discontinue immediately in patients who develop constipation or symptoms of ischemic colitis; pregnancy Category B

c. Constipation predominant

(1) Fiber supplements—psyllium, polycarbophil, methylcellulose (see "Constipation" section in this chapter)

(2) Osmotic laxative—lactulose, sorbitol, polyethylene glycol, magnesium hydroxide (see "Constipation" section in this chapter)

(3) Lubiprostone (see "Constipation" section in this chapter)

3. Patient education

a. Appropriate implementation of the nonpharmacologic measures

b. Reassurance of the relative benign nature of disorder

c. Need for reevaluation if symptoms progress or change

- Referral—onset in those older than 50 years; presence of symptoms suggestive of organic disease/alarm symptoms

Appendicitis

- Definition—inflammation of the wall of the vermiform appendix that may result in perforation with subsequent peritonitis
- Etiology/incidence
  1. Etiology
     a. Based on operative findings, classified as simple, gangrenous, or perforated
     b. Acute appendicitis secondary to obstruction due to fecal material, lymphoid hyperplasia, foreign bodies, or parasites with secondary bacterial infection
     c. Gangrene and perforation develop within 24–36 hours; perforation results in release of luminal contents into peritoneal cavity
  2. Incidence—occurs in all age groups; highest incidence in males 10–30 years of age
- Signs and symptoms—classic sequence of symptoms
  1. Pain is initial symptom; begins in epigastrum or periumbilical area
  2. Anorexia, nausea, or vomiting
  3. Pain localizes to RLQ after several hours
  4. Sense of constipation; infrequently diarrhea
- Physical findings
  1. Fever of 99–100°F (> 100°F may indicate peritonitis)
  2. Tenderness localized to McBurney's point; pain worsened and localized with cough
  3. Signs of peritoneal irritation—guarding, rigidity, and rebound tenderness RLQ
  4. Absent bowel sounds
  5. Positive psoas sign—pain with flexion at the hip against resistance or hyperextension
  6. Positive Rovsing's sign—RLQ pain elicited when LLQ is deeply palpated and pressure is released
  7. Positive obturator sign—pain with passive internal rotation of flexed right hip/knee
  8. Rectal examination may reveal tenderness/mass

- Differential diagnosis
  1. Ovarian (e.g., mittelschmerz, cyst)
  2. Ectopic pregnancy
  3. Pelvic inflammatory disease
  4. Pyelonephritis, calculi
  5. Gallbladder or pancreatic inflammation
  6. Gastroenteritis
- Diagnostic tests/findings
  1. White blood cell count—moderate leukocytosis 10,000–18,000/mm^3
  2. Urinalysis may demonstrate hematuria and pyuria
  3. Pregnancy test
  4. Ultrasound diagnostic in 85% of patients
  5. Focused appendix computerized tomography (FACT)—highly specific and sensitive but time and expense limit usefulness in routine diagnosis
- Management/treatment
  1. Nonpharmacologic—none
  2. Pharmacologic—none
  3. Patient education
     a. Need for emergency care if pain or other symptoms change during observation, evaluation period
     b. Postoperative care instructions
- Referral—immediate surgery consult for acute abdomen

Peptic Ulcer Disease (PUD)

- Definition—chronic mucosal ulcerative disorder involving the upper GI tract (stomach or duodenum); imbalance both in amount of acid–pepsin production and ability of gastric and duodenal mucosa to protect itself
- Etiology/incidence/risk factors
  1. Etiology
     a. Acid and pepsin activity overpower mucosal defenses to produce ulcers when mucosal defense is impaired by exogenous factors/*Helicobacter pylori*, and NSAIDs
     b. *H. pylori* is an established causative factor; 90–95% of duodenal ulcer patients and 70–80% of gastric ulcer patients infected with *H. pylori*
     c. *H. pylori* is a Gram-negative bacterium; produces urease that breaks down urea-forming ammonia and CO_2, allowing organism to control pH of its environment
     d. NSAIDs damage mucosa through a direct action and systemically by inhibiting endogenous prostaglandin synthesis; NSAID-related ulcers more likely to be gastric
  2. Incidence
     a. Estimated 5–10% of the general population
     b. Male/female ratio nearly equal
     c. Duodenal ulcers more common; peak incidence of gastric ulcers ages 55–65
  3. Risk factors
     a. Family history
     b. Cigarette smoking—delays healing and increases risk of recurrence
     c. Medications—corticosteroids, NSAIDs
     d. Alcohol use—delays healing and increases risk of recurrence

- Signs and symptoms
  1. Burning or deep epigastric pain that occurs 1–3 hours after meals; relieved by ingestion of food or antacids
  2. Pain commonly causes early morning awakening
  3. Other dyspeptic symptoms—nausea, vomiting, belching, bloating
  4. Symptomatic periods occur in clusters lasting a few weeks followed by symptom-free periods for weeks/months
  5. Gastric ulcer presentation more variable; food may make symptoms worse
  6. Complications—hemorrhage, perforation, obstruction
  7. Alarm symptoms for gastric cancer or complicated PUD
     a. Bloody or black stools
     b. Unintended weight loss
     c. Dysphagia
     d. Persistent, severe epigastric or stomach pain
     e. Bloody or coffee-ground-type vomit
- Physical findings
  1. Usually none in uncomplicated peptic ulcer disease
  2. Occasionally, well-localized epigastric tenderness
- Differential diagnosis
  1. Gastroesophageal reflux disease
  2. Nonulcer dyspepsia
  3. Gastric carcinoma
  4. Angina
- Diagnostic tests/findings
  1. Stool for occult blood
  2. *H. pylori* testing
     a. Unless indications for endoscopy, use serology to identify infection and stool antigen test or urea breath test to determine cure if indicated
        (1) Serologic test—ELISA detects IgG antibodies indicating current or past infection; may or may not revert to negative after treatment
        (2) Stool antigen test—reverts to negative within 5 days/few months after eradication of organism
        (3) Urea breath test—detects presence or absence of active infection
  3. CBC with differential
  4. Mucosal biopsy during endoscopy indicated if age older than 50 years, alarm symptoms, family history of gastric cancer, no improvement with treatment
- Management/treatment
  1. Nonpharmacologic
     a. Avoid aspirin and NSAIDs
     b. Smoking cessation
     c. Decrease alcohol intake
     d. Decrease intake of any identified irritants that make symptoms worse—coffee, caffeine, spicy foods
     e. Use stress management, relaxation techniques
  2. Pharmacologic
     a. Disease not due to *H. pylori*
        (1) Histamine 2 receptor antagonists (H_2RA) —cimetidine, ranitidine, nizatidine, famotidine
           (a) Drug action—inhibits acid secretion by blocking H_2 receptors in parietal cell

        (b) Side effects
           i. Headache, fatigue, dizziness
           ii. Minimal GI upset
        (c) Drug interactions—may alter absorption of certain drugs secondary to changes in gastric pH
        (d) Contraindications/precautions
           i. Severe renal insufficiency
           ii. Pregnancy Category B; not recommended while nursing
        (2) Proton pump inhibitors (PPIs)—omeprazole, lansoprazole, rabeprazole, pantoprazole, esomeprazole
           (a) Drug action—inhibits gastric acid secretion by altering the activity of the proton pump; virtual cessation of acid production
           (b) Side effects
              i. Headache
              ii. Nausea, abdominal pain, flatulence, constipation, diarrhea
           (c) Drug interactions—may interact with drugs that depend on gastric pH for absorption
           (d) Contraindications/precautions
              i. Omeprazole—pregnancy Category C; not recommended while nursing
              ii. Lansoprazole—pregnancy Category B; caution while nursing
     b. Ulcers caused by *H. pylori*—eradication of *H. pylori* to reduce risk of recurrent duodenal ulcer
        (1) PPI triple therapy—lansoprazole, amoxicillin, clarithromycin
        (2) Bismuth quadruple therapy—bismuth subsalicylate, metronidazole, tetracycline, plus PPI or H_2RA
        (3) Persistent *H. pylori* infection—re-treat with alternative combination
  3. Patient education
     a. Importance of positive lifestyle changes (e.g., smoking cessation, decreased alcohol consumption)
     b. Purpose, dosage, side effects of medications
     c. Importance of compliance with medication regimen
- Referral
  1. Patients with weight loss, dysphagia, anorexia, vomiting, hematemesis/melena; new-onset pain in patients older than 45 years
  2. If treatment for *H. pylori* fails second time, referral indicated
  3. Obtain surgical consultation for patients with evidence of bleeding, gastric outlet obstruction, or perforation

Viral Hepatitis

- Definition—a group of systemic infections involving the liver with common clinical manifestations caused by different viruses with distinctive epidemiologic patterns
- Etiology/incidence/risk factors
  1. Hepatitis A virus (HAV)
     a. Spread via fecal–oral route by person-to-person contact or eating/drinking contaminated food/water; spreads readily in households and child care centers

b. Mean incubation time 25 days; range 15 to 60 days; maximum infectivity 2 weeks before jaundice; acute onset

c. Infections in infancy/childhood generally mild without jaundice; adult infections can be severe

d. Self-limited; no carrier state or chronic liver disease results

e. Accounts for up to one-third of acute viral hepatitis cases

2. Hepatitis B virus (HBV)

a. Transmitted via percutaneous or mucosal contact with infectious blood or body fluids (saliva, vaginal secretions, semen) by parenteral, sexual, perinatal exposure

b. Mean incubation time 75 days; range 28 to 160 days

c. Spectrum of illness ranging from asymptomatic seroconversion to acute illness; fulminant hepatitis results in less than 1%

d. Up to 10% infected as adults and 90% infected as neonates become chronic carriers; increased risk of cirrhosis, hepatocellular carcinoma

3. Hepatitis C virus (HCV)

a. Transmitted most efficiently via large or repeated percutaneous exposure to infected blood through transfusion prior to 1992 or IV drug use; transmitted much less frequently through occupational, sexual, or perinatal exposures; most common chronic bloodborne infection in the United States

b. Mean incubation time 50 days; range 2 to 22 weeks; onset insidious

c. Acute disease often mild in adults; asymptomatic in children

d. Up to 80% of infected individuals develop chronic hepatitis; 20–30% eventually develop cirrhosis or hepatocellular carcinoma

4. Hepatitis D virus (HDV)

a. An incomplete virus that requires the helper function of HBV to replicate

b. Transmitted via percutaneous or mucosal exposure to infectious blood as a coinfection with HBV or superinfection in person with HBV

c. Incubation period for superinfection is 2–8 weeks

d. Contributes to severity of HBV infection

e. Suspect superinfection with HDV in patient who presents with fulminant hepatitis and chronic HBV

5. Hepatitis E virus (HEV)

a. Spread via fecal–oral route

b. Endemic in developing countries

c. Mean incubation time 27 days; range 2 to 9 weeks

d. More common in children and young adults; infection during pregnancy can lead to liver failure

e. No risk of chronicity or carcinoma

6. Miscellaneous viral causes

a. Herpes simplex virus

b. Epstein-Barr virus

c. Cytomegalovirus

- Signs and symptoms—all viral types produce very similar syndromes; severity of illness can vary widely

1. Phase 1—incubation

a. Asymptomatic

b. Weeks to months

2. Phase 2—preicteric (prodromal)

a. 3 to 10 days in length

b. Malaise, fatigue

c. Anorexia, nausea, vomiting

d. "Flu-like" aches, headache

e. Skin rash

f. Change in sense of smell or taste; aversion to cigarettes

3. Phase 3—icteric

a. 1 to 4 weeks in length

b. RUQ pain

c. Dark-colored urine

d. Clay-colored stools

e. Jaundice of skin, sclera, nail beds

4. Phase 4—convalescence

a. May last weeks to months

b. Chronic disease develops in certain types

c. Hepatitis B, C, D may be fatal; HEV 30% mortality rate in pregnant women

- Physical findings

1. Rash—maculopapular and urticarial lesions

2. Low-grade fever

3. Jaundice

4. Hepatomegaly

5. Splenomegaly

- Differential diagnosis—noninfectious causes of hepatitis (e.g., hepatotoxic drugs, alcohol)

- Diagnostic tests/findings

1. Viral serologies (see **Table 9-4**)

2. Urinalysis—positive for protein, bilirubin

3. Liver function tests

a. Marked elevation—alanine aminotransferase (ALT) and aspartate aminotransferase (AST)

b. Mild elevation of alkaline phosphatase

c. Normal serum bilirubin or mild bilirubinemia

- Management/treatment

1. Nonpharmacologic

a. Activity as tolerated; avoid strenuous activities or contact sports

b. Hydration

c. Maintain adequate caloric intake and balanced diet; small feedings may be better tolerated

d. Discontinue all but essential medications

e. Avoid alcohol

2. Pharmacologic

a. Antiemetics if indicated for nausea—trimethobenzamide (Tigan)

(1) Drug action—acts centrally to inhibit the medullary chemoreceptor trigger zone

(2) Side effects—drowsiness, dizziness, blurred vision, hypotension

(3) Drug interactions—potentiates alcohol, other CNS depressants

(4) Contraindications/precautions—pregnancy Category C; not recommended while nursing

b. Chronic hepatitis B

■ **Table 9-4   Serologic Diagnosis and Markers of Active or Chronic Hepatitis**

Test Name	HAV	HBV	HCV	HDV
HAV IgM antibody	+ current or recent infection	N.A. (not applicable)	N.A.	N.A.
HAV total antibody	+ indicates immunity in absence of + HAV IgM	N.A.	N.A.	N.A.
HBV surface antigen	N.A.	+ acute & chronic infection	N.A.	+ with HBV/HDV coinfection or superinfection
HBV surface antibody	N.A.	+ resolution and immune	N.A.	N.A.
HBV core IgM antibody	N.A.	+ acute infection, resolves 4-6 months	N.A.	+ with HBV/HDV coinfection or superinfection
HBV e antigen	N.A.	+ resolving infection or response to therapy	N.A.	N.A.
HBV DNA		+ active infection	N.A.	+ with HBV/HDV coinfection or superinfection
HCV antibody	N.A.	N.A.	+ late in acute & in chronic infection	N.A.
HCV RNA	N.A.	N.A.	+ confirms current infection	N.A.
HDV antibody	N.A.	N.A.	N.A.	+ with positive HBV surface antigen, current or past HBV/HDV coinfection or superinfection
HDV IgM antibody	N.A.	N.A.	N.A.	+ with positive HBV surface antigen, current or past HBV/HDV coinfection or superinfection Negative, resolved HDV infection

(1) Antiviral treatment indicated for active viral replication (sustained presence of HBeAg and HBV DNA), elevated ALT levels, and histologic evidence of chronic liver injury

(2) Agents approved for treatment of chronic HBV—interferon alfa, lamivudine, entecavir, adefovir dipivoxil, telbivudine

c. Chronic hepatitis C—peginterferon in combination with ribavirin

d. Prevention

  (1) HAV

    (a) Immune globulin—recommended for travelers going to countries for longer than 6 months where HAV is endemic; give as prophylaxis within 2 weeks of known exposure

    (b) HAV vaccine

  (2) HBV

    (a) HBIG—give as prophylaxis to infants born to HBsAg-positive women; give within 14 days of sexual exposure

    (b) HBV vaccine

3. Patient education

  a. Careful disposal of infected wastes

  b. Scrupulous hand washing, food-handling techniques

  c. Need for prophylactic immunization of contacts, household members

  d. Safer sexual practices

  e. Avoidance of blood contamination—no sharing toothbrushes, razors, needles

  f. Laboratory follow-up

    (1) Monitor aminotransferase at 1- to 4-week intervals during acute illness

    (2) Monitor HBsAg and anti-HBsAg until anti-HBs present

• Referral

1. Fulminant disease—patients presenting with altered mental state

2. Chronic HBV patients who require treatment

3. HCV—early identification/referral important because evidence suggests that early treatment reduces risk of chronic infection

Cholecystitis

- Definition
  1. Gallstones/cholelithiasis
  2. Biliary colic is most common symptom of cholelithiasis and results from transient obstruction of the cystic duct by a stone
  3. Acute cholecystitis is the most common complication of cholelithiasis and develops when a gallstone(s) obstructs the cystic duct, resulting in distention and inflammation of the gallbladder; secondary bacterial infection occurs in about 50% of cases
- Etiology/incidence/risk factors
  1. Etiology
     a. Gallstones may be result of imbalance in bile components
     b. About 85–95% of gallstones are composed primarily of cholesterol
     c. Pigment stones are composed of calcium bilirubinate; less common
  2. Incidence—gallstones occur in 10–15% of the U.S. population
     a. Majority of patients with gallstones have asymptomatic disease
     b. About 20% of asymptomatic patients develop symptoms over a period of 20 years; majority present with biliary pain rather than biliary complication
  3. Risk factors for cholelithiasis
     a. Female gender
     b. Advanced age
     c. Obesity
     d. Multiparity, pregnancy
     e. Rapid weight loss
     f. Hypertriglyceridemia
     g. Medications/oral contraceptives
- Signs and symptoms
  1. Biliary colic—presenting symptom in more than 90% of patients
     a. Severe, steady pain localized to the epigastrum or RUQ; may radiate to back or scapula
     b. Pain is precipitated by spasm of a dilated cystic duct obstructed by gallstone(s)
     c. Attacks of biliary colic more common at night
     d. Pain typically has a sudden onset and may last 3 hours; may be accompanied by nausea/vomiting
  2. Acute cholecystitis
     a. Pain similar to biliary colic but lasts longer; associated with nausea/vomiting and fever
     b. Symptoms of local inflammation and systemic toxicity
     c. Pain shifts from epigastrum to RUQ; sequence secondary to visceral pain from ductal impaction by stones progressing to inflammation of the gall bladder with parietal pain
     d. Most patients have had previous attacks of biliary colic
- Physical findings—acute cholecystitis
  1. Fever
  2. Murphy's sign—inspiratory arrest secondary to pain during deep palpation of right subcostal region; relatively specific finding
  3. Gallbladder distended and palpable
  4. Jaundice
  5. Localized tenderness may be only finding in elderly patients; pain and fever may be absent
- Differential diagnosis
  1. Appendicitis
  2. Pancreatitis
  3. Ruptured ectopic pregnancy or ovarian cyst
  4. Peptic ulcer disease
- Diagnostic tests/findings
  1. Ultrasound
     a. Has a 95% sensitivity for detecting stones in the gallbladder; detects bile duct stones in only 50% of cases
     b. Best noninvasive imaging technique to diagnose acute cholecystitis; findings include thick gallbladder wall, gallbladder distension, sludge in the lumen, peri-cholecystic fluid
  2. Hepatobiliary scintigraphy—can confirm/exclude diagnosis of acute cholecystitis with high degree of sensitivity/specificity
  3. Endoscopic retrograde cholangiopancreatography (ERCP)—best study for diagnosis of bile duct stones
  4. Computerized tomography (CT)/MRI—comparable to ERCP in terms of diagnostic accuracy
  5. Leukocytosis with a "left shift" observed in acute cholecystitis; serum aminotranferases, alkaline phosphatase, bilirubin, and amylase may also be elevated
  6. Elevation of serum bilirubin and alkaline phosphatase with bile duct stones
  7. Amylase greater than 1000 U/dL indicates acute pancreatitis
- Management/treatment
  1. Expectant management for patients with asymptomatic gallstones
  2. Elective cholecystectomy for most patients with symptomatic cholelithiasis
  3. Acute cholecystitis managed with hospital admission; early cholecystectomy once patient is stable
  4. Bile duct stones should be removed whether symptomatic or not because of high rate of complications

Gastroesophageal Reflux Disease (GERD)

- Definition
  1. *Gastroesophageal reflux* refers to movement of gastric contents from the stomach into the esophagus
  2. *GERD* refers to symptomatic clinical condition or histologic alteration that results from episodes of reflux
  3. When esophagus is repeatedly exposed to refluxed material for prolonged periods of time, inflammation of esophagus can occur
  4. Complications—esophagitis; strictures; Barrett's esophagus, which carries a 10% risk of progression to adenocarcinoma
- Etiology/incidence/risk factors
  1. Etiology
     a. Contributing factors include reflux of caustic gastric contents, a breakdown in defense mechanism of esophagus, and a functional abnormality that results in reflux
     b. Most common etiology is prolonged esophageal acid exposure due to transient lower esophageal relaxations

c. Less common mechanisms include pathologically weak lower esophageal sphincter (LES) tone, hiatal hernia, esophageal motility disorder, Zollinger–Ellison syndrome, and delayed gastric emptying

2. Incidence
   a. Approximately 20% of adults report reflux symptoms that occur at least weekly
   b. Approximately 1% of adults with GERD have Barrett's esophagus

3. Risk factors
   a. Foods that lower LES pressure—high fat, chocolate, peppermints
   b. Foods that irritate esophageal mucosa—citrus fruits, spicy tomato drinks
   c. Drugs that lower LES pressure—calcium channel blockers, progesterone
   d. Cigarette smoking, alcohol
   e. Pregnancy
   f. Obesity

- Signs and symptoms
   1. "Heartburn"—retrosternal burning sensation radiating upward
   2. Acid regurgitation—effortless return of gastric contents into pharynx
   3. Symptoms usually occur postprandially
   4. Symptoms aggravated by reclining, straining, bending, or stooping
   5. Atypical symptoms
      a. Odynophagia—burning, squeezing pain with swallowing
      b. Dysphagia—sensation of food lodged in the chest secondary to stricture
      c. Globus sensation—sensation of lump in the throat
   6. Extraesophageal symptoms
      a. Hoarseness
      b. Chronic cough
      c. Asthma/reactive airway disease
      d. Hiccups
      e. Dental disease
      f. Nausea

- Physical findings
   1. Usually normal examination
   2. Occasionally epigastric tenderness with palpation

- Differential diagnosis
   1. Cardiac chest pain
   2. Peptic ulcer disease
   3. Infectious esophagitis—viral, fungal
   4. Medication-induced esophagitis—antibiotics
   5. Esophageal/gastric malignancy
   6. Hepatobiliary disease

- Diagnostic tests/findings
   1. Diagnosis of GERD based on clinical findings and confirmed by response to therapy
   2. Diagnostic evaluation if symptoms chronic or refractory to therapy or if esophageal complications suspected
      a. Endoscopy
         (1) Useful for diagnosis of complications—esophagitis, strictures, Barrett's esophagus

         (2) Indications
            (a) Dysphagia or odynophagia
            (b) Weight loss
            (c) Evidence of GI bleeding or iron-deficiency anemia
            (d) Screen for Barrett's if 10 years or more of GERD symptoms
      b. Upper GI may demonstrate structural problems; evaluation of dysphagia
      c. Ambulatory esophageal pH monitoring—best test to establish abnormal acid reflux

- Management/treatment
   1. Nonpharmacologic
      a. Weight loss if obese
      b. Smoking cessation
      c. Elevate head of bed (HOB); sleep on wedge-shaped bolster
      d. Avoid recumbency for 3 hours postprandially
      e. Reduce fat to no more than 30% of calories
      f. Reduce consumption of alcohol, chocolate, colas, coffee, peppermint, citrus juices, tomato products
   2. Pharmacologic
      a. Commercially available antacids and antirefluxants/alginic acid are useful for mild symptoms
         (1) Drug action
            (a) Neutralizes acids
            (b) Produces foaming neutral barrier to reflux
         (2) Side effects—diarrhea, constipation
         (3) Drug interactions—reduces absorption of tetracycline, possibly other drugs
         (4) Contraindications/precautions—impaired renal function
      b. H_2-receptor antagonists (acid reducers)—effective treatment for less severe GERD (see "Peptic Ulcer Disease (PUD)" section earlier in this chapter)
      c. Proton pump inhibitors (acid suppressant agents)—most effective agents for healing esophagitis and preventing complications (see "Peptic Ulcer Disease (PUD)" section in this chapter)
   3. Patient education—lifestyle modifications

- Referral
   1. Symptoms of dysphagia, weight loss, blood loss, obstructive symptoms including nausea/vomiting, early satiety, anorexia
   2. Long-standing or refractory cases
   3. Candidates for surgical intervention

Hematologic Disorders

Anemias

- Definition
   1. Abnormally low hemoglobin concentration (< 12 g/dL for women, 13 g/dL for men) (de Benoist, B., McLean, E., Egli, I., & Cogswell, M., 2008) or inadequate red blood cell (RBC) population
   2. Numerous diverse causes

3. Usually classified according to RBC size—mean corpuscular volume (MCV)

    a. Microcytic anemia (MCV < 80 fL) (e.g., iron-deficiency anemia, thalassemia trait)

    b. Macrocytic anemia (MCV > 100 fL) (e.g., B_{12} deficiency, folate deficiency, liver disease, hypothyroidism)

    c. Normocytic anemia (MCV 80–100 fL) (e.g., anemia of chronic disease, hemolysis/hemoglobinopathy/sickle cell disease, renal failure)

- Etiology/incidence—commonly encountered anemias

1. Iron-deficiency anemia (IDA)

    a. Etiology

        (1) Blood loss—GI overt/occult, menorrhagia

        (2) Inadequate dietary intake of iron-rich foods—most common in infants and adolescents, vegetarians

        (3) Metabolic demands in excess of intake—pregnancy, lactation

    b. Incidence

        (1) Most common form of anemia; represents 25% of all anemia cases

        (2) Affects 10–15% of premenopausal women

    c. Risk factors

        (1) Female gender

        (2) Menorrhagia

        (3) Pregnancy

2. Anemia of chronic disease

    a. Etiology

        (1) A hypoproliferative anemia associated with underlying chronic disorders such as infections, inflammatory disorders, and malignancy

        (2) Reduced production and response to erythropoietin; decreased RBC life span

        (3) Defect in iron reutilization

    b. Incidence—second most common anemia

3. Vitamin B_{12}–deficiency anemia

    a. Etiology

        (1) B_{12} deficiency alters DNA synthesis

        (2) B_{12} deficiency develops secondary to lack or relative deficiency of intrinsic factor that leads to impaired vitamin B_{12} absorption (pernicious anemia)

            (a) Autoimmune reaction involving gastric parietal cells

            (b) History of gastrectomy

        (3) Rarely secondary to nutritional deficiency of vitamin B_{12}

    b. Incidence—regarded as a disorder affecting older persons of northern European descent; likely underrecognized in other populations

    c. Risk factors

        (1) Usually presents around age 60, familial tendency

        (2) Both sexes equally affected

        (3) Strict vegan diet

        (4) Recent gastric surgery

4. Folic acid–deficiency anemia

    a. Etiology

        (1) Folic acid deficiency alters synthesis of DNA and RBC maturation

        (2) Folic acid deficiency due to

            (a) Malabsorption syndromes

            (b) Increased demand—pregnancy, infancy

            (c) Inadequate intake—alcoholics, elderly

        (3) Certain drugs decrease folic acid levels—oral contraceptives, Dilantin (phenytoin)

    b. Incidence

        (1) Found in all races and age groups

        (2) Most common megaloblastic anemia in pregnancy

    c. Risk factors

        (1) Pregnancy

        (2) Alcoholism

5. Sickle cell anemia

    a. Etiology

        (1) A chronic hemolytic anemia characterized by sickle-shaped RBCs

        (2) Autosomal recessive genetic disorder

            (a) Hgb S develops instead of Hgb A

            (b) Individual is homozygous for Hgb S

    b. Incidence

        (1) Homozygous Hgb S in an estimated 0.5% African Americans

        (2) Heterozygous trait in an estimated 8% of African Americans; essentially asymptomatic carrier state

        (3) Most common hemoglobinopathy in the United States

    c. Risk factors

        (1) African American race

        (2) Lower frequency in persons of Mediterranean ancestry

- Signs and symptoms

1. Iron-deficiency anemia

    a. Asymptomatic unless severe, then nonspecific

    b. Fatigue, generalized weakness

    c. Dyspnea on exertion

    d. Headaches

    e. Pica

2. Anemia of chronic disease

    a. Symptoms common to all anemias—fatigue, weakness, exertional dyspnea, light headedness, anorexia

    b. Other signs and symptoms related to specific underlying disease

3. Vitamin B_{12}–deficiency anemia

    a. None at first, insidious onset

    b. Fatigue, weakness, lightheadedness

    c. Dyspnea, palpitations

    d. GI disturbances—anorexia, bloating, diarrhea

    e. Sore tongue

    f. Neurologic—paresthesias, ataxia

    g. Loss of taste and smell

4. Folate-deficiency anemia—signs and symptoms similar to vitamin B_{12}–deficiency anemia, except there is no neurologic involvement

5. Sickle cell anemia

    a. Often none during remissions

    b. Vaso-occlusive crises—precipitating factors include infection, physical or emotional stress, blood loss, pregnancy, surgery, high altitudes

        (1) Malaise, chills

(2) Pain, especially in bones, abdomen, chest, lower legs

(3) Headaches, epistaxis, vomiting

(4) Difficulty walking

- Physical findings
  1. Iron-deficiency anemia
     a. Often none
     b. Skin or conjunctival pallor
     c. Glossitis, stomatitis
     d. Tachycardia with/without systolic flow murmur
     e. Tachypnea
     f. Nail changes
        (1) Spoon shaped (koilonychia)
        (2) Brittle, easily split
     g. Hair thinning, breaking
  2. Anemia of chronic disease
     a. Ill appearance
     b. Signs of precipitating illness
  3. Vitamin B_{12}–deficiency anemia
     a. Skin pale, occasionally jaundiced
     b. Stomatitis; glossitis; smooth, beefy-red tongue
     c. Tachycardia, arrhythmias, systolic flow murmur
     d. Organomegaly—hepatomegaly, splenomegaly
     e. Neurologic
        (1) Ataxia, positive Romberg test
        (2) Hyperactive reflexes
        (3) Peripheral loss of sensation, decreased vibratory sense, impaired proprioception
        (4) Changes in mental state with possible wide range of expression—mild confusion to acute psychosis
  4. Folate-deficiency anemia
     a. Pallor
     b. Tachycardia, tachypnea
     c. Malnourished appearance
     d. No neurologic findings
  5. Sickle cell anemia
     a. In crises
        (1) Temperature, pulse, respirations elevated
        (2) Hypotension
        (3) Pallor, cyanosis secondary to poor oxygenation
        (4) Scleral jaundice
        (5) Decreased skin turgor
     b. Chronic findings due to anemia, vaso-occlusive events, end-organ damage
        (1) Cardiomegaly
        (2) Skin ulcers, especially on lower extremities
        (3) Osteomyelitis
        (4) Retinopathy
        (5) Renal disease—hematuria
- Differential diagnosis
  1. Iron-deficiency anemia
     a. Anemia of chronic disease
     b. Thalassemia trait
     c. Sideroblastic anemia
  2. Anemia of chronic disease—diagnosis of exclusion
     a. Iron-deficiency anemia
     b. Anemia of renal disease

3. Vitamin B_{12}–deficiency anemia
   a. Nutritional deficiency
   b. Malabsorption
   c. Chronic alcoholism
   d. Chronic gastritis (*H. pylori* infection)
   e. Folic acid deficiency
4. Folate-deficiency anemia
   a. Pernicious anemia
   b. Medication, toxins
5. Sickle crises
   a. Appendicitis
   b. Acute cholecystitis
   c. Pneumonia

- Diagnostic tests/findings
  1. World Health Organization standard for anemia diagnosis
     a. Hemoglobin 13 g/dL or less in men (approximately 38% hematocrit)
     b. Hemoglobin 12 g/dL or less in women (approximately 35% hematocrit)
  2. Severe anemia (symptomatic) generally less than 25% hematocrit (Hct)
  3. Iron-deficiency anemia—hypochromic microcytic RBCs
     a. RBC changes in early disease may be mild
     b. MCV less than 80 fL
     c. Increased red cell width (RDW)
     d. Serum ferritin less than 10 mg/L
        (1) Levels reflect iron stores; single most useful test for diagnosing IDA
        (2) Ferritin is an acute-phase reactant; may be elevated in inflammatory disease
     e. Decreased reticulocyte count
  4. Anemia of chronic disease—normochromic-normocytic early in course, becomes microcytic
     a. Anemia is typically mild; hematocrit remains around 30%
     b. Low serum iron levels; normal or increased total iron binding capacity TIBC
     c. Normal or increased serum ferritin
  5. Vitamin B_{12}–deficiency anemia—megaloblastic-macrocytic anemia
     a. MCV greater than 100 fL
     b. Serum B_{12} decreased, less than 100 pg/mL
     c. Peripheral blood smear—RBCs of widely varying size (anisocytosis) and shape (poikilocytosis)
     d. Serum methylmalonic acid and homocysteine levels elevated
     e. Schilling test or assay for anti-intrinsic factor antibody
        (1) Obtain if vitamin B_{12} deficiency detected
        (2) Helps distinguish lack of intrinsic factor from malabsorption
  6. Folate deficiency—megaloblastic-macrocytic anemia
     a. MCV greater than 100 fL
     b. Serum folate less than 3 ng/mL; normal serum vitamin B_{12}
     c. Elevated homocysteine level; normal methylmalonic acid level
  7. Sickle cell anemia
     a. Hgb of 7–9 g/dL; Hct 20–30%
     b. Mild leukocytosis—12,000 to 15,000/mm^3

c. Reticulocytosis 10–25%

d. Irreversibly sickled cells on peripheral smear

e. Platelets may be elevated

f. Sickledex used for screening—sickle cells present in patients with disease and trait

g. Hemoglobin electrophoresis—Hgb S/85–95% in sickle cell anemia; Hgb S/40% in sickle cell trait

- Management/treatment

1. Iron-deficiency anemia—identify the cause of iron deficiency and correct it
   a. Nonpharmacologic
      (1) Diet with increased iron content
      (2) Hemoglobin monitoring schedule
         (a) Check 3 weeks after initiation of treatment; recheck in 6–8 weeks
         (b) Ongoing monitoring every 3 months until stable
   b. Pharmacologic
      (1) Ferrous sulfate—may need to continue therapy 4–6 months to replenish iron stores; may discontinue when serum ferritin exceeds 50 mg/L
         (a) Drug action—replenishes depleted iron stores; incorporated into hemoglobin; allows the transportation of oxygen via hemoglobin
         (b) Side effects
            i. Nausea, vomiting, GI upset
            ii. Black stools
            iii. Constipation
         (c) Drug interactions
            i. Antacids, calcium supplements inhibit iron absorption
            ii. Inhibits tetracycline absorption
         (d) Contraindications/precautions
            i. Hemochromocytosis
            ii. Caution in elderly adults
            iii. Caution with peptic ulcer

2. Anemia of chronic disease
   a. Nonpharmacologic—treatment of underlying disorder; transfusion if severe anemia
   b. Pharmacologic—none; iron, folate, and vitamin B_{12} have not been shown to be effective

3. Vitamin B_{12}–deficiency anemia
   a. Nonpharmacologic—none
   b. Pharmacologic
      (1) Vitamin B_{12}/cyanocobalamin—dose IM daily for 1 week, then weekly until Hct is normal, then monthly for life
      (2) Cyanocobalamin nasal gel—weekly dosing; alternate maintenance therapy
      (3) Drug action—required for hematopoiesis
      (4) Side effects
         (a) Manifested with parenteral use—local stinging, burning at injection site; urticaria, itching; pulmonary edema, anaphylaxis
         (b) Manifested with intranasal use—headache, nausea, rhinitis

(5) Drug interactions—ethanol decreases vitamin B_{12} absorption; decreased response with concomitant chloramphenicol, neomycin

(6) Contraindications/precautions—hypersensitivity to cobalt

4. Folate-deficiency anemia
   a. Nonpharmacologic—increased dietary sources of folic acid: legumes, leafy green vegetables, fruits, and liver
   b. Pharmacologic—folic acid
      (1) Drug action—cofactor in biosynthesis of nucleic acids needed for RBC synthesis
      (2) Side effects
         (a) Allergic reactions—skin rash, urticaria, itching
         (b) Gastrointestinal—nausea, bloating, flatulence, foul taste in mouth
         (c) CNS—sleep disturbances, irritability, confusion
      (3) Drug interactions
         (a) Oral contraceptives increase risk of folic acid deficiency
         (b) Corticosteroids increase folic acid requirements
         (c) Sulfonamides decrease absorption of folic acid

5. Sickle cell anemia
   a. Nonpharmacologic
      (1) Treat all infections aggressively
      (2) Maintain hydration, oxygenation
   b. Pharmacologic—maintained continuously on folic acid supplement
   c. Therapy during crisis
      (1) Hydration and adequate oxygenation
      (2) Analgesics for pain control
      (3) Antibiotics for associated infections

6. Patient education
   a. Iron-deficiency anemia
      (1) Take iron with meals to alleviate GI distress; taking with orange juice or other vitamin C source will enhance absorption
      (2) Dietary counseling to improve iron intake and overall nutrition
      (3) Need for follow-up blood monitoring
   b. Vitamin B_{12}–deficiency anemia—need for monthly supplementation
   c. Folate-deficiency anemia
      (1) Folate maintenance dosage
      (2) Avoid overcooking folate-rich foods
   d. Sickle cell anemia
      (1) Consider genetic counseling
      (2) Crises avoidance
         (a) Maintain good nutrition
         (b) Avoid temperature extremes
         (c) Immunizations for pneumococcus and influenza
      (3) Routine evaluation of body systems every 3 to 6 months

- Referral

1. Evaluation of suspected GI blood loss
2. Sickle cell crisis
3. Evaluation of resistant cases

Immunologic Disorders

Human Immunodeficiency Virus (HIV) Infection

- Definition
  1. HIV infection produces a spectrum of diseases progressing from a clinically latent or asymptomatic state to a state of profound immunosuppression with acquired immune deficiency syndrome (AIDS) as a late manifestation
  2. Stages of HIV infection
     a. Transmission/primary HIV infection
     b. Acute HIV infection/seroconversion
     c. Asymptomatic infection/clinically latent period with or without persistent generalized lymphadenopathy (PGL)
     d. Early symptomatic infection; previously referred to as "AIDS-related complex"
     e. AIDS, specific clinical conditions present or CD4+ cell count less than 200 cells/mm^3
     f. Advanced HIV infection, characterized by CD4+ cell count less than 50 cells/mm^3
- Etiology/incidence
  1. Etiology
     a. HIV virus transmitted through direct contact with blood, blood products, other body fluids
     b. Methods of transmission include—sexual contact, sharing needles, blood transfusions, babies born to HIV-infected mothers, occupational exposure
  2. Incidence (Centers for Disease Control and Prevention [CDC], 2013a; 2014)
     a. Prevalence of HIV infection in United States estimated to be 1,144,500, including 15.8% undiagnosed infections
     b. One in four individuals living with HIV is female
     c. Incidence in United States has remained stable overall in recent years with approximately 50,000 new diagnosed HIV infections each year
     d. Incidence in women decreased 21% from 2008 to 2011
     e. Heterosexual contact responsible for 84% of new HIV infections in women
     f. Black females remain disproportionately affected representing 64% of new HIV infections in women in 2010
  3. Risk factors
     a. Unprotected or traumatic sexual activity (e.g., multiple partners or partners with other partners, anal intercourse, lack of condom use)
     b. Intravenous drug use, sharing needles
     c. Infant of HIV-positive mother (vertical transmission)—15–25% if woman does not receive antiretroviral therapy during pregnancy
        (1) Risk of transmission may be reduced to less than 1% if pregnant woman receives multiagent antiretroviral therapy and has undetectable viral load at delivery
        (2) Risk of transmission greater with maternal CD4+ counts of less than 200 cells/mm^3
     d. Transfusion of blood or blood products, artificial insemination, organ transplant recipient prior to 1985

     e. Healthcare worker or service worker exposed to blood or body fluids (e.g., needle stick injury, splash)
- Signs and symptoms
  1. Acute HIV infection and seroconversion
     a. Moderate "flu-like" syndrome 2 to 4 weeks after inoculation
     b. Fever, diarrhea, headache, oral lesions on palate, lethargy, muscle/joint pain, rash lasting 2 to 4 weeks
     c. Self-limited; patients who seek care often misdiagnosed
     d. Seroconversion usually in 6–12 weeks; may take up to 6 months
  2. HIV disease progression—asymptomatic infection
     a. 12 weeks to 8 or more years; period of intense battle by immune system
     b. Influenced by general physical condition, age, mitigating drug therapy
        (1) Risk of progression correlates with length of seroconversion illness
        (2) Early HIV detection improves opportunity for successful antiviral therapy
  3. Early symptomatic HIV infection
     a. Usually occurs in 8 to 10 years; immune system begins to weaken
     b. Constitutional symptoms
        (1) Fatigue, headache, arthralgia, myalgia
        (2) Weight loss, anorexia, diarrhea
        (3) Fevers, night sweats, chills
     c. Occurrence of opportunistic infections
  4. Advanced disease/AIDS
     a. Usually occurs in 10 to 11 years
     b. Severe infections
  5. Opportunistic infections
     a. Caused by a spectrum of pathogens that rarely cause disease in healthy people; most occur when CD4+ count is less than 200 cells/mm^3
     b. May be the reactivation of a previous pathogen; may have atypical presentation
     c. Causative agents include bacterial, fungal, viral, and parasitic infections
        (1) Candidiasis—mouth, vagina, penis, esophagus, large intestine, skin
        (2) Toxoplasmosis
        (3) Malignancies
        (4) Kaposi's sarcoma
        (5) Lymphoma—late manifestation of HIV
        (6) Invasive squamous cell carcinoma—cervix, vulva, anus secondary to human papillomavirus (HPV)
        (7) *Pneumocystis* (*carinii*) *jiroveci* pneumonia (PCP)—major AIDS-defining diagnosis
        (8) Tuberculosis
        (9) *Mycobacterium avium* complex (MAC)—occurs in late-stage HIV infection
- Physical findings—related to immunocompromised status
  1. Early findings
     a. Lymphadenopathy
     b. Dermatologic abnormalities—seborrheic dermatitis, folliculitis

c. Oral lesions—aphthous ulcers, herpes simplex labialis, thrush, oral hairy leukoplakia

2. As disease progresses, more frequent skin disorders, oral lesions, infections

- Differential diagnosis
  1. Lymphomas
  2. Pneumonia
  3. Tuberculosis
  4. Chronic fatigue syndrome
  5. Mononucleosis
- Diagnostic tests/findings
  1. Diagnosis
     a. Enzyme-linked immunosorbant assay (ELISA)—positive for HIV antibodies (highly sensitive)
        (1) Conducted in laboratory or as rapid test at testing site
        (2) Performed with blood or oral fluid (not saliva)
        (3) False negative may occur if conducted during window period; average is 25 days from exposure to identifiable antibodies; 97% will be positive by 3 months after exposure
        (4) All positive tests must be followed with a confirmatory test
     b. Follow-up confirmatory tests are highly specific
        (1) Indirect immunofluorescence assay (Western blot) detects antibodies
        (2) Antibody differentiation test distinguishes HIV-1 from HIV-2
        (3) HIV-1 nucleic acid test looks for virus directly
     c. Home HIV tests are available—rapid test using oral fluids; test with finger blood stick sample sent to laboratory
     d. Antigen tests—can directly detect virus
        (1) Nucleic acid testing—use in patients suspected of having acute retroviral syndrome
        (2) HIV blood culture
        (3) p24 antigen detects presence of HIV protein
        (4) RNA PCR assay and branched DNA (bDNA) assay; measure amount of HIV RNA in plasma
  2. Initial and interim laboratory tests for women with established HIV infection—stage HIV infection, screen for comorbidities, establish baselines before treatment with antiretroviral (ARV) medications, monitor response to therapy (U.S. Department of Health and Human Services [U.S. DHHS], 2011)
     a. Complete blood count with differential and platelets every 3–6 months
     b. Chemistry panel with electrolytes, renal function, liver function tests every 3–6 months
     c. Lipid profile, fasting glucose, urinalysis with protein and creatinine—baseline and before start ARV therapy
     d. RPR or VDRL every 6–12 months
     e. Varicella, cytomegalovirus serology—baseline
     f. Hepatitis A, B, C—baseline and as indicated
     g. Toxoplasmosis—as indicated
     h. TB testing every 6–12 months
     i. Chest radiography—as indicated
     j. Pap test—every 6 months first year after diagnosis and annually thereafter
     k. Chlamydia and gonorrhea tests every 6–12 months

l. Quantitative plasma HIV ribonucleic acid (RNA) every 3–6 months
   (1) Useful for predicting progression of disease by indicating viral load
   (2) Monitoring response to antiviral therapy

m. CD4+ cell count every 3–6 months
   (1) Indicative of immune status, predictor of disease progression
   (2) Complements viral load assay
   (3) Normal is 800 to 1050 cells/mm^3
   (4) Patients with CD4+ of 200 cells/mm^3 or less are likely to have symptoms or an AIDS-defining condition

n. Drug resistance testing (genotype, phenotype)—test for possible ARV medication resistance

- Management/treatment
  1. Nonpharmacologic
     a. Symptom management
     b. Laboratory monitoring
     c. Nutrition counseling—identify and address symptoms that may affect appetite, chewing, swallowing; support overall health and immune system function
  2. Pharmacologic (see **Table 9-5**)
     a. Antiretroviral therapy for HIV suppression
        (1) Highly active antiretroviral therapy (HAART)—combining three or four drugs is the standard of care for treatment of HIV infection
        (2) Goal to reduce HIV RNA to minimal levels for as long as possible (undetectable level < 500 copies/mL)
        (3) Decisions regarding need to change therapy based on measured antiviral effect per HIV RNA levels
        (4) HIV mutates rapidly
           (a) HIV can mutate rapidly from a drug-sensitive form to a drug-resistant form
           (b) Treatment with a combination of drugs to minimize development of resistance
        (5) Treatment modification called for when HIV RNA levels fail to reach less than 500 copies/mL after 6 months of therapy
     b. Antiretroviral drug classes
        (1) Nucleoside reverse transcriptase inhibitors (NRTIs)
        (2) Nonnucleoside reverse transcriptase inhibitors (NNRTIs)
        (3) Protease inhibitors (PIs)
        (4) Nucleotide reverse transcriptase inhibitors
     c. HIV treatment in pregnancy is discussed elsewhere
  3. Patient education
     a. Natural history of HIV infection
     b. Explain modes of transmission
        (1) Discuss lifelong ability to transmit virus
        (2) Teach effective ways to reduce fluid exchange
           (a) Breastfeeding contraindicated
           (b) Encourage "safe sex" practices; condom use, limiting number of partners
           (c) Eliminate needle sharing
     c. Emphasize behaviors that protect/enhance immune system
        (1) Maintain immunizations
           (a) Hepatitis B and A
           (b) Pneumococcal vaccine (repeat in 5 years)

■ **Table 9-5   Antiretroviral Therapy for HIV Suppression (representative list)**

Drug	Action	Side-effects	Interactions	Contraindications / Precautions
Nucleoside reverse transcriptase inhibitors (NRTI) zidovudine (AZT, ZDV) didanosine (ddI) zalcitabine (ddC) stavudine (d4T) lamivudine (3TC)	Faulty version of building blocks needed for HIV to make copies of itself; stalls virus reproduction	AZT—reversible bone marrow toxicity - anemia, leukopenia, GI effects, muscle pain, fatigue ddI—pancreatitis d4T/ddC—peripheral neuropathy 3TC—headache, fatigue, GI effects, minimal toxicity	Caution with other nephrotoxic, cytotoxic myelosuppressive drugs; antagonized by rifampin	Monitor closely for hematologic toxicity and opportunistic infections; Benefits of antiretroviral therapy in prevention of mother-to-child transmission generally outweigh potential for adverse effects; in United States breastfeeding by HIV-positive mother is not recommended; only a few antiretroviral drugs have been studied for concentrations in breast milk
Nonnucleoside reverse transcriptase inhibitors (NNRTI)— efavirenz, nevirapine, delavirdine	Binds to and disables reverse transcriptase, protein HIV needs to make copies of itself	Mild to moderate skin rash, nausea, dizziness, headache, impaired concentration, vivid dreams, insomnia (efavirenz)	Metabolized by and can induce/inhibit cytochrome P450 enzymes; drug interactions can occur with PIs and many other drugs	Monitor liver, renal functions; See NRTI information on use in pregnancy and breastfeeding
Protease inhibitors (PIs)— amprenavir, indinavir, nelfinavir ritonavir, saquinavir, lopinavir/ ritonavir	Disables protease, protein HIV needs to make copies of itself	GI effects; fat redistribution, lipid abnormalities, increased transaminase levels Indinavir—kidney stones	Metabolized by cytochrome P450 enzymes; drug interactions common; avoid rifampin	Impaired hepatic function; monitor blood, liver and hyperglycemia See NRTI information on use in pregnancy and breastfeeding

(c) Influenza (annually)

(d) Tetanus-diphtheria vaccine, Tdap vaccine if not done previously, booster every 10 years

(e) HPV vaccine

(f) Live vaccines contraindicated if severe immunosuppression (CD4 count < 200 cells/mm^3)

(2) Stop tobacco, alcohol, street drug use

(3) Follow nutritious diet, use clean food preparation techniques

(4) Reduce/manage stress

(5) Exercise as tolerated

(6) Avoid infectious individuals and high-risk environments (e.g., child care settings, work settings such as hospitals)

(7) Avoid or eliminate exposure to pets, especially dogs, cats, or birds

(8) Control travel exposures

d. Drug regimens, interactions, and resistance—importance of adherence to medication schedule, CD4$^+$ monitoring

e. HIV and pregnancy implications—encourage antiviral medication to reduce vertical transmission

f. Contraception

(1) Barrier methods reduce transmission

(a) Condoms—male or female for vaginal or anal penetrative acts

(b) Dental dams or plastic film for oral contact

(c) Stress need for consistent barrier use in addition to other contraception

(2) Oral contraceptives and depomedroxyprogesterone acetate (DMPA) injections—not contraindicated; limited data indicate antiretroviral drugs have potential to either increase or decrease bioavailability of contraceptive hormones

(3) Spermicides—controversy regarding role in possible increase in vaginal susceptibility

(4) Intrauterine contraception (IUC)—not contraindicated if HIV positive or if has AIDS but is clinically well on antiretroviral therapy

- Referral
  1. All cases initially for full evaluation
  2. Monitoring and titration of medications
  3. Evaluation of new symptomatology

Systemic Lupus Erythematosus (SLE)

- Definition—chronic, inflammatory, multisystem disorder of the immune system characterized by periods of remission and exacerbation; course of disease unpredictable and highly variable
- Etiology/incidence/risk factors
  1. Etiology
     a. An autoimmune disorder—abnormal immune response creates antibodies to normal tissue
     b. Associated with reaction to some medications—chlorpromazine, hydralazine, isoniazid, methyldopa
     c. Criteria for diagnosis; 4 of 11 criteria to make diagnosis (Petri, 2005)
        (1) Malar rash
        (2) Discoid rash
        (3) Photosensitivity
        (4) Oral ulcers
        (5) Arthritis involving two or more peripheral joints
        (6) Serositis—pleuritis, pericarditis, or peritonitis
        (7) Renal disorder involving proteinuria or cellular casts
        (8) Neurologic disorder involving seizures or psychoses
        (9) Hematologic disorders—hemolytic anemia, leukopenia, thrombocytopenia
        (10) Positive ANA (antineutrophil antibody) test
        (11) Positive other immunologic test—anti-double-stranded DNA (anti-dsDNA), anti-Smith (anti-Sm), LE (lupus erythematosus) cell preparation, false-positive syphilis serology
  2. Incidence/prevalence
     a. Approximately 5 per 100,000 individuals each year in United States
     b. Primarily affects women of childbearing age
     c. Approximately 250,000 definitive cases of SLE in United States
     d. Prevalence much higher in African American women (1 in 250) and Hispanic women (100 in 100,000) than in Caucasian women (12–39 in 100,000)
  3. Risk factors
     a. African American or Hispanic descent
     b. First-degree relative with SLE
     c. Cigarette smoking, other environmental exposures
- Signs and symptoms
  1. Early symptoms—vague, nonspecific, frequently misdiagnosed
  2. Constitutional—fever, fatigue, weight loss
  3. Arthralgia, arthritis
  4. Photosensitivity
  5. Headache, seizures
- Physical findings
  1. Malar rash—erythematous, flat or raised rash over malar eminences
  2. Discoid rash—erythematous raised patches with scaling
  3. Alopecia

  4. Mucosal ulcers
  5. Pleurisy
  6. Pericarditis
- Differential diagnosis
  1. Contact dermatitis, eczema
  2. Rheumatoid arthritis
  3. Infectious processes
  4. Chronic fatigue syndrome
- Diagnostic tests/findings
  1. Positive ANA
  2. Anti-dsDNA, anti-Sm, LE cell prep, biologic false-positive VDRL
  3. CBC—anemia, leukopenia, lymphopenia, thombocytopenia
  4. Serum creatinine to assess kidney function
  5. Urinalysis to determine presence of hematuria, cellular casts, and proteinuria
  6. Antiphospholipid antibodies (anticardiolipin IgG or IgM or lupus anticoagulant); 30–50% of individuals with SLE have positive antiphospholipid antibodies
- Management/treatment
  1. Nonpharmacologic
     a. Modest physical activity
     b. Protection from direct sunlight
     c. Proper diet and nutrition—low fat, low cholesterol, adequate vitamin D and calcium
  2. Pharmacologic
     a. Some drugs may induce or aggravate symptoms
     b. Treatment is generally symptomatic and variable
     c. Nonsteroidal anti-inflammatory drugs (NSAIDs)—may control associated fever, arthralgias, but not fatigue, malaise, major organ system involvement
     d. Corticosteroids—low-dose topical or injection for skin lesions; higher doses oral or IV for major organ involvement
     e. Hydroxychloroquine
        (1) Drug action—antimalarial drug; may help treat lupus rashes and joint symptoms; evidence that may decrease flares and organ damage with long-term use
        (2) Side effects
           (a) Irreversible retinopathy, corneal edema
           (b) Neuromuscular dysfunction
           (c) Pruritus, rash, skin pigmentation
           (d) Blood dyscrasias
        (3) Drug interactions
           (a) Hepatotoxic drugs
           (b) Dermatotoxic drugs
        (4) Contraindications/precautions
           (a) Hepatic dysfunction, alcoholism
           (b) Psoriasis
           (c) Pregnancy Category C; not recommended while nursing
  3. Patient education
     a. Sunscreen, protective clothing to avoid UV light
     b. Relaxation, stress reduction
     c. Individualized exercise/rest program
     d. Prompt treatment of infections

e. Effective contraception
  (1) Many women with SLE are good candidates for most contraceptive methods
  (2) Combination hormonal contraceptives are Category 4, progestin-only contraceptives Category 3, and LNG-IUS Category 3 if positive or unknown antiphospholipid antibodies; associated with higher risk for both arterial and venous thrombosis
  (3) Initiation but not continuation of DMPA or copper IUC is Category 3 if have severe thrombocytopenia
f. Careful supervision of obstetric care
  (1) Increased risk for premature delivery, spontaneous abortion, intrauterine fetal death, intrauterine growth restriction, pregnancy-induced hypertension, venous thromboembolism, postpartum hemorrhage
  (2) Exacerbation of symptoms may occur—usually mild to moderate in severity
  (3) Pregnancy outcomes best when mother has been in remission for at least 6 months prior to pregnancy and has normal renal function
g. Avoidance of surgery, dental procedures when SLE symptoms present
h. Immunizations
  (1) Pneumococcal vaccine, meningococcal vaccine, annual influenza vaccine
  (2) Live vaccines not advisable
i. Vitamin D supplementation
- Referral
  1. Evaluation of new symptoms, exacerbations
  2. When invasive procedures are indicated
  3. Social services, family or individual counseling regarding chronic disease coping strategies

Rheumatoid Arthritis (RA)

- Definition—an autoimmune disorder characterized by symmetric, erosive destruction of synovial tissues resulting in deformity and loss of joint function; may involve extra-articular manifestations
- Etiology/incidence
  1. Etiology
    a. Exact etiology unknown
    b. Complex of factors likely
      (1) Genetic
      (2) Environmental—viral, bacterial trigger suspected
      (3) Hormonal—controversial
    c. Criteria for diagnosis; score-based algorithm with total score of 6 out of 10 needed in 4 categories (A–D) for classification of patient as having definite RA (American College of Rheumatology, 2010)
      (1) A. Joint involvement—score 0–5 dependent on number and size of joints with clinical synovitis (stiffness, swelling)
      (2) B. Serology—score 0–3 dependent on negative, positive, and level of rheumatoid factor (RA) and anticitrullinated protein antibody (ACPA)

      (3) C. Acute phase reactants—score 0–1 dependent on normal/abnormal C-reactive protein (CRP) and/or erythrocyte sedimentation rate (ESR)
      (4) D. Duration of symptoms—score 0–1 with 1 point if has had symptoms for 6 or more weeks
    d. The 2010 criteria do not include presence of rheumatoid nodules, radiographic erosive changes, and symmetric arthritis because these may not be present in early RA
  2. Incidence
    a. Prevalence—approximately 1% of the population
    b. Occurs twice as often in women as in men; typically presents between 30 and 50 years of age
    c. Genetic predisposition
- Signs and symptoms
  1. Morning stiffness in joints lasting more than 1 hour
  2. Joint pain, constant or recurring; insidious development over weeks to months
  3. Joint warmth and redness; functional impairment
  4. Fatigue, weakness, anorexia, low-grade fever, malaise may precede arthritic symptoms
- Physical findings
  1. Soft tissue swelling—most frequently in metacarpophalangeal (MCP) and proximal interphalangeal (PIP) joints; usually symmetric
  2. Deformity of involved joints
  3. Limited range of motion in affected joint
  4. Subcutaneous nodules
  5. Lymphadenopathy
  6. Splenomegaly
  7. Ocular disease—scleritis
  8. Entrapment neuropathies
- Differential diagnosis
  1. Polymyalgia rheumatica
  2. Osteoarthritis
  3. Systemic lupus erythematosus
  4. Ankylosing spondylitis
  5. Reiter's syndrome
- Diagnostic tests/findings
  1. Rheumatoid (antibody) factor—can be isolated in 70–80% of patients and/or anticitrullinated protein antibody
  2. Elevated erythrocyte sedimentation rate and/or C-reactive protein
  3. Radiography—joint erosion, narrowing of joint space—may not be evident in early disease
- Management/treatment—reduce joint inflammation, manage pain, prevent joint destruction
  1. Nonpharmacologic
    a. Physical therapy, occupational therapy, hydrotherapy
    b. Rest
    c. Exercise
    d. Assistive devices
      (1) Footwear—orthotics
      (2) Canes, crutches
      (3) Splints, braces
    e. Surgery—synovectomy, arthroscopy

2. Pharmacologic
   a. Nonsteroidal anti-inflammatory drugs (NSAIDs)—use for short-term therapy until disease-modifying antirheumatic drugs take effect
      (1) Agents
         (a) Ibuprofen, naproxen, diclofenac
         (b) Meloxicam, etodolac, nabumetone
         (c) COX-2 inhibitors—celecoxib, rofecoxib, valdecoxib
      (2) Drug action—analgesic and anti-inflammatory effects
      (3) Side effects
         (a) GI effects—dyspepsia, gastric and duodenal ulceration, perforation and bleeding; selective COX-2 inhibitors have less upper GI toxicity
         (b) Renal toxicity
         (c) CNS toxicity—dizziness, anxiety, drowsiness, confusion
      (4) Drug interactions—may decrease effectiveness of diuretics, beta blockers, ACE inhibitors; may increase toxicity of lithium and methotrexate
      (5) Contraindications/precautions—aspirin allergy; pregnancy Category C, but contraindicated third trimester; not recommended while nursing
   b. Corticosteroids—use for short-term therapy until disease-modifying antirheumatic drugs take effect
   c. Nonbiologic disease-modifying antirheumatic drugs (DMARDs)—no analgesic effects; can control symptoms and may delay progression of disease
      (1) Hydroxychloroquine—moderately effective for mild RA (see "Systemic Lupus Erythematosus (SLE)" section earlier)
      (2) Sulfasalazine
         (a) Side effects—nausea, anorexia, rash; hepatitis, leukopenia, agranulocytosis
         (b) Drug interactions—reduces absorption of digoxin, folic acid
         (c) Contraindication/precautions—intestinal or urinary obstruction; pregnancy Category B; not recommended in nursing mothers
      (3) Methotrexate
         (a) Side effects—stomatitis, anorexia, nausea, abdominal cramps, increased aminotransferase activity
         (b) Drug interactions—avoid other hepatotoxic drugs, live virus vaccines
         (c) Contraindications/precautions—immunodeficiency, blood dyscrasias, alcoholism, chronic liver disease; pregnancy Category X; not recommended in nursing mothers
      (4) Leflunomide
         (a) Side effects—diarrhea, elevated liver enzymes, alopecia, rash
         (b) Drug interactions—may increase levels of diclofenac, ibuprofen; caution with other hepatotoxic drugs
         (c) Contraindications/precautions—hepatic impairment; pregnancy Category X; not recommended in nursing mothers
   d. Biologic agent DMARDs—initial treatment for severe RA or when have toxicity, failure or intolerance of other DMARDs
      (1) Drug agents
         (a) Infliximab—only approved for use with methotrexate
         (b) Adalimumab and etanercept may be used as monotherapy or with methotrexate or other DMARDs
      (2) Drug action—blocks activity of proinflammatory cytokines or their effect; reduces symptoms and slows progression of joint erosion
      (3) Side effects—headache, aseptic meningitis, infection, infusion reactions (fever, urticaria, dyspnea, hypotension), and exacerbation of congestive heart failure (CHF)
      (4) Drug interactions—specific drug interaction studies have not been conducted
      (5) Contraindications/precautions—CHF, active infection, live vaccines; pregnancy Category B; not recommended in nursing mothers
3. Patient education
   a. Safety issues—footwear, balance, transport, walking
   b. Discussion of long-term, chronic nature of disease, support network helpful
   c. Etiology—genetic component, noncontagious
   d. Episodic nature of disease
   e. Pain control techniques—relaxation, drug therapy, rest, appropriate exercise
- Referral
1. Physical therapy, occupational therapy
2. Surgical procedures

Endocrine Disorders

Diabetes

- Definition
1. A heterozygous group of metabolic diseases characterized by hyperglycemia resulting from defects in insulin secretion, insulin action, or both
2. Types
   a. Type 1—absolute insulin deficiency
   b. Type 2—combination of resistance to insulin action and inadequate compensatory insulin secretory response
   c. Gestational diabetes mellitus (GDM)—glucose intolerance diagnosed during pregnancy; excludes high-risk women found to have diabetes at initial prenatal visit using standard criteria
   d. Diabetes secondary to other causes
      (1) Genetic defects in beta-cell function/insulin action
      (2) Diseases of the pancreas or other endocrinopathies in which excess hormones antagonize insulin action (e.g., growth hormone, cortisol, glucagon, epinephrine)
      (3) Drug, chemical, or viral infection induced
   e. Metabolic syndrome—group of metabolic components, synergistic in nature that can lead to cardiovascular disease—abdominal obesity, insulin resistance and hyperglycemia, elevated triglycerides and low HDL, hypertension, and proinflammatory state

3. Complications
   a. Macrovascular
      (1) Coronary artery disease
      (2) Myocardial infarction; sudden cardiac death
      (3) Cerebrovascular disease
      (4) Peripheral vascular disease
      (5) Intestinal ischemia
      (6) Renal artery stenosis
   b. Microvascular
      (1) Retinopathy
      (2) Nephropathy
      (3) Peripheral neuropathy—parasthesias and glove and stocking neuropathy
      (4) Autonomic neuropathy—gastroparesis and sexual dysfunction (e.g., decreased vaginal lubrication, decreased frequency of orgasm, impotence, retrograde ejaculation)
   c. Depression—three- to fourfold increase in prevalence of depression in patients with type 1 or type 2 diabetes
- Etiology/prevalence/risk factors
   1. Type 1
      a. Caused by autoimmune destruction of the pancreatic beta cells that produce insulin
         (1) Genetic predisposition, a hypothetical triggering event, and immunologically mediated beta cell destruction
         (2) Typically begins in childhood or adolescence, but can occur in adults of any age, rarely obese when present with this type of diabetes
      b. Manifested by absolute insulin deficiency that results in elevation of blood glucose, breakdown of fats and proteins
      c. Predisposition to development of ketoacidosis—this may be first manifestation of type 1 diabetes or first appear in presence of infection or other stress
   2. Type 2
      a. Characterized by impaired insulin secretion, peripheral insulin resistance, and increased hepatic glucose production
      b. Typically occurs in those older than age 45 years, those who are overweight and sedentary, and those with a family history of diabetes
      c. Racial/ethnic groups at increased risk—Native Americans, Hispanics, African Americans
   3. Gestational diabetes mellitus (GDM)
      a. Function of hormonal/metabolic demands of pregnancy; usually regresses after parturition
      b. 50% risk of developing diabetes within 5 years if insulin was required for control of GDM; 60% risk of developing disease within 10 to 15 years if dietary management was sufficient
   4. Prediabetes—impaired fasting glucose (IFG) and impaired glucose tolerance (IGT)
      a. Hyperglycemia not sufficient to meet diagnostic criteria for diabetes
      b. Categorized as IFG if identified by fasting blood glucose or IGT if identified by oral glucose tolerance test in the 2-hour sample
      c. Both categories are risk factors for diabetes and cardiovascular disease

   5. Prevalence in the general population estimated at 6–8% of individuals older than 40 years
      a. Type 1 accounts for approximately 10% of diagnosed cases
      b. Type 2 prevalence is estimated at more than 14 million cases, many undiagnosed
- Signs and symptoms
   1. "Classic" symptoms—polyuria, polydipsia, polyphagia
   2. Weight loss
   3. Fatigue and/or weakness
   4. Persistent/recurrent vaginal candidiasis; candidal balanitis
   5. Vision changes, blurred vision
   6. Type 2 often asymptomatic in early stages
- Physical findings
   1. Early
      a. Thin, decreased weight/type 1; overweight, obese/type 2
      b. Hypertension/type 2
      c. Skin infections—frequent or slow to heal
   2. With more advanced disease
      a. Skin—ulcerations of feet and legs; loss of hair lower legs and toes
      b. Eyes—retinopathy/microaneurysms, exudates, neovascularization; cataracts, glaucoma
      c. Cardiovascular—diminished or absent peripheral pulses; orthostatic hypotension/ominous finding
      d. Neurologic—sensory loss; diminished/absent deep tendon reflexes
- Differential diagnosis
   1. Type 1 versus type 2
   2. Pancreatic disease
   3. Cushing's syndrome
   4. Secondary effects of drug therapy—corticosteroids, thiazide diuretics
- Diagnostic tests/findings
   1. Criteria for diagnosis of diabetes type 1 and type 2 (American Diabetes Association [ADA], 2011)
      a. Diabetes can be diagnosed in any one of four ways; must be confirmed on a subsequent day unless also has classic symptoms of hyperglycemia or hyperglycemic crisis
         (1) Fasting plasma glucose 126 mg/dL or greater; fasting defined as no caloric intake for at least 8 hours; or
         (2) An oral glucose tolerance test (OGTT) value of 200 mg/dL or greater in the 2–hour sample; using glucose load of the equivalent of 75 g glucose dissolved in water
         (3) Hemoglobin A_{1c} 6.5% or greater
         (4) Random plasma glucose 200 mg/dL or greater with classic symptoms of hyperglycemia or hyperglycemic crisis
      b. Criteria for diagnosis of prediabetes
         (1) Impaired fasting glucose—fasting plasma glucose of 100–125 mg/dL
         (2) Impaired glucose tolerance—results of oral glucose tolerance test of 140–199 mg/dL in the 2-hour sample
      c. Criteria for diagnosis of GDM (ADA, 2011)—75-g OGTT at 24–28 weeks in women not previously diagnosed with overt diabetes with any of these values exceeded—fasting 92 mg/dL, 1 hour 180 mg/dL, 2 hour 153 mg/dL

2. Criteria for screening asymptomatic adults (fasting plasma glucose, 2-hour 75-g OGTT, or HgbA$_{1c}$) include (ADA, 2014):
   a. Anyone older than 45 years at 3-year intervals
   b. Consider testing younger than 45 years or more frequent screening in adults who are overweight or obese (BMI 25 or greater) with one or more additional risk factors:
      (1) Physical inactivity
      (2) First-degree relative with diabetes (parent, sibling)
      (3) Member of a high-risk race/ethnic population
      (4) Delivered infant of greater than 9 pounds or history of GDM
      (5) Hypertension
      (6) HDL cholesterol of 35 mg/dL or less and/or triglyceride level of 250 mg/dL or more
      (7) Cardiovascular disease
      (8) HbA$_{1c}$ 5.7%, IFG or IGT on previous testing
      (9) Polycystic ovarian syndrome
      (10) Other conditions associated with insulin resistance (e.g., severe obesity, acanthosis nigricans)
3. Criteria for screening pregnant and postpartum women (ADA, 2014)
   a. Screen for undiagnosed type 2 diabetes at initial prenatal visit in women with risk factors using standard diagnostic criteria
   b. Screen at 24–28 weeks with 75-g OGTT in women not previously diagnosed with overt diabetes
   c. Screen women with GDM for persistent diabetes at 6–12 weeks postpartum using OGTT and standard diagnostic criteria
   d. Screen women with GDM every 3 years for diabetes or prediabetes
4. Recommended glycemic goals for nonpregnant patients (ADA, 2014)
   a. Preprandial capillary plasma glucose 70 to 130 mg/dL
   b. Peak postprandial capillary glucose (1 to 2 hours after beginning meal) less than 180 mg/dL
   c. HgbA$_{1c}$—less than 7%
5. Tests helpful in identifying associated risk factors and complications include:
   a. Lipid profile, liver function tests, serum creatinine with calculated GFR
   b. Testing for urine albumin excretion with spot urine albumin to creatinine ratio
   c. TSH in type 1 diabetes, dyslipidemia, women age 50 years or older

- Management/treatment
1. Clinical trials have demonstrated that glycemic control is associated with decreased rates of microvascular complications; epidemiologic studies support reduction in cardiovascular disease (ADA, 2014)
2. Nonpharmacologic—types 1 and 2
   a. Home glucose determinations to monitor glycemic control daily
   b. Diet
      (1) Evidence inconclusive on percentage of calories to come from carbohydrates, protein, and fat
      (2) Individualized diabetes nutrition therapy is needed to achieve treatment goals with registered dietician
      (3) Reduced caloric intake while maintaining healthful eating for weight loss as needed
   c. Regular aerobic exercise
      (1) Improves blood glucose control
      (2) Reduces cardiovascular risk factors
      (3) Contributes to weight loss
   d. Aggressively manage additional cardiovascular risk factors
      (1) Blood pressure goal of less than 125/75 mm Hg
      (2) LDL cholesterol of less than 70 mg/dL
      (3) Smoking cessation
   e. Refer type 2 diabetics at time of diagnosis and type 1 diabetics within 3–5 years for eye examination; annually thereafter
   f. Perform comprehensive foot examination annually; examination should include use of a Semmes-Weinstein monofilament, tuning fork, and a visual examination
   g. Annual influenza vaccination; pneumococcal vaccination
   h. Diabetes self-management education (DSME) and diabetes self-management support (DSMS) according to national standards from American Diabetes Association (ADA)
3. Pharmacologic
   a. Insulin—type 1 diabetes, may be combined with oral medications for type 2 diabetes if needed
      (1) Insulin products
         (a) Rapid acting (lispro, aspart, glulisine)—onset less than 0.5 hour, peak 0.5–2.5 hours, duration 5 hours or less
         (b) Short acting (regular)—onset 0.5–1 hour, peak 2–5 hours, duration 4–8 hours
         (c) Intermediate acting (NPH or combination NPH and regular)—onset 0.5–1.5 hours, peak 4–12 hours, duration 14–24 hours
         (d) Long acting (glargine, detemir)—onset 1–2 hours, constant with no peak, duration 24 hours
      (2) Multiple dose insulin (MDI) 3–4 injections per day of both basal (long acting) and prandial (rapid acting) insulin or insulin pump therapy
      (3) Match prandial insulin to carbohydrate intake, premeal blood glucose, and anticipated activity
      (4) For most patients (especially with hypoglycemia) use insulin analogs; analogs are insulin types that have been chemically modified to act faster or slower than the human insulin (e.g., rapid or long acting)
      (5) For patients with frequent nocturnal hypoglycemia and/or hypoglycemia unawareness consider use of sensor-augmented low glucose suspend threshold pump
   b. Oral hypoglycemic agents—type 2 diabetes (see **Table 9-6**)
      (1) May consider management with diet and exercise first; if glucose intolerance persists, begin oral agent
      (2) Metformin is preferred initial oral agent unless contraindicated or not tolerated
      (3) If glycemic control not achieved within 3 months with metformin monotherapy, add second oral agent from different class; if still not controlled after 3 months, add third agent (oral or long-acting insulin)

▪ **Table 9-6 Oral Medications Used to Treat Type 2 Diabetes Mellitus (representative list)**

Drug	Action	Side-effects	Interactions	Contraindications/Precautions
Biguanides - metformin Preferred initial agent for Type 2 diabetes in non-pregnant individual if tolerated and not contraindicated	Decreases hepatic glucose production and intestinal absorption of glucose; increases peripheral glucose uptake and utilization May be used as monotherapy or as combination therapy	Anorexia, nausea, diarrhea, abdominal bloating; lactic acidosis—serious, rare	Effects potentiated by cimetidine, ranitidine, nifedipine, digoxin, trimethoprim, alcohol	Renal disease or dysfunction, metabolic acidosis, high risk for lactic acidosis No evidence of harm to fetus; low concentration levels in breast milk; compatible with breastfeeding (Briggs & Freeman, 2015)
Sulfonylureas 1st generation— chlorpropamide, tolbutamide 2nd generation— glipizide, glyburide, glimepiride	Stimulates insulin secretion from pancreatic beta cells May be used as monotherapy or as combination therapy	Hypoglycemia, weight gain, photosensitivity, GI upset, cholestatic jaundice	Several drugs may potentiate or reduce hypoglycemic effect	Ketoacidosis, impaired renal, hepatic function; 1st generation sulfonylureas associated with teratogenic risk in animal studies, no controlled human data in pregnancy, neonatal hypoglycemia has been reported; 2nd generation sulfonylureas lower maternal to fetal transfer; limited data indicate low concentration levels of sulfonylureas in breast milk, consider monitoring infant glucose levels
Dipeptidyl peptidase-4 inhibitors – sitagliptin, linagliptin	Inhibits degradation of incretin GLP-1 with subsequent increase of insulin release from pancreas; action in response to elevated glucose May be used as monotherapy or as combination therapy	Nasopharyngitis, headache, GI discomforts, arthralgia	Several drugs may reduce effects; beta blockers may prolong hypoglycemia	Contraindicated for type 1 diabetes; caution with renal function impairment No evidence of fetal harm in animal studies, no controlled human data in pregnancy; no data on excretion in breast milk; compatibility with breastfeeding is probable (Briggs & Freeman, 2015)

Drug	Mechanism/Use	Adverse effects	Interactions	Cautions/Pregnancy/Lactation
Glucagon like peptide 1 (GLP-1) receptor agonists/ Incretin mimetic – exenatide, liraglutide. Subcutaneous injection rather than oral medication	Binds to GLP-1 receptor, stimulates production and secretion of insulin. May be used as monotherapy or as combination therapy	GI upset, hypoglycemia, jittery feeling, dizziness, headache	Increased risk for hypoglycemia in combination with meglitinides or sulfonylurias	Contraindicated for type 1 diabetes; caution with renal function impairment, GI disorders. No evidence of fetal harm in animal studies, no controlled human data in pregnancy; no data on excretion in breast milk
Alpha-glucosidase inhibitors— Aacarbose, miglitol	Delays absorption of carbohydrates, inhibits metabolism of sucrose to glucose and fructose. Not used as monotherapy	Flatulence, diarrhea, abdominal discomfort (symptoms decrease over time); increases in AST, ALT	Digestive enzymes, intestinal absorbents decrease effect; may decrease effects of digoxin, propranolol	Inflammatory bowel disease, or any intestinal disease causing disordered digestion or absorption. No evidence of fetal harm in animal studies, no controlled human data in pregnancy; limited data indicate poorly excreted into breast milk
Meglitinides— repaglinide	Stimulates insulin release from pancreas. May be used as monotherapy or as combination therapy	Hypoglycemia, headache, dizziness	Several drugs may potentiate or reduce hypoglycemic effect	Caution in hepatic impairment. No evidence of fetal harm in animal studies, no controlled human data in pregnancy; no data on excretion in breast milk
Thiazolidinediones— rosiglitazone, pioglitazone	Improves insulin sensitivity, glucose uptake in muscle and adipose tissue; inhibits gluconeogenesis. May be used as monotherapy or as combination therapy	Edema, headache, myalgia, initial increase in LDL and HDL	Several drugs may potentiate or reduce hypoglycemic effect	Hepatotoxicity—monitor LFTs at start of therapy, q 2 mo, first year; congestive heart failure. No evidence of teratogenicity in animal studies, no controlled human data in pregnancy; no data on excretion in breast milk

(4) If still not controlled within 3–6 months, move to complex insulin strategy usually in combination with one or two oral medications

c. Use aspirin therapy in female diabetic patients who have a history of cardiovascular disease, are age 60 years or older with one or more additional cardiovascular risk factors; consider if younger than age 60 with multiple cardiovascular risk factors (ADA, 2014)

4. Patient education—diabetes self-management education (DSME) and support

a. Family involvement in care, medication instruction

b. Safety concerns, especially compensation for neuropathies

c. Ensure compliance with drug regimen

(1) Appropriate injection technique for insulin

(2) Importance of regular dosing, oral or parenteral

d. Blood glucose monitoring

(1) Routine schedule and glycemic target values

(2) Aseptic technique for blood sampling

(3) Medication dosage calculation based on blood glucose

e. Risk factor management and screening

(1) Smoking cessation if appropriate

(2) Annual comprehensive eye examination with ophthalmologist

(3) Foot care

(4) Dental hygiene and annual examination

(5) Nutritional counseling with registered dietitian

f. Preconception counseling emphasizing optimal glucose control, folic acid supplementation, early prenatal care, precautions in pregnancy concerning oral diabetes medication

g. Contraception counseling

(1) Most contraceptive methods can be used by women who have diabetes without complications

(2) Combination hormonal contraceptives contraindicated (Category 4) if diabetes with nephropathy, retinopathy, neuropathy, other vascular disease or longer than 20 years' duration

(3) DMPA not recommended unless other acceptable methods are not available or acceptable (Category 3) if diabetes with nephropathy, retinopathy, neuropathy, other vascular disease or longer than 20 years' duration

h. Hypoglycemia causes, symptoms, management

(1) Cause—side effect of insulin or oral medications for diabetes, skipped or delayed meals or snacks, increased physical activity, alcohol intake especially on empty stomach

(2) Symptoms

(a) Caused by alteration in brain and CNS function because of lowered glucose levels—mild, moderate, severe dependent on blood glucose level

(b) Mild—hunger, weakness, shakiness, sweating, difficulty concentrating, irritability, palpitations

(c) Moderate—increased irritability, inability to complete tasks, some changes in mental status

(d) Severe—confusion, drowsiness, progression to unconsciousness

(3) Management

(a) Take simple carbohydrates—4 ounces fruit juice or regular soft drink, 5–6 pieces hard candy, tablespoon honey, 3–4 glucose tablets; test blood glucose in 10–15 minutes; if less than 60 mg/dL, take more simple carbohydrates

(b) Administration of subcutaneous glucagon by caregiver or family member if not able to swallow/unconscious

(c) Wear medical identification bracelet or necklace

(d) Keep simple carbohydrates in car if driving

i. Hyperglycemia causes, symptoms, management

(1) Cause—insulin deficiency precipitated by acute illness, injury, infection, lack of adherence to or errors in treatment, other medications

(2) Symptoms

(a) Early symptoms may include increased thirst, frequent urination, headache, blurred vision, fatigue, difficulty concentrating

(b) Progressive symptoms with diabetic ketoacidosis may include fruity breath, abdominal pain, nausea and vomiting, dehydration, changes in consciousness

(3) Management—medical emergency—insulin, hydration, electrolyte repletion

• Referral

1. All newly diagnosed cases for complete medical evaluation

2. Evaluation of suspected or developing complications

Hyperthyroidism

• Definition—a hypermetabolic syndrome affecting all body systems characterized by excess circulating thyroid hormone

• Etiology/incidence

1. Etiology

a. Graves' disease

(1) Comprises 90% of cases

(2) Autoimmune condition; excess synthesis and secretion of thyroid hormone caused by antibodies that stimulate thyroid-stimulating hormone (TSH) receptors

b. Toxic multinodular goiter—accounts for most cases in middle-aged and elderly adults

c. Toxic adenoma/solitary autonomous nodule—single hyperfunctioning nodule surrounded by suppressed thyroid tissue

d. Thyroiditis—group of inflammatory diseases

(1) Inflammation causes disruption of the follicles resulting in release of preformed thyroid hormone

(2) Usually self-limited

(3) Phases—thyrotoxicosis, transient euthyroid, hypothyroid, recovery

(4) Classification of thyroiditis

(a) Subacute lymphocytic—autoimmune process

i. Postpartum thyroiditis

ii. Painless/sporadic thyroiditis

(b) Subacute granulomatous/de Quervain's thyroiditis—likely viral in origin and generally preceded by URI

2. Incidence
   a. Annual incidence 0.05–1% in general adult population
   b. Hyperthyroidism is 5–10 times more common in females than in males
   c. Postpartum thyroiditis occurs in 8–10% of women within 1 year of delivery; increased incidence with diabetes or high microsomal antibody titers before pregnancy
- Signs and symptoms—nonspecific, affecting all body systems; reflect increased stimulation from excess thyroid hormone
   1. Increased appetite, weight loss
   2. Irritability, nervousness, sleep disturbance
   3. Heat intolerance, sweating
   4. Fatigue, exertional shortness of breath
   5. Palpitations, chest pain
   6. Diarrhea
   7. Menstrual irregularities, amenorrhea, infertility
   8. Eye irritation, vision changes, double vision (Graves')
   9. Proximal muscle weakness, tremor
- Physical findings
   1. Thyroid gland—enlarged/diffuse or asymmetric nodularity
   2. Neuromuscular system—hyperreflexia, tremor, muscle wasting
   3. Dermatologic system—skin moist, smooth
   4. Cardiovascular system—tachycardia, systolic flow murmur, atrial fibrillation in elderly adults
   5. Eyes—lid retraction
   6. Gastrointestinal system—increased bowel sounds
   7. Graves' disease
      a. Symmetrical and moderate thyroid enlargement/bruit
      b. Exophthalmos/proptosis and pretibial myxedema (nonpitting thickening of skin)
   8. Toxic multinodular goiter—asymmetric nodularity
   9. Toxic adenoma—single nodule surrounded by suppressed thyroid tissue
   10. Thyroiditis—slight enlargement; tender with subacute granulomatous thyroiditis
- Differential diagnosis
   1. Neoplasm—because of associated weight loss and weakness
   2. Psychological disorders—panic disorder
- Diagnostic tests/findings
   1. Ultrasensitive serum thyroid-stimulating hormone (TSH)
      a. Most effective initial test for diagnosis
      b. Low or undetectable in response to excess circulation thyroid hormone
   2. Free T_4 usually elevated
   3. Serum T_3 elevated—useful when T_4 normal, TSH low, and patient is symptomatic
   4. Antithyroid peroxidase (anti-TPO) may be detected in Graves' disease
   5. Radioactive iodine (RAI) scan with uptake if clinical presentation is not diagnostic of Graves' disease or in the presence of thyroid nodularity, contraindicated during pregnancy
      a. Scan/anatomic definition
      b. RAI uptake/hyper- versus hypofunction
         (1) Uptake diffusely increased in Graves'
         (2) Uptake decreased in thyroiditis
         (3) Hot nodule with little uptake in rest of gland in toxic adenoma

- Management/treatment
   1. Treatment depends on cause, severity, patient's age, goiter size, comorbid conditions, and treatment desires
   2. Goal is to correct hypermetabolic state with fewest side effects and lowest incidence of hypothyroidism
   3. Antithyroid drugs—propylthiouracil (PTU), methimazole
      a. Drug action
         (1) Blocks multiple steps in the synthesis of thyroid hormone
         (2) Permanent remission in half of patients and one-fourth of these hypothyroid in 15–20 years
         (3) Clinically euthyroid in 4–8 weeks
      b. Side effects
         (1) Dermatitis, myalgias
         (2) Leukopenia—monitor CBC
         (3) Agranulocytosis—cannot be predicted; instructions to notify healthcare provider if fever or sore throat
         (4) Hepatocellular damage—monitor liver function tests (LFTs)
         (5) Drug interactions—potentiates oral anticoagulants
         (6) Contraindications/precautions—pregnancy Category D, PTU preferred over methimazole because PTU predominantly protein bound so less able to cross placenta in significant amounts, also lower breast milk concentration; monitor FT_4 every 2 to 4 weeks and use lowest doses to maintain euthyroid; methimazole contraindicated while nursing
      c. RAI therapy
         (1) Drug action
            (a) Damages functioning thyroid tissue
            (b) Reduces symptoms in 6–12 weeks
         (2) Side effects
            (a) Long-term hypothyroidism; 70% of patients at 10 years
            (b) May exacerbate ophthalmopathy in the short term
         (3) Contraindications—pregnancy or lactation; use contraception for 6–12 months following RAI administration
      d. Beta blockers—propranolol, atenolol (see Table 9-1)
         (1) Decrease signs and symptoms by blocking sympathetic nervous system
         (2) Indicated for symptomatic relief until more specific therapy initiated
      e. Management of thyroiditis—often no treatment required
         (1) Beta blockers for symptomatic treatment of thyrotoxicosis
         (2) Subacute granulomatous thyroiditis
            (a) NSAIDs for pain/inflammation
            (b) Prednisone for extreme cases (see Table 9-3)
   4. Patient education
      a. Medication regimens, side effects
      b. Signs/symptoms of thyroid storm—an exaggeration of signs and symptoms of hyperthyroidism; acute, life-threatening exacerbation of hyperthyroidism that is a medical emergency
      c. Avoid pregnancy for 6–12 months after RAI administration to avoid fetal thyroid ablation and possible gonadal chromosomal damage secondary to radiation effect on ovaries

- Referral
  1. Evaluation for treatment options
  2. Ophthalmologist referral for ophthalmopathy
  3. Surgical referral for patients with obstructive symptoms

Hypothyroidism

- Definition—a metabolic syndrome affecting all organ systems characterized by deficient levels of circulating thyroid hormone
- Etiology/incidence/risk factors
  1. Etiology
     a. Primary thyroid failure
        (1) Hashimoto's thyroiditis—chronic autoimmune thyroiditis
        (2) Previous radioactive iodine treatment, surgery
     b. Secondary—pituitary or hypothalamic disease
     c. Transient
        (1) Subacute granulomatous thyroiditis/de Quervain's
        (2) Subacute lymphocytic thyroiditis/postpartum and sporadic painless
  2. Prevalence estimated 1–3% of general population
     a. Increasing prevalence with age and in women
     b. Women older than 50 years have estimated 5% prevalence
  3. Risk factors
     a. Age older than 50 years
     b. Female-to-male ratio is 8–10:1
     c. History of autoimmune disease
     d. Family or personal history of thyroid disease
- Signs and symptoms—often subclinical; reflect slowed physiologic functioning of all organ systems
  1. Weakness, lethargy
  2. Skin changes—dry or coarse skin, skin pallor; coarse hair
  3. Slow speech, forgetfulness, depression
  4. Cold sensation, decreased sweating
  5. Eyelid, facial edema
  6. Constipation
  7. Irregular menses—menorrhagia, amenorrhea; infertility
- Physical findings—depend on severity, duration of deficiency, and rapidity of development
  1. Thyroid gland may be atrophic, normal, or goitrous
  2. Neuromuscular system—diminished relaxation phase of reflexes, carpal tunnel syndrome, hearing loss
  3. Dermatologic system—skin cool, dry; hair dry, brittle; generalized hair loss, especially outer third of eyebrows
  4. Cardiovascular system—bradycardia; edema, especially periorbital, anemia
  5. Gastrointestinal system—mild weight gain, diminished bowel sounds
  6. Endocrine system—galactorrhea
  7. Mentation may be slowed and may appear lethargic and expressionless
- Differential diagnosis
  1. Primary versus secondary
  2. Clinical depression
  3. Antithyroid drugs—lithium
- Diagnostic tests/findings
  1. TSH—elevated in primary hypothyroidism
  2. Free T_4—decreased

3. Decreased TSH and FT_4 in secondary hypothyroidism
4. Antithyroid peroxidase (anti-TPO), Hashimoto's thyroiditis
5. Women with positive TPO antibodies (even when euthyroid) have increased risk for recurrent miscarriage with or without infertility
6. Other lab findings may include an elevated cholesterol level and mild normocytic, normochromic anemia
- Management/treatment
  1. Most patients with primary hypothyroidism will need lifelong thyroid hormone therapy
  2. Levothyroxine
     a. Drug action—synthetic T_4
        (1) T_4 converted to T_3; administration of T_4 produces both hormones
        (2) Half-life 6 days; slow rate of achieving steady state
        (3) Adjust dose every 6 weeks until TSH normalizes
        (4) Considered safe in pregnancy and lactation—increase number of doses from 7 to 9 each week during pregnancy and monitor TSH levels
     b. Side effects—symptoms of hyperthyroidism/excess replacement
     c. Drug interactions
        (1) Potentiates sympathomimetics
        (2) Monitor antihyperglycemics, oral anticoagulants
     d. Contraindications
        (1) Thyrotoxicosis
        (2) Acute MI
        (3) Uncorrected adrenal insufficiency
  3. Treatment of subclinical hypothyroidism elevated TSH in presence of normal thyroid hormone levels (American Association of Clinical Endocrinologists and American Thyroid Association, 2012)
     a. Majority will progress to clinical hypothyroidism
     b. Treat if TSH greater than 10 μIU/mL
     c. Treat if TSH between 5 and 10 μIU/mL and elevated anti-TPO titers, symptoms of hypothyroidism, goiter, or depression
     d. Treat if TSH between 5 and 10 μIU/mL and pregnant, attempting to conceive, or if experiencing infertility
  4. Patient education
     a. Medication use and doses; need for long-term therapy
     b. Danger of increasing medication too rapidly or taking more than prescribed
     c. Preconception counseling—untreated hypothyroidism during pregnancy may adversely affect maternal and fetal outcomes; early prenatal care and close monitoring of TSH and T_4 levels for adjustments in medication are important
- Referral—all secondary cases for evaluation

Musculoskeletal Disorders

Low Back Pain (LBP)

- Definition—acute (< than 3 months), chronic, or recurrent pain occurring in the lumbosacral spine region; pain may be localized or radiate to the extremities

- Etiology/incidence/risk factors
  1. Etiology
     a. No specific identifiable cause in up to 85% of cases; lumbosacral strain results from stretching, tearing of muscles, tendons, ligaments, and fascia due to trauma or repetitive mechanical stress
     b. Herniated intervertebral disc causing nerve root compression resulting in pain below the knee and other neurologic signs and symptoms
     c. Spinal stenosis—soft tissue or bony encroachment of the spinal canal and nerve roots
  2. Incidence
     a. One of the top 10 reasons for visit to primary care provider
     b. Estimated 60–85% of individuals experience at least one episode
     c. Women and men equally affected
     d. Chronic LBP comprises about 2% of all cases
  3. Risk factors—acute LBP
     a. Repetitive motion
     b. Poor body mechanics
     c. Sedentary lifestyle; poor strength of abdominal and back muscles
- Signs and symptoms
  1. Lumbosacral strain
     a. Pain located in the back, buttocks, or one or both thighs
     b. Pain aggravated by standing/flexion; relieved with rest/reclining
  2. Herniated intervertebral disc
     a. Characterized by radicular pain; paresthesias may occur in distribution of involved nerve root
     b. Most common disc ruptures involve the L5 or S1 nerve roots
        (1) L5 root/L4–5 disc—pain/numbness lateral calf
        (2) S1 root/L5–S1 disc—pain buttocks, lateral leg, and malleolus; numbness lateral foot and posterior calf
  3. Spinal stenosis—pain precipitated by walking or standing upright; relieved by sitting or leaning forward
- Physical findings
  1. Lumbosacral strain
     a. Increased pain with flexion
     b. Negative straight leg raise (SLR); normal neurologic exam
  2. Herniated intervertebral disc
     a. Increased pain with flexion
     b. Positive SLR—radicular pain when leg is passively raised 30–60°
     c. L5 root—weakness of dorsiflexion of great toe; decreased sensation anterior/medial dorsal foot
     d. S1 root—weakness of plantar flexion/tip-toe walking; diminished/absent Achilles reflex; decreased sensation lateral foot
  3. Spinal stenosis—assessment of lower extremities for loss of hair, color, and pulses to differentiate spinal stenosis from vascular insufficiency
- Differential diagnosis
  1. Cauda equina syndrome
     a. Surgical emergency because of impingement on the cauda equina

b. Characterized by saddle anesthesia, bladder or bowel incontinence, muscle weakness
     c. Immediate magnetic resonance imaging and referral to neurosurgery
  2. Fracture
     a. Major trauma such as motor vehicle accident or fall from high place
     b. Risks: ≥ 50 years of age, osteoporosis
  3. Osteoporosis/compression fracture—may be precipitated by minor trauma or lifting
  4. Neoplasm
     a. Constitutional symptoms, no relief with bed rest, chronic pain, urinary retention
     b. Risks: ≥ 50 years of age, history of cancer
  5. Infection—chills, fever, IV drug user, recent bacterial infection, immunosuppression, comorbidities
- Diagnostic tests/findings
  1. Indicated in the presence of "red flags"—fever, chills, weight loss, recent onset bladder/bowel dysfunction, lower extremity sensory or neurologic deficit
  2. Radiograph of lumbosacral spine
     a. Generally not necessary in acute phase—3–6 weeks duration
     b. Suspicion of fracture
     c. Suspicion of malignancy—patient older than 50 years; persistent bone pain unrelieved by bed rest; history of malignancy
  3. MRI or CT
     a. Severe persistent symptoms despite conservative treatment
     b. Suspected disc herniation
- Management/treatment
  1. Nonpharmacologic
     a. Encourage continuation of daily activities rather than bed rest
     b. Local application of heat, warm baths
     c. Prescribe physical therapy program to improve strength and conditioning
     d. Low-stress aerobic exercise—walking, biking, swimming
  2. Pharmacologic
     a. Nonsteroidal anti-inflammatory drugs (NSAIDs) (see "Acute Otitis Media" section earlier in this chapter)—ibuprofen, naproxen, etodolac
     b. Muscle relaxant—cyclobenzaprine
        (1) Drug action—reduces tonic somatic motor activity in the brain stem
        (2) Side effects—somnolence, dry mouth
        (3) Drug interactions—hypertensive crisis with MAOIs; potentiates alcohol and other CNS depressants
        (4) Contraindications/precautions—acute post-MI, arrhythmias; pregnancy Category B; precaution in nursing mothers
  3. Patient education
     a. Avoid bed rest
     b. Weight loss if indicated to reduce lordosis
     c. Good body mechanics; proper lifting
     d. Appropriate exercises

e. Signs of deterioration
   (1) Loss of bladder control
   (2) Numbness or weakness in groin or rectal area
   (3) Pain extending down leg past knee
f. Reassurance
   (1) Excellent prognosis for complete resolution of acute LBP episodes
   (2) Recurrence likely at variable intervals
- Referral
  1. Urgently refer patients to neurosurgery with symptoms suggestive of cauda equina or cord compression
  2. Symptoms suggestive of spinal infection or malignancy
  3. Neurologic consultation if back pain remains severe after 4–6 weeks of conservative treatment or findings of neurologic deficits

Osteoarthritis

- Definition
  1. Noninflammatory joint disease characterized by degeneration of articular cartilage with new bone formation at articular surface
  2. Most commonly involved joints are distal and proximal interphalangeals of hands, hips, knees, and cervical and lumbar spine
  3. Primary—no obvious cause
  4. Secondary—occurring in damaged or abnormal joints
- Etiology/incidence/risk factors
  1. Etiology
     a. Progressive degeneration and loss of articular cartilage and subchondral bone
     b. Bone ends thicken and osteophytes or spurs form where the ligaments and capsule attach to the bone
     c. Variable synovial inflammation results
  2. Incidence
     a. Radiographic evidence in 80% of adults by age 60
     b. Clinical osteoarthritis affects approximately 25% of adults
  3. Risk factors
     a. Increasing age
     b. Female gender
     c. Obesity
     d. Major joint trauma
     e. Repetitive joint stress
     f. Congenital and developmental joint defects
     g. Metabolic and endocrine disorders
- Signs and symptoms
  1. Gradual onset of joint pain, tenderness, and limited movement
  2. Pain aggravated by joint use and subsides with rest
  3. Morning joint stiffness or stiffness following a period of inactivity, lasting generally less than 30 minutes
  4. Symptoms often asymmetrical
- Physical findings
  1. Decreased range of motion
  2. Effusions of involved joint(s) with minimal local warmth and no erythema
  3. Enlargement of distal interphalangeal (DIP) joints—Heberden's nodes; enlargement of proximal interphalangeal (PIP) joints—Bouchard's nodes
  4. Crepitus with joint motion

- Differential diagnosis
  1. Rheumatoid arthritis
  2. Infectious arthritis
  3. Tendonitis/bursitis syndromes
  4. Crystal-induced arthritis—gout, pseudogout
  5. Fracture
- Diagnostic tests/findings
  1. Radiography
     a. Will not demonstrate deterioration of cartilage
     b. Four cardinal radiologic features
        (1) Narrowed joint space
        (2) Sclerosis of subchondral bone
        (3) Bony cysts
        (4) Osteophytes
  2. Diagnostic joint fluid aspiration
     a. Indicated if joint effusion
     b. Synovial fluid analysis—white blood cell (WBC) count with differential; culture; evaluation for crystals
     c. Findings in osteoarthritis—WBC count less than 2000 cells/mL; negative culture; negative for crystals
  3. Laboratory—normal in primary osteoarthritis
     a. Rheumatoid factor (RF)/antinuclear antibodies (ANA)—if arthritis is inflammatory and symmetrical in distribution to exclude rheumatoid arthritis or systemic lupus erythematosus (SLE)
     b. Erythrocyte sedimentation rate—elevated in many autoimmune, inflammatory, infectious diseases
     c. CBC—if an inflammatory or infectious arthritis suspected
- Management/treatment
  1. Nonpharmacologic
     a. Appliances (e.g., canes, crutches, orthotics)
     b. Exercise
        (1) Aerobic
        (2) Resistance training
        (3) Muscle strengthening
     c. Yoga
     d. Supervised heat and cold therapy
     e. Weight loss if indicated
     f. Transcutaneous electrical nerve stimulation (TENS)
     g. Massage
     h. Acupuncture
     i. Rest during exacerbations
  2. Pharmacologic
     a. Supplements
        (1) Glucosamine sulfate
        (2) Chondroitin sulfate
     b. Nonopioid analgesics
        (1) Acetaminophen
        (2) Tramadol
     c. Nonsteroidal anti-inflammatory drugs (NSAIDs) as described for LBP
        (1) Nonselective cyclooxygenase inhibitors:
           ○ Ibuprofen
           ○ Naproxen
           ○ Aspirin
           ○ Indomethacin
        (2) Cyclooxygenase-2 inhibitor

d. Opioid analgesics
e. Topical analgesics
   (1) Capsaicin cream
   (2) Diclofenac
f. Intra-articular injection
   (1) Glucocorticoids—beneficial in patients with inflammation, effusion, or substantial pain
   (2) Synovial fluid analog—sodium hyaluronate/hylan G-F20; usefulness documented in knee joints; safety in other joints not documented
3. Patient education
   a. Symptomatic relief techniques (e.g., cold, heat, immobilization, rest)
   b. Medication regimens and precautions
- Referral
   a. Physical therapy, exercise
   b. Need for joint injection
   c. Surgery consultation—joint replacement

Osteoporosis

- Definition—disease characterized by low bone mass and structural deterioration of bone tissue, leading to bone fragility and an increased susceptibility to fractures of the hip, spine, and wrist (National Institute of Health, 2012)
- Etiology/incidence
1. Combination of factors including nutrition, genetics, level of physical activity, age of menopause, and estrogen status
2. According to the National Health and Nutrition Examination Survey III (NHANES III), 10 million Americans have osteoporosis
3. Approximately one out of every two Caucasian women and one in five men will experience a fracture related to osteoporosis (U.S. DHHS, 2004)
4. Most common fracture sites are vertebrae, femur, and dorsal forearm. In older population, these fractures may lead to chronic pain, disability, and even death (National Osteoporosis Foundation, 2014)
5. Conditions, diseases, and medications that cause or contribute to osteoporosis and fractures include but are not limited to (National Osteoporosis Foundation, 2014)
   a. Advanced age
   b. Female gender
   c. Lifestyle
      (1) Low calcium intake
      (2) Alcohol (intake of 3 or more drinks/day)
      (3) Current cigarette smoking (active or passive)
      (4) Vitamin D insufficiency
      (5) High salt intake
      (6) Inadequate physical activity, immobilization
      (7) Falling, prior history of osteoporotic fracture
      (8) Thinness, low BMI
   d. Genetic disorders
      (1) Cystic fibrosis
      (2) Ehlers–Danlos
      (3) Gaucher's disease
      (4) Hemochromatosis
      (5) Marfan syndrome
      (6) Osteogenesis imperfecta
      (7) Parental history of hip fracture
   e. Hypogonadal states
      (1) Androgen insensitivity
      (2) Anorexia nervosa and bulimia
      (3) Athletic amenorrhea
      (4) Hyperprolactenemia
      (5) Panhypopituitarism
      (6) Premature ovarian failure
      (7) Turner's and Klinefelter's syndromes
   f. Endocrine disorders
      (1) Adrenal insufficiency
      (2) Cushing's syndrome
      (3) Diabetes mellitus
   g. Medications
      (1) Glucosteroids—long term use
      (2) Aromatase inhibitors
      (3) Certain anticonvulsants
      (4) Excessive thyroxine doses
      (5) Cytotoxic agents
      (6) Gonadotropin-releasing agonists or analogues
- Signs and symptoms
1. Often a silent disease
2. Backache
3. Spontaneous fracture or collapse of vertebrae
- Physical findings
1. Loss of height
2. Kyphosis
3. Fractures—spine, hip, wrist
- Differential diagnosis
1. Malignancy—bone neoplasms, metastatic carcinoma, multiple myeloma
2. Osteomalacia
3. Paget's disease
4. Secondary causes of osteoporosis include:
   a. Hyperparathyroidism
   b. Hyperthyroidism
   c. Cushing's syndrome
- Diagnostic tests/findings
1. Bone mineral density (BMD) tests
   a. World Health Organization definitions based on bone mass measurement in women include:
      (1) Normal—BMD within 1 standard deviation (SD) of a young normal adult; T-score above –1
      (2) Osteopenia (low bone mass)—BMD between 1 and 2.5 SD below that of a young normal adult; T-score between –1 and –2.5
      (3) Osteoporosis—BMD 2.5 SD or more or below that of a young normal adult; T-score at or below –2.5
   b. Dual-energy X-ray absorptiometry (DXA)—most widely used; quick; radiation exposure one-tenth of standard chest radiograph; body sites measured—hip, spine, wrist; BMD testing at one or more of these body sites with DXA required for densitometric diagnosis of osteoporosis
   c. Other bone densitometry technologies and measurement at peripheral body sites (e.g., finger, heel) may be used to predict fracture risk but are not diagnostic

2. Standard radiography—20–30% bone loss must occur for osteoporosis detection; used to detect osteoporotic fractures
3. Laboratory tests if indicated to rule out secondary causes of osteoporosis—parathyroid hormone (PTH) level, TSH, dexamethasone suppression test, and urine cortisol level for Cushing's syndrome
4. Biochemical markers for bone turnover (urine and serum) can aid in risk assessment and as an additional monitoring tool during treatment
5. Vertebral fracture assessment (VFA)—vertebral imaging available on most modern DXA machines, can perform VFA at time of BMD assessment; vertebral fracture is consistent with diagnosis of osteoporosis independent of BMD results; consider VFA for women who are:
   a. Age 70 or older if BMD T-score is at or below - 1.0
   b. Age 65 to 69 if BMD T-score is at or below – 1.5
   c. Postmenopause with low trauma fracture during adulthood, historical height loss of 4 cm or more, prospective height loss of 2 cm or more, recent or ongoing long term glucocorticoid treatment
6. Fracture risk algorithm (FRAX)—developed to calculate 10-year probability of hip fracture and 10-year probability of a major osteoporotic fracture taking into account femoral neck BMD and clinical risk factors; used to make decisions concerning preventive medications for postmenopausal women with osteopenia

- Management/treatment
  1. Nonpharmacologic—prevention and treatment
     a. Adequate intake of calcium and vitamin D
     b. Regular weight-bearing exercise
        (1) 30 minutes 3 to 4 times each week
        (2) Walking, stair climbing, dancing, tai-chi, jogging
     c. Regular muscle-strengthening exercise—lifting weights, swimming
     d. Avoidance of tobacco use and alcohol abuse
     e. Fall prevention strategies—correct impaired vision, assess medications for potential to cause orthostatic hypotension, supportive low-heeled shoes, assistive devices if needed (cane, walker), home safety measures
  2. Pharmacologic
     a. Consider pharmacologic treatment for postmenopausal women presenting with any of the following (National Osteoporosis Foundation, 2014):
        (1) Hip or vertebral fracture
        (2) T-score of –2.5 or less at the femoral neck or spine after appropriate evaluation to exclude secondary causes
        (3) T-score between –1.0 and –2.5 at femoral neck or spine and 10-year probability of hip fracture of 3% or greater; or a 10-year probability of major osteoporotic-related fracture of 20% or greater based on U.S.-adapted WHO algorithm
     b. Estrogen/hormone therapy (HT)—may be considered short term (5 years) for prevention if needs treatment for vasomotor symptoms and/or vulvovaginal atrophy; not approved for treatment of existing osteoporosis
     c. Bisphosphonates—alendronate/risedronate—indicated for prevention and treatment; ibandronate—oral form approved for prevention and treatment, intravenous form approved for treatment; zoledronic acid—intravenous form approved for treatment
        (1) Drug action—osteoclast-mediated bone resorption inhibitor—bone formation exceeds bone resorption, leading to progressive gains in bone mass
        (2) Side effects—GI upset, abdominal pain, esophagitis, musculoskeletal pain, headache, osteonecrosis of jaw (rare), atypical femoral fracture (rare)
        (3) Drug interactions—antacids and calcium interfere with absorption
        (4) Contraindications/precautions—esophageal stricture, inability to stand/sit upright for at least 30 minutes, hypocalcemia, renal disease, measure serum calcium and creatinine prior to starting medication, check serum creatinine before each ibandronate injection; pregnancy risk Category C
        (5) Client instructions
           (a) Take with 8 oz of water in the morning at least 30 minutes before any beverage, food, or medication
           (b) Do not lie down for at least 30 minutes and until the first food of the day
           (c) May take acetaminophen prior to zoledronic acid injection to reduce risk of postinjection arthralgia, headache, myalgia, fever
     d. Estrogen agonist/antagonist (formerly known as selective estrogen receptor modulators [SERM])—raloxifene—indicated for prevention and treatment
        (1) Drug action—estrogen-like effects on bones and lipid metabolism; lacks estrogen-like effect on uterus and breasts
        (2) Side effects—hot flashes, leg cramps, venous thromboembolic events (rare)
        (3) Drug interactions—may antagonize warfarin
        (4) Contraindications—women who are pregnant or may become pregnant; active or history of venous thromboembolic events; do not give with estrogen- or cholesterol-lowering medication
     e. Denosumab—indicated for treatment of postmenopausal women with osteoporosis at high risk for fracture, if have failed or are intolerant to other therapy, if receiving adjuvant aromatase inhibitor therapy for breast cancer; subcutaneous administration by healthcare professional every 6 months
        (1) Drug action—receptor activator of nuclear factor-B ligand (RANKL) inhibitor, inhibits osteoclasts
        (2) Side-effects—back, arm, leg, and muscle pain; high cholesterol; cystitis; hypocalcemia; skin infections; rash; osteonecrosis of jaw (rare); atypical femoral fracture (rare)
        (3) Drug interactions—increased risk of osteonecrosis of jaw with concomitant use of corticosteroids or chemotherapy; increased infection risk with concomitant use of immunosuppressants
        (4) Contraindications—hypocalcemia, pregnancy Category X

f. Calcitonin—indicated for treatment only
   (1) Drug action—directly inhibits bone resorption of calcium; administered as a nasal spray or injection
   (2) Side effects—nasal spray—rhinitis, GI upset; injection—GI upset, local inflammation, rash, flushing
   (3) Drug interactions—none reported
   (4) Contraindications—hypersensitivity to salmon calcitonin, pregnancy risk Category C
g. Parathyroid hormone—PTH (1–34), teriparatide—approved for treatment if high risk for fracture
   (1) Drug action—anabolic bone-building agent, parathyroid hormone; administered as subcutaneous injection
   (2) Side effects—leg cramps, dizziness
   (3) Drug interactions—none reported
   (4) Contraindications/precautions—avoid if increased risk of osteosarcoma, prior radiation of skeleton, bone metastases, hypercalcemia
h. Monitoring pharmacologic therapy effectiveness
   (1) Baseline BMD before onset of therapy
   (2) Repeat test every 2 years; more frequently if warranted by certain clinical situations
   (3) Urine/serum biochemical markers of bone formation or resorption may be used as adjunct to monitor response to therapy—variable results and precision error limit usefulness; changes must be large to be clinically meaningful
3. Patient education
   a. Adequate calcium and vitamin D intake
   b. Weight-bearing and muscle-strengthening exercises
   c. Avoidance of tobacco and excessive alcohol
   d. Fall prevention strategies
   e. Medication use

Fibromyalgia

- Definition
  1. A syndrome characterized by chronic fatigue, generalized, widespread musculoskeletal pain and stiffness associated with the finding of characteristic tender points of pain on physical examination
  2. Criteria for the classification of fibromyalgia—American College of Rheumatology (Wolfe, et al., 2010)
     a. Widespread pain index (WPI) 7 or greater and symptom severity (SS) scale score of 5 or greater or WPI 3-6 and SS scale score 9 or greater
     b. Symptoms present at similar level for at least 3 months
     c. Exclusion of other disorder that would otherwise explain pain
     d. WPI—note the number of areas in which patient has pain over the last week (0-19)
     e. SS scale score—presence and severity of fatigue, waking unrefreshed, cognitive symptoms over the past week (0-12)
- Etiology/incidence
  1. Etiology—unknown, but classified as a rheumatic disease; several causal mechanisms postulated
     a. Physical or mental stress
     b. Sleep disturbances
     c. Decreased serotonin levels
     d. Metabolic factors
     e. Viral infection—Epstein-Barr virus, cytomegalovirus, herpes virus, enteroviruses
  2. Incidence—unknown in general population because of misdiagnosis, self-treatment
     a. More common in women, with a 9:1 female:male ratio
     b. Most common in 30- to 50-year-olds
- Signs and symptoms
  1. Multiple, specific areas of muscle tenderness ("trigger points")
  2. Fatigue, sleep disturbances
  3. Muscle weakness and generalized aching
  4. Pain typically worsens with cold
  5. Paresthesias
  6. Headaches
  7. Anxiety, stress
  8. Depression
- Physical findings
  1. Pain on digital palpation of characteristic tender points
  2. Normal muscle strength, range of motion
- Differential diagnosis
  1. Chronic fatigue syndrome
  2. Rheumatoid arthritis
  3. SLE
  4. Somatization and depression
- Diagnostic tests/findings
  1. Unnecessary unless a coexisting condition is suspected
  2. Erythrocyte sedimentation rate normal; excludes inflammatory conditions
- Management/treatment
  1. Nonpharmacologic
     a. Low-impact exercise (e.g., walking, swimming, tai-chi, yoga)
     b. Supervised heat and cold therapy
     c. Massage, relaxation therapy
     d. Biofeedback
     e. Hypnotherapy
     f. Strength training
     g. Acupuncture
  2. Pharmacologic
     a. FDA-approved drugs to treat fibromyalgia (Food and Drug Administration, 2014):
        (1) Pregabalin
        (2) Selective serotonin-norepinephrine reuptake inhibitors (SNRI)- duloxetine hydrochloride, milnacipran HCL
           (a) Drug action—mechanism by which these drugs reduce pain for people with fibromyalgia is unknown; data suggest that these drugs possibly affect the release of neurotransmitters
           (b) Side effects—nausea, dry mouth, dizziness, somnolence, other central nervous system effects
           (c) Contraindications/precautions—avoid abrupt cessation; pregnancy Category C; not recommended in nursing mothers
     b. Tramadol—not recommended as first treatment
        (1) Drug action—centrally acting analgesic; creates a weak bond to opioid receptors and inhibits reuptake of both norepinephrine and serotonin

(2) Side effects—drowsiness, dizziness, headache, nausea, and constipation

(3) Drug interactions—seizure risk with other agents that lower threshold/MAOIs, SSRIs; potentiated with alcohol and other CNS depressants

(4) Contraindications/precautions—abuse potential; pregnancy Category C; not recommended in nursing mothers

c. Over-the counter analgesics

(1) Acetaminophen

(2) Nonsteroidal anti-inflammatory drugs (NSAIDs)

i. Naproxen

ii. Ibuprofen

3. Patient education

a. Reassurance regarding benign course of condition

b. Supportive care for chronic pain

- Referral—physical therapy, rheumatologist

Strains/Sprains

- Definition—musculoskeletal injury of varying degrees
1. *Strain* refers to injury to muscle or tendon
2. *Sprain* refers to stretching or tearing of ligaments
- Etiology/incidence/risk factors
1. Etiology
    a. Overuse of the muscle–tendon unit by stretching, tearing, hyperextension, forceful contraction
    b. Acute injury
    c. Chronic overuse as seen in sports injury, repetitive motion
2. Incidence—unknown because of frequent self-treatment, but common presenting complaint in primary care practice
3. Risk factors
    a. Increased physical activity
    b. New physical exercise program
    c. Overweight
- Signs and symptoms
1. Pain at site of injury
2. Strain
    a. Temporary weakness
    b. Pain with stretch of muscle
    c. Pain and spasm with more severe strains
3. Sprain
    a. Marked swelling
    b. Loss of function
- Physical findings
1. Strain—temporarily reduced range of motion, muscle strength
2. Sprain
    a. Contusion, hemorrhage
    b. Reduced range of motion, muscle strength
    c. Joint instability in severe sprain or ruptured ligament
- Differential diagnosis
1. Other overuse syndromes—tendonitis, shin splints
2. Fracture
- Diagnostic tests/findings
1. Radiograph to rule out fractures—negative for bony abnormality in strains/sprains
2. MRI

- Management/treatment
1. Nonpharmacologic
    a. "RICE"—initial therapeutic strategy
       (1) *R*est or immobilization of injured part
       (2) *I*ce or application of cold
       (3) *C*ompression, elastic wrap
       (4) *E*levation of affected area
    b. Application of heat 24 to 36 hours after injury
    c. Topical heat-generating liniments for symptomatic relief
2. Pharmacologic
    a. Usually none indicated, not curative
    b. NSAIDs as for acute LBP
3. Patient education
    a. Physical training progression to avoid repeat injury
    b. Stretching and warm-up exercises
    c. Appropriate footwear, protective gear for exercise
- Referral
1. Physical therapy for stretching and strengthening program
2. Consult orthopaedic surgeon if no response to conservative management

---

Neurologic Disorders

Headaches

- Definition
1. Headache/cephalgia is defined as diffuse pain in various parts of the head
2. Primary headaches—migraine, tension, cluster headaches are not directly related to a specific underlying cause or secondary to another problem, and not showing any red flag signs and symptoms
3. Secondary headaches are the result of identifiable structural or physiologic pathology
- Etiology/incidence/risk factors
1. Etiology
    a. Primary headaches—90–98% of headaches presenting in primary care
       (1) Migraine headache
          (a) Current understanding suggests genetic basis
          (b) Those genetically predisposed inherit a nervous system that is more sensitive/easily aroused to a variety of internal/external factors—hormonal fluctuations, weather changes, diet, psychosocial disruptions
          (c) Changes in serotonin activity result in release of vasoactive mediators; mediators produce an inflammatory response adjacent to cerebral blood vessels accompanied by vasodilation
          (d) The dilated vessels and inflammatory response stimulate the trigeminal nerve to transmit impulses to the brain resulting in migraine headache
       (2) Tension headache
          (a) Pathophysiology poorly understood; formerly attributed to contraction of the muscles of the scalp and neck

(b) Recent theories suggest tension headaches may involve changes in the intracranial neurotransmitter and vascular systems similar to migraine

(c) Symptom complex resulting from several simultaneous processes—muscle tension, psychological stress, neurovascular changes

(3) Cluster headache

  (a) Secondary to serotonergic neurologic dysfunction

  (b) Clustering of attacks suggests involvement of circadian pacemakers of the anterior hypothalamus

  (c) Tearing and nasal stuffiness suggests abnormality in autonomic nervous system

b. Secondary headaches

(1) Vascular disorders—subarachnoid, cerebral, cerebellar hemorrhage; acute ischemic cerebrovascular disorder; AV malformation; temporal arteritis; arterial hypertension (HTN)

(2) Nonvascular intracranial disorders—neoplasm; infection; low cerebrospinal fluid pressure/post lumbar puncture; benign intracranial HTN/pseudotumor cerebri

(3) Traumatic—concussion and postconcussion; hematoma/subdural and epidural

(4) Metabolic disorders—hypoxia, hypercapnia, hypoglycemia

(5) Substances that act as triggers—medications; foods/monosodium glutamate (MSG), alcohol; exposures/carbon monoxide; rebound/caffeine, analgesics

(6) Extracranial structures—eyes/glaucoma, refractive errors; sinusitis; temporomandibular joint dysfunction; neck/cervical disk disease; trigeminal neuralgia

(7) Systemic—infection; allergies/pollen; hormonal

2. Incidence

a. Migraine

(1) Reported in up to 15–17% of women; 5% of men

(2) Estimated 10% of adults affected

b. Tension—most common form of headache

c. Cluster—relatively rare incidence compared to other types; six times more common in males

3. Risk factors—primary headache syndromes

a. Migraine headaches—female gender, family history

b. Tension headaches—overuse of headache medications

c. Cluster headaches—male, middle-aged or older

- Signs and symptoms

1. Migraine

a. Types

(1) Migraine with aura/classic migraine

  (a) Aura consists of focal neurologic symptoms that may precede or accompany headache

  (b) Usually visual phenomenon; flashing lights, zigzag/jagged lines, difficulty focusing

  (c) May have a premonitory phase, occurring hours or days before the headache

(2) Migraine without aura/common migraine—accounts for 75% of migraines

(3) Complicated migraine—basilar/hemiplegic migraine

b. Phases

(1) Prodrome—occurs 24 hours prior to onset of headache: fatigue, euphoria, difficulty concentrating, irritability

(2) Aura

(3) Early and late stages of migraine

(4) Postdrome—individual feels "wiped out," fatigued, "hung over"

c. Triggers

(1) Stress

(2) Hormonal changes

(3) Certain foods, caffeine, alcohol, skipping meals

(4) Fatigue, oversleeping

(5) Medications

(6) Changes in weather or barometric pressure

d. Location—unilateral tendency

e. Duration—4–72 hours

f. Character

(1) Moderate to severe intensity; inhibits daily activities

(2) Characterized as throbbing, pounding

g. Associated symptoms—nausea, vomiting, photophobia, phonophobia, fatigue

h. Frequency—recurrent, variable from two to three per year to two to three per week

2. Tension headache

a. Onset—gradual

b. Location—diffuse, bilateral, generalized

c. Duration—variable, hours to days

d. Character

(1) Mild to moderate severity; generally able to continue with daily activities

(2) Dull, pressure, constant, vise-like

e. Associated symptoms—fatigue, irritability, difficulty concentrating, neck and shoulder spasm

f. Frequency

(1) Episodic—less than 15 days per month

(2) Chronic—must be present 15 days or more a month for at least 6 months

3. Cluster headaches

a. Onset

(1) Abrupt

(2) Often nocturnal, awakens patient; often recurs at same time of day

b. Location

(1) Unilateral

(2) During a series, pain remains on same side

(3) Retro-orbital, sometimes radiating

c. Duration—usually 30 to 45 minutes

d. Character—intense, severe

e. Associated symptoms—facial pain, ptosis of the affected side, lacrimation, nasal congestion

f. Frequency—occurs in clusters lasting a few weeks with remission lasting weeks to months

- Physical findings

1. General appearance indicates discomfort

2. Neurologic assessment normal in primary headaches—occasional temporary focal neurologic findings with migraine

3. Blood pressure, vital signs normal
4. Cluster headache—unilaterally constricted pupil, nasal discharge

- Differential diagnosis—"red flags" suggesting secondary causes
1. Headache beginning after 50 years of age—temporal arteritis, mass lesion
2. Sudden onset, worst headache—subarachnoid hemorrhage
3. Headaches increasing in severity/frequency—mass lesion, subdural hematoma, medication overuse
4. Focal neurologic signs/papilledema
5. Headache subsequent to head trauma—intracranial hemorrhage, subdural/epidural hematoma, posttraumatic headache
6. Systemic illness/fever—meningitis/encephalitis

- Diagnostic tests/findings
1. None indicated when examination is consistent with primary headache syndromes
2. Erythrocyte sedimentation rate on all patients with new onset older than 40 years to rule out temporal arteritis
3. CT/MRI
   a. Indicated if persistent focal neurologic findings or history of trauma
   b. CT preferred to identify acute hemorrhage
   c. MRI more sensitive in identifying pathologic intracranial changes
   d. Magnetic resonance angiography if aneurysm suspected—history of exertional headaches

- Management/treatment
1. Nonpharmacologic
   a. Regular sleep and meal schedules
   b. Daily exercise
   c. Avoiding known triggers
2. Pharmacologic
   a. Migraine
      (1) Abortive therapy
         (a) First-line therapy—mild-to-moderate intensity
            i. NSAIDs, acetaminophen
            ii. Combination analgesics—acetaminophen 250 mg/aspirin 250 mg/caffeine 65 mg—1 tablet(s) every 6 hours, not to take more than 8 tablets/day
         (b) First-line therapy—moderate-to-severe intensity—triptans
            i. Agents—sumatriptan, zolmitriptan, naratriptan, rizatriptan, almotriptan, frovatriptan; available in oral, nasal, subcutaneous SC forms
            ii. Drug action—selective serotonin agonists
            iii. Side effects—tightness of the throat/chest, flushing, numbness, tingling, dizziness; side effects tend to abate with time
            iv. Drug interactions—should not be used within 24 hours of another triptan or any ergotamine-containing drug
            v. Contraindications/precautions—coronary artery disease, hypertension; pregnancy Category C; caution in lactation
         (c) Second line—ergotamines
            i. Agents—ergotamine, dihydroergotamine/parenteral and nasal spray
            ii. Drug action—nonspecific serotonin agonist and vasoconstrictor
            iii. Side effects—nausea/vomiting (premedicate with antiemetic), tachycardia, vasoconstriction
            iv. Drug interactions—do not give with triptan
            v. Contraindications/precautions—coronary artery disease, hypertension; pregnancy Category X; not recommended while nursing
      (2) Prophylactic therapy—consider in patients who experience more than two severe headaches per month, need acute treatment medication more than two times per week, or are unable to tolerate abortive agents
         (a) Beta blocker—propranolol/timolol (see Table 9-1)
         (b) Calcium channel blockers—verapamil (see Table 9-1)
         (c) Antiepileptic agents—valproic acid (see **Table 9-7**)
   b. Tension
      (1) Episodic
         (a) NSAIDs, acetaminophen (see "Acute Otitis Media" section earlier in this chapter)
         (b) Caffeine, butalbital, acetaminophen (Fioricet) and caffeine, aspirin (Fiorinal)
            i. Drug action—butalbital is a barbiturate; muscle relaxant at lower doses, hypnotic at higher doses
            ii. Side effects—drowsiness, lightheadedness, nausea, vomiting
            iii. Drug interactions—potentiation with alcohol, CNS depressants
            iv. Contraindications/precautions—hepatic impairment; pregnancy Category C; not recommended in nursing mothers
      (2) Chronic
         (a) Tricyclic antidepressants (TCAs)—amitriptyline, nortriptyline
            i. Action—increases synaptic concentration of serotonin and norepinephrine in CNS
            ii. Side effects—sedation, dry mouth, blurred vision, constipation, abnormal cardiac conduction, dysrhythmias
            iii. Drug interactions—additive anticholinergic effects
            iv. Contraindications—with MAOI, impaired liver function; pregnancy Category C; not recommended while nursing
         (b) Selective serotonin reuptake inhibitors—less effective than TCAs (see "Major Depressive Disorder (MDD)" section in this chapter)
3. Patient education
   a. Signs indicating need for emergency treatment
      (1) Acute fever with headache
      (2) Abnormal mental status or personality changes

■ **Table 9-7 Commonly Used Anti-epileptic Drugs (AED) (representative list)**

Drug	Action	Side-effects	Interactions	Contraindications
Phenytoin	Stabilizes membranes and prevents spread of seizure from hyperactive focus	Nystagmus, drowsiness, ataxia, diplopia, gingival hyperplasia, hirsutism, low folate level	Antagonizes oral contraceptives, digoxin, oral anti-coagulants; potentiated by benzodiazepines, estrogens, H₂-blockers; other AED	Heart block, sinus bradycardia May be teratogenic to fetus
Carbamazepine	Delays recovery of sodium channels from their inactivated state; inhibits sustained repetitive firing	Sedation, GI upset, ataxia, blurred vision, skin rash, aplastic anemia	Increased plasma levels with CYP3A4 inhibitors-INH, macrolides; decreased plasma levels with CYP3A4 inducers-phenytoin	History of bone marrow depression Associated with neural tube defects and cleft palate in fetus
Valproic acid	Increased brain levels of neurotransmitter GABA, which has an inhibitory effect on seizures	Nausea, vomiting, sedation, blood dyscrasias	Potentiates phenobarbital, phenytoin	Liver disease or dysfunction; human teratogen associated with neural tube defects, mental and physical growth defects
Clonazepam	Enhances GABA action; depresses nerve transmission in motor cortex	Fatigue, sedation, behavior changes—aggressiveness and confusion	Potentiates CNS depression with alcohol; antagonized by phenytoin, carbamazepine	Liver disease; acute angle-closure glaucoma; human data suggest low risk in pregnancy
Topiramate	Enhances GABA action	Drowsiness, dizziness, ataxia, fatigue, visual disorders	Potentiates CNS depression with alcohol; potentiates phenobarbital, phenytoin; antagonized by carbamazepine, phenobarbital, phenytoin, valproic acid, verapamil	Acute myopia and secondary angle-closure glaucoma, hepatic or renal impairment, kidney stones; human and animal data suggest risk, birth defects increased when combined with other antiepileptics; avoid during 1st trimester
Gabapentin	Exact mechanism unknown; possibly increases GABA concentrations in some regions of the brain	Somnolence, dizziness, ataxia, fatigue	Not metabolized in humans; excreted unchanged in urine; no pharmacokinetic interaction with other AED; caution with cimetidine use due to decrease of glomerular filtration rate	Convulsions. In pregnancy, limited human data exists, but animal data suggest risk to fetus. However, benefits of therapy appear to outweigh potential risk to fetus
Lamotrigine	Exact mechanism unknown; possible effects on voltage-sensitive sodium channels	Skin rash, may be severe; fever, malaise, flu-like symptoms, drowsiness, visual disturbance, headache, nausea and vomiting, hallucination	Metabolism of lamotrigine may be inhibited by valproate resulting in increased concentrations of lamotrigine; carbamazepine, phenytoin, or phenobarbital increase elimination of lamotrigine	Angioedema, lymphadenopathy, facial edema, hepatic dysfunction (rare), agitation, confusion. In pregnancy, human data suggests risk to fetus

(3) Sudden onset; worst headache experienced

(4) Neurologic symptoms (e.g., projectile emesis, visual disturbances)

b. Self-medication for abortive therapy, injections

c. Education regarding nonpharmacologic management—avoidance of precipitating factors

- Referral
1. Focal neurologic findings
2. Specific secondary diagnosis is suspected
3. Chronic headaches develop new features
4. New headaches in individuals older than 50 years

Seizure Disorders

- Definition
1. Sudden change in body functioning with or without loss of consciousness due to an abnormal discharge of neurons
   a. Think of seizure as positive phenomenon, such as movement versus negative phenomenon, such as paralysis in transient ischemic attack (TIA)
   b. Where the discharge arises and how far it spreads determine what the seizure looks like clinically
2. Classification of seizures
   a. Partial seizures occur within localized regions of the brain; result of a localized physiologic or structural abnormality in the brain
      (1) Simple partial—consciousness not impaired
      (2) Complex partial—consciousness impaired
      (3) Partial with secondary generalization
   b. Generalized seizures arise from both sides of the brain simultaneously
      (1) Tonic-clonic (formerly "grand mal")
      (2) Absence (formerly "petit mal")
      (3) Myoclonic
      (4) Atonic
- Etiology/incidence
1. Etiology
   a. First step in evaluation of suspected seizure is to determine whether event was a seizure
   b. Once event identified as a seizure, need to determine whether epilepsy or secondary to another medical problem—hypoxia, hypoglycemia, infection, fever, toxic substance abuse
   c. Epilepsy is characterized by recurrent seizures; can be secondary to inherited or acquired factors
      (1) Head injury
      (2) Brain tumor
      (3) Cerebrovascular events
      (4) Idiopathic
2. Incidence
   a. Recurrence rate widely variable, linked to etiology
   b. Complex partial seizures most common adult type
   c. Absence seizures most common in childhood
3. Risk factors
   a. Inherited neurologic disease
   b. History of trauma

c. In persons with known seizure disorders
   (1) Sleep deprivation
   (2) Unusual stresses
   (3) Menstruation
   (4) Medications/drugs
- Signs and symptoms
1. Partial seizures
   a. Simple partial
      (1) Lasts 5–10 seconds
      (2) No loss of consciousness; no postseizure confusion
      (3) Symptoms reflect focal area of brain affected
         (a) Jerking or shaking in one area of body; may progress as focus spreads along cortical motor strip
         (b) Somatosensory symptoms
         (c) Visual or auditory symptoms
         (d) Autonomic symptoms—sweating, epigastric discomfort
         (e) Psychic symptoms
   b. Complex partial
      (1) Duration—5–10 seconds; 1–2 minutes; rarely more than 5 minutes
      (2) Loss of consciousness; postseizure confusion
      (3) Blank stare followed by an automatism (e.g., lip smacking, picking at clothing, purposeless walking)
2. Generalized seizures—always involve loss of consciousness
   a. Tonic-clonic seizures (grand mal)
      (1) Tonic phase—all skeletal muscles contract and patient falls
      (2) Clonic phase
         (a) Repetitive motor activity of all extremities that may last 2–3 minutes
         (b) As clonic phases abate muscles become flaccid and incontinence can occur
      (3) Postictal period
         (a) Consciousness may not return for 10–15 minutes
         (b) Confusion, headache, and fatigue may last from hours to days
   b. Absence "petit mal" seizure
      (1) Duration—5–10 seconds; may cluster
      (2) Manifest with blank stare, eye blinking
      (3) No postseizure confusion
   c. Myoclonic seizure
      (1) Quick, involuntary muscle jerks lasting a few seconds involving one body part or entire body
      (2) May accompany other generalized seizures; common to specific epilepsy syndromes
   d. Atonic
      (1) Sudden loss of postural tone causing patient to fall
      (2) Often associated with other seizure types; common in Lennox–Gastaut syndrome
- Physical findings
1. Often no physical findings
2. Focus physical examination on cardiovascular and neurologic systems
   a. Normal neurologic examination found in patients with idiopathic seizures
   b. Focal neurologic findings—brain lesion

- Differential diagnosis
  1. Vascular events (e.g., transient ischemic attack (TIA), classic migraine)
  2. Syncope
  3. Hyperventilation/anxiety attacks
  4. Narcolepsy
  5. Psychogenic spells (e.g., transient global amnesia)
- Diagnostic tests/findings
  1. Electrolytes, glucose, BUN/creatinine, LFTs, calcium, magnesium
  2. Toxicology screen
  3. CBC
  4. Lumbar puncture if infection is a consideration
  5. CT can detect bleeding or gross structural lesions
  6. MRI is study of choice; more sensitive and specific for evaluating structural lesions and brain parenchyma
  7. EEG
     a. Used to establish presence and type of epilepsy
     b. Initial EEG abnormal in only 40% of patients with probable epilepsy
- Management/treatment
  1. Nonpharmacologic—avoidance of triggers
  2. Pharmacologic (see Table 9-7)
     a. Principles
        (1) Goal—complete suppression of seizures
        (2) Initial treatment—single drug
        (3) Blood levels should be monitored periodically
        (4) When adding a second drug, maintain the first drug, titrating dosages after second drug reaches therapeutic levels
        (5) Treatment withdrawal should not be considered until seizure-free for a minimum of 2 years
     b. Pharmacologic management by seizure type
        (1) Partial seizures—carbamazepine, phenytoin, topiramate
        (2) Generalized seizures
            (a) Tonic-clonic seizures—phenytoin, carbamazepine, valproic acid, topiramate
            (b) Absence—valproic acid, ethosuximide
            (c) Myoclonic—valproic acid, clonazepam
            (d) Atonic—clonazepam
  3. Patient education
     a. Pregnancy and contraception
        (1) Impact on seizure frequency, severity variable
        (2) Teratogenic effects of seizure medications
        (3) Decreased oral contraceptive efficacy with many antiseizure medications; select backup or alternative method
     b. Safety issues regarding recurrent seizures
        (1) Activity limitations (e.g., driving)
        (2) Possible need for protective wear
        (3) Household hazards identification and modification
     c. Medication schedules and side effects
- Referral
  1. All clients with first-time seizures
  2. Uncontrolled seizures
  3. For EEG and interpretation

  4. Suspected underlying metabolic disease, neural lesion
  5. Pregnancy care

Dermatologic Disorders

Acne

- Definition—a common self-limited disease that presents with a variety of lesions, including open and closed comedones, papules and pustules, nodules, and cysts
- Etiology/incidence/risk factors
  1. Etiology
     a. Primary cause is obstruction of the pilosebaceous follicle
     b. Characterized by plugging of the hair follicle with abnormally cohesive desquamated cells, sebaceous gland hyperactivity, proliferation of bacteria (*P. acnes*), and inflammation
     c. Obstruction of follicle leads to development of noninflammatory acne—closed comedones/white heads and open comedones/black heads
     d. Proliferation of *P. acnes*/rupture of follicle wall results in inflammatory acne with papules, pustules, nodules, cysts
  2. Incidence
     a. Affects up to 90% of teens; 15% have moderate to severe acne
     b. May persist to older than 40 years in some, especially women
  3. Risk factors
     a. Aggravated by stress, hormonal cycling
     b. Use of topical steroids
     c. Contact with irritant oils or cosmetics
     d. More common and more severe in males
- Signs and symptoms
  1. Erythematous lesions, sometimes tender
  2. May be episodic, cyclic in severity
  3. Distribution and severity tend to be similar in family members
- Physical findings
  1. Lesions occur primarily on the face, but neck, shoulders, chest, and back may be involved
  2. Mild—open and closed comedones without inflammation
  3. Moderate—comedones with papules and pustules
  4. Severe—comedones, papules and pustules with nodules, cysts, and scarring
- Differential diagnosis
  1. Rosacea
  2. Pyoderma
  3. Drug eruptions
  4. Underlying endocrine disease—polycystic ovarian syndrome, Cushing's syndrome
  5. Folliculitis
  6. Perioral dermatitis
- Diagnostic tests/findings—none indicated
- Management/treatment
  1. Nonpharmacologic—cleansing
  2. Pharmacologic
     a. Mild acne—topical medications
        (1) Benzoyl peroxide
            (a) Drug action—antibacterial and comedolytic properties

(b) Side effects
   i. Skin irritation
   ii. Allergic dermatitis
   iii. May bleach clothing/bed linens, hair
(c) Drug interactions—PABA sunscreens may temporarily discolor skin
(d) Contraindications/precautions
   i. Avoid eyes, mouth, mucous membranes
   ii. Pregnancy Category C; precaution in nursing mothers

(2) Retinoic acid derivatives—tretinoin/cream, gel, lotion, and microspheres; adapalene gel/solution; tazarotene gel
(a) Drug action—comedolytic agent
(b) Side effects—local irritation, erythema, scaling
(c) Drug interactions—concomitant use with benzoyl peroxide may cause skin irritation
(d) Contraindications/precautions
   i. Avoid UV light, sun, extreme weather
   ii. Do not use with eczema
   iii. Pregnancy Category C; not recommended while nursing

(3) Azelaic acid
(a) Drug action—antibacterial and normalizes keratinization
(b) Side effects
   i. Local irritation, itching, contact dermatitis
   ii. Depigmentation
(c) Drug interactions—none identified
(d) Contraindications/precautions—pregnancy Category B; caution in nursing mothers

b. Moderate acne—topical antibiotics
(1) Topical antibiotics—clindamycin, erythromycin
(a) Drug action—bactericidal effects
(b) Side effects
   i. Local irritation
   ii. Folliculitis
(c) Drug interactions—additive effect with other topical agents
(d) Contraindications/precautions
   i. Avoid eyes, mucous membranes
   ii. History of regional enteritis, ulcerative or antibiotic-induced colitis/clindamycin
   iii. Pregnancy Category B/C; not recommended while nursing

(2) Oral medications—tetracycline, doxycycline, minocycline; erythromycin, azithromycin
(a) Drug action (tetracycline and its derivatives)—antibacterial and anti-inflammatory effect
(b) Side effects
   i. GI effects
   ii. Photosensitivity
   iii. Yeast infections
(c) Drug interactions—reduced absorption with antacids
(d) Contraindications/precautions—pregnancy Category D; not recommended in nursing mothers

(3) Oral contraceptives—some have FDA approval for treatment of moderate acne in women who also desire contraception; all with low androgenic or antiandrogenic progestin are likely effective
(a) Drug action—antiandrogenic/decreases free testosterone available for metabolism in sebaceous glands
(b) Side effects
   i. Nausea, vomiting
   ii. Minor bleeding irregularities, headaches
   iii. Hypertension
   iv. Thromboembolic events
(c) Drug interactions—antagonized by hepatic enzyme inducing drugs (e.g., griseofulvin, rifampin)
(d) Contraindications
   i. Thromboembolic disorders
   ii. Known or suspected estrogen-dependent neoplasm
   iii. History of cardiovascular or cerebrovascular disease
   iv. Pregnancy Category X; not recommended in nursing mothers

c. Severe acne—isotretinoin
(1) Drug action—decreases size and secretion of sebaceous glands, normalizes follicular keratinization, inhibits *P. acnes*, and modulates the inflammatory response
(2) Side effects
(a) Liver function test abnormalities
(b) Anemia, depression
(c) Skin and mucosal dryness
(d) Tendonitis
(e) Lipid abnormalities, pancreatitis
(3) Drug interactions
(a) Tetracyclines may increase incidence of pseudotumor cerebri
(b) Avoid alcohol
(c) Vitamin A
(4) Contraindications/precautions—pregnancy Category X; not recommended while nursing

3. Patient education
a. Use of mild cleansers, noncomedogenic moisturizers, sunscreen
b. "Hands off" policy to avoid secondary infection, scarring
c. Importance of avoiding pregnancy if using isotretinoin
- Referral—severe acne; may refer patients requiring treatment with isotretinoin

Contact Dermatitis

- Definition—skin inflammation due to irritants (irritant contact dermatitis) or allergens (allergic contact dermatitis)
- Etiology/risk factors
1. Etiology
a. Irritant contact dermatitis
(1) Eczematous response that is nonallergic caused by irritants, including chemicals, dry and cold air, and friction
(2) May occur acutely, more commonly occurs after chronic exposure

b. Allergic contact dermatitis
(1) A manifestation of cell-mediated hypersensitivity; causes delayed reaction on first exposure
(2) *Rhus* plant antigens (poison oak, poison ivy) will result in clinical eruption in 12–72 hours and within minutes on reexposure
(3) Other common allergic sensitizers include nickel (jewelry), rubber compounds (gloves), cosmetics, topical medications

2. Risk factors
a. Irritant contact dermatitis
(1) Everyone at risk; people vary in response
(2) Frequent exposure; chronic exposure
b. Allergic contact dermatitis—genetically predisposed reaction

- Signs and symptoms
1. Report of recent exposure (within 24 hours) to known allergens; exposure to irritants
2. Pruritus

- Physical findings
1. Irritant contact dermatitis
a. Mild irritants cause erythema, dryness, fissuring
b. Chronic exposure may cause oozing, weeping lesions
2. Allergic contact dermatitis
a. Classic lesions are vesicles and blisters on erythematous base
b. Linear eruption is the hallmark of most plant dermatoses
3. Distribution often provides clues to diagnosis

- Differential diagnosis
1. Atopic dermatitis, eczema
2. Tinea
3. Scabies/pediculosis
4. Herpes simplex/herpes zoster

- Diagnostic tests/findings
1. Usually none indicated
2. Negative potassium hydroxide (KOH) preparation of skin scraping
3. Patch testing with suspected allergens in difficult cases

- Management/treatment
1. Nonpharmacologic
a. Compresses, soaks (e.g., Burow's solution, Epsom salts)
b. Lubricants—lubricating ointments, petrolatum, no creams
2. Pharmacologic
a. Topical corticosteroids—intermediate potency for mild/moderate dermatitis; hydrocortisone for face/groin
(1) Drug action—anti-inflammatory effect
(2) Side effects
(a) Local irritation
(b) Epidermal and dermal atrophy
(3) Drug interactions—none identified
(4) Contraindications/precautions
(a) Avoid prolonged use on large areas
(b) Pregnancy Category C; not recommended while nursing
b. Systemic steroids for widespread or severe dermatitis (see Table 9-3)

c. Antihistamines—allergic pruritus
(1) Hydroxyzine
(a) Drug action—antihistamine
(b) Side effects—drowsiness, dry mouth
(c) Drug interactions—potentiates CNS depression with alcohol, other CNS depressants
(d) Contraindications—early pregnancy; nursing mothers
(2) Cetirizine (see Table 9-2)
3. Patient education
a. Avoidance of allergens
b. Protective garments, gloves

Skin Cancer

- Definition—malignant neoplasms arising in skin cells
- Etiology/incidence/risk factors
1. Etiology
a. Basal cell carcinoma (BCC)
(1) Slow growing, rarely metastasizes, but may cause extensive local tissue damage
(2) Tumor arises in basal layer of epidermis; causes include chronic sun exposure and genetic predisposition
b. Squamous cell carcinoma (SCC)
(1) Directly attributable to sun exposure or chronic irritation
(2) 60% occur at site of previous actinic keratoses
(3) Low tendency for metastasis
c. Malignant melanoma (MM)
(1) Arises from cells of the melanocyte system; begins either de novo or develops from preexisting lesion
(2) Initially grows superficially and laterally; enters vertical growth phase with potential to metastasize
2. Incidence
a. Basal cell approximately 75% all skin cancers, affects about 1 million people per year in the United States
b. Squamous cell second most common skin cancer in whites; most common skin cancer in blacks
c. Malignant melanoma represents 1% of skin cancers; 77% of skin cancer deaths
3. Risk factors
a. Nonmelanoma skin cancers
(1) Cumulative sun exposure; higher incidence in outdoor workers
(2) White race; fair complexion that burns easily/tans poorly
(3) Advancing age
(4) Male gender
(5) Previous history of skin cancer
b. Malignant melanoma
(1) History of changing mole
(2) Family and/or personal history of melanoma
(3) History of nonmelanoma skin cancer
(4) Atypical nevus syndrome
(5) Fair complexion; tendency to sunburn

- Signs and symptoms
1. Basal cell—painless, slow-growing lesion on sun-exposed areas
2. Squamous cell

a. Lesions seen in sun-exposed areas or skin damaged by burns or chronic inflammation; lower lip lesions common; but can also be found on the face, scalp, ears, neck, arms, hand, genitalia

b. A skin lesion that does not heal

3. Malignant melanoma
    a. Changing nevus; change in color, diameter increase, or border change
    b. Pruritus is early symptom
    c. Bleeding, ulceration, discomfort are late signs
    d. Location of melanoma commonly on skin but also found in eyes, ears, mucosal membranes of the mouth and genitals

- Physical findings
    1. Basal cell—several clinical variants; nodular basal cell most common
        a. Waxy, semitranslucent nodule with rolled borders
        b. Central ulcerations; telangectasias
    2. Squamous cell
        a. Red/reddish brown plaque/nodule
        b. Surface is scaly/crusted with erosions or ulcerations
    3. Malignant melanoma—tends to have *Asymmetry*, *Border* irregularity, *Color* variations, and *Diameter* greater than 6 mm (ABCD)
        a. Superficial spreading type/70%—prolonged horizontal growth phase; vertical growth occurs later
        b. Nodular—raised, pigmented (blue, black, dark brown, gray) nodules with normal surrounding skin
        c. Acral lentiginous—found on palms, soles, nail beds, mucous membranes
        d. Lentigo melanoma—occurs in preexisting lentigo maligna

- Differential diagnosis
    1. Common melanocytic nevus
    2. Seborrheic keratosis
    3. Dermatofibroma

- Diagnostic tests/findings—biopsy

- Management/treatment
    1. Nonpharmacologic/pharmacologic
        a. Excision and biopsy of lesions
        b. Basal cell carcinoma/squamous cell carcinoma—treatment options
            (1) Mohs' micrographic surgery—gradual lesion excision using serial frozen section analysis and mapping of excised tissue until tumor-free plane reached
            (2) Cryotherapy
            (3) Curettage with electrodesiccation/freezing
            (4) 5-FU or imiquimod
        c. Malignant melanoma
            (1) Excision of lesion
            (2) Lymph node dissection
            (3) Adjunctive therapy—chemotherapy, radiation, excision of metastasis
            (4) Long-term follow-up
    2. Patient education—focused on prevention
        a. Reduce exposure
            (1) Avoid sun exposure
            (2) Use of sunscreen with sun protective factor (SPF) of 15 or greater
            (3) Protective clothing
            (4) Educate regarding risk of tanning salons
        b. Educate regarding the acronym ABCD; useful reminder of the clinical features that should raise suspicion of melanoma in a pigmented lesion
        c. Total cutaneous examination (TCE)—recommended annually for populations with risk factors
            (1) Complete visual inspection of skin, scalp, hands, and feet for any suspicious lesions
            (2) Include questions regarding risk, exposures, family history
            (3) Best preventive practice to reduce mortality
        d. Self-examination for lesions, changing nevi

- Referral for ongoing care (chemotherapy, immunotherapy)

Tinea/Dermatophytosis

- Definition
    1. Superficial fungal infection caused by dermatophytes and yeasts
    2. Dermatophytes require keratin for growth; infection restricted to hair, superficial skin, and nails
    3. Classified according to involved anatomic location
        a. Tinea capitis—scalp; mainly affects children
        b. Tinea corporis—body
        c. Tinea cruris—upper inner thigh/spares scrotum
        d. Tinea pedis—toe webs; soles/heels
        e. Tinea unguium—toenails more frequently involved than fingernails

- Etiology/incidence/risk factors
    1. Etiology
        a. *Microsporum*, *Trichophyton*, *Epidermophyton* species
        b. Transmission via contact with infected persons, fomites (shoes, towels, shower stalls), animals, or soil
    2. Incidence
        a. Scalp infections more common in children
        b. Tinea cruris and tinea pedis—both more common in men than in women; and both types of tinea are usually associated with each other
        c. Intertriginous infections common in young adults
        d. Tinea pedis clinically apparent in 5–10% of population
    3. Risk factors
        a. Tinea capitis—overcrowding and poor hygiene
        b. Tinea cruris—hot, humid conditions, occlusive clothing
        c. Tinea unguium—aging, diabetes, poorly fitting shoes

- Signs and symptoms
    1. May be asymptomatic
    2. Itching, burning variable

- Physical findings
    1. Classic presentation is a lesion with central clearing surrounded by an advancing, red, scaly, elevated border
    2. Scalp lesions characterized by hair loss/scaling
    3. Maceration, especially intertriginous lesions
    4. Involved nails are yellowish/thickened with subungual debris

- Diagnostic tests/findings
    1. Potassium hydroxide (KOH) microscopy positive for hyphae
    2. Fungal culture for specific identification

3. Wood's lamp of limited usefulness; most dermatophytes currently seen in United States do not fluoresce

- Management/treatment
  1. Nonpharmacologic
     a. Careful nail and skin care
     b. Keep area dry, absorbent clothing
  2. Pharmacologic
     a. Topical antifungals—tinea corporis, tinea cruris, tinea pedis
        (1) Azoles—clotrimazole, econazole, ketoconazole, miconazole
            (a) Drug action—fungicidal activity
            (b) Side effects—pruritus, irritation, stinging
            (c) Drug interactions—none identified
            (d) Contraindications/precautions—pregnancy Category C; not recommended in nursing mothers
        (2) Allylamines—naftifine, terbinafine, butenafine
            (a) Drug action—fungicidal activity
            (b) Side effects—burning, stinging, irritation, dryness
            (c) Drug interactions—none identified
            (d) Contraindications/precautions—pregnancy Category B; precaution in nursing mothers
     b. Oral antifungals—tinea capitis, tinea unguium
        (1) Griseofulvin
            (a) Drug action—interferes with fungal microtube formation by disrupting mitosis and cell division
            (b) Side effects—headache, nausea, vomiting, diarrhea, photosensitivity
            (c) Drug interactions—reduces effectiveness of oral contraceptives
            (d) Contraindications/precautions—porphyria, hepatocellular failure, avoid use during pregnancy, particularly during organogenesis; precaution in nursing mothers (Briggs & Freeman, 2015)
        (2) Itraconazole
            (a) Drug action—decreases ergosterol synthesis, inhibiting cell membrane formation
            (b) Side effects—GI upset, rash, fatigue, headache, dizziness, edema; hepatitis reported/monitor LFTs
            (c) Drug interactions—inhibits drug-metabolizing enzymes/CYP3A4; may increase levels of other drugs
            (d) Contraindications/precautions—hepatic dysfunction; pregnancy Category C; not recommended in nursing mothers
        (3) Terbinafine
            (a) Drug action—inhibits enzyme activity in fungi; inhibits synthesis of ergosterol
            (b) Side effects—GI disturbances, headaches; rare LFT abnormalities
            (c) Drug interactions—potentiated by cimetidine; antagonized by rifampin
            (d) Contraindications/precautions—liver or renal disease; pregnancy Category B; not recommended in nursing mothers
  3. Patient education
     a. Keep skin dry as possible, especially intertrigal spaces
     b. Wear loose, clean, absorbent clothing
     c. Contagious nature of condition

Psychosocial Problems

Stress

- Definition—Selye's theory of stress response and adaptation describes a continuum related to stress
  1. Eustress or good stress—degree of stress that is motivating and viewed as positive for the individual
  2. Distress—point at which stress becomes psychologically or physically debilitating
- Etiology/incidence
  1. Major life events—marriage, divorce, job change, death of a family member
  2. Chronic situations—poverty, illness of self or family member, abuse
  3. Acute situations—acute pain, sudden threats to safety
  4. Environmental conditions—noise, pollution, overcrowding
  5. Daily hassles—minor events that occur on a regular basis
- Signs and symptoms
  1. Irritability, anxiety, depression, chronic worrying
  2. Decreased productivity, sleep disturbances, appetite changes, loss of libido
  3. Vague or nonspecific physical complaints—headaches, nausea, diarrhea, chest pain, muscle tension
- Physical findings
  1. Muscle tension
  2. Increase in blood pressure
- Differential diagnosis
  1. Depression
  2. Anxiety disorders
  3. Other medical conditions that could account for signs and symptoms
- Diagnostic tests/findings—none
- Management/treatment
  1. Eliminate or modify stressors—assertiveness training, time management, positive thought strategies, communication skills
  2. Relaxation techniques—guided imagery, muscle relaxation exercises, biofeedback, massage, meditation, use of humor, physical exercise

Anxiety

- Definition—*DSM-IV-TR* lists several psychiatric syndromes of which anxiety is a primary component; interference with everyday function must be present to classify anxiety as a psychiatric syndrome
  1. Generalized anxiety disorder (GAD)
     a. Persistent, excessive, incapacitating worry over life events occurring more days than not, for at least 6 months
     b. Anxiety and worry are associated with three or more of the following symptoms—restlessness, easily fatigued, difficulty concentrating, irritability, muscle tension, sleep disturbance
  2. Panic attack
     a. Period of intense fear or discomfort, develops abruptly and peaks within 10 minutes

b. At least four of the following symptoms must be present—palpitations, sweating, trembling, sensation of shortness of breath/smothering, choking sensation, chest pain, nausea/abdominal distress, dizziness/lightheadedness, derealization, fear of losing control, sense of impending doom, paresthesias, chills/hot flashes

3. Panic disorder

    a. Recurrent, unexpected panic attacks—not due to substance abuse, medical condition, or other mental disorder

    b. At least one attack followed by at least 1 month of one more of the following:

        (1) Persistent concern about having other panic attacks

        (2) Worry about implications of attack and its consequences

        (2) Significant change in behavior related to attacks

    c. May occur with or without agoraphobia

4. Agoraphobia—anxiety about, or avoidance of, places or situations in which the ability to leave suddenly may be difficult in the event of having a panic attack

5. Specific phobia—anxiety elicited by a discrete stimulus such as heights or specific animals; individual recognizes that the fear is excessive or unreasonable

6. Social phobia—fear of one or more social and performance situations that is excessive or incapacitating; individual recognizes the fear is excessive or unreasonable

7. Post-traumatic stress disorder (PTSD)—persistent anxiety lasting more than 1 month following an extremely traumatic event; symptoms may not start until several days or weeks after the event

    a. Exposure to a traumatic event in which experienced, witnessed, or was confronted with event that involved actual or threatened death, serious injury, or threat to physical integrity of others

    b. Traumatic event persistently reexperienced through at least one of the following ways:

        (1) Intrusive distressing recollections of event

        (2) Distressing dreams

        (3) Feeling as if traumatic event was recurring

        (4) Psychological distress when exposed to cues symbolizing event

        (5) Physiologic reaction on exposure to cues symbolizing event

    c. Avoidance of stimuli associated with trauma and numbing of general responsiveness

    d. Persistent symptoms of increased arousal

8. Acute stress disorder (ASD)—similar to PTSD but more immediate and of shorter duration; lasts minimum of 2 days and maximum of 4 weeks, occurs within 4 weeks of traumatic event

9. Obsessive-compulsive disorder (OCD)—characterized by obsessions that cause marked anxiety or distress and/or by compulsions that serve to neutralize the anxiety

- Etiology/incidence/prevalence

1. One of the most prevalent of all psychiatric disorders

2. Prevalence varies with specific phobia most common (25%), social phobia (13%), PTSD (7.8%; 12% in women, 20% in victims of war trauma), GAD (5%), panic disorder (3.5%)

3. Disrupted modulation of the central nervous system with several neuroregulators implicated in the cause of anxiety (e.g., dopamine, serotonin, norepinephrine)

4. May be a genetic predisposition

- Signs and symptoms—vary with the particular anxiety disorder

- Physical findings

1. Physical findings may be present with an acute anxiety attack

2. Tachycardia, increased respirations, elevated BP

3. Restlessness

4. Diaphoresis

5. Muscle tension

- Differential diagnosis

1. Medical conditions that may account for symptoms of anxiety—cardiac arrhythmias, mitral valve prolapse, angina, pulmonary embolism, hypoglycemia, hyperthyroidism, asthma, chronic obstructive pulmonary disease, Cushing's disease, pheochromocytoma

2. Medication-induced symptoms of anxiety—steroids, anticholinergics, sympathomimetics, digoxin, thyroxine

3. Drug abuse or withdrawal

4. Other psychological disorders—depression, bipolar disorder

- Diagnostic tests/findings

1. May be done to exclude other medical conditions suggested by history/physical

2. TSH, urine toxicology, electrocardiogram, complete blood count, metabolic panel

- Management/treatment

1. Nonpharmacologic—psychotherapy/cognitive behavioral therapy

2. Pharmacologicc

    a. Benzodiazepines for short-term management if needed for severe impairment until acceptable reduction of symptoms is achieved with SSRIs and /or cognitive behavioral therapy, lorazepam, diazepam, clonazepam, alprazolam

        (1) Drug action—produce an antianxiety effect by enhancing the action of the neurotransmitter gamma-aminobutyric acid at the cortical and limbic areas of the brain

        (2) Side effects—sedation, impaired concentration, anterograde amnesia; dependence; abuse potential

        (3) Drug interactions—potentiates the effect of other CNS depressants, including alcohol; may be potentiated by use with cimetidine

        (4) Contraindications/precautions—pregnancy Category D, risk of rebound anxiety with withdrawal of alprazolam because of short half-life

    b. SSRIs—paroxetine, venlafaxine, sertraline (see "Major Depressive Disorder (MDD)" section in this chapter)—best tolerance and response rates for GAD, panic disorder, PTSD, OCD, social anxiety disorder

    c. Serotonin and norepinephrine reuptake inhibitors (SNRIs)—duloxetine, venlafaxine (see "Major Depressive Disorder (MDD)" section in this chapter)

    d. Buspirone—nonbenzodiazepine antianxiety agent

        (a) Drug effect—partial agonism or mixed agonism/antagonism at $5-HT_{1A}$ receptors

        (b) Side effects—nausea, dizziness, headache, restlessness

(c) Drug interactions—hypertensive crisis with MAOIs; cytochrome P-450 effect

(d) Contraindications/precautions—pregnancy Category B

3. Client education

a. Caution about potential for physical/psychological dependence with use of benzodiazepines

b. Caution against use of alcohol or other CNS depressants with benzodiazepines

c. Discuss the use of relaxation techniques and effective coping mechanisms

d. Reassurance that effective treatment is available, but patience required until the right combination of modalities is found

Major Depressive Disorder (MDD)

- Definition (*DSM-IV-TR*)—at least five of the symptoms listed must be present most of the day, nearly every day for 2 weeks and no. 1 or no. 2 must be present for a diagnosis of major depression
  1. Sad or depressed mood most of the day, every day
  2. Loss of interest in usual activities
  3. Fatigue, weight gain/loss, sleep disturbance, difficulty concentrating, feelings of worthlessness/guilt, psychomotor retardation/agitation, suicidal ideation
- Etiology/incidence/prevalence/risk factors
  1. Lifetime prevalence of clinically significant MDD is 16%; women affected 2–3 times more than men
  2. First major depressive episode usually occurs in adolescence or early adulthood
  3. Bimodal curve of prevalence—one peak in late 20s and early 30s and a second peak around 65 to 70 years of age
  4. Theories include biologic, sociologic, and neuroendocrine etiologies
  5. Risk factors for depression include:
     a. Prior incident of major depression
     b. Family history of depression
     c. Severe or chronic illness/chronic pain
     d. History of early trauma, abuse, neglect, deprivation
     e. Current high stress burden (e.g., marital or family problems, abuse)
     f. Postpartum period
  6. 15% of depressed individuals attempt suicide
  7. Risk factors for suicide include:
     a. Prior attempt/family history of suicide attempt
     b. Male gender
     c. Substance abuse/family history of substance abuse
     d. Living alone
     e. Medical illness
     f. Hopelessness
     g. Psychosis or panic disorder
     h. Advanced age
     i. Violence or impulsivity
- Signs and symptoms
  1. As listed in definition
  2. Vague pain, headaches, GI complaints, sexual complaints
  3. Substance abuse or dependence

- Physical findings
  1. Poor eye contact, tearful, downcast
  2. Inattention to appearance/hygiene
  3. Slow, monotone speech
  4. Psychomotor retardation or agitation
  5. Impaired cognitive reasoning
- Differential diagnosis
  1. Adjustment disorder following a stressor event
  2. Bereavement or grief reaction
  3. Dysthymia
     a. Chronic low-grade depressive symptoms for 2 or more years
     b. Insufficient number and intensity of symptoms to qualify as MDD
     c. Often accompanies chronic, disabling medical disorders
  4. Other psychiatric syndromes
  5. Medical disorders—thyroid disorders, sleep apnea, Parkinson's disease, multiple sclerosis
  6. Medications—corticosteroids, antihypertensives, benzodiazepines, chemotherapeutic drugs and others
- Diagnostic tests/findings
  1. Laboratory/diagnostic tests may be done to exclude other diagnostic possibilities
     a. CBC
     b. TSH
     c. Glucose
  2. Screening tools—depression assessment scales
     a. Ask patients to rate severity or frequency of various symptoms
     b. Beck Depression Inventory, Zung Self-Rating Depression Scale, Geriatric Depression Scale, Edinburgh Postnatal Depression Scale
- Management/treatment
  1. Nonpharmacologic—psychotherapy, regular exercise, light therapy for seasonal affective disorder (subtype of MDD), neuromodulation techniques (e.g., electroconvulsive therapy, vagus nerve stimulation); hospitalization may be required for severe depression or if client has suicidal ideation
  2. Pharmacologic
     a. Selective serotonin reuptake inhibitors (SSRIs) have replaced tricyclic antidepressants (TCAs) as the drugs of choice because of their improved tolerability and safety if taken in overdose
        (1) Agents—fluoxetine, sertraline, paroxetine, citalopram, escitalopram
        (2) Drug action—block reuptake of serotonin, enhancing serotonin neurotransmission
        (3) Side effects—anxiety, insomnia/hypersomnia, headache, nausea, anorexia, sexual dysfunction
        (4) Drug interactions—use with MAO inhibitors may cause hypertensive crisis; CY P-450 drug–drug interactions
        (5) Contraindications/precautions—not to be used in conjunction with MAO inhibitors; screen patients for symptoms of bipolar disorder before prescribing to avoid precipitating a manic episode; pregnancy Category C; caution in nursing mothers

b. Selective serotonin and norepinephrine reuptake inhibitors (SNRIs)
   (1) Agents—venlafaxine, duloxetine
   (2) Drug action—inhibits both serotonin and norepinephrine reuptake
   (3) Side effects—nausea, dizziness, insomnia, somnolence, dry mouth, constipation, sexual dysfunction
   (4) Drug interactions—MAO inhibitors, tryptophan, other SSRIs or SNRIs, CYP1A2 inhibitors, other
   (5) Contraindications/precautions—not to be used in conjunction with MAO inhibitors; uncontrolled narrow-angle glaucoma; pregnancy Category C, caution in nursing mothers
c. Other classes of antidepressants
   (1) Mirtazapine—stimulates release of norepinephrine and serotonin; side effects include fatigue, dizziness, orthostatic hypotension, transient sedation, and weight gain; contraindications/precautions: pregnancy Category C, caution in nursing mothers
   (2) Bupropion—decreases reuptake of dopamine in the CNS; major side effects include agitation, headache, and nausea; no sexual side effects; contraindications/precautions: contraindicated with seizure disorders, eating disorders, pregnancy Category C, caution in nursing mothers
d. Once full remission achieved, continue therapy for 6 to 12 months; for second episode continue therapy for 1 to 2 years; a third episode requires indefinite maintenance

3. Client education
   a. SSRIs—usually taken in morning to reduce incidence of insomnia
   b. Antidepressants should be started slowly and dose increased to a therapeutic level that alleviates symptoms
   c. An adequate trial period and close follow-up are essential for successful treatment
   d. Caution concerning use of medications with alcohol
   e. Encourage use of support systems, effective coping mechanisms

- Referral
  1. Patients requiring referral to a psychiatrist include those with suicidal ideation or severe depression; bipolar disorder; atypical depression, substance abuse, treatment resistance
  2. Referral to a licensed counselor should be offered to most patients with depression

Domestic Violence/Intimate Partner Violence (IPV)

- Definition—a pattern of coercive and controlling behavior that occurs in an intimate adult relationship; four main types—physical violence, sexual violence, threats of physical or sexual violence, psychological/emotional violence
- Etiology/incidence/prevalence
  1. 1 in 4 women has been the victim of severe physical violence by an intimate partner in her lifetime
  2. One-third of female murder victims age 12 and older are killed by an intimate partner, IPV is a leading cause of homicides and injury-related deaths during pregnancy (Office for the Prevention of Domestic Violence, 2012)
  3. Intimate partner violence is the single most common reason women go to emergency rooms
  4. 12% of teenagers and more than 20% of college students have experienced dating violence
  5. Pregnant women may be at increased risk for initiation or escalation of abuse
  6. Associated impacts on pregnancy include preterm delivery, low birth weight, delayed prenatal care, substance abuse
  7. 80% of women who have experienced intimate partner violence suffer significant short- or long-term psychological impacts, including PTSD, depression, fear of intimacy, inability to trust others, low self-esteem, sleep disturbances, suicidal behavior, substance abuse
  8. Gastrointestinal and gynecologic disorders, headaches, sexual dysfunction, and chronic pain syndromes are common in women who have experienced intimate partner violence
- Signs and symptoms
  1. History of frequent visits to emergency room
  2. Evidence of current or old injuries
  3. Delay in reporting an injury/explanation of cause inconsistent with injury
  4. Depression, anxiety, post-traumatic stress reactions, low self-esteem
  5. History of suicide attempts or ideation
  6. Alcohol or drug abuse
  7. Vague or nonspecific physical complaints
  8. Late/sporadic prenatal care or other health care
  9. Controlling partner/increased anxiety in presence of partner
  10. Behavioral problems in children who are witnessing the abuse
  11. Cycle of violence—tension building, serious battering incident, honeymoon phase
- Physical findings
  1. Facial lacerations
  2. Injuries to breasts, back, abdomen, and genitalia
  3. Bilateral injuries to arms/legs
  4. Obvious patterns—bite marks, hand grip, cigarette burns
  5. Injuries during pregnancy
  6. Recurrent or chronic injuries
- Differential diagnosis
  1. Accidental injuries
  2. Self-inflicted injuries
- Diagnostic tests/findings—none
- Management/treatment
  1. Routine assessment for abuse in all women
  2. Danger assessment—suicide or homicide
  3. Safety plan—where to go in an emergency or dangerous situation; what to do during violent incidents; what items/documents will be needed for a comfortable and safe escape
  4. ABCDEs of intervention
     a. *Alone*—assure the woman that she is not alone in being a victim of domestic violence
     b. *Belief*—let the woman know that you believe that no one deserves to be hurt or threatened in a relationship
     c. *Confidential*—assure the woman that the information she shares is confidential

d. *Document*—record any findings that may be helpful to the woman at a later date; use accurate description of incident and/or threats in patient's own words; include all pertinent physical examination findings with body map and/or photographs, with woman's permission

e. *Educate*—provide information about available resources, dangers of escalating violence, and safety plans

5. Referrals
   a. Shelters
   b. Legal assistance
   c. Counseling

6. Mandatory reporting—laws vary in each state

Sexual Violence

- Definition—any sexual act that is forced against someone's will; may be physical, verbal, or psychological
  1. 4 types of sexual violence (CDC, 2002)
     a. Completed sex act—sexual assault that involves penetration, however slight, of the labia by the penis; legal definitions of rape vary from state to state but typically include the use of force, threat, or coercion and lack of consent by the victim in relation to sexual intercourse
     b. An attempted (but not completed) sex act
     c. Abusive sexual contact—intentional touching, directly or through clothing of genitalia, anus, groin, breast, inner thigh, or buttocks of any person
     d. Noncontact sexual abuse—does not involve physical contact; examples include voyeurism, exposure to exhibitionism, pornography, sexual harassment, threats of sexual violence
  2. Legal terminology—varies from state to state
     a. Sexual assault—force, threats, or coercion to engage in any unwanted sexual contact; includes contact or penetration of the intimate parts (sexual organs, anus, groin, buttocks, and breasts)
     b. Rape—sexual assault that involves penetration, however slight, of the labia by the penis; legal definitions of rape vary from state to state but typically include the use of force, threat, or coercion and lack of consent by the victim in relation to sexual intercourse
- Etiology/incidence
  1. Sexual violence occurs in all age, race, ethnic, and cultural groups
  2. Approximately 18% of women in United States have experienced a completed or attempted act of sexual violence in their lifetime; majority perpetrated by an acquaintance rather than a stranger
- Signs and symptoms—sexual assault
  1. Genital injury may or may not be present and is often difficult to visualize
  2. Typical findings include lacerations, ecchymosis, abrasions, erythema, and edema in areas of assault
  3. Rape trauma syndrome describes the symptoms that occur in most survivors of sexual assault
     a. Acute phase—lasts a few days to a few weeks

(1) Emotional responses may be expressed or controlled ranging from anger, fear, anxiety, and restlessness to a calm, composed, subdued affect

(2) Physical responses include general soreness and soreness in the areas of assault; gastrointestinal and genitourinary symptoms; sleep disruption and nightmares; and sexual disruption

   b. Reorganization phase—wide range of emotions and physical responses with the purpose of reorganizing life after the assault

4. Post-traumatic stress disorder (PTSD) occurs in 30–65% of sexual assault survivors—see "Anxiety" section earlier in this chapter for diagnostic criteria

- Physical findings
  1. Physical findings may be minimal or not apparent until a day or more after the assault
  2. Lacerations, ecchymosis, abrasions, erythema, edema in areas of assault
  3. Colposcopic examination may be used to assist in evaluation
- Differential diagnosis
  1. Accidental injuries
  2. Violence—nonsexual
- Diagnostic tests/findings
  1. Forensic evidence collection technique and requirements may vary from state to state—most states supply evidence collection kits that contain instructions and collection materials
  2. Sexually transmitted infection (STI) and HIV testing is not recommended as part of routine care of sexual assault survivor
- Management/treatment
  1. Comprehensive care for sexual assault victim is often provided by a multidisciplinary team that includes a sexual assault nurse examiner (SANE), victims' advocate, and law enforcement
  2. Triage and immediate treatment of any life-threatening injuries
  3. Attention to emotional needs of the victim
  4. Collection of evidence per state and agency protocol
  5. Prophylactic treatment for STIs—chlamydia, gonorrhea, trichomoniasis
  6. Initiate hepatitis B vaccination series if has not had previously
  7. Prophylactic treatment for HIV—decision based on risk as a result of type of sexual contact, vaginal lacerations, multiple assailants, HIV prevalence in geographic area
  8. Offer emergency contraception if pregnancy is a concern
  9. Discuss need for chlamydia and gonorrhea testing in 1–2 weeks if not treated prophylactically, along with testing for HIV and syphilis at 6 weeks, 3 months, and 6 months
  10. Referrals
      a. Legal and social service referrals
      b. Counseling for survivor and family
  11. Screen all female patients for history of sexual violence

Eating Disorders

- Definitions
  1. Anorexia nervosa—*DSM-IV* criteria for diagnosis include:
     a. Refusal to maintain body weight at or above a minimal normal weight for age and height, body weight less than 85% of what expected

b. Intense fear of gaining weight even though underweight

c. Disturbed body image

d. Amenorrhea or the absence of at least three consecutive menstrual cycles when otherwise expected

2. Bulimia nervosa—*DSM-IV* criteria for diagnosis include:

a. Recurrent episodes of binge eating

b. Recurrent, inappropriate compensatory behavior to prevent weight gain (self-induced vomiting; misuse of laxatives, diuretics or enemas; strict dieting or fasting; excessive exercise)

c. Binge eating and inappropriate compensatory behaviors occur on the average at least twice a week for at least 3 months

d. Persistent overconcern with body shape and weight

- Etiology/incidence/prevalence/risk factors

1. Anorexia nervosa

a. Etiology—biologic, psychological, social, and family factors

b. About 1% of female adolescents have anorexia

c. Age of onset—early to late adolescence

d. 10–20% mortality due to cardiac arrest or suicide

e. Risk factors include:

(1) Female gender

(2) Parent or sibling with eating disorder

(3) Career choice or aspiration that stresses thinness, perfection, or self-discipline

(4) A difficult transition or loss (leaving home for college, breakup of an important relationship)

2. Bulimia nervosa

a. Etiology—biologic, psychological, social, and family factors

b. Age of onset—late adolescence to early adulthood

c. Occurs in 4% of college-age women

d. Mortality rate lower than with anorexia nervosa

e. 30–80% of bulimics have history of anorexia nervosa

- Signs and symptoms

1. Anorexia nervosa—fatigue, cold intolerance, muscle weakness and cramps, dizziness, fainting spells, bloating, amenorrhea, social isolation, excessive concerns about weight, compulsive exercising, odd food rituals, depression

2. Bulimia nervosa—menstrual irregularities, depression, anxiety, impulsive behaviors (shoplifting, alcohol or drug abuse, unsafe sexual behaviors), lack of meaningful relationships, excessive concerns about weight, requests for diet pills, diuretics, or laxatives

- Physical findings

1. Anorexia nervosa—emaciation, dry skin, fine body hair (lanugo), muscle wasting, peripheral edema, bradycardia, arrhythmias, hypotension, delayed sexual maturation, stress fractures

2. Bulimia—erosion of tooth enamel, calluses on dorsal surface of hands from inducing vomiting, swollen parotid glands, cardiac arrhythmias if syrup of ipecac used

- Differential diagnosis

1. Gastrointestinal disorders

2. Malignancies

3. Depression

4. Other psychiatric disorders

- Diagnostic tests/findings

1. Anorexia—mild anemia, elevated BUN, cholesterol, and liver function tests, electrolyte imbalance, low serum estrogen, abnormal ECG

2. Bulimia—electrolyte imbalance, abnormal ECG

3. Rating instruments—Eating Attitudes Test, Eating Disorders Inventory, Body Shape Questionnaire

- Management/treatment

1. Outpatient treatment—individual/group/family therapy, nutritional counseling, treatment of any medical complications, treatment of any associated mood disorders

2. Pharmacologic—SSRI fluoxetine approved for treatment of bulimia

3. Hospitalization is indicated if any of the following apply:

a. Weight is less than 75% of ideal body weight

b. Client is suicidal

c. Rapid, persistent decline in oral intake or weight despite intensive outpatient interventions

d. Electrolyte or metabolic abnormalities, hematemesis, orthostatic hypotension, heart rate < 40 beats per minute (BPM) or > 110 BPM, inability to sustain core body temperature

4. Pregnancy considerations—individuals with anorexia nervosa may have fertility problems; pregnant individuals with eating disorders will require special nutritional management to ensure adequate weight gain and nutrient intake

Addictive Disorders (Alcohol and Drugs)

- Definitions

1. Substance dependence (*DSM-IV* criteria)—maladaptive pattern of substance use leading to significant impairment or distress with at least three of the following occurring within a 12-month period:

a. Tolerance

b. Withdrawal syndrome or use of substance to relieve withdrawal symptoms

c. Substance taken in larger amounts or over a longer period of time than intended

d. Persistent desire or unsuccessful attempts to cut down use

e. Significant amount of time spent obtaining, consuming, or recovering from substance

f. Important social or occupational activities reduced because of substance use

g. Persistent use despite knowledge of social, psychological, or physical problems caused by its use

2. Substance abuse (*DSM-IV* criteria)—maladaptive pattern of use leading to a significant impairment or distress with at least one of the following within a 12–month period:

a. Recurrent substance use resulting in a failure to fulfill major role obligations (work, school, home)

b. Recurrent use in situations where use is physically hazardous (driving while intoxicated)

c. Recurrent substance abuse–related legal problems

d. Continued use despite knowledge of having a persistent or recurring social or interpersonal problem that is caused or worsened by the substance use

e. Symptoms have never met the criteria for substance dependence

- Etiology/incidence/prevalence/risk factors
  1. Genetic, cultural, biochemical, behavioral, and psychological factors have all been considered in the etiology of substance dependence
  2. 3–8% of women will experience alcohol dependence at some point in lifetime
  3. 30% of general population engages in risky or unhealthy alcohol drinking
  4. Other drugs of abuse include opioids, depressants, stimulants, hallucinogens, and marijuana
  5. Substance abuse is involved in more than 50% of domestic violence and in 50% of driving accident fatalities
  6. Risk factors
     a. First-degree relative with alcohol dependence
     b. Psychiatric disorders—major depressive disorder, generalized anxiety disorder, panic disorder, attention deficit disorder, schizophrenia
     c. Risk factors for adolescent drug use
        (1) Individual—alienation, rebelliousness, friends engaged in problem behavior, favorable attitude toward the problem behavior
        (2) Community—availability of drugs, transitions and mobility, low neighborhood attachment and community disorganization, extreme economic deprivation
        (3) Family—history of the problem behavior, family conflict
        (4) School—early and persistent antisocial behavior, academic failure beginning in late elementary school, lack of commitment to school
- Signs and symptoms
  1. Alcoholism
     a. Frequent falls/minor injuries, blackouts, legal or marital problems, depression, vague GI complaints, sleep disorders, withdrawal symptoms, seizures
     b. The National Institute on Alcohol Abuse and Alcoholism (NIAAA) recommends asking all clients if they ever drink alcohol, and if the answer is yes, ask about maximum number of drinks on any occasion in past month, how many drinks they have on a typical day when they drink, and how many days per week they drink to identify hazardous drinkers
     c. CAGE is one of several screening tools used to assess a drinking problem
        (1) Have you ever felt you should *cut down* on your drinking?
        (2) Have people *annoyed* you by criticizing your drinking?
        (3) Have you ever felt bad or *guilty* about your drinking?
        (4) Have you ever had a drink first thing in the morning to steady your nerves or get rid of a hangover (*eye-opener*)?

2. Signs and symptoms of depressant (benzodiazepine, barbiturate) abuse—euphoria, apathy, violent or bizarre behavior
3. Signs and symptoms of stimulant (cocaine, amphetamine) abuse—anxiety, euphoria, violent or bizarre behavior, hallucinations, nausea/vomiting

- Physical findings
  1. Alcoholism—hepatomegaly, tremors, peripheral neuropathy, ataxia, confusion, impairment of recent memory
  2. Depressants—psychomotor retardation, slurred speech, lack of coordination, tremors
  3. Stimulants—diaphoresis, hypertension, tachycardia, hyperactive deep tendon reflexes (DTR), pupil dilation, tremors, seizures
- Differential diagnosis
  1. Psychiatric disorders that could account for the signs and symptoms (e.g., depression, anxiety disorders, schizophrenia)
  2. Medical conditions that could account for the signs and symptoms (e.g., endocrinopathies, seizure disorders, head injury)
- Diagnostic tests/findings
  1. Blood alcohol level may be elevated
  2. Elevated gamma glutamyl transferase (GGT) indicates heavy or chronic alcohol use
  3. Urine toxicology tests for other drugs of abuse
  4. Consider other laboratory and diagnostic tests based on risk factors and clinical presentation
- Management/treatment
  1. Follow federal and state laws regarding protection of confidentiality for persons receiving alcohol and drug abuse treatment services and treatment of minors for alcohol and drug abuse without parental consent
  2. Detoxification—outpatient or inpatient
  3. Addiction counseling
  4. Maternal/infant complications, and management of substance abuse in pregnancy are discussed elsewhere
  5. Prevention of relapse
     a. Alcoholics Anonymous, Narcotics Anonymous
     b. Pharmacologic agents—short-term adjuncts to psychosocial treatment
        (1) Naltrexone—alcohol craving is reduced in about one-half of patients
        (2) Disulfiram—creates a toxic response when patient consumes alcohol
        (3) Acamprosate—antagonizes glutamate receptors, restores chemical balance between excitatory and inhibitory neurotransmitters, prescribed to help in maintaining alcohol abstinence
     c. Family involvement—counseling, Al-Anon, Ala-Teen, Nar-Anon
     d. Employee assistance programs

Questions

Select the best answer.

1. A systolic heart murmur present in an asymptomatic pregnant woman is likely:
   a. Due to valvular disease
   b. Associated with history of rheumatic fever
   c. A physiologic (innocent) murmur
   d. To intensify with Valsalva maneuver

2. Which of the following, if left untreated, may progress to squamous cell carcinoma?
   a. Keratosis pilaris
   b. Seborrheic keratosis
   c. Actinic keratosis
   d. Lichen planus

3. Which of the following is *not* a finding in asthma?
   a. Shortened expiratory phase
   b. Wheezing
   c. Tachypnea, dyspnea
   d. Diminished lung sounds

4. Which of the following is consistent with a diagnosis of mild persistent asthma?
   a. Symptoms fewer than twice a week
   b. Daily symptoms
   c. Symptoms 3–6 days of the week
   d. Nocturnal symptoms less than twice per month

5. Approximately what percentage of tuberculosis infections cause active disease?
   a. 75%
   b. 60%
   c. 30%
   d. 10%

6. Which of the following is considered a positive PPD reaction?
   a. A 35-year-old healthy individual with a tuberculin reaction of 5 mm who has been in close contact with a TB-infected person
   b. A 45-year-old individual who was recently released from 1 year of incarceration with a tuberculin reaction of 5 mm
   c. A 28-year-old individual who has no risk factors with a tuberculin reaction of 10 mm
   d. A 40-year-old individual who has recently immigrated from a country with high TB prevalence with a tuberculin reaction of 5 mm

7. Which of the following is *not* an anticipated symptom of active TB infection?
   a. Tachycardia
   b. Chest pain
   c. Weight loss
   d. Night sweats

8. Which cohort is most frequently affected by migraine headache?
   a. Teenagers
   b. Males and females equally
   c. Females
   d. Postmenopausal women

9. Referral for neurologic evaluation of headaches is indicated when:
   a. New headaches occur in an individual older than 50
   b. There is a family history of stroke
   c. Focal neurologic deficits precede headache episodes
   d. New "triggers" are identified in migraine pattern

10. Important nonpharmacologic treatments for acute low back pain do *not* include:
    a. Continuation of daily activities
    b. Heat application
    c. Strength-building exercises
    d. Bed rest

11. Osteoarthritis may be distinguished from rheumatoid arthritis by:
    a. The severity of pain reported
    b. Asymmetry of involvement
    c. The joints involved
    d. Length of time symptoms have been in evidence

12. "RICE" therapy refers to:
    a. A nonpharmacologic therapy plan for muscle injuries
    b. A bland diet therapy for nausea and vomiting
    c. A weight loss plan
    d. A combination therapy for peptic ulcer disease

13. A 46-year-old female presents with complaints of worsening low back pain after lifting a heavy object the previous day. She has a history of intermittent low back pain in the last year, but notes the pain is now radiating down her right leg. No complaints of trouble with urination or bowel movements. On exam, there is decreased range of motion of the spine in all planes. Straight leg raising at 35 degrees is positive on the right. Achilles tendon reflex on the right is diminished compared to the left with decreased sensation over the right lateral foot. The most likely etiology of this patient's symptoms is:
    a. Rupture of the Achilles tendon
    b. Cauda equina syndrome
    c. Herniated disc involving L5 root
    d. Herniated disc involving the S1 root

14. A 27-year-old female presents with moderate sore throat, runny nose, cough, and general malaise for the past 2 days. Physical examination reveals temperature of 99.8°F, mild pharyngeal erythema, and no exudates. Appropriate management includes:
    a. CBC with differential
    b. Rapid strep antigen test
    c. Saline gargles
    d. Antibiotic treatment

15. Risk of vertical transmission of the HIV virus has been reduced by:
    a. Artificial rupture of membranes at 38 weeks
    b. Antiretroviral treatment of infants
    c. Stopping maternal therapy in pregnancy in order to reduce CD4+ counts
    d. Antiretroviral therapy during pregnancy

16. The confirmatory test for HIV infection is:
    a. Enzyme-linked immunosorbent assay (ELISA)
    b. Quantitative plasma HIV RNA
    c. CD4+ lymphocyte count
    d. Western blot

17. An important principle of antiretroviral therapy is:
    a. Response to drug therapy is monitored with CD4+ counts
    b. Monotherapy is recommended
    c. Response to drug therapy is monitored by HIV RNA levels
    d. Therapy should be started when symptoms first appear

18. A 34-year-old female presents with a 2-month history of a nonproductive cough associated with shortness of breath. She complains of fatigue and has noted an intermittent fever for the past 6 weeks. Significant cervical, inguinal, and axillary lymphadenopathy is noted. Her HIV test is positive. Chest X-ray shows a bilateral infiltrate, and she is diagnosed with pneumocystis pneumonia (PCP). HIV infection produces a spectrum of disease. This patient's symptoms place her in which stage of HIV infection?
    a. Acute HIV infection
    b. Asymptomatic infection
    c. Early symptomatic infection
    d. AIDS

19. For the client described in the previous question, INH prophylaxis would be recommended if her PPD was:
    a. ≥ 5 mm
    b. ≥ 10 mm
    c. ≥ 15 mm
    d. ≥ 20 mm

20. Risk factors for systemic lupus erythematosus (SLE) include all but which of the following?
    a. Female gender
    b. Reproductive age group
    c. First-degree relative with SLE
    d. Caucasian race

21. Diagnosis of SLE is made by:
    a. Abnormal antinuclear antibodies (ANA) titer
    b. Presence of at least four combined signs, symptoms, and laboratory findings
    c. Presence of a specific hematologic disorder on a single occasion
    d. Identification of an immunologic disorder such as abnormal anti-DNA

22. Systemic lupus erythematosus is usually characterized by:
    a. Periods of exacerbation and remission
    b. Slow, steady disease progression
    c. Initial symptoms of typical skin eruptions
    d. Remission in pregnancy

23. Which of the following is *not* suspect in the etiology of rheumatoid arthritis?
    a. Genetic factors
    b. Environmental factors
    c. Hormonal factors
    d. Joint trauma

24. The World Health Organization standard for anemia diagnosis in women is:
    a. Hemoglobin < 10 g/dL
    b. Hemoglobin < 11 g/dL
    c. Hemoglobin < 12 g/dL
    d. Hemoglobin < 13 g/dL

25. Otitis media is suspected when deep ear pain develops concurrent with or following:
    a. An acute allergic reaction
    b. An asthma attack
    c. An upper respiratory infection
    d. Persistent headache

26. A patient presents with moderate scratchy sensation in her right eye and a watery discharge that started about 24 hours ago. She states she is just getting over a cold. Appropriate treatment would include:
    a. Antibiotics
    b. Comfort measures only
    c. Mast cell stabilizer
    d. Topical antihistamine

27. Antibiotic treatment should be initiated for the patient with sinusitis who has:
    a. Increased pain when bends over or with sudden head movement
    b. Symptoms that have worsened again within 10 days of improvement
    c. Symptoms that started within the first week of onset of an upper respiratory infection
    d. Yellow/green nasal discharge

28. A 21-year-old female presents with symptoms suggestive of infectious mononucleosis. Which of the following does *not* support the diagnosis?
    a. Pharyngitis
    b. Positive monospot/heterophile antibody test
    c. CBC with atypical lymphocytes
    d. Cough

29. The group most often affected by infectious mononucleosis is:
    a. Prepubertal children
    b. Women of reproductive age
    c. Females at any age
    d. Teens to early twenties

30. The most common reason for painless rectal bleeding with defecation is:
    a. External hemorrhoids
    b. Internal hemorrhoids
    c. Rectal polyps
    d. Colorectal cancer

31. A 21-year-old female complains of intermittent abdominal pain, bloating, and loose stools 3–4 times a month for the past 3 months. Which of the following additional information would lead you toward a diagnosis of irritable bowel syndrome?
    a. Abdominal pain is relieved with defecation
    b. Antacids relieve the pain
    c. She is awakened at night by need to defecate
    d. She has noted a small amount of bright red blood in the loose stools

32. For the client described in the previous question, initial management of symptoms may include:
    a. Alosetron
    b. Fiber supplements
    c. Lubiprostone
    d. Trial of elimination of dairy products

33. African American women are at increased risk for:
    a. Systemic lupus erythematosus
    b. Skin cancer
    c. Iron-deficiency anemia
    d. Tinea corporis

34. Appendicitis typically presents with which of the following?
    a. High fever as the initial symptom
    b. Pain beginning in the right-lower quadrant (RLQ)
    c. Diarrhea as the initial symptom
    d. Pain in periumbilical area followed by localization to the RLQ

35. Peptic ulcer disease associated with presence of *H. pylori* can be diagnosed by:
    a. Visualization of *H. pylori* on Gram-stained preparation
    b. Negative urea breath analysis
    c. Negative urease assay via endoscopy
    d. Serology positive for *H. pylori* antibodies

36. Initial laboratory evaluation of a patient presenting with symptoms suggestive of acute viral hepatitis should include:
    a. IgG anti-HAV
    b. HBsAg and IgM anti-HBc
    c. IgM anti-HAV
    d. HbsAg, IgM anti-HBc, and IgM anti-HAV

37. The primary goal of pharmacologic therapy for acute viral hepatitis B is:
    a. Prevention of secondary infection
    b. Relief of symptoms
    c. Reduction of infectivity
    d. Prevention of complications

38. Most gallstones are composed of:
    a. Precipitated bile salts
    b. Precipitated calcium salts
    c. Cholesterol
    d. Pigments

39. A 45-year-old female presents with right-upper quadrant (RUQ) pain that radiates to the right infrascapular area. The pain is described as colicky and was precipitated by eating pizza. Onset of the symptom was a few hours ago, and the pain is beginning to ease. There was associated nausea and vomiting. The initial study of choice in this patient is:
    a. Plain abdominal radiograph
    b. Ultrasound
    c. Computerized tomography (CT)
    d. Percutaneous transhepatic cholangiogram

40. Among the following causes of viral hepatitis, which of the following is most likely to lead to chronic infection and is the most common reason for liver transplantation?
    a. Hepatitis A
    b. Hepatitis B
    c. Hepatitis C
    d. Hepatitis D

41. Patients with acute cholecystitis should be advised:
    a. To undertake strict weight reduction diets if obese
    b. Of the likelihood of recurrence
    c. That immediate surgery is a recommended treatment
    d. Of the availability of lithotripsy as a highly successful treatment

42. A 35-year-old overweight female presents with intermittent heartburn for several months. The use of Tums antacid provides temporary relief. During the past week, she has been awakened during the night with a burning sensation in her chest. She is not taking any other medications and has no major health problems. What additional information would support a diagnosis of gastroesophageal reflux disease (GERD) as the cause of her symptoms?
    a. She has occasional nausea and vomiting
    b. She often notes coughing during the night and a bad taste in her mouth
    c. The pain is usually relieved by eating
    d. Constipation has been a chronic problem and she uses laxatives twice a week

43. Your patient in the previous question denies weight loss, dysphagia, and dark, tarry stools. What is your next step?
    a. Order an endoscopic exam
    b. Start her on H₂ receptor blockers
    c. Tell her to eat a snack before bedtime
    d. Refer her to a gastroenterologist

44. Assuming a diagnosis of GERD, you would advise that:
    a. She probably has a hiatal hernia causing the reflux
    b. She will likely require surgery
    c. She should avoid dairy products
    d. High-fat foods and chocolate will likely aggravate the problem

45. The laboratory diagnosis of diabetes mellitus can be determined by:
    a. Fasting plasma glucose ≥ 126 mg/dL
    b. A 2-hour postprandial glucose ≥ 126 mg/dL
    c. HbA₁c > 5.5%
    d. Random glucose ≥ 150 mg/dL

46. A 26-year-old female presents with complaint of watery diarrhea, abdominal cramping, and nausea that started a few days after she returned from a trip to Mexico. She has not noted any blood in her stools and has no fever. You suspect traveler's diarrhea. The most common causative agent is:
    a. *E. coli*
    b. *Giardia lamblia*
    c. Norwalk virus
    d. *Staphylococcus*

47. A 40-year-old patient started taking nicotinic acid and simvastatin 1 week ago as part of the management of her dyslipidemia. She reports facial flushing and itching shortly after taking her medications every day. Appropriate advice would include:
    a. Discontinue the nicotinic acid because this is an allergic reaction
    b. Take aspirin about 30 minutes before taking the nicotinic acid
    c. Take one medication in the morning and the other in the evening
    d. Take both medications after a full meal each day

48. The condition comprising 90% of hyperthyroidism is:
    a. Graves' disease
    b. Thyroiditis
    c. Toxic goiter
    d. Adenoma

49. Infiltrative ophthalmopathy (exophthalmos) is unique to which of the following disorders?
    a. Graves' disease
    b. Hashimoto's thyroiditis
    c. Toxic multinodular goiter
    d. Papillary thyroid carcinoma

50. Which of the following test results would be expected with primary hyperthyroidism?
    a. Low serum TSH and elevated free T_4
    b. Low serum TSH and low free T_4
    c. High serum TSH and elevated free T_4
    d. High serum TSH and low free T_4

51. A patient with a history of radioactive iodine treatment for Graves' disease presents with fatigue, weight gain, and dry skin. You would expect this patient to have which of the following laboratory findings?
    a. Low T_3, low TSH, high total T_4
    b. Low TSH, high total T_4, normal free T_4
    c. High TSH, low free T_4
    d. High TSH, high free T_4

52. A 35-year-old female was diagnosed with Hashimoto thyroiditis and placed on 0.1 mg of levothyroxine. After 1 week of treatment, the patient states that she still feels fatigued. How would you manage this patient?
    a. Increase the dose of levothyroxine to 0.125 mg
    b. Schedule an appointment this week to have a TSH drawn
    c. Add propranolol to the regimen
    d. No change in levothyroxine is indicated at this time

53. A factor *not* associated with exacerbations of facial acne is:
    a. Hormonal cycling
    b. Stress
    c. Fried foods
    d. Cosmetics

54. The most important point to stress with female patients using isotretinoin for acne is:
    a. Possibility of hematologic disturbances
    b. Rare occurrence of pseudotumor cerebri
    c. Necessity for highly effective contraception
    d. Avoiding alcohol while on this drug

55. An 18-year-old presents with open and closed comedones and a few scattered papules. The most appropriate first-line treatment would be:
    a. Topical antibiotics
    b. Oral tetracycline
    c. Tretinoin cream (Retin-A)
    d. Isotretinoin (Accutane)

56. The most common form of skin cancer is:
    a. Squamous cell
    b. Basal cell
    c. Malignant melanoma
    d. Basal cell nevus syndrome

57. A 60-year-old presents with a pearly, translucent smooth papule with rolled edges and surface telangiectasias on her forehead. She notes that it has been there for at least a year but has recently increased in size. The lesion most likely represents which of the following?

    a. Squamous cell carcinoma
    b. Basal cell carcinoma
    c. Seborrheic keratosis
    d. Malignant melanoma

58. Education for the woman with systemic lupus erythematosus (SLE) should include which of the following?
    a. She should not use hormonal contraception
    b. She should receive annual live attenuated influenza vaccine
    c. If she becomes pregnant, a C-section will be planned to avoid stress of labor
    d. She should use sunscreen and protective clothing when outdoors

59. Which of the following is *not* a risk factor for malignant melanoma?
    a. Hispanic ethnicity
    b. Multiple pigmented nevi
    c. Severe childhood sunburn
    d. Family history

60. A 20-year-old female presents with two annular lesions with a scaly border and central clearing on her trunk. The lesions have been present for 1 week and are mildly pruritic. What is the most likely diagnosis?
    a. Psoriasis
    b. Pityriasis rosea
    c. Tinea versicolor
    d. Tinea corporis

61. A 20-year-old female presents with complaint of itching, red eye with a sticky, yellow discharge that started in one eye yesterday afternoon and this morning is in both eyes. She states no fever or other symptoms. The most likely diagnosis is:
    a. Allergic conjunctivitis
    b. Bacterial conjunctivitis
    c. Chemical exposure conjunctivitis
    d. Viral conjunctivitis

62. The most common reason for lumbosacral back pain is:
    a. Herniated disc
    b. Muscle strain
    c. Neoplasm
    d. Arthritis

63. A 28-year-old female presents with complaints of low back pain after helping a friend move 2 days ago. She denies any radiation of the pain, numbness, or tingling in the lower extremities or problems with elimination. On physical exam, mild paravertebral muscle spasm is noted with decreased range of motion of the spine. There are no focal neurologic findings. Appropriate management would include:
    a. Radiograph of the lumbosacral spine
    b. Bed rest for 3–4 days
    c. NSAIDs
    d. Referral to neurologist

64. The frequency of sickle cell crises may be reduced by:
    a. Activity restrictions
    b. Oxygen therapy
    c. Aggressive treatment of infections
    d. High-protein diet

65. Which of the following is an expected finding in tinea unguium?
    a. Hair loss in affected areas
    b. Negative KOH slide preparation
    c. Yellowish, thickened nails
    d. Crusted ulcerations

66. Approximately 10% of those infected with hepatitis B virus become chronic carriers of the disease, a state putting them at risk for:
    a. Hepatocellular carcinoma
    b. Mononucleosis
    c. Gall bladder disease
    d. Chronic immunocompromised status

67. Your patient's blood work returns with a positive hepatitis B surface antigen (HbsAg). This suggests:
    a. Chronic liver disease
    b. Previous infection with hepatitis B virus
    c. Acute or chronic infection with hepatitis B virus
    d. Recent vaccination

68. General principles of drug therapy for hypertension include setting blood pressure goals and initial blood pressure–lowering medication based on all of the following *except*:
    a. Age
    b. Chronic kidney disease
    c. Diabetes
    d. Obesity

69. Management of constipation should include:
    a. Routine use of stool softeners
    b. Bulk-forming agents for acute constipation
    c. Hyperosmolar laxatives (sorbitol) as initial treatment for chronic constipation
    d. Saline laxatives (milk of magnesia) for acute constipation

70. A 38-year-old female presents with complaint of fever, chills, a cough, and dyspnea on exertion. She has no chronic health problems and has been healthy over the past year. Physical examination findings include fever of 100.8°F, heart rate 88 beats per minute, and respiratory rate 24 breaths per minute. Signs and symptoms that would lead to a diagnosis of a viral rather than bacterial pneumonia would include:
    a. Blood-streaked mucoid sputum
    b. Pleuritic chest pain
    c. Rales that clear with coughing
    d. Reported spikes in temperature to above 102°F

71. You suspect that the patient in the previous question does have viral community-acquired pneumonia. Appropriate management would include:
    a. Comfort measures with antibiotics if symptoms persist more than 5 days
    b. Ordering a sputum culture before any antibiotic treatment
    c. Treatment with azithromycin
    d. Treatment with levofloxacin

72. Which of the following most likely suggests a secondary cause of hypertension?
    a. BMI greater than 30
    b. Abdominal bruit
    c. Total cholesterol greater than 280
    d. Enlarged spleen

73. Choices of initial antihypertension medication for a 45-year-old African American female with hypertension but otherwise healthy may include:
    a. Angiotensin-converting enzyme (ACE) inhibitor
    b. Angiotensin II receptor blockers (ARBs)
    c. Calcium channel blocker (CCB)
    d. Potassium-sparing diuretic

74. A 21-year-old comes to the clinic with complaint of amenorrhea. She also complains of feeling cold all of the time. Physical examination reveals an underweight female with heart rate of 58 beats per minute and blood pressure 96/52 mm Hg. Pregnancy test is negative. Which of the following additional findings would contribute to a diagnosis of anorexia nervosa?
    a. Currently on probation for shoplifting
    b. Fine body hair on extremities
    c. Migraine headaches
    d. Swollen parotid glands

75. Common physical findings with allergic rhinitis include:
    a. Facial tenderness
    b. Inflamed nasal mucosa
    c. Nasal crease
    d. Purulent nasal discharge

76. The recommended initial test for deep vein thrombosis (DVT) in a symptomatic patient is:
    a. Plasma D-dimer
    b. Contrast venography
    c. Antithrombin III
    d. Duplex ultrasound

77. Which of the following is *not* a recommended treatment for superficial thrombophlebitis?
    a. Compression with an ace wrap
    b. Elevation of affected limb
    c. Heparin
    d. Nonsteroidal anti-inflammatory drugs (NSAIDs)

78. The National Cholesterol Education Program recommends hyperlipidemia screening every _____ years beginning at age 20.
    a. 5
    b. 3
    c. 2
    d. 1

79. A 44-year-old female presents with type 2 diabetes and hyperlipidemia. Which of the following should be your main treatment goal?
    a. HDL > 40 mg/dL
    b. LDL cholesterol < 100 mg/dL
    c. Total cholesterol < 200 mg/dL, LDL cholesterol < 100 mg/dL
    d. Triglycerides < 250 mg/dL

80. A 50-year-old female patient presents with complaint of severe pain that started in her upper mid abdomen that now is worse in the right-upper quadrant (RUQ) of her abdomen. She has also had nausea and vomiting. On deep palpation of her RUQ, she momentarily holds her breath on inspiration. You suspect:
    a. Appendicitis
    b. Acute cholecystitis
    c. Pancreatitis
    d. Peptic ulcer disease

81. A microcytic anemia with a low serum ferritin is likely secondary to:
   a. Anemia of chronic disease
   b. Iron deficiency
   c. Hypersplenism
   d. Thalassemia minor

82. The use of statins for pharmacologic therapy of hyperlipidemia is:
   a. Category B use in pregnancy
   b. Category C use in pregnancy
   c. Category D use in pregnancy
   d. Category X use in pregnancy

83. Of the following signs and symptoms, fibromyalgia most commonly presents with:
   a. Abrupt onset of proximal muscle weakness
   b. Widespread musculoskeletal pain and tender points
   c. Effusion of involved joints with mild local warmth
   d. Subcutaneous nodules

84. Secondary causes for high blood cholesterol do *not* include:
   a. Hypertension
   b. Obstructive liver disease
   c. Medication-induced states
   d. Hypothyroidism

85. A systolic click preceding a mid to late systolic murmur is most likely caused by which of the following?
   a. Aortic stenosis
   b. Mitral valve prolapse
   c. Mitral valve stenosis
   d. Idiopathic hypertrophic subaortic stenosis

86. Which of the following is *not* a common finding with an innocent murmur?
   a. Heard best with patient supine
   b. Increases with increased cardiac output
   c. Increases with Valsava maneuver
   d. Most frequently heard during systole

87. The leading killer of women in the United States is:
   a. Coronary heart disease
   b. Lung cancer
   c. Ovarian cancer
   d. Violence

88. Virchow's triad defines the clinical origin of most venous thrombi and includes all of the following factors *except*:
   a. Stasis
   b. Endothelial damage
   c. Deposition of cholesterol plaques
   d. Hypercoagulability

89. A patient presents with signs and symptoms suggestive of a superficial phlebitis. Physical findings in this patient would include:
   a. Tenderness in the area of the involved vein
   b. Edema of the involved extremity
   c. Pale, cool skin in the area of involved vein
   d. Palpable venous cord

90. In the United States, the most common cause of community-acquired bacterial pneumonia is:
   a. *Streptococcus pneumoniae*
   b. *Streptococcus pyogenes*
   c. *Haemophilus influenzae*
   d. *Legionella pneumophilia*

91. A 24-year-old female with asthma classified as mild persistent is considering pregnancy. She currently uses an albuterol metered dose inhaler and the inhaled corticosteroid budesonide. Advice concerning her asthma and pregnancy should include:
   a. Exacerbations during pregnancy are common but will not harm the fetus/infant
   b. It is safer to be treated for asthma during pregnancy than to have symptoms and exacerbations
   c. Oral corticosteroids should be initiated prior to conception so that asthma is well controlled in early pregnancy
   d. The medications she is currently using are contraindicated during pregnancy

92. American College of Rheumatology (2010) criteria for a diagnosis of rheumatoid arthritis include:
   a. Fever
   b. Elevated erythrocyte sedimentation rate
   c. Joint erosion on radiography
   d. Symmetrical joint involvement

93. Your patient is experiencing 3–4 migraine headaches per month. You decide to begin prophylactic medication. Which of the following is recommended for migraine headache prophylaxis?
   a. Ergotamine
   b. Propranolol (beta blocker)
   c. Sumatriptan
   d. SSRI

94. Which of the following is true concerning the treatment of rheumatoid arthritis?
   a. NSAIDs and corticosteroids are important for long-term management
   b. The main mechanism of action of disease-modifying anti-rheumatic drugs (DMARD) is analgesia
   c. Nonbiologic and biologic DMARDs may be combined if monotherapy is not effective
   d. Methotrexate is the preferred DMARD for use by pregnant women with RA

95. Metabolic syndrome is defined as having at least three of a set of five risk factors. One of these risk factors for women is:
   a. Blood pressure 150/90 mm Hg or higher
   b. HDL-C 40 mg/dL or less
   c. Triglycerides 200 mg/dL or higher
   d. Waist circumference greater than 35 inches

96. Acute otitis media is characterized by all of the following physical examination findings *except*:
   a. Distorted light reflex
   b. Obscured bony landmarks
   c. Erythema of the ear canal
   d. Preauricular lymphadenopathy

97. Laboratory tests supportive of a diagnosis of infectious mononucleosis include all of the following *except*:
   a. Elevated basophils and eosinophils
   b. Presence of heterophil antibodies
   c. Elevated liver enzymes
   d. GABHS on throat culture

98. Secondary causes of seizures include:
    a. Syncope
    b. Hyperventilation
    c. Narcolepsy
    d. Toxic substance abuse

99. The most common type of seizure disorder in adults is:
    a. Clonic-tonic
    b. Partial
    c. Complex partial
    d. Grand mal

100. Macrocytic anemias include:
    a. Anemia of chronic disease
    b. Vitamin B_{12}–deficiency anemia
    c. Iron-deficiency anemia
    d. Sickle cell anemia

101. A 52-year-old menopausal female client smokes one pack of cigarettes per day and has a history of a deep vein thrombosis in her leg 2 years ago. She has a BMD T-score of –1.75. Which of the following medications would be the most appropriate for this client to prevent osteoporosis?
    a. Alendronate
    b. Calcitonin
    c. Estrogen
    d. Raloxifene

102. Which of the following statements is correct concerning bone mineral density (BMD) testing?
    a. Test results are most predictive of bone fracture when done on an annual basis
    b. The T-score compares BMD of the client with an age-matched normal adult
    c. BMD T-scores should be combined with bone X-ray to confirm osteoporosis
    d. Treatment decisions based on T-scores may vary according to risk factors

103. A 40-year-old female has complaints of chronic backache and has been diagnosed to have a vertebral compression fracture. She also has hirsutism, facial acne, and red-purple abdominal striae. An appropriate initial test for a possible secondary cause for osteoporosis in this client would be:
    a. Dexamethasone suppression test
    b. Parathyroid hormone level
    c. Protein electrophoresis
    d. Thyroid function tests

104. Client instructions for taking alendronate should include:
    a. Take medication with breakfast
    b. Take medication at bedtime
    c. Take medication on an empty stomach
    d. Take medication with an antacid

105. One of the most significant laboratory tests for evaluating an individual for chronic or heavy alcohol use is a/an:
    a. ALP
    b. BUN
    c. CBC
    d. GGT

106. Which of the following is a characteristic finding with stimulant abuse, but not depressant abuse?
    a. Euphoria
    b. Pupil dilation
    c. Tremors
    d. Violent behavior

107. Two months after being raped, a client tells you she cannot concentrate on her schoolwork and is having nightmares about the experience. These symptoms indicate that she:
    a. Is still in the acute phase of rape trauma syndrome
    b. Is going through normal reorganization following a rape
    c. Is experiencing post-traumatic stress disorder
    d. Now has a generalized anxiety disorder

108. A client who has been experiencing fatigue, insomnia, difficulty concentrating, and feelings of worthlessness for the past 2 weeks would meet the *DSM-IV* criteria for a major depressive disorder if she also has:
    a. Loss of interest in her usual activities
    b. Psychomotor retardation
    c. Psychosomatic complaints
    d. Suicidal ideation

109. Contraceptive counseling for a 24-year-old female with diabetes who has no complications or other health problems should include:
    a. Combination hormonal contraceptives are contraindicated
    b. Progestin-only methods are a better choice than are those containing estrogen
    c. She can use any of the long-acting reversible contraceptives
    d. She should complete her childbearing by age 30 and consider sterilization

110. A 24-year-old female client with major depression tells you that she feels like her life is falling apart with no hope of improving. She recently lost her job, had to move out of her apartment, and now lives with her sister. Her risk factors for a suicide attempt include:
    a. Age between 20 and 30 years
    b. Female gender
    c. Current living situation
    d. Sense of hopelessness

111. A client tells you that she has experienced chest tightness, difficulty breathing, and dizziness whenever she rides on the city bus. She has been trying to find other transportation because she is very fearful about these symptoms recurring. Her symptoms best fit a description of:
    a. Acute stress disorder
    b. Panic disorder with agoraphobia
    c. Obsessive-compulsive disorder
    d. Social phobia

112. The most common type of anxiety disorder is:
    a. Generalized anxiety disorder
    b. Specific phobia
    c. Panic disorder
    d. Post-traumatic stress disorder

113. Which of the following statements concerning bulimia is correct?
    a. Age of onset is usually early adolescence
    b. Amenorrhea is usually present
    c. Mortality rate is higher than for anorexia nervosa
    d. Impulsive behavior is a common characteristic

114. Major side effects of SSRIs include:
    a. Anticholinergic effects
    b. Nausea
    c. Orthostatic hypotension
    d. Urinary retention

115. A 35-year-old female with a history of generalized anxiety disorder requests a refill of alprazolam. You are concerned about risks associated with long-term use. Which of the following represents an alternative medication?
    a. Buspirone (Buspar)
    b. Clonazepam (Klonopin)
    c. Bupropion (Wellbutrin)
    d. Citalopram (Celexa)

116. A behavior that fits the criteria for substance dependence but not for substance abuse is:
    a. Loss of a job related to substance use
    b. Driving while intoxicated
    c. Continuing to drink despite family's objections
    d. Unsuccessful attempts to cut down use

117. Physical findings that help the clinician to make a diagnosis of bulimia would include:
    a. Erosion of tooth enamel
    b. Hypotension

    c. Presence of lanugo
    d. Stress fractures

118. Which of the following statements concerning rape is correct?
    a. All of the states have now established the same legal definition for rape
    b. The majority of rapes are committed by acquaintances of the victim
    c. The most common emotional response of the victim in the acute phase is anger
    d. The clinician is responsible for determining whether a rape has actually occurred

119. The recommended initial pharmacologic agent for type 2 diabetes is:
    a. Insulin
    b. Metformin
    c. Sulfonylurea
    d. Thiazolidinedione

120. Severe exacerbations in an individual with intermittent (step 1) asthma are appropriately treated with:
    a. Mast-cell stabilizers
    b. Short-acting inhaled B_2 agonists
    c. Systemic corticosteroids
    d. Theophylline

Answers with Rationales

1. c. A physiologic (innocent) murmur
   Pregnant women may have grade 1 or 2 systolic murmurs due to physiologic increased cardiac output.

2. c. Actinic keratosis
   Sixty percent of squamous cell carcinoma occurs at site of previous actinic keratosis.

3. a. Shortened expiratory phase
   Physical respiratory findings in asthma include hyperresonance with percussion, wheezing, prolonged expiratory phase, and diminished breath sounds, tachypnea, and dyspnea.

4. c. Symptoms 3–6 days of the week
   Symptoms 3–6 days of the week with nocturnal symptoms 3–4 times a month is classified as mild persistent asthma.

5. d. 10%
   The asymptomatic state (latent TB infection) may last months to years with 10% going on to develop active TB.

6. a. 35-year-old healthy individual with a tuberculin reaction of 5 mm who has been in close contact with a TB-infected person
   A 5-mm or greater skin reaction on PPD test is considered positive in individuals who are HIV positive, immunocompromised, with abnormal chest radiograph findings consistent with healed TB lesions, or in recent close contacts with a TB-infected person.

7. a. Tachycardia
   Individuals with active TB may have generalized symptoms of night sweats, fever, malaise, weakness, anorexia and weight loss, and pulmonary symptoms of productive cough, hemoptysis, chest pain, and dyspnea.

8. c. Females

An estimated 10% of adults are affected by migraines. Migraines are reported in 15–17% of women and 5% of men.

9. a. New headaches occur in an individual older than 50
   Referral is indicated for the following individuals: focal neurologic findings, specific secondary diagnosis is suspected, chronic headaches develop new features, new headaches in individuals older than 50 years.

10. d. Bed rest
    Nonpharmacologic interventions for managing lower back pain include continuation of daily activities rather than bed rest, in addition to local application of heat, warm baths, physical therapy program to improve strength and conditioning, and low-stress aerobic exercise—walking, biking, swimming.

11. b. Asymmetry of involvement
    Symptoms for osteoarthritis commonly present in asymmetrical fashion, while rheumatoid arthritis and systemic lupus erythematosus are inflammatory and symmetrically distributed.

12. a. A nonpharmacologic therapy plan for muscle injuries
    "RICE" is the mnemonic to remember the initial therapeutic strategy for muscle injuries. It stands for:
    *R*est or immobilization of injured part
    *I*ce or application of cold
    *C*ompression, elastic wrap
    *E*levation of affected area

13. d. Herniated disc involving the S1 root
    A herniated disc is characterized by radicular pain; paresthesias may occur in distribution of involved nerve root. Most common disc ruptures involve the L5 or S1 nerve roots. S1 root/L5–S1 disc involves pain in the buttocks, lateral leg, and malleolus and numbness in lateral foot and posterior calf.

14. c. Saline gargles

Symptomatic relief measures are appropriate for this individual. Rapid streptococcal antigen test is recommended for adult with pharyngitis that meets two or more of the following criteria: fever, lack of cough, tonsillar exudates, tender anterior cervical adenopathy.

15. d. Antiretroviral therapy during pregnancy

The risk of vertical transmission of the HIV virus from HIV-positive mother to infant may be reduced to less than 1% if mother receives multiagent antiretroviral therapy and has undetectable viral load at delivery.

16. d. Western blot

Confirmatory tests are highly specific for detecting HIV antibodies and are indicated if the individual has a positive HIV screening test. The indirect immunofluorescence assay (Western blot) is a commonly used confirmatory test.

17. c. Response to drug therapy is monitored by HIV RNA levels

HIV RNA levels are useful for predicting progression of disease by indicating viral load and are used to monitor antiretroviral therapy.

18. d. AIDS

Pneumocystis (*carinii*) *jiroveci* pneumonia (PCP) is an opportunistic infection that rarely occurs in healthy people. Most opportunistic infections occur in HIV-infected individuals with a CD4+ count less than 200 cells/mm³. PCP is a major AIDS-defining diagnosis.

19. a. ≥ 5 mm

A 5-mm or greater skin reaction on PPD test is considered positive in individuals who are HIV positive, immunocompromised, with abnormal chest radiograph findings consistent with healed TB lesions, or in recent close contacts with a TB-infected person.

20. d. Caucasian race

Risk factors for systemic lupus erythematosus (SLE) include being of African American or Hispanic descent or having a first-degree relative with SLE.

21. b. Presence of at least four combined signs, symptoms, and laboratory findings

The American College of Rheumatology has set the SLE diagnostic criteria to include the presence of at least 4 of 11 criteria. Criteria include presence of specific dermatologic symptoms; arthritis; serositis; renal, neurologic, and hematologic conditions; positive ANA test; and other immunologic positive tests.

22. a. Periods of exacerbation and remission

SLE is a chronic, inflammatory, multisystem disorder of the immune system characterized by periods of remission and exacerbation with the course of disease unpredictable and highly variable.

23. d. Joint trauma

The exact etiology of rheumatoid arthritis (RA) is unknown. The cause is likely a complex including genetic, environmental, and perhaps hormonal factors.

24. c. Hemoglobin < 12 g/dL

According to the World Health Organization, anemia is defined as < 12 g/dL for women and <13 g/dL for men.

25. c. An upper respiratory infection

Eustachian tube dysfunction secondary to URI (often viral) or allergies causes edema and congestion that impedes flow of middle ear secretions; accumulation of secretions promotes growth of pathogens.

26. b. Comfort measures only

Viral conjunctivitis usually has an acute onset, mild symptoms in one or both eyes, and a watery discharge. It is may be associated with an upper respiratory infection and is self-limited. Cold compresses and liquid tears may offer relief of symptoms.

27. b. Symptoms that have worsened again within 10 days of improvement

Antibiotic treatment for acute sinusitis should be initiated if signs and symptoms are present 10 or more days after onset of upper respiratory symptoms or if symptoms improve and then within 10 days they worsen again.

28. d. Cough

The classic triad of symptoms for mononucleosis is fever, sore throat, and swollen lymph nodes (particularly the anterior and posterior cervical chain). A monospot/heterophile antibody test will usually be positive within 1 to 2 weeks after onset of symptoms. The CBC will show lymphocytic leukocytosis with 10% of cells atypical.

29. d. Teens to early twenties

Most clinically apparent mononucleosis infections occur in individuals 10 to 30 years old, with a peak rate in ages 15 to 19 years old.

30. b. Internal hemorrhoids

Internal hemorrhoids originate above the anorectal line, are covered by nonsensitive rectal mucosa, and are usually painless. They may present with bright red bleeding during defecation.

31. a. Abdominal pain is relieved with defecation

Abdominal pain and bloating are often relieved at least temporarily with defecation in patients with irritable bowel syndrome (IBS). IBS is not characterized by symptoms that awaken the patient at night or by blood in the stools.

32. d. Trial of elimination of dairy products

A 2-week trial of lactose-free, fructose-free, or sorbitol-free foods (one at a time) may be considered to rule out food intolerance in a patient who has bloating, gas, abdominal distention, and diarrhea. Alosetron should be limited to use in women with severe chronic diarrhea–predominant IBS not responsive to conventional therapy. Lubiprostone and fiber supplements may be appropriate for the patient with constipation-dominant IBS.

33. a. Systemic lupus erythematosus

The prevalence of SLE is much higher in African American women (1 in 250) and Hispanic women (100 in 100,000) than in Caucasian women (12–39 in 100,000).

34. d. Pain in periumbilical area followed by localization to the RLQ

Pain is the initial symptom in appendicitis beginning in the epigastrum or periumbilical area and localizing to the RLQ after several hours.

35. d. Serology positive for *H. pylori* antibodies

A serologic ELISA test detects IgG antibodies, indicating current or past infection with *H. pylori*. It may or may not revert to negative after treatment. A positive urea breath test indicates presence of active *H. pylori* infection.

36. d. HBsAg, IgM anti-HBc, and IgM anti-HAV

HBsAg is positive with acute and chronic hepatitis B infection. IgM anti-HBc is positive in the acute stage of hepatitis B infection, and IgM anti-HAV is positive in the acute stage of hepatitis A infection.

37. b. Relief of symptoms

Nonpharmacologic treatment for acute hepatitis B infection includes activity as tolerated, hydration, adequate caloric intake in small feedings, discontinuation of all but essential medications, and avoidance of alcohol. Antiemetics may be indicated for nausea.

38. c. Cholesterol

Approximately 85–95% of gallstones are composed primarily of cholesterol.

39. b. Ultrasound

This patient's symptoms are consistent with acute cholecystitis. Ultrasound has a 95% sensitivity in detecting stones in the gallbladder. It is the best noninvasive imaging technique to diagnose acute cholecystitis.

40. c. Hepatitis C

Up to 80% of patients with hepatitis C will develop chronic hepatitis; 20–30% eventually develop cirrhosis or hepatocellular carcinoma.

41. c. That immediate surgery is a recommended treatment

Acute cholecystitis is managed with hospital admission and early cholecystectomy once the patient is stable.

42. b. She often notes coughing during the night and a bad taste in her mouth

Acid regurgitation with GERD is most common when reclining, straining, bending, or stooping. This can cause coughing and a bad taste in the mouth.

43. b. Start her on H_2 receptor blockers

GI referral and diagnostic evaluation are needed if symptoms are chronic or refractory to therapy, if esophageal complications are suspected, or if the patient has dysphagia, weight loss, or evidence of GI bleeding. H_2 receptor blockers inhibit acid secretions and are effective for less severe GERD.

44. d. High-fat foods and chocolate will likely aggravate the problem

High-fat foods, chocolate, and peppermint decrease lower esophageal pressure, making reflux more likely.

45. a. Fasting plasma glucose ≥ 126 mg/dL

Criteria for diagnosis of diabetes includes any of the following: fasting plasma glucose ≥ 126 mg/dL, 2-hour postprandial glucose ≥ 200 mg/dL, HbA_{1c} ≥ 6.5%, or random glucose ≥ 200 mg/dL with classic symptoms of hyperglycemia or hyperglycemic crisis.

46. a. *E. coli*

The most common causative agent for traveler's diarrhea is *E. coli*.

47. b. Take aspirin about 30 minutes before taking the nicotinic acid

A common side effect of nicotinic acid is flushing and pruritus. This side effect is decreased when the patient takes 325 mg of aspirin or 200 mg ibuprofen 30–60 minutes prior to taking the nicotinic acid.

48. a. Graves' disease

Graves' disease represents 90% of hyperthyroidism. This is an autoimmune condition with excess synthesis and secretion of thyroid hormone caused by antibodies that stimulate TSH receptors.

49. a. Graves' disease

Hyperthyroidism caused by Graves' disease is characterized by exophthalmos.

50. a. Low serum TSH and elevated free T_4

Low TSH is a result of excess circulation of thyroid hormone (T_4, T_3) with hyperthyroidism.

51. c. High TSH, low free T_4

Radioactive iodine treatment for Graves' disease usually results in long-term hypothyroidism—70% of patients at 10 years.

52. d. No change in levothyroxine is indicated at this time

Levothyroxine has a half-life of 6 days and a slow rate of achieving steady state. Adjust dose every 6 weeks until TSH normalizes.

53. c. Fried foods

Factors that can exacerbate acne include stress, hormonal cycling, use of topical steroids, and contact with irritant oils or cosmetics.

54. c. Necessity for highly effective contraception

Isotretinoin is labeled Category X and should not be used in pregnancy because of its detrimental effects to the fetus.

55. c. Tretinoin cream (Retin-A)

Tretinoin cream is an effective comedolytic agent that is applied topically to affected areas.

56. b. Basal cell

Basal cell carcinoma is the most common skin cancer, comprising approximately 75% of all skin cancers, and it affects nearly 1 million people per year in the United States.

57. b. Basal cell carcinoma

Basal cell carcinoma has several clinical variants; nodular basal cell is most common. Basal cell carcinoma presents as waxy, semitranslucent nodules with rolled borders that may have central ulcerations and telangiectasias. They are slow-growing lesions.

58. d. She should use sunscreen and protective clothing when outdoors

Photosensitivity is a characteristic of systemic lupus erythematosus. Malar skin rash and rash on other exposed body parts may occur with sun exposure. Sun exposure may also exacerbate disease activity.

59. a. Hispanic ethnicity

Risk factors for malignant carcinoma include history of changing mole, family and or personal history of melanoma, history of nonmelanoma skin cancer, atypical nevus syndrome, fair complexion, tendency to sunburn.

60. d. Tinea corporis

Classic presentation of tinea is a lesion with central clearing surrounded by an advancing, red, scaly, elevated border. If the tinea is found on the body, it is classified as tinea corporis.

61. b. Bacterial conjunctivitis
    Bacterial conjunctivitis has an acute onset with itchy sensation/discomfort and mucopurulent discharge beginning in one eye and spreading to the other eye.

62. b. Muscle strain
    Lumbosacral strain results from stretching or tearing of muscles, tendons, ligaments, and fascia due to trauma or repetitive mechanical stress.

63. c. NSAIDs
    Lower back pain is located in the back, buttocks, or one or both thighs. Pain is usually aggravated by standing/flexion and relieved with rest/reclining. There is increased pain with flexion and negative straight leg raise (SLR) with a normal neurologic exam. A radiograph of the lumbosacral spine or a referral to the neurologist is not necessary at this time. Bed rest is not recommended for treatment of lower back pain. NSAIDs would be an appropriate management for this patient.

64. c. Aggressive treatment of infections
    Precipitating factors for vaso-occlusive crises include infection, physical or emotional stress, blood loss, pregnancy, surgery, and high altitudes. Aggressive treatment of infections may prevent a crisis for the patient with sickle cell disease.

65. c. Yellowish, thickened nails
    Tinea unguium is characterized by toenails being more frequently involved than fingernails and nails that are yellowish/thickened.

66. a. Hepatocellular carcinoma
    Up to 10% of hepatitis B–infected adults and 90% of those infected as neonates become chronic carriers with increased risk of cirrhosis and hepatocellular carcinoma.

67. c. Acute or chronic infection with hepatitis B virus
    Positive hepatitis B surface antigen (HBsAg) indicates acute or chronic infection with hepatitis B virus. Positive IgM anti-HBc indicates acute infection and disappears in 3–13 months.

68. d. Obesity
    General principles of drug therapy for hypertension include setting blood pressure goals and initiating blood pressure–lowering medication based on age, diabetes, and chronic kidney disease.

69. d. Saline laxatives (milk of magnesia) for acute constipation
    Saline laxatives draw water into the intestinal lumen, causing fecal mass to soften and swell; swelling stretches the intestinal lumen and simulates peristalsis.

70. b. Pleuritic chest pain
    Community-acquired pneumonia typically presents with symptoms of fever, chills, cough, pleuritic chest pain, and dyspnea with exertion. Physical examination findings include tachycardia, tachypnea, rales that do not clear with cough, and rhonchi that may clear with cough. Dullness to percussion and diminished breath sounds may be found in affected lobes. Spikes in fever and blood-tinged mucoid or purulent sputum may be seen with bacterial community-acquired pneumonia.

71. c. Treatment with azithromycin
    Recommended first-line treatment of community-acquired pneumonia whether viral or bacterial is empiric antimicrobial therapy with an advanced generation macrolide such as azithromycin. If the patient has risk factors for drug-resistant

Streptococcus pneumoniae (DRSP), the recommended antibiotic is a respiratory fluoroquinilone.

72. b. Abdominal bruit
    Secondary hypertension may be the result of renal artery stenosis. An abdominal bruit may indicate renal artery stenosis.

73. c. Calcium channel blocker (CCB)
    Initial management of hypertension in African Americans of all ages without diabetes or chronic kidney disease is a thiazide-type diuretic or calcium channel blocker (CCB), alone or in combination

74. b. Fine body hair on extremities
    Physical examination findings with anorexia nervosa include emaciation, dry skin, fine body hair (lanugo), muscle wasting, peripheral edema, bradycardia, arrhythmias, hypotension, delayed sexual maturation, and stress fractures.

75. c. Nasal crease
    A common physical finding with perennial allergic rhinitis is a horizontal crease along the lower bridge of the nose from the patient pushing nose upward and backward because of itching and nasal discharge.

76. d. Duplex ultrasound
    Duplex ultrasound has good sensitivity and specificity for diagnosis of a patient who has intermediate to high probability of deep vein thrombosis (DVT). A negative test, however, does not rule out DVT in the symptomatic patient, so other follow-up tests are needed.

77. c. Heparin
    Treatment for superficial thrombophlebitis includes elevation of the affected limb, compression with an ace wrap, and nonsteroidal anti-inflammatory drugs (NSAIDs).

78. a. 5
    The National Cholesterol Education Program recommends a fasting lipoprotein profile (total cholesterol, LDL-C, HDL-C, triglycerides) every 5 years in patients 20 years or older.

79. b. LDL cholesterol < 100 mg/dL
    Treatment goals for hyperlipidemia are based on risk factors. Diabetes is considered a coronary heart disease (CHD) risk equivalent. The treatment goal for an individual who has hyperlipidemia and clinically manifested CHD or a CHD risk equivalent is an LDL-C of less than 100 mg/dL.

80. b. Acute cholecystitis
    Symptoms of acute cholecystitis include pain that starts in the epigastrum and then moves to the RUQ accompanied with nausea and vomiting. The patient with acute cholecystitis will have a stop in inspiratory effort because of the sharp increase in pain (Murphy's sign) when the RUQ is palpated.

81. b. Iron deficiency
    Diagnostic findings for iron-deficiency anemia include hypochromic microcytic RBCs, MCV less than 80 fL, increased red cell width (RDW), a low serum ferritin less than 10 mg/L, and decreased reticulocyte count.

82. d. Category X use in pregnancy
    The use of HMG-CoA reductase inhibitor (statin) medications for management of hyperlipidemia is contraindicated in pregnancy.

83. b. Widespread musculoskeletal pain and tender points
Fibromyalgia is a syndrome characterized by chronic fatigue, generalized, widespread musculoskeletal pain and stiffness associated with the finding of characteristic tender points of pain on physical examination.

84. a. Hypertension
Secondary causes for high blood cholesterol include obesity, disease processes such as endocrine and metabolic disorders, obstructive liver disease, and renal disorders. Medications such as corticosteroids, thiazide diuretics, and beta blockers may also cause high cholesterol.

85. b. Mitral valve prolapse
A mid or late systolic click is usually caused by mitral valve prolapse. A late systolic murmur may be present if there is mitral valve regurgitation.

86. c. Increases with Valsalva maneuver
Innocent murmurs are usually soft (grade 1 or 2), medium-pitch, systolic murmurs. They are heard best with the patient supine and disappear with standing or straining. They increase with increased cardiac output, for example, pregnancy, exercise, or fever.

87. a. Coronary heart disease
Coronary heart disease is the cause of death of one out of every three women each year.

88. c. Deposition of cholesterol plaques
The origin of most venous thrombi lies in Virchow's triad—endothelial damage, stasis, and hypercoagulability.

89. a. Tenderness in the area of the involved vein
Localized area of edema, erythema, and tenderness of the involved vein in an extremity are suggestive of superficial phlebitis.

90. a. *Streptococcus pneumoniae*
The most common cause of bacterial community-acquired pneumonia is *Streptococcus pneumoniae*.

91. b. It is safer to be treated for asthma during pregnancy than to have symptoms and exacerbations
Asthma exacerbations during pregnancy increase the risk for perinatal mortality, preterm birth, and low-birth-weight infants. First-line treatment during pregnancy includes the short-acting inhaled B_2 agonist albuterol and the inhaled corticosteroid budesonide.

92. b. Elevated erythrocyte sedimentation rate
The 2010 American College of Rheumatology criteria for diagnosis use a score-based algorithm that includes joint involvement (stiffness, swelling), serology (rheumatoid factor, anticitrullinated protein antibody), and acute phase reactants (C-reactive protein, erythrocyte sedimentation rate), and duration of symptoms).

93. b. Propranolol (beta blocker)
For patients who experience more than two severe headaches per month, who need acute treatment medication more than two times per week, or who are unable to tolerate abortive agents, consider prophylactic therapy: beta blockers such as propranolol/timolol, calcium channel blockers, or antiepileptic agents.

94. c. Nonbiologic and biologic DMARDs may be combined if monotherapy is not effective

DMARDs are the preferred therapy for long-term management of rheumatoid arthritis. Methotrexate, a nonbiologic DMARD, is pregnancy Category X.

95. d. Waist circumference greater than 35 inches
Metabolic syndrome is defined as presence of at least three of five risk factors. For women these include abdominal obesity/waist circumference greater than 35 inches, triglycerides 150 mg/dL or greater, HDL-C less than 50 mg/dL, blood pressure 130/85 or greater, and fasting glucose 110 mg/dL or greater.

96. c. Erythema of the ear canal
Common physical examination findings with otitis media include full or bulging tympanic membrane with absent or obscured landmarks, distorted light reflex, and preauricular or cervical lymphadenopathy.

97. d. GABHS on throat culture
Group A beta-hemolytic streptococci (GABHS) may be a secondary infection for consideration but is not diagnostic of mononucleosis.

98. d. Toxic substance abuse
In persons with known seizure disorders, possible causes include sleep deprivation, unusual stresses, menstruation, medications, and drugs, including toxic substances.

99. c. Complex partial
Complex partial seizures are the most common adult type of seizures. Absence seizures are most common in childhood.

100. b. Vitamin B_{12}–deficiency anemia
Macrocytic anemia (MCV > 100 fL) is found in people with vitamin B_{12} deficiency, folate deficiency, liver disease, and hypothyroidism.

101. a. Alendronate
Alendronate is indicated for prevention and treatment of osteoporosis. Given the patient's history of cigarette smoking and DVT, she is not the best candidate for estrogen/hormone therapy because of the possible increased risk of a thromboembolic event. Calcitonin is indicated for treatment only and not for prevention.

102. d. Treatment decisions based on T-scores may vary according to risk factors
Pharmacologic treatment is considered for postmenopausal women presenting with any of the following: hip or vertebral fracture; T-score of –2.5 or less at the femoral neck or spine after appropriate evaluation to exclude secondary causes; T-score between –1.0 and –2.5 at femoral neck or spine and 10-year probability of hip fracture of 3% or greater; or a 10-year probability of major osteoporotic-related fracture of 20% or greater based on U.S.-adapted WHO algorithm.

103. a. Dexamethasone suppression test
Laboratory tests used to rule out secondary causes of osteoporosis include parathyroid hormone (PTH) level, TSH, dexamethasone suppression test, and urine cortisol level for Cushing's syndrome.

104. c. Take medication on an empty stomach
Client instructions for taking alendronate include the following: take medication with 8 oz of water in the morning at least 30 minutes before any beverage, food, or medication and avoid lying down for at least 30 minutes and until the first food of the day.

105. d. GGT
    An elevated gamma glutamyl transferase (GGT) level may indicate heavy or chronic alcohol use.
106. b. Pupil dilation
    Signs and symptoms of both depressant and stimulant abuse may include euphoria, violent or bizarre behavior, and tremors. Pupil dilation may be seen with stimulant use.
107. c. Is experiencing post-traumatic stress disorder
    Post-traumatic stress disorder (PTSD) occurs in 30–65% of sexual assault survivors. PTSD is persistent anxiety lasting more than 1 month following an extremely traumatic event. Inability to concentrate and nightmares are characteristic of PTSD.
108. a. Loss of interest in her usual activities
    Loss of interest in usual activities and/or sad or depressed mood most of the day, every day, are required for diagnosis of major depressive disorder along with a complex of symptoms that may include fatigue, insomnia, difficulty concentrating, feelings of worthlessness, and others.
109. c. She can use any of the long-acting reversible contraceptives
    Women with uncomplicated diabetes of less than 20 years' duration can use any of the available contraceptive methods, including long-acting reversible contraceptives such as intra-uterine contraception, progestin-only injections, and progestin-only implants. Combination hormonal contraceptives are also acceptable choices.
110. d. Sense of hopelessness
    Risk factors for suicide in the individual with major depressive order include but are not limited to sense of hopelessness, substance abuse/family history of substance abuse, prior suicide attempt/family history of suicide attempt, living alone, medical illness, advanced age, and male gender.
111. b. Panic disorder with agorophobia
    Agorophobia is an anxiety disorder that includes avoidance of places or situations in which the ability to leave suddenly may be difficult in the event of having a panic attack. The recurrence of these panic attacks and fear related to their possible occurrence are considered panic disorder.
112. b. Specific phobia
    Anxiety is one of the most prevalent of all psychiatric disorders. Specific phobia is the most common at 25%, social phobia at 13%, PTSD at 12% in women, general anxiety disorder at 5%, and panic disorder at 3.5%.
113. d. Impulsive behavior is a common characteristic

Age of onset of bulimia nervosa is late adolescence to early adulthood. Mortality rate is lower than for anorexia nervosa. Impulsive behaviors such as shoplifting, alcohol and drug abuse, and unsafe sexual behaviors are characteristic of bulimia nervosa.
114. b. Nausea
    Side effects of selective serotonin reuptake inhibitors (SSRIs) include anxiety, insomnia/hypersomnia, headache, nausea, anorexia, and sexual dysfunction.
115. a. Buspirone (Buspar)
    Buspirone (Buspar) is a nonbenzodiazepine antianxiety agent with less abuse and dependence potential than alprazolam, a benzodiazepine.
116. d. Unsuccessful attempts to cut down use
    Substance abuse is a maladaptive pattern of use leading to significant impairment or distress in at least one of the following within a 12-month period—failing to fulfill major role obligations, use in situations where use is physically hazardous, substance-abuse-related legal problems, continued use despite knowledge of social and interpersonal problems caused or worsened by the substance use, and symptoms that do not meet criteria for substance dependence. Persistent desire or unsuccessful attempts to cut down is one of the criterion for a diagnosis of substance dependence.
117. a. Erosion of tooth enamel
    Erosion of tooth enamel may occur in the individual with bulimia nervosa as a result of frequent induced vomiting that exposes enamel to gastric acid.
118. b. The majority of rapes are committed by acquaintances of the victim
    The majority of rapes are perpetuated by an acquaintance rather than a stranger. *Rape* is a legal term and its definition may vary in different states but typically includes the use of force, threat, or coercion and lack of consent by the victim in relation to sexual intercourse. Initial response of the victim/survivor may range from calm to anxious to angry.
119. b. Metformin
    Metformin is the preferred initial oral agent for treatment of type 2 diabetes unless contraindicated or not tolerated.
120. c. Systemic corticosteroids
    Severe exacerbations (peak flow < 60%) of asthma may require the use of a short course of oral steroids for 5–10 days.

Bibliography

American Academy of Dermatology. (2011). Guidelines of care for the management of primary cutaneous melanoma. *Journal American Academy of Dermatology, 65*(15), 1032–1047. doi:10.1016/j.jaad.2011.04.031.

American Association of Clinical Endocrinologists and American Thyroid Association. (2012). *Clinical practice guidelines for hypothyroidism in adults: Cosponsored by the American Association of Clinical Endocrinologists and the American Thyroid Association.* Retrieved from http://www.thyroid.org/thyroid-guidelines/hypothyroidism/

American College of Obstetricians and Gynecologists. (2013). *Hypertension in pregnancy*. Washington, DC: Author.

American Diabetes Association. (2011). Diagnosis and classification of diabetes mellitus. *Diabetes Care, 34*(Suppl. 1), S62–S69.

American Diabetes Association. (2014). Standards of medical care in diabetes—2014. *Diabetes Care, 37*(Suppl. 1), S14–S80.

American Heart Association Statistics Committee and Stroke Subcommittee. (2014). Heart disease and stroke statistics: 2014 update. *Circulation, 129*, e28–e292.

American Psychiatric Association. (2013). *Diagnostic and statistical manual of mental disorders* (5th ed.). Arlington, VA: Author.

American Rheumatology Association. (2010). *2010 rheumatoid arthritis classification.* Retrieved from http://www.rheumatology.org/ACR/practice/clinical/classification/ra/ra_2010.asp

American Thyroid Association and American Association of Clinical Endocrinologists. (2011). *Hyperthyroidism and other causes of thyrotoxicosis: Management guidelines of the American Thyroid Association and American Association of Clinical Endocrinologists.* Retrieved from http://www.thyroid.org/thyroid-guidelines/hyperthyroidism/Bailey, A., & Bernsetein, C. (2013). *Pain in women: A clinical guide.* New York: NY: Springer Science and Business Media. doi:10.1007/978-1-4419-7113-5_3

Berger, T. G. (2014). Chapter 6. Dermatologic disorders. In Papadakis, M. A., McPhee, S. J., & Rabow, M. W. (Eds.), *CURRENT medical diagnosis and treatment 2014.* Retrieved from http://accessmedicine.mhmedical.com/content.aspx?bookid=330&Sectionid=44291008

Bickley, L., & Szilagyi, P. (2013). *Bates' guide to physical examination and history taking* (11th ed.). Philadelphia, PA: Lippincott Williams & Wilkins.

Briggs, G. G., & Freeman, R. K. (2015). *Drugs in pregnancy and lactation: A reference guide to fetal and neonatal risk.* Philadelphia, PA: Lippincott Williams & Wilkins.

Buttaro, T., Trybulski, J., Bailey, P., & Sandberg-Cook, J. (2013). *Primary care: A collaborative approach* (4th ed.). St. Louis, MO: Mosby.

Centers for Disease Control and Prevention. (2002). *Sexual violence surveillance: Uniform definitions and recommended data elements.* Retrieved from http://www.cdc.gov/violenceprevention/pdf/sv_surveillance_definitionsl-2009-a.pdf

Centers for Disease Control and Prevention. (2013a). *HIV surveillance report, 2011.* Retrieved from http://www.cdc.gov/hiv/topics/surveillance/resources/reports/

Centers for Disease Control and Prevention. (2013b). *Intimate partner violence: Consequences.* Retrieved from http://www.cdc.gov/violenceprevention/intimatepartnerviolence

Centers for Disease Control and Prevention. (2014). *HIV among women.* Retrieved from http://www.cdc.gov/hiv/risk/gender/women/facts/index.html

Committee on Drugs. (2001). The Transfer of Drugs and Other Chemicals into Human Milk. *Pediatrics, 108*(3). Retrieved from http://pediatrics.aappublications.org/content/108/3/776.full.html

Crofford, L. J. (2013). *Fibromyalgia.* American College of Rheumatology. Retrieved from http://www.rheumatology.org/Practice/Clinical/Patients/Diseases_And_Conditions/Fibromyalgia/

Cronholm, P., Fogarty, C., Ambuel, B., & Harrison, S. (2011). Intimate partner violence. *American Family Physician, 83*(10), 1165–1172.

de Benoist, B., McLean, E., Egli, I., & Cogswell, M. (Eds.). (2008). *Worldwide prevalence of anaemia 1993–2005: WHO global database of anaemia.* In Geneva, Switzerland: World Health Organization. Retrieved from http://whqlibdoc.who.int/publications/2008/9789241596657_eng.pdf

Duncan, C., Watson, D., & Stein, A. (2008). Diagnosis and management of headache in adults: Summary of SIGN guideline. *British Medical Journal, 337,* a2329. doi:http://dx.doi.org/10.1136/bmj.a2329.

Ernst, D., & Lee, A. (Eds.). (2014). *Nurse practitioner's prescribing reference.* New York, NY: Prescribing Reference.

Ferri, F. (2014). *Ferri's 2014 clinical advisor.* St. Louis, MO: Mosby.

Food and Drug Administration. (2014). *Living with fibromyalgia, drugs approved to manage pain.* Retrieved from http://www.fda.gov/downloads/ForConsumers/ConsumerUpdates/ucm107805.pdf

Garber, J., Cobin, R., Gharib, H., Hennessey, J., Klein, I., Mechanick, J. I., . . . Woeber, K. (2012). Clinical practice guidelines for hypothyroidism in adults: Cosponsored by the American Association of Clinical Endocrinologists and the American Thyroid Association. *Endocrinology Practice, 18*(6), 989–1028.

Gilmore, B., & Michael, M. (2011). Treatment of acute migraine headache. *American Family Physician, 83*(3) 271–280. Retrieved from http://www.aafp.org/afp/2011/0201/p271.html

Hackely, B., Kriebs, J., & Rousseau, M. (2007). *Primary care of women: A guide for midwives and women's health providers.* Burlington, MA: Jones & Bartlett Learning.

Hainer, B., & Matherson, E. (2013). Approach to acute headache in adults. *American Family Physician, 87*(10), 682–687.

International Headache Society. (2013). The international classification of headache disorders, 3rd edition (beta version). *Cephalalgia, 33*(9), 629–808. doi:10.1177/0333102413485658.

James, P., Oparil, S., Carter, B., Cushman, W., Dennison-Himmelfarb, C., Handler, J, ...Ortiz, E. (2014). 2014 evidence-based guidelines for the management of high blood pressure in adults: Report from the panel members appointed to the eighth joint national committee (JNC 8). *Journal of the American Medical Association, 311*(5):507-520.

Jefferson, J. W. (2005). Lamotrigine in psychiatry: Pharmacology and therapeutics. *Central Nervous System Spectrums, 10*(3), 224–232. Retrieved from http://www.cnsspectrums.com/aspx/article_pf.aspx?articleid=283

King, T., & Brucker, M. (2011). *Pharmacology for women's health.* Sudbury, MA: Jones and Bartlett.

Knutsen-Larson, S., Dawson, A., Dunnick, C., & Dellavalle, R. (2012). Acne vulgaris: Pathogenesis, treatment, and needs assessment. *Dermatologic Clinics, 30*(1), 99–106. doi:http://dx.doi.org/10.1016/j.det.2011.09.001.

Lacy, B., Weiser, K., & De Lee, R. (2009). The treatment of irritable bowel syndrome. *Therapeutic Advances in Gastroenterology, 2*(4), 221–238.

Longstreth, R., Thompson, W., Chey, W., Houghton, L., Mearin, F., & Spiller, R. (2006). Functional bowel patterns. *Gastroenterology, 130*(5), 1480-1491.

Mandell, L., Wunderink, R., Anzueto, A., Bartlett, J., Campbell, G., Dean, N. C., . . . Whitney, C. G. (2007). Infectious Diseases Society of America/American Thoracic Society consensus guidelines on the management of community-acquired pneumonia in adults. *Clinical Infectious Disease, 44,* S27–72.

Mann, J. D., & Coeytaux, R. R. (2012). Chapter 10: Headache. In D. Rakel (Ed.), *Intgerative medicine* (3rd ed.). St. Louis, MO: Saunders. Retrieved from http://www.mdconsult.com/das/book/pdf/439358770-5/978-1-4377-1793-8/4-u1.0-B978-1-4377-1793-8..00010-8..DOCPDF.pdf?isbn=978-1-4377-1793-8&eid=4-u1.0-B978-1-4377-1793-8..00010-8..DOCPDF

National Heart, Lung, and Blood Institute. (2001). *Third report of the National Cholesterol Education Program Expert Panel on Detection, Evaluation, and Treatment of High Cholesterol in Adults* (Adult Treatment Panel III). (NIH Publication No. 01-3095). Bethesda, MD: Author.

National Heart, Lung, and Blood Institute. (2003). *Seventh report of the Joint National Committee on Prevention, Detection, Evaluation, and Treatment of High Blood Pressure.* (NIH Publication No. 03-5233). Bethesda, MD: Author.

National Heart, Lung, and Blood Institute. (2007). *Expert panel report 3: Guidelines for the diagnosis and management of asthma.* (NIH Publication No. 08-4051). Bethesda, MD: Author.

National Institute of Health Osteoporosis and Related Bone Diseases National Resource Center. (2012). Osteoporosis Overview, Retrieved from: http://www.niams.nih.gov/Health_Info/Bone/Osteoporosis/overview.pdf

National Osteoporosis Foundation. (2014). *Clinician's guide to prevention and treatment of osteoporosis.* Washington, DC: Author.

Office for the Prevention of Domestic Violence. (2012). *National data on intimate partner violence.* Retrieved from http://www.opdv.state.ny.us/statistics/nationaldvdata/nationaldvdata.pdf

Papadakis, M., McPhee, S., & Rabow, M. (2014). *CURRENT medical diagnosis and treatment 2014* (53rd ed.). New York, NY: McGraw-Hill Medical.

Petri, M. (2005). Review of classification criteria for systemic lupus erythematosus. *Rheumatic Diseases Clinics of North America*, *31*(2), 245-54.Rakel, D. (2012). *Integrative medicine* (3rd ed.). St. Louis, MO: Saunders. doi:10.1016/B978-1-4377-1160-8.10033-8.

Rose, M. A., & Kam, P. C. A. (2002). Gabapentin: Pharmacology and its use in pain management. *Anaesthesia*, *57*(5), 451–462. doi:10.1046/j.0003–2409.2001.02399.x.

Royal Pharmaceutical Society of Great Britain. (2014). Lamotrigine. Micromedex. Truven Health Analytics. Retrieved from http://www.micromedexsolutions.com/micromedex2/librarian/ND_T/evidencexpert/ND_PR/evidencexpert/CS/B00375/ND_AppProduct/evidencexpert/DUPLICATIONSHIELDSYNC

/6A7531/ND_PG/evidencexpert/ND_B/evidencexpert/ND_P/evidencexpert/PFActionId/evidencexpert.IntermediateToDocumentLink?docId=18658-r&contentSetId=30&title=Lamotrigine&servicesTitle=Lamotrigine&topicId=null

Schuiling, K., & Likis, F. (2013). *Women's gynecologic health* (2nd ed.). Burlington, MA: Jones & Bartlett Learning.

Tharpe, N., Farley, C., & Jordan, R. (2013). *Clinical practice guidelines for midwifery and women's health* (4th ed.). Burlington, MA: Jones & Bartlett Learning.

U.S. Department of Health and Human Services. (2004). *Bone health and osteoporosis: A report of the surgeon general.* Rockville, MD: Author.

U.S. Department of Health and Human Services. (2011). *Guide for HIV/AIDS clinical care.* Rockville, MD: Author.

U.S. Department of Health and Human Services, Office of the Surgeon General. (2012). *The Surgeon General's report on bone health and osteoporosis: What it means to you.* Rockville, MD: Author. Retrieved from http://www.niams.nih.gov/Health_Info/Bone/SGR/SGRBoneHealth_Eng.pdf

Wasserman, A. (2011). Diagnosis and management of rheumatoid arthritis. *American Family Physician*, *84*(11), 1245–1251.

Wilbur, J., & Shian, B. (2012). Diagnosis of deep venous thrombosis and pulmonary embolism. *American Family Physician*, *86*(10), 913–919.

Wolfe, F., Clauw, D., Fitzcharles, M., Goldenberg, D., Katz, R., Mease, P, ...Yunus, M. (2010). The American College of Rheumatology preliminary diagnostic criteria for fibromyalgia and measurement of symptom severity. *Arthritis Care & Research*, *62*(5), 600-610.

World Health Organization. (2004). *WHO scientific group on the assessment of osteoporosis at primary health care level: Summary meeting report.* Geneva, Switzerland: World Health Organization. Retrieved from http://www.who.int/chp/topics/Osteoporosis.pdf

10

Professional Issues

Beth M. Kelsey and Kimberly K. Trout

© Kheng Guan Toh/ShutterStock, Inc.

Advanced Practice Registered Nurse (APRN)

- Definition—a registered nurse who meets the following criteria:
  1. Completes an accredited graduate-level program preparing him or her for one of four recognized APRN roles and a population focus
  2. Passes a national certification examination that measures APRN role and population competencies and maintains certification
  3. Possesses advanced clinical knowledge and skills preparing him or her to provide direct care to patients as well as a component of indirect care
  4. Builds on competencies of the registered nurse (RN) by demonstrating greater breadth and depth of knowledge and greater synthesis of data to perform more complex interventions with greater role autonomy
  5. Is educationally prepared to assume responsibility and accountability for health promotion/maintenance, assessment, diagnosis, and management of patient problems, which includes use and prescription of pharmacologic and nonpharmacologic interventions
  6. Has clinical experience of sufficient depth and breadth to reflect the intended license
  7. Obtains a license to practice as an APRN in one of the four APRN roles (APRN Consensus Workgroup & National Council of State Boards of Nursing APRN Advisory Committee, 2008)
- The four APRN roles:
  1. Certified Nurse Practitioner (CNP)
     a. Definition—licensed, independent practitioner who provides primary and/or specialty health care in ambulatory, acute, and long-term care settings for individuals, families, and groups. CNPs practice autonomously and in collaboration with other healthcare professionals to assess, treat, and manage patients' health problems and needs (American Academy of Nurse Practitioners, 2013a)

b. Practice
   (1) As a primary care provider (PCP), provides care that is integrated and accessible
   (2) Emphasizes health promotion, disease prevention
   (3) Professionally, practice is autonomous, collaborative, and evidence based
   (4) Functionally, practice is defined by state law, regulations, and clinical privileges
   (5) Diagnoses, treats, and manages health problems
   (6) Teaches and counsels individuals, families, and groups
   (7) Clinical roles include researcher, consultant, and patient advocate
   (8) Professional roles include mentor, educator, researcher, and administrator
   (9) Maintains accountability for care of patients and decisions reached
c. Core competencies of nurse practitioner practice (National Organization of Nurse Practitioner Faculties, 2012)
   (1) Scientific Foundation
   (2) Leadership
   (3) Quality
   (4) Practice Inquiry
   (5) Technology and Information Literacy
   (6) Policy
   (7) Health Delivery System
   (8) Ethics
   (9) Independent Practice
d. Education
   (1) Master's degree, post-master's certificate, or Doctorate of Nursing Practice (DNP)
   (2) Includes extensive clinical experience supervised by qualified preceptors within a population focus
   (3) Curriculum—APRN
      (a) Master's-level core courses that include foundational curriculum content considered essential for all students pursuing a master's degree in nursing regardless of functional focus (e.g., nursing theory, organizational and systems leadership, quality

improvement and safety, health policy and advocacy, interprofessional collaboration, clinical prevention and population health, ethics, research, legal issues, economics)

(b) APRN direct care core content that includes advanced health assessment, pathophysiology, pharmacology, clinical diagnosis and management, health promotion, and disease prevention

(c) Additional courses with content specific to the nurse practitioner population focus (family/individual across the life span, adult–gerontology, women's health–gender specific, neonatal, pediatrics, psychiatric–mental health); includes extensive supervised clinical hours

(d) Nurse practitioner (NP) programs are accredited within schools of nursing by two organizations: the National League for Nursing Accrediting Commission (NLNAC) or the Commission on Collegiate Nursing Education (CCNE)

(4) Curriculum—Women's Health Nurse Practitioner (WHNP) specific

(a) The Association of Women's Health, Obstetric, and Neonatal Nurses (AWHONN) and National Association of Nurse Practitioners in Women's Health (NPWH) (2014) jointly provide guidelines for women's health nurse practitioner practice and education

(b) Content includes—general health assessment, gynecology, childbearing and pregnancy care, primary care health issues, male reproductive health needs/problems, clinical pharmacology/pharmacokinetics/pharmacodynamics, health maintenance and disease prevention, professional role

e. Certification—WHNP

(1) To be eligible to take the certification examination offered for the Women's Health NP, the student must have graduated from an accredited master's degree, postmaster's certificate, or DNP program in the women's health population focus

(2) Women's Health Nurse Practitioner certification is provided by the National Certification Corporation (NCC)

f. Certification maintenance—must be renewed every 3 years through one of the following mechanisms:

(1) Professional development certification maintenance program—take the NCC specialty assessment evaluation, which covers topics that reflect major content areas tested on the certification examination; results determine the topics and amount of continuing education required (15 to 50 hours includes 5 hours for taking the assessment)

(2) Complete 50 continuing education hours covering all core certification knowledge competency areas

(3) Retake the certification examination

2. Certified Nurse-Midwife (CNM)

a. Definition—licensed, independent healthcare provider who provides a full range of primary healthcare services for women from adolescence to beyond menopause to include gynecologic and family planning services; preconception care; care during pregnancy, childbirth, and the postpartum period; care of the normal newborn during the first 28 days of life; and treatment of male partners for sexually transmitted infections (American College of Nurse–Midwives [ACNM], 2011)

b. Practice

(1) As a primary healthcare provider, provides care that is integrated and accessible to women and families

(2) Practice is autonomous or collaborative and evidence based

(3) Provides health promotion, disease prevention, counseling, and education across the life span

(4) Diagnoses, treats, and manages common health problems

(5) Focuses on childbearing, newborn care, postpartum care, family planning, and gynecologic care

(6) Accepts accountability for care provided

(7) Of the various models of practice, private practice in a midwifery group provides the most autonomy

(8) Site of practice is in all places where women's health care is needed, including the home

c. Hallmarks of Midwifery (ACNM, 2012a)

(1) Recognition of menarche, pregnancy, birth, and menopause as normal physiologic and developmental processes

(2) Advocacy of nonintervention in normal processes in the absence of complications

(3) Incorporation of scientific evidence into clinical practice

(4) Promotion of woman- and family-centered care

(5) Empowerment of women as partners in health care

(6) Facilitation of healthy family and interpersonal relationships

(7) Promotion of continuity of care

(8) Health promotion, disease prevention, and health education

(9) Promotion of a public healthcare perspective

(10) Care to vulnerable populations

(11) Advocacy for informed choice, shared decision making, and the right to self-determination

(12) Integration of cultural humility

(13) Incorporation of evidence-based complementary and alternative therapies in education and practice

(14) Skillful communication, guidance, and counseling

(15) Therapeutic value of human presence

(16) Collaboration with other members of the interprofessional healthcare team

d. Education

(1) Master's degree, post-master's certificate, or DNP

(2) Includes extensive clinical experience supervised by qualified preceptors

(3) Some programs do not require nursing and prepare the graduate as a midwife rather than nurse–midwife

e. Curriculum—based on American College of Nurse–Midwives (ACNM) Core Competencies (ACNM, 2012a) that include the following components:

(1) Hallmarks of Midwifery—art and science of midwifery

(2) Midwifery care: Professional responsibilities

(3) Midwifery care: Midwifery management process

(4) Midwifery care: Fundamentals

(5) Midwifery care of women

(6) Midwifery care of the newborn

f. Certification

(1) American Midwifery Certification Board (AMCB) certifies both nurse–midwives (CNMs) and non-nurse–midwives (CMs)

(2) To be eligible to take the certification exam of the AMCB, the student must graduate from a program accredited by the Accreditation Commission on Midwifery Education (ACME)

(3) ACME accredits both nurse–midwife and non-nurse–midwife programs

g. Certification maintenance—must be renewed every 5 years through one of the following two mechanisms:

(1) Complete three AMCB Certificate Maintenance Modules during the 5-year certification cycle—one in each of the three areas of practice: Antepartum and Primary Care of the Pregnant Woman; Intrapartum, Postpartum, and Newborn; and Gynecology and Primary Care for the Well-Woman; and obtain 20 contact hours (2.0 CEUs) of ACNM or Accreditation Council for Continuing Medical Education (ACCME) Category 1 approved continuing education units; the Certificate Maintenance Modules completed cannot count toward the required 20 contact hours (2.0 CEUs). Up to 10 contact hours can be earned for precepting nurse–midwifery/midwifery students from an ACME-accredited program

(2) Take the current AMCB Certification Examination no sooner than the fourth year of the current 5-year certification cycle and obtain 20 contact hours (2.0 CEUs) of ACNM or ACCME Category 1 approved continuing education units

3. Certified Registered Nurse Anesthetists (CRNAs) (American Association of Nurse Anesthetists, 2013)

a. Definition—an advanced practice nurse who provides anesthesia and care for patients before, during, and after surgical procedures in which anesthesia is administered; the CRNA provides anesthetics to patients in every care setting and for every type of surgery or procedure

b. Practice

(1) Provides preanesthetic preparation and evaluation

(2) Manages anesthesia induction, maintenance, and emergence

(3) Provides postanesthesia care

(4) Provides perianesthetic and clinical support functions

c. Education

(1) Master's degree or DNP

(2) Curriculum is governed by Council on Accreditation of Nurse Anesthesia Educational (COE) Programs Standards

(3) Programs are accredited by COE

(4) National certification is required through Council on Certification of Nurse Anesthetists

(5) Must earn continuing education credits to maintain certification

4. Clinical Nurse Specialist (CNS) (National Association of Clinical Nurse Specialists, 2010)

a. Definition—APRN with role of integrating care across the health–illness continuum and through three spheres of influence: patient, nurse, system

b. Practice

(1) Direct care functions include expert practitioner, role model, patient advocate, and educator

(2) Indirect care functions include change agent, consultant or resource person, liaison person, and innovator

c. Education

(1) Master's degree, post-master's certificate, or DNP

(2) Curriculum includes core courses in nursing theory, organizational theory, ethics, legal issues, healthcare delivery and CNS role, and population focused courses/supervised clinical experience

(3) CNS programs are accredited within schools of nursing by two organizations: the National League for Nursing Accrediting Commission (NLNAC) or the Commission on Collegiate Nursing Education (CCNE)

(4) Certification is available for population foci through the American Nurses' Credentialing Center (ANCC)

Trends and Issues

- Patient Protection and Affordable Care Act (ACA)

1. Federal statute signed into law in March 2010 with goals of increasing quality and affordability of health insurance and lowering the uninsured rate by expanding public and private insurance coverage and reducing healthcare costs for individuals and the government

2. ACA includes numerous provisions to take effect between 2010 and 2020

3. Significant healthcare reforms, most of which have taken effect as of 2014, include:

a. Insurers cannot deny coverage to individuals because of preexisting conditions

b. Insurers must offer the same premium rate to all applicants of same age and geographical location without regard to gender or preexisting conditions (except tobacco use)

c. Minimum standards for health insurance policies have been established

d. All individuals must have health insurance through employer, Medicaid, Medicare, or other public insurance programs or must secure an approved private insurance policy; federal subsidies are provided to help individuals with low incomes to comply with mandate

e. Children may remain on parent's health insurance plan until age 26

f. Medicaid eligibility has been expanded to include individuals and families with incomes up to 133% of poverty level, including adults without disabilities or dependent children

g. The State Children's Health Insurance Program (CHIP) enrollment process has been simplified

h. Medicare reimbursement has been restructured to change from fee for service to bundled payments—a single payment is made to a hospital or provider group for a defined episode of care (e.g., hip replacement) rather than individual payments to individual service providers

i. Health insurance exchanges will commence operation in every state as online marketplaces where individuals and small businesses can compare policies and buy insurance (with government subsidy if eligible)

j. Specific preventive services must be covered without a deductible or copayment, including but not limited to:
   (1) Childhood and adult immunizations
   (2) Well-woman visits
   (3) Mammograms
   (4) Gestational diabetes screening
   (5) Sexually transmitted infection counseling
   (6) HIV screening and counseling
   (7) FDA-approved contraceptive methods (with some religious exemptions)
   (8) Breastfeeding support and supplies
   (9) Domestic violence screening and counseling

- Primary health care

1. Definition—provision of integrated, accessible healthcare services by clinicians who are accountable for addressing a large majority of personal healthcare needs, developing sustained partnerships with patients, and practicing within the context of family and community (Institute of Medicine, 1996)

2. Terms used by Institute of Medicine (IOM) to define primary care:

   a. Integrated—comprehensive, coordinated care, focused on particular needs of patient, clinician continuity, patient record continuity, effective communication of information

   b. Accessible—elimination of geographic, cultural, language, reimbursement barriers to care

   c. Accountable—clinician and system accountability for services provided

   d. Majority of personal healthcare needs—competency to manage most healthcare needs, use of consultation and referral as needed, sustained relationship between clinician and patient over time

   e. Context of family and community—understanding of the circumstances of the patient that affect health and healthcare outcomes, awareness of community health trends, use of specific health promotion/disease prevention strategies within this context

3. Primary healthcare providers include family physicians, general internal medicine physicians, pediatricians, obstetricians/gynecologists, nurse–midwives, and nurse practitioners

4. WHNPs and nurse–midwives are educationally prepared and qualified to be providers of primary care within their population focus

5. Issues related to APRN ability to engage in full scope of practice as primary care providers include:
   a. Nurse practice act regulations
   b. Prescriptive authority statutes
   c. Reimbursement policies

- Healthy People 2020 (U.S. Department of Health and Human Services, n.d.)

1. Origin is the 1979 Healthy People: The Surgeon General's Report on Health Promotion and Disease Prevention

2. Followed by Healthy People initiatives each decade in 1990, 2000, and 2010

3. Purpose of Healthy People 2020—provide science-based, 10-year national objectives for improving the health of all Americans; establish benchmarks and monitor progress

4. Four overarching goals:

   a. Attain high-quality, longer lives free of preventable disease, disability, injury, and premature death

   b. Achieve health equity, eliminate disparities, and improve health of all groups

   c. Create social and physical environments that promote good health for all

   d. Promote quality of life, healthy development, and healthy behaviors across all life stages

- Baby-Friendly Hospital Initiative (BFHI)

1. Launched by World Health Organization (WHO) and United Nations Children's Fund (UNICEF) in 1991

2. Purpose—encourage and recognize birthing hospitals and centers that offer an optimal level of care for infant feeding and mother–baby bonding

3. Qualifications to receive a Baby-Friendly designation include:

   a. Implementation of the Ten Steps to Successful Breastfeeding

   b. Compliance with the International Code on Marketing Breast-milk Substitutes

4. Ten Steps to Successful Breastfeeding

   a. Have a written breastfeeding policy that is routinely communicated to all healthcare staff

   b. Train all healthcare staff in the skills necessary to implement this policy

   c. Inform all pregnant women about the benefits and management of breastfeeding

   d. Help mothers initiate breastfeeding within 1 hour of birth

   e. Show mothers how to breastfeed and how to maintain lactation, even if they are separated from their infants

   f. Give infants no food or drink other than breast milk, unless medically indicated

   g. Practice rooming in—allow mothers and infants to remain together 24 hours a day

   h. Encourage breastfeeding on demand

   i. Give no pacifiers or artificial nipples to breastfeeding infants

   j. Foster the establishment of breastfeeding support groups and refer mothers to them on discharge from the hospital or birth center

5. International Code on Marketing Breast-milk Substitutes

   a. No advertising of breast milk substitutes to families

b. No free samples or supplies in the healthcare system

c. No promotion of products through healthcare facilities, including no free or low-cost formula

d. No contact between marketing personnel and mothers

e. No gifts or personal samples to health workers

f. No words or pictures idealizing artificial feeding, including pictures of infants, on the labels or product

g. Information to health workers should be scientific and factual only

h. All information on artificial feeding, including labels, should explain the benefits of breastfeeding and the costs and hazards associated with artificial feeding

i. Unsuitable products should not be promoted for babies

j. All products should be of high quality and take account of the climate and storage conditions of the country where they are used

- Institute of Medicine (2011): *The Future of Nursing: Leading Change, Advancing Health*
  1. Robert Wood Johnson Foundation and Institute of Medicine partnered to assess and respond to the need to transform the nursing profession partially in response to enactment of the Affordable Care Act
  2. Report was presented in 2010 with four key messages:
     a. Nurses should practice to the full extent of their education and training
     b. Nurses should achieve higher levels of education and training through an improved education system that promotes seamless academic progression
     c. Nurses should be full partners with physicians and other health professionals in redesigning health care in the United States
     d. Effective workforce planning and policymaking require better data collection and an improved information infrastructure
  3. Recommendations in regard to each of the key messages were presented
- Doctorate in Nursing Practice (DNP)
  1. Practice-focused rather than research-focused nursing doctoral degree
  2. DNP Essentials established by AACN (American Association of Colleges of Nursing [AACN], 2006) for curricular elements and competencies
  3. Entry into DNP program may be after completion of baccalaureate nursing degree (BS to DNP) or master's nursing degree (MS to DNP)
  4. Program length varies depending on BS-to-DNP/MS-to-DNP program type as well as APRN role and population focus
  5. Requires a minimum of 1000 hours of supervised postbaccalaureate clinical experience
  6. American Association of Colleges of Nursing (AACN) 2004 position statement calls for DNP degree to be required for entry into advanced nursing practice by 2015
  7. Currently, school accrediting bodies, APRN certification agencies, and state nursing boards are not requiring a DNP degree for advanced practice registered nursing practice

- Consensus Model
  1. Completed by APRN Consensus Work Group and National Council of State Boards of Nursing APRN Advisory Committee in 2008
  2. Purpose—development of a national regulatory model for APRNs with relevant definitions, roles, and titles to be used and population foci
  3. Defines four essential components for regulation (LACE)
     a. *Licensure*—the granting of authority to practice
     b. *Accreditation*—formal review and approval by a recognized agency of educational degree programs in nursing
     c. *Certification*—formal recognition of the knowledge, skills, and experience demonstrated by the achievement of standards identified by the profession
     d. *Education*—formal preparation of APRNs in graduate-degree granting or postgraduate certificate programs
  4. Four APRN roles—nurse anesthetist, nurse–midwife, clinical nurse specialist, nurse practitioner
  5. Six population foci—family/individual across life span, adult–gerontology, neonatal, pediatrics, women's health–gender specific, psychiatric–mental health
  6. Education, certification, and licensure of individual must be congruent in terms of role and population focus
  7. APRNs may specialize (e.g., palliative care, critical care) but cannot be certified or licensed solely within a specialty area
  8. Identifies titles to be used by APRN
  9. State boards of nursing will be solely responsible for licensing APRNs
  10. Implementation of model is occurring incrementally in states; target date for full implementation is 2015

Professional Components of Advanced Practice Registered Nursing

- Scope of practice
  1. Definition—legal authority granted to a profession to provide and be reimbursed for services
  2. Defines what APRN can do with patients, what he or she can delegate, and when collaboration with others is required
  3. Scope may differ depending on APRN role—clinical nurse specialist, nurse anesthetist, nurse–midwife, nurse practitioner
  4. Based on state laws promulgated by the various nurse practice acts and rules and regulations for APRN—varies from state to state
- Nurse practice acts
  1. Definition—legislative enactments that define the practice of nursing, give guidance within the scope of practice issues, and set standards for practice; passage through state legislatures makes these the law under which nursing is practiced
  2. Regulated state by state
  3. Authorizes state boards of nursing to establish statutory authority for the licensure of registered nurses, including APRNs
  4. Authorizes state boards of nursing to establish a scope of practice, determine disciplinary actions, and regulate its practice via legislative statutes

5. Licensure statutes limit practice to individuals with specific qualifications as defined by law

6. Registration and certification statutes provide a definition and limit as to who may use title, without restraint of practice

7. May authorize prescriptive authority

8. Regulations reflect a trend to increase APRN authority and autonomy

- Licensure
   1. Definition—process by which a government agency authorizes individuals to practice a profession or occupation by validating that the individual has attained the required degree of competency as prescribed by law to protect the public welfare
   2. State law governs the requirement for holding a professional license in the state
   3. All states require the APRN to hold a state RN license; currently, not all states require a separate APRN license
   4. CNMs are licensed through Boards of Nursing, Boards of Medicine, or Boards of Midwifery/Nurse–Midwifery
   5. CMs may receive license to practice in New Jersey, New York, and Rhode Island through Boards of Medicine, Boards of Midwifery, or State Health Department; CMs are also able to receive authorization to practice in Delaware and Missouri

- Certification
   1. Definition—the formal process by which a private agency or organization certifies (usually by examination) that an individual has met standards as specified by that profession (Hamric, Hanson, Tracy, & O'Grady, 2014)
   2. National certification examinations provide a consistent standard that must be met by the APRN to demonstrate competency for an advanced level of practice in her or his role
   3. Almost all states require national certification for nurse practitioners and nurse–midwives
   4. Maintenance of a particular level of competence following initial certification is required

- Prescriptive authority
   1. Definition—legal authority to prescribe medications or devices
   2. Authority is contained in state nurse or midwifery practice acts or in other statutes and varies from state to state
   3. May require approval of state board of medicine, midwifery, public health, or pharmacy
   4. Requires completion of an advanced pharmacology course and continuing education hours to maintain prescribing status
   5. May require a collaborative practice agreement and/or written protocols
   6. May obtain federal Drug Enforcement Administration (DEA) registration number, depending on scope of state law

- Independent and collaborative management of care
   1. Independent—care of women within the provider's scope of practice, based on knowledge, skills, and competencies
   2. Consultation—seeks advice or opinion of a physician or other member of the healthcare team while the NP/nurse–midwife retains primary responsibility for the woman's care
   3. Referral—the process by which the provider directs the client to a physician or another healthcare professional for management of a particular problem or aspect of the client's care
   4. Collaboration—NP/nurse–midwife and physician or other healthcare professional jointly manage the care of a woman who has developed complications, the goal of which is to share authority while providing quality care within each individual's scope of practice

- Hospital privileges
   1. Definition—authorization granted to a practitioner by the healthcare network or a component of the network to provide specific in-patient care services within defined limits based on the practitioner's qualifications and current competence
   2. Hospitals may have levels of privileges determining extent of decision making permitted by the provider (e.g., review records, admit patients, write orders)
   3. Often it is the medical staff governing body that decides which other providers may have hospital privileges and at what level based on an application and review process
   4. ACNM (2006) Principles for Credentialing and Privileging of CNMs and CMs include:
      a. Bylaws and guidelines of hospitals/healthcare organizations should reflect the scope of practice of CNMs/CMs as defined by national standards and state laws
      b. Clinical practice guidelines should be the mechanism used to determine circumstances under which consultation or management by a physician is required
      c. Bylaws and guidelines should be written to ensure the midwife is accountable for care provided and should avoid requirements that create vicarious liability of other healthcare professionals
      d. Bylaws and guidelines should not require routine physician co-signature on CNM/CM notes or orders in medical record
      e. Requirements for credentialing, privileging, and reprivileging of physicians and midwives should be equivalent
      f. Requirements for continuous professional practice evaluation should be consistent for procedures performed by both midwives and physicians, and midwives should be included in development of such guidelines
      g. A broad definition of medical or professional staff that does not designate categories of providers should be used
      h. Delineation of CNM/CM privileges should clearly state that they can admit and discharge patients and should provide a mechanism for recognizing expanded practices distinguished from the standard privileges granted to midwives

- Standards of practice
   1. Definition—overarching statements that the nursing profession uses to describe the responsibilities of its members to provide safe and competent care
   2. APRNs are held to standards of practice promulgated both by the nursing profession and standards determined by professional organizations representing their role and population focus
   3. American Association of Nurse Practitioners (2013b) *Standards of Practice for Nurse Practitioners* include:
      a. Process of care—assessment, diagnosis, development of treatment plan, implementation of plan, follow-up, and evaluation of patient status
      b. Care priorities—patient and family education, facilitation of patient participation in self-care, promotion of optimal health, provision of continually competent care, facilitation of entry into healthcare system, promotion of a safe environment

    c. Interdisciplinary and collaborative responsibilities

    d. Accurate documentation of patient status and care

    e. Responsibility as patient advocate

    f. Quality assurance and continued competence

    g. Adjunct roles of nurse practitioners—e.g., mentor, educator, researcher, consultant, manager

    h. Research as basis for practice

4. American College of Nurse–Midwives (2011) *Definition of Midwifery and Scope of Practice of Certified Nurse Midwives and Certified Midwives* includes that midwifery care:

    a. Is provided by qualified practitioners

    b. Occurs in a safe environment within the context of the family, community, and a system of health care

    c. Supports individual rights and self-determination within boundaries of safety

    d. Is composed of knowledge, skills, and judgments that foster the delivery of safe, satisfying, and culturally competent care

    e. Is based on knowledge, skills, and judgments that are reflected in written practice guidelines and are used to guide the scope of midwifery care and services provided to clients

    f. Is documented in a format that is accessible and complete

    g. Is evaluated according to an established program for quality management that includes a plan to identify and resolve problems

    h. May be expanded beyond the ACNM core competencies to incorporate new procedures that improve care for women and their families

- Standards of care

  1. Definition—also called practice guidelines; define a standard of appropriate care; used in legal decisions about care provided

  2. Standards of care are evidence based and continuously evolving

  3. APRNs are responsible to remain up to date on these standards/guidelines

  4. Examples of sources of practice guidelines include Agency for Healthcare Research and Quality (AHRQ), Centers for Disease Control and Prevention (CDC), professional medical and nursing specialty organizations

- Professional organizations

  1. Purposes and benefits of membership

    a. Purposes of professional nursing organizations

      (1) Promote and set high standards for health care

      (2) Enhance the identity, visibility, and practice of its members

      (3) Provide a collective voice to promote the profession of nursing and the APRN role

    b. Individual benefits

      (1) Membership within a community of like providers who share commonalities specific to their specialty areas

      (2) Networking availability through participation in local, regional, and national meetings, alliances, and coalitions

      (3) Legislative representation, support, and participation at all levels

      (4) Continuing education programs to attain/maintain clinical competency

      (5) May provide consultation and assistance in securing federal scholarship and loans for continuation of study

      (6) Receipt of organizational publications

      (7) Listings of employment opportunities

      (8) Professional recognition of excellence in practice and research

  2. Organizational activities

    a. Provides, fosters, and facilitates leadership for and among members

    b. Disseminates information relevant to practice

    c. Monitors and influences laws and regulations

    d. Produces position papers communicating organizational perspectives on issues of concern

    e. Establishes practice competencies and standards and may offer continuing education resources

    f. Enhances the visibility of the members through marketing, public relation efforts

    g. May construct and maintain a national database of all provider activities

    h. Encourages and supports research efforts

  3. Professional organizations relevant to women's health nurse practitioners and nurse–midwives include but are not limited to:

    a. American College of Nurse–Midwives (ACNM)

    b. National Association of Nurse Practitioners in Women's Health (NPWH)

    c. Association of Women's Health, Obstetrics, and Neonatal Nurses (AWHONN)

- Reimbursement—third-party payers

  1. Medicare—federal program that provides health insurance for those older than 65 years or disabled; not income dependent; four parts—A, B, C, and D

    a. Part A—hospital insurance

      (1) No fee for enrollment—covered by payroll taxes; cost-sharing may include deductibles and coinsurance

      (2) Automatic enrollment at age 65 or if eligible for Social Security disability insurance

      (3) Covers inpatient hospital services, skilled nursing facilities, hospice, home health care

    b. Part B—supplementary medical insurance if eligible for Part A

      (1) Pay monthly premium

      (2) Covers provider services, outpatient coverage, diagnostics, and durable medical equipment

      (3) Some preventive services are mandated to be covered with no deductible or copay

    c. Part C—Medicare Advantage Plan

      (1) Available through participation in coordinated care or private fee-for-service plans and medical savings accounts

      (2) Covers same services as Part B

    d. Part D—Prescription drug coverage

      (1) Pay monthly premium

      (2) May include deductible or copay

    e. APRN qualifications to be a Medicare provider

      (1) Current RN and APRN license to practice in state in which services rendered

      (2) National certification in an advanced practice nurse role

      (3) Master's degree in nursing

(4) National Provider Identifier (NPI) number—obtained from Centers for Medicare and Medicaid Services (CMS)

f. Fee-for-service Medicare—APRN submits bills to local Medicare carrier agent for each visit or procedure; NP reimbursed at 85% of physician fee for same service; CNM reimbursed at 100%

g. Capitated Medicare—fee paid to healthcare provider, per patient, per month, for care of Medicare patient enrolled in managed care organization (MCO); APRN applies to MCO to be on panel of providers

h. "Incident to" services—services are billed at 100% under supervising physician's National Provider Identifier (NPI) number; physician must be present in office suite; does not include APRN seeing patient for an initial visit or subsequent visit with a new problem; physician must demonstrate ongoing participation in the management of the patient's care; limits APRN autonomy and professional visibility

2. Medicaid—federal program administered by the states to cover mandated healthcare costs for eligible low-income individuals and families

a. Pregnant women and children younger than 6 years of age with family incomes up to 133% of the federal poverty level

b. Children who are younger than age 19, in families whose income is at or below poverty level

c. Childless adults who qualify on basis of poverty

d. Adults with short-term (1 year or less) disability and who qualify on basis of poverty

e. General coverage includes:
   (1) Hospital and provider services
   (2) Laboratory and radiologic services
   (3) Nursing home and home healthcare services
   (4) Prenatal and postpartum care
   (5) Preventive services
   (6) Medically necessary transportation
   (7) States may opt to cover additional services

f. Reimbursement—determined by states
   (1) Operates as a vendor payment program with broad discretion in determining methodology at the state level
   (2) Providers must accept Medicaid payment rates as payment in full
   (3) Omnibus Budget Reconciliation Act (OBRA) (1989)
      (a) Mandated Medicaid reimbursement for Pediatric Nurse Practitioner (PNP), Certified Nurse-Midwife (CNM), and Family Nurse Practitioner (FNP)
      (b) Must practice within scope of state law and are not required to be under supervision or association with a physician
      (c) Level of payment determined by states, with usual range of 70–100% of physician fee schedule, and may bill Medicaid directly
      (d) States have option of including other NPs for reimbursement
      (e) States can apply for "Medicaid waivers" to enroll patients covered by Medicaid in MCOs
      (f) APRN must apply to state Medicaid agency to be a fee-for-service provider; must apply to the MCO to be included on provider panel

   (4) Payment to hospitals
      (a) Based on predetermined fee schedule for projected cost of care
      (b) States are mandated to make additional payments to hospitals with "disproportionate share hospital" (DSH) adjustments for disproportionate numbers of Medicaid recipients
      (c) APRN not paid directly for inpatient services
      (d) All other forms of insurance must be exhausted before Medicaid will cover expenses

3. Children's Health Insurance Program (CHIP)—federal program with set proportion matched by state funds to extend insurance to children not income eligible for Medicaid but who cannot afford health insurance

a. Three different mechanisms used by states
   (1) Expanded Medicaid programs
   (2) Separate child health insurance plans
   (3) Combination plans

4. Indemnity (private) insurance companies—insurance company that pays for medical care of its insured but does not deliver health care
   (1) Pay on a per-visit, per-procedure basis
   (2) Fee schedules are negotiated between provider and insurance company; usually based on usual and customary charges for the local area
   (3) APRN direct reimbursement by indemnity insurance companies varies from state to state
   (4) APRN must apply to the insurance company for provider status
   (5) APRN must submit billing form to insurance company for reimbursement

5. Managed care organizations (MCOs)—an MCO is an insurer that provides both healthcare services and payment for services
   a. Financial arrangements determined prospectively under terms of contract and include prospective pricing, service bundling, price discounts/discounted fees for services to certain populations and for coverage of specific conditions
   b. Types of managed care plans include:
      (1) Health maintenance organization (HMO)—patient is assigned or chooses a primary care provider who manages total care and must make referrals for patient to see a specialist and for nonemergency hospital admissions
         (a) Healthcare providers are paid a preset amount in advance for all services the insured population is projected to need over a period of time
         (b) Capitation—a method that pays providers for services; a per-member-per-month basis is a common form of prepayment; incentive to provider to contain costs of care provided
      (2) Preferred provider organization (PPO)—MCO contracts with independent providers for negotiated fee-for-service; patient can choose provider; PPO guarantees a certain volume of business to hospitals and providers in return for negotiated discount in fees
      (3) Point-of-service plan (POS)—utilizes some of features of both HMO and PPO; patients may choose to see whichever provider they want either in the network

plan or out of the network, although they pay more for out-of-network care

c. If APRN is employee of a group practice, someone within the group negotiates terms of MCO contract for the group

d. If APRN is in private practice, he or she applies to the MCO to be a provider and negotiates terms of contract

e. Not all MCOs currently recognize APRNs as primary care providers

Healthcare Delivery Systems

- Traditional health care
  1. Emphasizes independent providers
  2. Characteristics
     a. Providers chosen by patient with little, if any, influence from third-party payer
     b. Provider reimbursed by patient and insurers in fee-for-service arrangement
     c. Insurers reimburse according to usual, customary, and reasonable system
- Integrated delivery systems/managed care organizations (MCOs)
  1. A health delivery system that strives to provide high-quality, cost-effective care through a coordination of health services provided by a variety of caregivers; shifting emphasis from a fee-for-service strategy to one in which the network of providers assumes some degree of responsibility for both provision and cost of care
  2. Characteristics
     a. Varying levels of care that are coordinated into a seamless system
     b. Capitated system of payment/prospective pricing
        (1) Financial risk assumed by provider
        (2) Unit of value is cost per member per month (PMPM), determined in advance by contract (prospectively)
        (3) To remain financially solvent, target population should be healthy, which means that they consume the least dollars for care provided
     c. Low-cost, high-quality service with emphasis on health promotion
     d. Service bundling, where complementary care can be offered as a package, further reduces costs

Ethical and Legal Issues and Principles

- Ethics and the law
  1. Law is founded on rules that guide a society, regardless of personal views and values
  2. Ethical values are affected by moral, philosophical, and individual interpretation
  3. These areas intertwine, creating dilemmas in the provision of health/medical care
  4. MORAL model of ethical decision making:
     a. *M*anage the dilemma—define issues, consider options, identify players
     b. *O*utline the options—examine these fully

c. *R*esolve the dilemma—apply basic ethical principles to each option

d. *A*ct by applying the chosen option

e. *L*ook back and evaluate the entire process

- Ethical principles in health care
  1. Autonomy—individuals have the right to self-determine the course of treatment they find most acceptable and with whom information may be shared
  2. Beneficence—the actions one takes as a healthcare professional should promote good
  3. Nonmaleficence—the actions one takes as a healthcare professional should do no harm
  4. Veracity—the healthcare professional should be truthful when giving individuals information about their healthcare needs
  5. Fidelity—the healthcare professional should keep one's promises or commitments made in the therapeutic relationship
  6. Justice—the healthcare professional should advocate for fair and equal treatment for all individuals
- Legal liability and risk management in providing care
  1. Malpractice—failure of the healthcare professional to exercise the degree of skill and learning commonly applied by the average prudent, reputable member of the profession; falls under tort law
  2. Tort law—a branch of civil law (rather than criminal law) that concerns legal wrongs committed by one person against another; an act that causes harm to body or property and for which the injured party is seeking monetary damages; includes assault, battery, intentional infliction of emotional distress, negligence
     a. Intentional tort—a volitional or willful act, with expressed intent to bring harm to the affected person; forms the foundation for consent for treatment requirements (see "Consent" later in this section)
        (1) Assault—intentional threat by word or act to unlawfully touch or strike a person, coupled with apparent ability, and causing fear in that person that such an act is imminent
        (2) Battery—actual, intentional, and unlawful touching or striking of another person against the will of the other
        (3) False imprisonment—unlawful restraint or detention against the will of the individual
        (4) Intentional infliction of emotional distress—intentional infliction of emotional or mental distress that results in mental reaction such as anguish, grief, or fright to another person
     b. Negligence tort—involves an act of negligence; conduct lacking in due care; carelessness; doing something any reasonable, prudent person would not do
        (1) Most malpractice suits are based on negligence; requires the following four elements to be present:
           (a) Duty—the responsibility to act in accordance with a standard of care
           (b) Breach of duty—violation or deviation from the standard of care
           (c) Causation—determination of whether the injury is the result of negligence
           (d) Damages—must be actual harm to the person or property

3. Breach of confidentiality—may be an intentional tort, negligence tort, basis of disciplinary action by state health professional regulation board, or violation of state or federal law

4. Consent—a legal action given by a patient to undergo particular treatments and/or procedures; informed consent—agreement to do something or to allow something to happen only after all the relevant facts are disclosed

   a. Most states have legislation regarding what types of tests, treatments, or procedures require written informed consent and who is authorized to provide informed consent for a minor, incompetent, or incapacitated person

   b. Components of a written informed consent generally include description of procedure/treatment/test, potential risks and benefits, and alternatives with documentation that the patient is acting voluntarily, has received full disclosure, and is competent to act

   c. Refusal of treatment—the inherent right of conscious and mentally competent individuals to refuse any form of treatment either personally or through their representative; includes Do Not Resuscitate (DNR) orders, refusal for extraordinary care, and implementation of supportive-care-only guidelines

   d. Withdrawal of treatment—the decision to terminate treatment that has been initiated after securing informed consent from a patient or the patient's representative, with the legal basis for decision and subsequent care as noted in refusal of treatment

5. Coworker incompetence—a legal obligation exists for a licensed professional to assist, relieve, or report any coworker who through substandard care or impairment places the health and welfare of patients at risk; official processes relevant to continued practice are determined through agencies and state boards, based on practice act regulations

6. Health Insurance Portability and Accountability Act (HIPAA)

   a. Purpose of HIPAA privacy rule provisions (implemented in 2003)—assure that individual's health information is properly protected while allowing the flow of information needed to promote high-quality health care and to protect the public's health and well-being

   b. Definitions

      (1) Covered entity—the privacy rule applies to health plans, healthcare clearinghouses, and any healthcare provider who transmits health information in electronic form in connection with transactions

         (a) Health plan—individual and group plans that provide or pay the cost of medical care

         (b) Healthcare clearinghouse—billing services, community health management systems

         (c) Healthcare provider—institutions (e.g., hospitals, health networks) and direct care providers who electronically transmit health information in connection with transactions for which U.S. Department of Health and Human Services (U.S. DHHS) has established privacy standards (e.g., claims, benefit eligibility inquiries, referral authorization requests)

      (2) Protected health information (PHI)—all individually identifiable health information held or transmitted by a covered entity in any form—electronic, paper, oral; pertains even if individual is deceased

   c. Required disclosures by covered entities include:

      (1) To individuals (or their personal representatives) specifically when they request access to or an accounting of disclosures of their PHI

      (2) To U.S. DHHS when it is undertaking a compliance investigation or enforcement of action

   d. Permitted disclosures by covered entities include but are not limited to:

      (1) The individual who is the subject of the PHI

      (2) The entity's own treatment, payment, and healthcare operation activities

      (3) Informal permission that clearly gives the individual the opportunity to agree or object and if the healthcare provider exercises professional judgment that the use or disclosure of PHI is determined to be in the best interest of the individual

      (4) Public health interests (e.g., communicable disease reporting, abuse or neglect reporting, serious threat to health or safety)

   e. Notice of privacy practices—each covered entity (with certain exceptions) must provide a notice to all patients of its privacy practices, including individual rights and how to exercise them

   f. Administrative requirements—implement policies and procedures designed to comply with privacy rule, designate privacy official to monitor compliance

   g. Complaint process—informal review may resolve issue fully without formal investigation; if not, begin investigation; Office for Civil Rights enforces the privacy rule with potential monetary penalties and imprisonment depending on intent of violation

7. Risk management plan—demonstrates that the APRN is cognizant of risks, is taking reasonable steps to limit risk, and seeks to provide care consistent with best practice; includes practice policies and procedures to include but not limited to:

   a. Role and scope of practice

   b. Licensing and certification requirements

   c. Practice guidelines and standards

   d. Health record documentation standards and forms

   e. Informed consent policy and process

   f. Protection of privacy/confidentiality policy and process

   g. Collaborative practice relationships

   h. Provisions of practice coverage

   i. Peer review and outcomes-based evaluation processes

   j. Patient complaint or concern review process

8. Professional liability insurance

   a. Recommended that each clinician carry individual policy

   b. Types of coverage

      (1) Occurrence—covers event of malpractice that occurred during the policy period without regard to when the claims are reported; provides protections for each policy period indefinitely; broadest protection available

(2) Claims made—incident must happen and be reported while policy is in force; requires purchase of a tail policy to protect, once policy period ends

   c. Cost of insurance varies with APRN role and population focus

Evidence-Based Practice

- Definition—the conscientious, judicious, and explicit use of current best evidence in making decisions about the care of individual patients, incorporating both clinical expertise and patient values
  1. Models for implementing evidence-based practice generally include the following steps:
     a. Identification of a clinical problem or question
     b. Search for the best evidence
     c. Critical appraisal of the strength of evidence
     d. Recommendation for action (change, no change, further study)
     e. Implementation of the change if recommended
     f. Evaluation of change in relationship to desired outcomes
  2. Categories of strength of reviewed evidence from individual research and other sources
     a. Level I (A–D)—meta-analysis or multiple controlled studies
     b. Level II (A–D)—individual experimental study
     c. Level III (A–D)—quasi-experimental study
     d. Level IV (A–D)—nonexperimental study
     e. Level V (A–D)—case report or systematically obtained, verifiable quality, or program evaluation data
     f. Level VI—opinion of respected authorities; this level also includes regulatory or legal opinions
  3. Level I is the strongest rating per type of research; however, quality for any level can range from A to D and reflects basic scientific credibility of the overall study; A indicates a very well-designed study, D indicates the study has a major flaw that raises serious questions about the believability of the findings
  4. Methodologies for research
     a. Quantitative research—formative, objective, systematic study process to describe and test relationships and/or to examine cause-and-effect interactions among variables
     b. Qualitative research—systematic, interactive, subjective approach used to describe life experiences and give them meaning
- Major quantitative research study designs
  1. Descriptive—used to explore and describe phenomena in real-life situations, identify and describe variables within the phenomenon, develop conceptual and operational definitions for variables
  2. Correlational—used for systematic investigation of relationships between two or more variables to explain type (positive or negative) relationships but not to examine cause and effect
  3. Quasi-experimental—conducted to explain relationships, clarify why certain events happen, and examine causality between selected independent and dependent variables; limited control developed to provide alternative for examining causality in situations not conducive to experimental-level controls

4. Experimental—provides the greatest amount of control possible to examine probability and causality among selected independent and dependent variables for the purpose of predicting and controlling phenomena

- Major clinical categories of primary research and common types of studies used
  1. Therapy—tests the effectiveness of a treatment; randomized, double-blinded, placebo-controlled
  2. Diagnosis and screening—measures the validity and reliability of a test or evaluates the effectiveness of a test in detecting disease at a presymptomatic stage—cross-sectional survey
  3. Causation or harm—assesses whether a substance is related to the development of an illness or condition—cohort or case-control
  4. Prognosis—determines the outcome of a disease—longitudinal cohort study
  5. Systematic review—a summary of the literature that uses explicit methods to perform a thorough literature search and critical appraisal of individual studies and that uses appropriate statistical techniques to combine these valid studies
  6. Meta-analysis—a systematic review that uses quantitative methods to summarize results
- Research terminology
  1. Reliability—represents the consistency of the measure obtained in a study
  2. Internal validity—extent to which the effects detected in a study are a true reflection of reality and not the result of the effects of extraneous variables
  3. External validity—extent to which study findings can be generalized beyond the sample used in the study
  4. Generalization—extends the implications of the findings from the sample studied to a larger population or from the situation studied to a larger situation
  5. Replication—reproducing or repeating a study to determine whether similar findings will be obtained
- Ethics in research
  1. Protection of human rights in research includes:
     a. Self-determination
     b. Privacy
     c. Autonomy
     d. Confidentiality
     e. Fair treatment
     f. Protection from discomfort and harm
  2. Components of informed consent for study participants:
     a. Purpose of study
     b. Role of the participant
     c. Risks and discomforts
     d. Benefits
     e. Alternatives
     f. Assurance of anonymity and/or confidentiality
     g. Any compensation for participation
     h. Explanation that participation is voluntary and can refuse to participate without any penalty
     i. Option to withdraw
     j. Offer to answer questions
     k. Institutional review—committee of researcher's peers examines the study for ethical concerns

3. Drug research trials—FDA investigational new drug regulations for clinical study has three phases
   a. Phase I clinical evaluation—first testing of new drug compound to establish tolerance of healthy human subjects at different doses, define pharmacologic effects at anticipated therapeutic levels, study absorption, distribution, metabolism, excretion in humans
   b. Phase II clinical evaluation—controlled studies on a small number of patients with the target disease or disorder to determine the drug's potential usefulness and short-term risks
   c. Phase III clinical evaluation—controlled and uncontrolled studies of the drug's safety and effectiveness in hospital and outpatient settings; gather information on the drug's effectiveness for specific indications, any adverse effects, best way to administer and use drug for purpose intended
   d. If drug is approved, the Phase III clinical trial information forms the basis for the content of the product label

Questions

Select the best answer.

1. Which of the following is *not* one of the six population foci for APRN established by the consensus model for APRN regulation?
   a. Critical care
   b. Neonatal
   c. Pediatrics
   d. Women's health

2. Which of the following statements concerning the Doctor of Nursing Practice (DNP) program is correct?
   a. It requires a minimum of 500 hours of supervised clinical experience
   b. Individuals must already be certified as an APRN before entry into the DNP program
   c. The program focus is on practice more so than research
   d. The DNP Essentials were developed by professional advanced practice nursing organizations

3. The Hallmarks of Midwifery would *not* allow for which of the following?
   a. Advocacy of regular use of technologic interventions
   b. Informed choice with participatory decision making
   c. Therapeutic value of human presence
   d. Recognition of women's life phases as normal, developmental processes

4. Prescriptive authority in all states requires that the APRN:
   a. Apply to the state medical licensing board
   b. Complete specified pharmacologic educational requirements
   c. Obtain a Drug Enforcement Administration (DEA) registration number
   d. Practice under a collaborative agreement with a physician

5. The nongovernmental validation of a nurse practitioner's or nurse–midwife's knowledge and acquired skills in a particular population focus is:
   a. Licensure
   b. Credentialing
   c. Certification
   d. Registration

6. The best source of information on APRN-specific requirements for prescriptive authority is:
   a. Federal Drug Enforcement Administration (DEA)
   b. Professional APRN organizations
   c. State boards of nursing
   d. State boards of pharmacy

7. The goal of an integrated system of healthcare/managed care organization is:
   a. Control of costs through member selection
   b. Reduction of costs through employment of fewer physicians
   c. To make available unlimited health services under one plan
   d. To provide low-cost, high-quality service

8. Which of the following best describes capitation as a financial strategy?
   a. Predetermined payment for services based on an accepted schedule of fees
   b. Predetermined fees set for usual and customary care
   c. Predetermined payment based on contractual per-member-per-month rate
   d. Predetermined rates negotiated monthly for each participating member

9. The purpose of HIPAA is to:
   a. Decrease the expenses and therefore the costs of healthcare delivery
   b. Improve the health system by standardizing the exchange of electronic data
   c. Reimburse providers and laboratories in a timely fashion
   d. Ensure that every person has ready access to appropriate health care

10. A covered entity under HIPAA may be any of the following *except*:
    a. Any health provider who transmits any health information electronically
    b. Any patient who has health records in a format that can be transmitted electronically
    c. Governmental agencies that license healthcare providers
    d. Insurance companies that pay for cost of medical care for patients

11. A goal of the privacy rule of HIPAA is to:
    a. Provide federal protections for privacy and preserve quality care
    b. Ensure that research subjects' privacy is maintained during the study
    c. Guarantee that the privacy of patients is protected at any cost
    d. Increase the level of confidentiality in Medicaid programs

12. One of the principal differences between Medicare Parts A and B is:
    a. Eligibility
    b. Rate of reimbursement

c. Monthly premium requirement for Part A

d. Monthly premium requirement for Part B

13. Managed care organization (MCO) characteristics include all of the following *except*:
    a. Capitated system of payment
    b. Opportunity for service bundling
    c. Payment to APRN restricted to "incident to" billing
    d. Some financial risk assumed by the provider

14. Nurse practitioners with Medicare provider status:
    a. Receive reimbursement at 85% of physician payment for services provided
    b. Must become a member of a managed care organization to receive reimbursement
    c. Can have more autonomy if they use "incident to" billing
    d. Can receive direct reimbursement under Medicare Part D

15. A National Provider Identifier (NPI) number can be obtained from:
    a. Centers for Medicare and Medicaid Services (CMS)
    b. Drug Enforcement Administration (DEA)
    c. Managed care organization (MCO)
    d. State board of nursing

16. All states are required to provide Medicaid to:
    a. Children younger than 19, in families whose income is below poverty level
    b. Families eligible for the federal Children's Health Insurance Program (CHIP)
    c. Individuals with long-term disabilities that have incomes below poverty level
    d. Individuals older than 65 years with a chronic medical condition who have incomes below poverty level

17. Which of the following statements concerning "incident to" billing is correct?
    a. It applies to both Medicare and Medicaid billing
    b. It can be used when APRN sees a patient for any visit other than the initial visit
    c. It promotes the visibility and status of advanced practice nurses
    d. It requires that the physician demonstrate ongoing involvement in the patient's care

18. Keeping one's promises or commitments is:
    a. Beneficence
    b. Fidelity
    c. Veracity
    d. Justice

19. To maintain AMCB certification the nurse–midwife must:
    a. Apply for renewal every 3 years
    b. Complete three maintenance modules plus 20 contact hours of continuing education every 5 years
    c. Document at least 1000 clinical hours as a midwife in the previous 3 years
    d. Take the certification examination every 5 years

20. During a malpractice hearing, an attorney describes the responsibility "to do no harm." The attorney is defining the ethical principle of:
    a. Justice
    b. Veracity

c. Fidelity

d. Nonmaleficence

21. A nurse practitioner or midwife fails to order a test that is clinically indicated. This omission is best described as:
    a. Maleficence
    b. Assault
    c. An intentional tort
    d. Negligence

22. A patient presents with an abnormal test result. The appropriate plan of care is to refer for additional testing, but the facility that performs the test has closed for the day. Rather than sending the patient to have the test performed at the hospital, the nurse practitioner or midwife in the practice orders the patient to report to the testing facility the next morning. During the evening, problems arise and the patient is admitted to the hospital with a negative outcome. This is an example of:
    a. An intentional tort
    b. A negligence tort
    c. Inappropriate cause for malpractice suit
    d. Withdrawal of treatment without consent

23. Placing an intrauterine contraceptive device in the uterus of an intellectually disabled patient who is not able to give informed consent may constitute:
    a. Assault
    b. Battery
    c. Intentional tort
    d. Paternalism

24. An elderly woman enters a nursing home following a broken hip and signs DNR orders and a statement that she does not want extraordinary care. She is:
    a. Exercising her right to refuse treatment
    b. Exercising her right to withdraw treatment
    c. Acting in a manner that should cause concern about her mental competence
    d. Lacking information needed to make an informed decision

25. A women's health nurse practitioner receives a call from an attorney, who tells her she is named in a suit related to an obstetric incident that occurred 4 years ago. When she calls the insurance company, she is told that the policy she had at that time will not cover her because the policy was:
    a. A claims made policy
    b. Tail insurance only
    c. An occurrence policy
    d. An HMO policy

26. Randomized controlled trials (RCTs) are most appropriate for what type of research study?
    a. Diagnosis and screening
    b. Therapy
    c. Causation or harm
    d. Prognosis

27. Which of the following types of research would receive the strongest rating for strength of evidence?
    a. Case report
    b. Experimental study
    c. Meta-analysis
    d. Quasi-experimental study

28. To maintain NCC certification the WHNP must:
    a. Apply for renewal every 5 years
    b. Complete a specialty assessment evaluation that determines the topics and number of hours of continuing education needed before the next renewal cycle
    c. Document at least 2000 clinical hours as a WHNP in the previous 5 years
    d. Take the certification examination every 5 years

29. According to the consensus model for APRN, what entity will be responsible for licensing APRNs?
    a. Advanced practice professional organizations
    b. Individual state boards of nursing
    c. National certification agencies
    d. National Council of State Boards of Nursing

30. A 24-year-old female with no children may have all of the following health insurance options under the Affordable Care Act *except*:
    a. Applying for Medicaid if she meets the income eligibility requirements
    b. Enrolling in the Children's Health Insurance Program (CHIP)
    c. Purchasing health insurance through a state health insurance exchange
    d. Remaining on her parent's health insurance plan

31. Under the Affordable Care Act, which of the follow individuals could be charged a higher premium by health insurance companies for coverage?
    a. 30-year-old pregnant female
    b. 32-year-old female smoker
    c. 40-year-old female with diabetes
    d. 62-year-old female with history of breast cancer

32. The quantitative research design in which the relationships between two or more variables are explained but cause and effect are not examined is:
    a. Correlational
    b. Descriptive
    c. Experimental
    d. Quasi-experimental

33. The A–D category applied to strength of evidence in research is based on:
    a. Ability to replicate the study with the same findings
    b. Quality of the design of the study
    c. Review by a panel of experts
    d. Type of research study design

34. Weighing yourself on the same scale 10 times in a row to see if you get the same weight each time is a measure of:
    a. External validity
    b. Generalization
    c. Internal validity
    d. Reliability

35. Which of the following statements is true concerning Phase III clinical evaluation in drug research trials?
    a. Drug absorption, distribution, metabolism, and excretion in humans are studied
    b. Drug is tested to establish tolerance in healthy subjects at different doses
    c. Drug is tested on small number of patients with the target disease to determine potential short-term risks
    d. Drug safety and effectiveness are evaluated with both controlled and uncontrolled studies

36. The Institute of Medicine definition of primary care is based on:
    a. Setting where care is provided
    b. Type of provider
    c. Context in which care is provided
    d. Ultimate oversight by physicians

37. The best place for the APRN to find comprehensive standards of practice related to her or his particular role and population focus is:
    a. National certification organization
    b. Professional organization representing the role and population focus
    c. State board of nursing
    d. School of nursing accreditation body

38. Which of the following hospital regulations would be against the principles for credentialing and privileging of CNMs and CMs established by the ACNM?
    a. Guidelines that ensure the midwife is accountable for care provided and that avoid placing liability on other healthcare professionals
    b. Mechanisms designated to determine the circumstances under which consultation or management by a physician is required
    c. Mechanisms for recognizing expanded practice procedures distinguished from standard privileges granted to midwives
    d. Requirements for credentialing, privileging, and reprivileging that focus on the difference in types of care provided by midwives and physicians

39. The CDC Sexually Transmitted Diseases Treatment Guidelines best fit the definition for:
    a. Expert opinion
    b. Scope of practice parameters
    c. Standard of care
    d. Standard of practice

40. The term used to indicate that the implications of the findings of a study with a particular population can be extended to a larger population is:
    a. Generalization
    b. External validity
    c. Internal validity
    d. Replication

Answers with Rationales

1. a. Critical care

   The six population foci are family/individual across the life span, adult–gerontology, neonatal, pediatrics, women's health–gender specific, psychiatric–mental health.

2. c. The program focus is on practice more so than research

   Entry into a DNP program may be after completion of baccalaureate nursing degree (BS-DNP) or master's nursing degree (MS-DNP). Programs require a minimum of 1000 hours of supervised postbaccalaureate clinical experience. The DNP Essentials were established by the American Association of Colleges of Nursing (AACN).

3. a. Advocacy of regular use of technologic interventions

   The Hallmarks of Midwifery include advocacy for nonintervention in normal processes in the absence of complications.

4. b. Complete specified pharmacologic educational requirements

   Individual states may require approval of the state board of medicine, although the majority of states have APRN prescriptive authority in nurse and midwifery practice acts. Some states, but not all, have a collaborative agreement requirement. DEA registration may be obtained depending on individual state scope of practice laws.

5. c. Certification

   Certification is the formal process by which a private agency or organization certifies (usually by examination) that an individual has met standards as specified by that profession. Almost all states require national certification for nurse practitioners and nurse–midwives.

6. c. State boards of nursing

   Authority for prescriptive authority is contained in state nurse or midwifery practice acts or in other statutes that vary from state to state. Additional approval may be required from other state boards.

7. d. To provide low-cost, high-quality service

   Integrated delivery systems/managed care organizations strive to provide high-quality, cost-effective care through coordination of services; there is a shift in emphasis from a fee-for-service strategy to one in which a network of providers assumes some responsibility for provision and cost of care.

8. c. Predetermined payment based on contractual per-member-per-month rate

   Capitated systems of payment/prospective pricing are set as cost per member per month (PMPM), determined in advance by contract (prospectively).

9. b. Improve the health system by standardizing the exchange of electronic data

   The purpose of the Health Insurance Portability and Accountability Act (HIPAA) is to ensure that individuals' health information is properly protected while allowing the flow of information needed to promote high-quality health care and to protect the public's health and well-being.

10. c. Governmental agencies that license healthcare providers

    HIPAA covered entities (those to whom the privacy rules apply) include health plans, healthcare clearinghouses, and any healthcare provider who transmits health information in electronic form in connection with transactions.

11. a. Provide federal protections for privacy and preserve quality care

    For the most part, HIPAA privacy rules apply to all protected health information (PHI). There are two situations in which a covered entity is required to share PHI and at least four situations in which the covered entity may be permitted to disclose PHI.

12. d. Monthly premium requirement for Part B

    Part B is supplementary medical insurance available to individuals for a monthly premium if they are eligible for Part A. Part B covers provider services, outpatient care, diagnostics, and durable medical equipment.

13. c. Payment to APRN restricted to "incident to" billing

    "Incident to" billing is for Medicare services provided by the APRN under the supervision of a physician and does not include initial visits or subsequent visits with a new problem.

14. a. Receive reimbursement at 85% of physician payment for services provided

    In fee-for-service Medicare, NPs are reimbursed at 85% and nurse–midwives at 100% of the physician fee for the same service.

15. a. Centers for Medicare and Medicaid Services (CMS)

    The APRN obtains a National Provider Identifier number from CMS.

16. a. Children younger than 19, in families whose income is below poverty level

    States must provide Medicaid coverage to the following groups if they meet specified income-eligibility requirements—pregnant women and children under age 6, children younger than 19, adults under 65 without dependent children, and adults with short-term disability.

17. d. It requires that the physician demonstrate ongoing involvement in the patient's care

    "Incident to" billing is for Medicare services provided by the APRN under the supervision of a physician and does not include initial visits or subsequent visits with a new problem. Billing as a Medicare provider rather than "incident to" promotes the visibility and status of APRNs.

18. b. Fidelity

    Fidelity is the ethical principle of the healthcare professional keeping one's promises or commitments made in a therapeutic relationship.

19. b. Complete three maintenance modules plus 20 contact hours of continuing education every 5 years

    AMCB certification must be renewed every 5 years with completion of three maintenance modules plus 20 contact hours of continuing education or retaking the AMCB certification examination (no sooner than 4th year of cycle) plus 20 contact hours of continuing education.

20. d. Nonmaleficence

Nonmaleficence is the ethical principle of the healthcare professional doing no harm in actions taken.

21. d. Negligence

Negligence is conduct lacking in due care; carelessness.

22. b. A negligence tort

A negligence tort involves conduct lacking in due care or careless conduct. Most malpractice cases are based on negligence.

23. b. Battery

Battery is the actual, intentional, and unlawful touching or striking of another person against the will of another.

24. a. Exercising her right to refuse treatment

Refusal of treatment is an inherent right of a conscious and mentally capable individual to refuse any form of treatment either personally or through the person's legal representative.

25. a. A claims made policy

With claims made policies, the incident must happen and be reported while the policy is in force to be covered.

26. b. Therapy

The clinical research category of therapy is that in which the effectiveness of a treatment is being tested. Randomized, double-blinded, placebo-controlled trials (RCTs) provide the strongest evidence for this category of clinical research.

27. c. Meta-analysis

Level I (meta-analysis or multiple controlled studies) is the strongest rating; however, quality may range from A to D, with A indicating a very well-designed study and D indicating the study has a major flaw that raises serious questions about the believability of the findings.

28. b. Complete a specialty assessment evaluation that determines the topics and number of hours of continuing education needed before the next renewal cycle

NCC certification must be renewed every 3 years with completion of a specialty assessment evaluation that determines the topics and number of hours of continuing education needed (15–50) before the next renewal cycle *or* completion of 50 continuing education hours covering all core certification knowledge areas *or* retaking the certification examination.

29. b. Individual state boards of nursing

According to the consensus model, state boards of nursing will be solely responsible for licensing APRNs.

30. b. Enrolling in the Children's Health Insurance Program (CHIP)

Under the ACA, a 24-year-old female without children would be eligible to remain on her parent's health insurance until age 26, to apply for Medicaid if her income is up to 133% of poverty level, or to purchase health insurance through a state health insurance exchange.

31. b. 30-year-old female smoker

Under the Affordable Care Act, a health insurance company may charge a higher premium for smokers. Insurance companies may not charge higher premiums based on gender, pregnancy, preexisting health condition, or history of a health condition.

32. a. Correlational

Correlational research study designs are used for systematic investigation of relationships between two or more variables to explain type (positive or negative) relationships, but not to examine cause and effect.

33. b. Quality of the design of the study

Categories of strength of evidence from research studies are based on a combination of the research design (Levels I–VI) used (e.g., meta-analysis, experimental) and the quality of the design of the study (Levels A–D) that affects believability of the findings.

34. d. Reliability

Reliability represents the consistency of a measure obtained in a study.

35. d. Drug safety and effectiveness are evaluated with both controlled and uncontrolled studies

Phase III clinical evaluation involves controlled and uncontrolled studies of the drug's safety and effectiveness in hospital and outpatient settings; gathers information on the drug's effectiveness for specific indications, any adverse effects, best way to administer and use drug for purpose intended; and forms basis of content of product label.

36. c. Context in which care is provided

The Institute of Medicine definition of primary care is provision of integrated, accessible healthcare services by clinicians who are accountable for addressing a large majority of personal healthcare needs, developing sustained partnerships with patients, and practicing within the context of family and community (Institute of Medicine, 1996).

37. b. Professional organization representing the role and population focus

Standards of practice are overarching statements that the nursing profession uses to describe the responsibilities of its members to provide safe and competent care. APRNs are held to standards of practice promulgated by the nursing profession and standards determined by professional organizations representing their role and population focus.

38. d. Requirements for credentialing, privileging, and reprivileging that focus on the difference in types of care provided by midwives and physicians

One of the ACNM principles for credentialing and privileging CNMs and NMs is that requirements for credentialing, privileging, and reprivileging should be equivalent.

39. c. Standard of care

Standards of care, also called practice guidelines, are evidence based, continuously evolving standards of appropriate care; sources include such entities as CDC, Agency for Healthcare Research and Quality (AHRQ), and professional medical and nursing specialty organizations.

40. a. Generalization

Generalization extends the implications of the findings of a study from the sample studied to a large population or from a situation studied to a larger situation.

Bibliography

Advanced Practice Registered Nurse Consensus Work Group and National Council of State Boards of Nursing APRN Advisory Committee. (2008). *Consensus model for APRN regulation: Licensure, accreditation, certification, and education.* Retrieved from http://www.aacn.nche.edu/education-resources/APRNReport.pdf

Ament, L. (2007). *Professional issues in midwifery.* Sudbury, MA: Jones and Bartlett.

American Association of Nurse Practitioners. (2013a). *Scope of practice for nurse practitioners.* Washington, DC: Author.

American Academy Association of Nurse Practitioners. (2013b). *Standards of practice for nurse practitioners.* Washington, DC: Author.

American Association of Colleges of Nursing. (2004). *AACN position statement on the practice doctorate in nursing.* Washington, DC: Author.

American Association of Colleges of Nursing. (2006). *The essentials of doctoral education for advanced nursing practice.* Washington, DC: Author.

American Association of Nurse Anesthetists. (2013). *Scope of nurse anesthesia practice.* Park Ridge, IL: Author.

American College of Nurse–Midwives. (2006). *Position statement: Principles for credentialing and privileging certified nurse–midwives and certified midwives.* Silver Spring, MD: Author.

American College of Nurse–Midwives. (2009). *Position statement: Midwifery certification in the United States.* Silver Spring, MD: Author.

American College of Nurse–Midwives. (2011). *Definition of midwifery and scope of practice of certified nurse–midwives and certified midwives.* Silver Spring, MD: Author.

American College of Nurse–Midwives. (2012a). *Core competencies for basic midwifery practice.* Silver Spring, MD: Author.

American College of Nurse–Midwives. (2012b). *Position statement: Mandatory degree requirements for midwives.* Silver Spring, MD: Author.

American College of Nurse–Midwives. (2012c). *Position statement: Midwives are primary care providers and leaders of maternity care homes.* Silver Spring, MD: Author.

American College of Nurse–Midwives. (2012d). *Standards for the practice of midwifery.* Silver Spring, MD: Author.

Association of Women's Health, Obstetric, and Neonatal Nurses and National Association of Nurse Practitioners in Women's Health. (2014). *The women's health nurse practitioner: Guidelines for practice and education* (7th ed.). Washington, DC: Author.

Baby-Friendly USA. *Baby-friendly hospital initiative in USA.* Retrieved from http://www.babyfriendlyusa.org/

Barker, A. (2009). *Advanced practice nursing: Essential knowledge for the profession.* Sudbury, MA: Jones and Bartlett.

Buppert, C. (2012). *Nurse practitioner's business practice and legal guide* (4th ed.). Burlington, MA: Jones & Bartlett Learning.

Grace, P. (2014). *Nursing ethics and professional responsibility* (2nd ed.). Burlington, MA: Jones & Bartlett Learning.

Grove, S., Burns, N., & Gray, J. (2013). *The practice of nursing research: Appraisal, synthesis, and generation of evidence* (7th ed.). St. Louis, MO: Saunders Elsevier.

Hamric, A., Hanson, C., Tracy, M., & O'Grady, E. (2014). *Advanced nursing practice: An integrative approach* (5th ed.). Philadelphia, PA: W. B. Saunders.

Institute of Medicine. (1996). *Primary care: American's health in a new era.* Washington, DC: National Academies Press.

Institute of Medicine. (2011). *The future of nursing: Leading change, advancing health.* Washington, DC: National Academies Press.

National Association of Clinical Nurse Specialists. (2010). *Clinical nurse specialists core competencies.* Retrieved from http://www.nacns.org/docs/CNSCoreCompetenciesBroch.pdf

National Organization of Nurse Practitioner Faculties. (2012). *Nurse practitioner core competencies.* Retrieved from http://c.ymcdn.com/sites/www.nonpf.org/resource/resmgr/competencies/npcorecompetenciesfinal2012.pdf

Office for Civil Rights. (2003). *Summary of the HIPAA privacy rule.* Washington, DC: U.S. Department of Health and Human Services.

U.S. Department of Health and Human Services. (n.d.). *Healthy people 2020.* Retrieved from http://www.healthypeople.gov/2020/default.aspx

Wynne, A., & Woo, T. (2012). *Pharmacotherapeutics for nurse practitioner prescribers* (3rd ed.). Philadelphia, PA: F.A. Davis.

Index

© Kheng Guan Toh/ShutterStock, Inc.

Note: Page numbers followed by *f* or *t* indicate materials in figures, or tables respectively.